Manual of Nursing Therapeutics

Applying Nursing Diagnoses to
Medical Disorders

Manual of Nursing Therapeutics

Applying Nursing Diagnoses to Medical Disorders

Pamela L. Swearingen, R.N.
Special Projects Editor

 Addison-Wesley Publishing Company, Inc.

Health Sciences Division, Menlo Park, California
Reading, Massachusetts • Don Mills, Ontario • Wokingham, UK
Amsterdam • Sydney • Singapore • Tokyo • Madrid
Bogotá • Santiago • San Juan

Sponsoring Editor • Nancy Evans
Production Coordinator • Glenda Epting
Cover Designer • George Omura
Interior Designer • Lorena LaForest

Library of Congress Cataloging in Publication Data
Swearingen, Pamela L.
  Manual of nursing therapeutics.
  Includes bibliographies and index.
  1. Nursing—Handbooks, manuals, etc.
2. Diagnosis—Handbooks, manuals, etc.
I. Title. [DNLM: 1. Nursing—handbooks.
2. Nursing Process—handbooks. WY 39 S974m]
RT48.S94 1986   610.73   85-28573
ISBN 0-201-12940-X

    EFGHIJKLMNOP-AL-898

The authors and publishers have exerted every effort to ensure that drug selection and dosage set forth in this text are in accord with current recommendations and practice at the time of publication. However, in view of ongoing research, changes in government regulation and the constant flow of information relating to drug therapy and drug reactions, the reader is urged to check the package insert for each drug for any change in the indications of dosage and for added warnings and precautions. This is particularly important where the recommended agent is a new and/or infrequently employed drug.

 Addison-Wesley Publishing Company
Health Sciences Division
2727 Sand Hill Road
Menlo Park, California 94025

Co-Authors

Janet Reiss Lederer, RN, MN
Patient Education Manager
El Camino Hospital
Mountain View, California

*Chapter 1/Respiratory Disorders; Chapter 9/
Reproductive Disorders:* Sections Two–
Four

Dennis G. Ross, RN, MSN, MAE, CNOR
Chairperson, Department of Nursing
Castleton State College
Castleton, Vermont;
Staff Nurse, Operating Room
Rutland Regional Medical Center
Rutland, Vermont

*Chapter 8/Musculoskeletal Disorders;
Chapter 4/Neurologic Disorders:* Co-
author, Section Three (I); *Appendix
One/Caring for Patients on Prolonged Bed Rest*

Carol Monlux Swift, RN, BSN
Nursing Coordinator
El Camino Hospital
Mountain View, California

Chapter 4/Neurologic Disorders: Sections
One–Six; *Appendix One/Caring for
Patients with Neurologic Problems;*
and Contributor, Caring for Patients
with Cancer and Other Life-
Disrupting Illnesses

Barbara L. Tueller, RN, MS, CCRN
Faculty, Department of
Medical-Surgical Nursing
Samuel Merritt College of Nursing
Oakland, California

*Chapter 2/Cardiovascular Disorders;
Chapter 7/Hematologic Disorders;
Appendix One/Contributor, Caring
for Preoperative and Postoperative
Patients*

Contributors

Deborah G. Althoff, RN, BSN, CNOR
Staff Nurse, Operating Room
Rutland Regional Medical Center
Rutland, Vermont

Chapter 8/Musculoskeletal Disorders:
Section Three (I); Contributor,
Section Three (II)

Lolita M. Adrien, RN, MS
Enterostomal Clinical Specialist
Home Health Care Services
Stanford University Hospital
Palo Alto, California

Chapter 6/Gastrointestinal Disorders: Co-
Author, Section Three; *Appendix One/*
Contributor, Caring for Patients with
Cancer and Other Life-Disrupting
Illnesses

Patricia A. Brown, RN, MS, PhD
Associate Professor
Marion A. Buckley School of Nursing
Adelphi University
Garden City, New York

Chapter 6/Gastrointestinal Disorders:
Section Two (I-V); *Appendix One/*
Contributor, Caring for Preoperative
and Postoperative Patients

Sue Forloines-Lynn, RN, BSN, CNSN
Nutrition Support Nurse
North Carolina Memorial Hospital
Chapel Hill, North Carolina

Chapter 6/Gastrointestinal Disorders: Co-
Author, Section Four; *Chapter 11/
Metabolic Disorders:* Co-Author,
Section Three

Mima M. Horne, RN, MSN
Staff Nurse, Dialysis Services
El Camino Hospital
Mountain View, California
Instructor, Nursing Continuing
Education
De Anza College
Cupertino, California

Chapter 3/Renal–Urinary Disorders:
Sections One–Four; *Chapter 5/
Endocrine Disorders:* Contributor,
Section Six

Susan Jackson, RN, MA
Head Nurse, Burn Unit
Santa Clara Valley Medical Center
San Jose, California

Chapter 10/Sensory Disorders: Co-Author,
Section Three

Patricia Ravitt Jansen, RN, BSN
Staff Development Instructor
El Camino Hospital
Mountain View, California

Chapter 3/Renal–Urinary Disorders:
  Sections Five–Seven; *Chapter 9/*
  Reproductive Disorders: Section Five

Karen M. Kawauchi, RN, MS
Assistant Director of Nursing
Nursing Education
Santa Barbara Cottage Hospital
Santa Barbara, California

Chapter 11/Metabolic Disorders:
  Section Two

Donna Kershner, RN, BSN
Staff Nurse, Medical-Surgical ICUs
Santa Clara Valley Medical Center
Santa Clara, California

Chapter 5/Endocrine Disorders:
  Sections One–Four

**Theresa LoCurto, RN, BSN, MBA,
CCRN**
Critical Care Clinical Coordinator/Staff
  Development
Santa Clara Valley Medical Center
San Jose, California

Chapter 10/Sensory Disorders: Co-Author,
  Section Three

Andrea Walsh Matz, RN, BSN
Staff Nurse, Phoenix Program
El Camino Hospital
Mountain View, California

Chapter 6/Gastrointestinal Disorders:
  Section Five (I–II); *Chapter 4/*
  Neurologic Disorders: Section Seven

Sheryl Michelson, RN, MS
Nursing Education Instructor
Stanford University Hospital
Stanford, California
Department of Nursing
University of Phoenix
Phoenix, Arizona

Chapter 10/Sensory Disorders:
  Section One

Julie Randolph Miller, RN, BSN
Staff Nurse III
El Camino Hospital
Mountain View, California

Chapter 6/Gastrointestinal Disorders:
  Section One; Section Two (VI–VIII);
  Section Five (III); *Appendix One/*
  Contributor, Caring for Preoperative
  and Postoperative Patients

Bonnie Raskin, RN, MSN, CCRN
Consultant, Nurse Educator;
Former Instructor
Santa Barbara City College
Santa Barbara, California

Chapter 11/Metabolic Disorders:
  Section One

Leigh W. Stedman, RN, BSN, CNSN
Nutrition Support Nurse
North Carolina Memorial Hospital
Chapel Hill, North Carolina

Chapter 6/Gastrointestinal Disorders: Co-
  Author, Section Four; *Chapter 11/*
  Metabolic Disorders: Co-Author,
  Section Three

Nancy Stotts, RN, MN, EdD
Assistant Professor, Department of
  Physiological Nursing
University of California, San Francisco
San Francisco, California

Chapter 10/Sensory Disorders: Section Two

Lorraine Walters, RN, BA
Medical Unit Staff Nurse
El Camino Hospital
Mountain View, California

Chapter 5/Endocrine Disorders: Sections
  Five and Six

Diane Wind Wardell, RN, MSN
Assistant Professor of Nursing
Thiel College
Greenville, Pennsylvania

Chapter 9/Reproductive Disorders:
  Section One

Rosemary Watt, RN, MS
Enterostomal Clinical Specialist
Stanford University Medical Center
Stanford, California

Chapter 6/Gastrointestinal Disorders: Co-
  author, Section Three; *Appendix One/*
  Contributor, Caring for Patients with
  Cancer and Other Life-Disrupting
  Illnesses

Contents

3 Renal–Urinary Disorders

4 Neurologic Disorders 145

5 Endocrine Disorders 219

6 Gastrointestinal Disorders 271

7 Hematologic Disorders 339

8 Musculoskeletal Disorders 365

Preface

Using a convenient pocket-sized format, **Manual of Nursing Therapeutics:** *Applying Nursing Diagnoses to Medical Disorders* offers nurses quick, easy access to clinical information formerly found only in medical–surgical textbooks or large manuals. It is the first pocket-sized reference to feature the application of nursing diagnoses and interventions to specific medical disorders. Written by clinical experts, it was designed to help both staff and student nurses plan and evaluate care of the adult medical–surgical patient. To provide a quick review and facilitate patient teaching, brief descriptions of pathophysiology, physical assessment, diagnostic testing, medical and surgical management, and patient–family teaching/discharge planning data are included.

Although many textbooks discuss nursing diagnosis, Carpenito, *Nursing Diagnosis: Application to Clinical Practice* (Lippincott, 1983) was used as our primary resource to ensure consistency throughout the manual. In addition to the approved list from North American Nursing Diagnosis Association (NANDA), we also used the nursing diagnosis "Alteration in respiratory function." We found that interventions and treatment for some nursing diagnoses, when applied to specific medical disorders, are, by necessity, interdependent with those made by physicians. Although some readers may question the use of nursing diagnoses that are not completely independent, we feel that it is unrealistic not to include them in a clinical manual and that to omit them could jeopardize patient safety. For example, although nurses cannot always treat or prevent a postoperative complication, their prompt assessment and reporting of the problem can prevent further injury to the patient.

Nursing diagnoses, interventions, and outcome criteria used for each medical disorder are not all-inclusive, but rather are those considered most important by the author. Additional, more generic information is discussed in Appendix One, which includes nursing diagnoses and interventions for preoperative and postoperative patients, patients on prolonged bed rest, neurologic patients, and patients with cancer and other life-disrupting illnesses. Appendix Two lists all the nursing diagnoses used in this manual, along with the related medical disorder and page number. Abbreviations that are used in the manual are found in Appendix Three; Appendix Four gives normal values for the laboratory tests that are discussed.

Finally, a word about the medical–surgical disorders that were selected: We chose those that are either commonly seen as primary admission diagnoses or seen frequently as secondary diagnoses in hospitalized patients. To control the number of pages and ensure a portable, pocket-sized reference, we did not include specific discussions of pediatric, critical care, mental health, or other specialized areas.

Manual of Nursing Therapeutics was designed to help students and staff nurses apply nursing diagnoses in the real world of the acute care hospital. Reviewers indicate that it achieves this objective. The ultimate judgment rests with the nurses who read and use the manual on a daily basis. We welcome comments on how we might enhance its usefulness in subsequent editions.

Acknowledgments

The co-authors, contributors, and I wish to thank the many individuals whose input was of value in the development of this manuscript, including the talented professionals at the Health Sciences Division of Addison-Wesley Publishing Company, especially Nancy Evans, Joanne Sipple Price, and Glenda Epting who helped tremendously. We also thank the following nurse specialists who reviewed specific chapters: Lolita M. Adrien, Cheryl Ashbaucher, Suzanne J. Axel, Cindi Bedell, Linda Belsky, Joyce M. Black, Joy Boarini, Barbara Boss, Marguerite Brady, Lora E. Burke, Kathryn Suggs Chance, Irene C. Cullin, Ursula Easterday, Jane Farrell, Christine Farris, Sheila Glennon, Mary Catherine Googe, Judy Harr, Phyllis Healy, Kay Holmes, Susan Hopper, Mima Horne, Cheri Howard, Virginia Kahn, Kimberly Keres, Leslie S. Kern, Donna Kershner, Parry J. Knauss, Marian Langer, Marianne Lillie, Deitra L. Lowdermilk, Esther Matassarin-Jacobs, Carolyn F. McCain, Mary Lou Muwaswes, Martha Orr, Kate O'Hare, Judith M. Petrick, Dorothy Pietras, Barbara B. Rosenblum, Vincent T. Rudan, Elizabeth Stokes, Charlene Strebel, Diana Sullivan, Joyce Waterman Taylor, Deborah M. Thorpe, Linda Winkler, and Kathleen S. Zadak, as well as Charles Christoph, RRT. We are also indebted to the following nurse educators and clinicians who read and critiqued the completed manuscript: Jane Hawks, Pam Jeffries, Avis McDonald, Kathy Pagana, Dennis Ross, and Betsy Todd. Finally, we wish to thank the following individuals who assisted us during the initial writing of the manuscript: Jean Lertola, RNC, MA; Francesco Marincola, MD; Edward E. Tueller, MD; and John Vaughn, ORT.

Pamela L. Swearingen
December, 1985

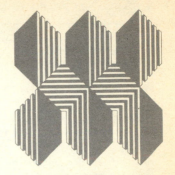

Respiratory Disorders

▶ Section One   **Acute Respiratory Disorders**

Acute respiratory disorders are short-term diseases or acute complications of underlying chronic conditions. They can occur once and respond to treatment or recur to further complicate an underlying condition.

I. Pneumothorax

Pneumothorax is a collection of gas or air in the pleural space. Risk factors include COPD, previous pneumothorax, chest injury, and positive pressure ventilation with high airway pressures. There are three types.

Spontaneous: Occurs when a small or large vesicle on the visceral pleura ruptures, usually from an unidentifiable cause. However, patients with chronic obstructive pulmonary disease (COPD) can develop a spontaneous pneumothorax from severe coughing, rupture of blebs, lung cancer, tuberculosis, lung abscess, or pulmonary infarction. Spontaneous pneumothorax also can occur after the insertion of a central line into the subclavian vein. This type is considered a closed pneumothorax in that the leak is closed to the atmosphere.

Traumatic: Results either from a traumatic injury to the chest wall such as a gunshot wound or stabbing, or artificially from a lung biopsy or thoracocentesis in which air enters the pleural space from the atmosphere (open pneumothorax).

Tension: Occurs when a tear in the pleura does not seal, resulting in a one-way valve effect: Air enters the pleura but cannot escape, causing an accumulation in the pleural space. This produces a shift in the affected lung and mediastinum toward the opposite side, potentially resulting in cardiovascular collapse. Tension pneumothorax is a *very dangerous* condition that can lead to death if left untreated.

A. Assessment

The clinical indicators vary somewhat depending on the type of pneumothorax.

Signs and Symptoms

☐ *Spontaneous or traumatic:* Sudden onset of sharp chest pain, dyspnea on exertion, coughing, restlessness, anxiety, feeling of chest tightness.

☐ *Tension:* Dyspnea, anxiety.

Physical exam

☐ *Spontaneous or traumatic:* Absent or diminished breath sounds on the affected side, decreased tactile fremitus, hyperresonance over the affected lung, and decreased thoracic movement on the affected side, depending on the size of the pneumothorax. Cyanosis and/or pallor appear as late signs.

☐ *Tension:* Decreased or absent breath sounds on the affected side, subcutaneous emphysema (crepitus), pallor, cool and clammy skin, neck vein distention, hypotension, tachycardia, cyanosis, and displaced trachea deviating toward the unaffected side. **Caution:** Tension pneumothorax is life threatening and requires immediate treatment.

B. Diagnostic Tests

1. <u>Chest x-ray:</u> Reveals the presence of air in the pleural space, determines the extent of the pneumothorax, and shows any shift in the mediastinum.

2. <u>ABGs:</u> Abnormal if there is a significant pneumothorax, in which case respiratory acidosis with hypoxemia will be present, showing a decrease in pH, decrease in Pao_2 and O_2 saturation, and an increase in $Paco_2$.

C. Medical Management and Surgical Interventions

Management is determined by the signs and symptoms in relationship to the extent of the pneumothorax. If the pneumothorax is small and corrects itself via reabsorption of the free air, medical intervention may be unnecessary.

1. **Oxygen therapy** if the pneumothorax is large and ABG results reveal a low Pao_2.

2. **Analgesics** for management of pain.

3. **Chest tube insertion** into the second or third anterior intercostal space. The tube is then connected to a closed chest drainage system or one-way flutter valve to remove air from the pleural space and facilitate lung re-expansion.

4. **Thoracocentesis** for a tension pneumothorax to remove air from the pleural space.

5. **Thoracotomy** to instill a pleural irritant, which causes the pleurae to adhere, preventing recurrence of the pneumothorax. This is performed when the pneumothorax has recurred on the same side three or four times, or when it has occurred on both sides.

D. Nursing Diagnoses and Interventions

Potential alteration in respiratory function related to blockage, air leak, or dislodging of chest tube

Desired outcome: Patient does not exhibit signs of respiratory dysfunction.

1. Maintain closed chest drainage system appropriately by ensuring patency and drainage, avoiding kinks in the tubing, securely taping connection sites, and monitoring fluid level in the collection chamber and water movement in the water seal chamber.

2. Be aware that fluctuations in the water seal chamber are normal until the lung re-expands. Bubbling is normal until the air leak begins to seal, but then it should lessen. If bubbling recurs (and the patient's respiratory status is normal), an air leak is present either at the chest tube insertion site or within the drainage collection system. A leak at the chest tube insertion site can be heard with auscultation. Reinforce the site with air-occlusive tape and notify MD of findings. A leak within the collection system necessitates exchanging the system for a new one.

3. **Do not clamp chest tube unless specifically prescribed.** Keep a sterile petrolatum (Vaseline) gauze pad at the bedside. If the chest tube becomes dislodged from the patient's body, remove the dressing and press the Vaseline gauze over the chest tube insertion site. Keep a small bottle of sterile water at the bedside so that if the chest tube becomes separated from the closed drainage system, the chest tube can be inserted into the water to maintain the closed system. A new sterile connector should be used to reconnect the chest tube to the drainage system.

Impaired gas exchange related to tissue hypoxia secondary to decreased lung capacity

Desired outcome: Patient demonstrates VS and ABG values within acceptable range.

1. Review ABG results, noting any changes in the Pao_2 and $Paco_2$. Report all ABG results to MD. A decreased Pao_2 occurs with hypoxemia and is indicative of the possible need for oxygen therapy; an increased $Paco_2$ occurs with hypoventilation.

2. Monitor for increased work of breathing, chest pain, cyanosis, and diminished or absent thoracic movement on the affected side.

3. To promote optimal air exchange, assist patient with attaining position of comfort, usually semi-Fowler's.

4. Encourage deep breathing and coughing in a controlled manner to help remove accumulated fluid in the pleural space and tracheobronchial tree and to enhance drainage.

5. Deliver oxygen as prescribed.

6. Report significant changes in respiratory status to MD.

Alteration in comfort: Pain related to pneumothorax and/or chest tube insertion

Desired outcome: Patient verbalizes a reduction in discomfort and does not exhibit signs of uncontrolled pain.

1. Assess patient for the presence of discomfort, and administer analgesics as prescribed.

2. Discuss the effectiveness of the pain management with the patient; document effective pain relief measures in the nursing care plan.

3. Premedicate patient a half-hour before coughing exercises and assist with changing positions and ambulating if necessary.

4. Teach patient to splint the affected side with pillows during coughing exercises.

5. Provide rest periods between care activities.

E. Patient–Family Teaching and Discharge Planning

Provide patient and SOs with verbal and written information for the following:

1. Potential for recurring pneumothorax and the need for immediate medical attention if it happens.

2. Medications, including name, purpose, frequency of administration, precautions, and potential side effects.

3. Importance of avoiding physical exertion until approved by MD.

4. Necessity for follow-up medical appointments; confirm time and date of next appointment if possible.

II. Pneumonia

Pneumonia is usually caused by bacteria or a virus. *Bacterial pneumonia* involves all or part of a lobe, whereas *viral pneumonia* appears throughout the lungs. Inflammation and edema occur first, and this leads to consolidation, in which the alveoli are filled with exudate. Patients who have had a recent cold or flu, chronic illness, or malnutrition have a predisposition for the development of pneumonia. *Aspiration pneumonia* is caused by the aspiration of gastric contents into the lungs, which produces severe inflammation.

A. Assessment

The severity of signs and symptoms is in direct proportion to the extent of the disease process.

Signs and symptoms: Fever and chills of sudden onset, chest pain, painful cough, malaise, diaphoresis, nausea and vomiting, diarrhea, herpes simplex, headache. **Note:** In elderly patients, symptoms may be absent or subtle.

Physical exam: Flaring of nostrils and grunting respirations during the expiratory phase, shallow and rapid respirations, crackles (rales) and bronchial sounds over areas of consolidation, decreased breath sounds, dullness over affected lung fields with percussion, increased fremitus over the affected area with palpation, elevated temperature, poor skin turgor, possible tachycardia, and circumoral cyanosis in the late stages. **Note:** Elderly patients might not cough or have a fever, but instead may present with a decreased appetite, lethargy, or confusion.

Risk factors: Recent URI, poor nutrition, COPD, exposure to pollutants, low activity level, fluid aspiration, smoking, cardiac failure.

B. Diagnostic Tests

1. <u>Chest x-ray:</u> Confirms the presence of pneumonia, showing vague haziness to consolidation in the affected lung fields.

2. <u>Sputum culture:</u> Determines the pathogen so that appropriate antibiotic treatment can be started. A culture is not helpful with viral pneumonia, however.

3. <u>WBC count:</u> Usually increased to 20,000–35,000.

4. <u>Blood culture:</u> Identifies the presence of infection and extent of the disease. It is positive in a third of all cases, and should be drawn before initiating antibiotic therapy.

5. <u>ABG results:</u> Depend on the progression of the disease. A decreased Pao_2 can occur, but an increased $Paco_2$ occurs rarely unless the patient also has COPD.

6. <u>EKG:</u> Often done to determine cardiac status.

C. Medical Management

1. **Oral and/or IV fluids:** To prevent dehydration.

2. **Oxygen therapy:** If indicated by ABG results or patient symptoms.

3. **Bed rest.**

4. **Pharmacotherapy**

   □ *Antipyretics:* To reduce temperature.

   □ *Antibiotics:* As determined by specific bacterial pathogen.

   □ *Antitussives:* In the absence of sputum production, if coughing is continuous and exhausting to patient.

5. **Percussion and postural drainage.**

6. **Hyperinflation therapy (IPPB):** For patients with inadequate inspiratory effort.

7. **Ventilator therapy:** For severe cases of pulmonary failure (usually occurs in ICU).

D. Nursing Diagnoses and Interventions

Ineffective airway clearance related to pain and fatigue secondary to lung consolidation

Desired outcome: Patient demonstrates effective airway clearance.

1. Assist patient with removing lung secretions by administering prescribed percussion and postural drainage. For optimal airway clearance, premedicate patient with analgesics a half-hour before the treatment, as necessary.

2. Enhance patient's ability and willingness to cough by demonstrating how to splint chest with a pillow or crossed arms.

3. Assess need for hyperinflation therapy (IPPB); if it is prescribed, administer as needed.

4. Inspect sputum for amount, color, and consistency, and document findings. Sputum will change in color from clear to white to yellow to green as the condition worsens.

5. If patient is on bed rest, arrange for turning q2h. If ambulatory, assist patient accordingly to facilitate movement of secretions.

6. Enhance deep breathing and coughing by assisting patient into position of comfort, usually semi-Fowler's.

7. Suction airway as needed.

Impaired gas exchange related to tissue hypoxia secondary to inflammatory process

Desired outcome: Patient demonstrates compliance with rest and exhibits VS and ABG values within acceptable range.

1. Assess patient's breathing status by noting chest movement and auscultating anterior, lateral, and posterior lung fields for breath sounds. Be alert to the presence of dyspnea, restlessness, tachycardia, or confusion.
2. Monitor and document VS q4h, assessing temperature rectally.
3. Review ABG results and report them to MD. Note changes in Pao_2: A decrease occurs with hypoxemia and is often indicative of the need for oxygen therapy.
4. Administer prescribed oxygen therapy as indicated.
5. During periods of fever, dyspnea, and fatigue, keep activity to a minimum.

Potential fluid volume deficit related to increased need secondary to infection and/or loss secondary to diaphoresis

Desired outcome: Patient does not exhibit signs of dehydration.

1. Monitor and document I&O and VS. Be alert to signs of decreased hydration such as poor skin turgor, hypotension, dried mucous membranes, tachycardia, weakened pulse, and thirst.
2. Encourage fluids to ensure adequate hydration, at least 2–3 L/day in the nonrestricted patient.
3. Provide oral hygiene, including lip and tongue care to moisten dried tissues and mucous membranes.

Activity intolerance related to fatigue secondary to inflammatory process

Desired outcome: Patient relates the attainment of optimal amounts of rest.

1. Pace activities to patient tolerance; ensure adequate rest periods.
2. If necessary, assist patient with ADLs and other activities such as ambulating to bathroom.
3. To ensure adequate rest, discourage SOs/staff from conversing at length with patient.
4. Involve patient and SOs in decisions regarding the pacing of activities.
5. Provide verbal support for activities that are accomplished.

Alterations in nutrition: Less than body requirements related to decreased intake secondary to anorexia

Desired outcome: Patient does not exhibit signs of malnutrition or weight loss.

1. If patient is SOB or otherwise uncomfortable, provide a liquid diet or frequent, small meals of foods that are easily swallowed. Request dietary supplements or a high-calorie diet.
2. If prescribed, administer parenteral nutrition.
3. Teach patient the importance of good nutrition.

E. Patient–Family Teaching and Discharge Planning

Provide patient and SOs with verbal and written information for the following:

1. Preventing fatigue by pacing activities and allowing for frequent rest periods.
2. Promoting adequate air exchange by coughing and deep breathing to remove secretions.
3. Avoiding exposure to individuals known to have colds or the flu.
4. Seeing MD for follow-up visits.

5. Need for patient and family to have yearly influenza vaccine.

6. Minimizing factors that can cause reinfection, including close living conditions, poor nutrition, and poorly ventilated living quarters and/or work environment.

7. Medications, including the name, purpose, dosage, schedule, precautions, and potential side effects.

III. Pleurisy

Pleurisy is the inflammation of the visceral and parietal pleurae of the lung. It develops suddenly and occurs as a complication of inflammatory pulmonary conditions such as pneumonia, tuberculosis, viral infections, or pulmonary abscess. The prognosis is good unless a chronic infection also develops. Pleurisy can lead to pleural effusion (see pp. 13–15).

A. Assessment

Signs and symptoms: Fever, malaise, pain with deep breath on inspiration or with coughing.

Physical exam of affected lung segment: Presence of pleural friction rub (squeaky, leathery sound) at the end of inspiration and/or beginning of expiration with auscultation; limited thoracic movement; dullness elicited with percussion. In addition, patients have shallow and rapid respirations and use accessory muscles with respirations.

History of: Recent URI, pulmonary emboli, heart failure, cancer.

B. Diagnostic Tests

Diagnosis is confirmed by the presence of a pleural friction rub with auscultation of the lung fields.

1. WBC: May be increased.

2. Culture and sensitivity of blood and sputum: May show presence of infection.

C. Medical Management

1. **Bed rest.**

2. **Oxygen therapy:** If required.

3. **Analgesics:** For pain relief.

4. **Antitussives:** For cough control.

5. **Nerve block:** In the presence of severe pain.

6. **Treatment of underlying condition** such as pneumonia (see p. 5) or tuberculosis (see p. 28).

D. Nursing Diagnoses and Interventions

Ineffective breathing patterns related to guarding secondary to pain at the affected lung site

Desired outcome: Patient's respiratory rate and depth are within acceptable limits.

1. Monitor and document respiratory rate and depth q4h. Auscultate anterior and posterior lung fields for breath sounds, noting presence of pleural friction rub.

2. Observe for and document increased work of breathing, including use of accessory muscles and flared nostrils.

3. To facilitate optimal breathing pattern, assist patient into a position of comfort, typically semi-Fowler's position.

4. Enhance air exchange by having patient utilize diaphragmatic breathing (see description, in point no. 5 under **Impaired gas exchange**, p. 26).
5. Encourage controlled coughing and deep breathing q2–4h; teach patient how to splint chest with coughing.
6. Provide prescribed oxygen therapy as indicated.
7. Be alert to signs of pleural effusion (see discussion, p. 14).
8. Report significant findings to MD.

Sleep pattern disturbance related to awakening secondary to pain and dyspnea

Desired outcome: Patient verbalizes the attainment of adequate amounts of rest.

1. Allow for rest periods between care activities. Ensure a restful environment.
2. Assist patient with ADLs.
3. Encourage visitors not to tire patient with long visits.
4. Involve patient in decisions regarding optimal pacing of activities.

E. Patient–Family Teaching and Discharge Planning

Provide patient and SOs with verbal and written information for the following:

1. Pacing activities to tolerance.
2. Recognizing symptoms of recurring pleurisy.
3. Avoiding exposure to individuals known to have URI or flu, which can cause recurrence or precipitate pneumonia.
4. Attaining positions of comfort such as sitting in a semi-Fowler's position and splinting affected side with pillows when sleeping.
5. Medications, including name of drug, rationale, route, schedule, precautions, and potential side effects.

IV. Pulmonary Embolism

A pulmonary embolus is a substance that plugs vessels in the pulmonary circulation, with or without damage to lung tissue. Usually the embolus is a blood clot, although air, fat, and amniotic fluid also can obstruct pulmonary circulation. A pulmonary embolism occurs suddenly, typically in the lower lobes. Its severity is determined by the number of clots and the degree of compromise to pulmonary circulation.

A. Assessment

Signs and symptoms: Dyspnea, sudden chest or shoulder pain, anxiety, nonproductive cough, restlessness, irritability, and syncope. Hemoptysis also can occur, but it is rare.

Physical exam: Hypotension, tachycardia, rapid and shallow respirations, distended neck veins. Auscultation over lung fields may reveal decreased breath sounds.

Risk factors: Recent deep-vein thrombosis of lower legs, immobilization secondary to fracture, prolonged periods of sitting or bed rest, use of oral contraceptives, obesity.

B. Diagnostic Tests

1. <u>Chest x-ray:</u> Usually normal but may show an elevated diaphragm, infiltrations, or dilated pulmonary arteries in the presence of significant disease.
2. <u>ABG results:</u> May reveal an elevated pH, decreased Pao_2, decreased $Paco_2$, respiratory alkalosis.
3. <u>EKG</u> (to rule out a myocardial infarction): May reveal tachycardia and/or right ventricular strain.

4. Lung scan (ventilation/perfusion scan): Visualizes pulmonary blood flow under fluoroscopy by injection of an isotope, or distribution of air by the inhalation of an isotope.

5. Fibrin split products test or fibrin degradation products test: Assesses for clotting abnormalities and measures the amount of fibrinogen available for clot formation. Elevation in this test indicates that clotting has taken place.

6. Hemogram (CBC without differential): Evaluates WBC, RBC, Hgb, mean corpuscular volume (MCV), mean corpuscular hemoglobin (MCH), and mean corpuscular hemoglobin concentration (MCHC).

7. Pulmonary angiogram: Determines the presence of filling defects in the pulmonary arteries. This is the most effective diagnostic tool, as it visualizes pulmonary vasculature by the injection of radiopaque dye into the pulmonary artery. **Caution:** Ensure that patient does not have dye allergies.

C. Medical Management and Surgical Interventions

1. **Oxygen therapy:** As indicated by ABG results and patient condition.

2. **Pharmacotherapy**

   □ *IV heparin:* Either continuous or intermittent, administered as soon as diagnosis is made. After 5 days the patient is started on *warfarin*, which is maintained for at least 1 month. Heparin is continued for the first 3–5 days of the warfarin administration because it takes that amount of time for warfarin to reach an effective level.

   □ *Streptokinase (a fibrinolytic agent):* Although not widely used, it may be administered in combination with heparin therapy.

   □ *Vasopressors:* May be used if shock is present secondary to excessive blood loss. The patient is transferred to an intensive care unit if shock occurs.

   □ *Analgesics:* For pain.

3. **Vena cava ligation:** To prevent clots from traveling to the heart and lungs.

4. **Pulmonary embolectomy:** To remove clots from the pulmonary circulation (used only as a secondary intervention). The use of fibrinolytic agents eliminates the need for this procedure.

D. Nursing Diagnoses and Interventions

Potential for injury related to increased risk of bleeding secondary to anticoagulant therapy

Desired outcomes: Patient does not exhibit signs of bleeding. Patient can verbalize knowledge of the side effects of anticoagulant therapy and measures that can prevent bleeding.

1. Review partial thromboplastin time (PTT) for heparin and prothrombin time (PT) for warfarin. Optimally, PTT will be 1½–2½ times normal, and PT will be 1½–2 times normal.

2. Monitor for and report any indications of bleeding to MD: melena, hematemesis, hematuria, hemoptysis, epistaxis, petechiae, and oozing around IV site. Test stool and urine daily for the presence of occult blood.

3. Unless mandatory, refrain from giving IM injections; use IV or PO route instead.

4. To prevent a hematoma or bleeding from the injection site, do not aspirate after needle insertion or massage the site after subcutaneous injection of heparin.

5. Have vitamin K available as an antidote for warfarin.

6. Correlate coagulation test results with anticoagulant dosage, documenting both on the Anticoagulant Flow Sheet and in the nurse's notes.

7. Check the following with another nurse before administering the anti-coagulant: drug name, dose, route, patient name, and time of administration.

8. Teach patient to use an electric razor and soft-bristled toothbrush.

9. Note in the nursing care plan and post a sign over the patient's bed to alert all personnel that the patient is on anticoagulant therapy.

10. Advise the patient about the following warfarin precautions:

   □ Do not omit dosages unless directed to by MD.

   □ Report any signs of bleeding to MD *stat*, such as bleeding gums, nose-bleeds, red or brown urine, red or black stools, bloody sputum, bruising, petechiae, excessive menstrual flow, faintness, weakness, or fever.

   □ Avoid activities that can result in bruises or trauma, such as going barefoot, engaging in contact sports, or using power tools or sharp objects. An intra-uterine device (IUD) should not be used while on this therapy because bleeding can be increased greatly.

   □ Avoid the use of OTC medications unless approved by MD, especially aspirin and salicylates, which inhibit platelet aggregation and predispose the anticoagulated patient to hemorrhage.

   □ Do not change dietary habits without first consulting nurse or MD. Increasing or decreasing dietary intake of vitamin K, a warfarin antagonist, may necessitate a dosage alteration.

   □ Keep appointments with MD or nurse for monitoring PT levels.

See "Pneumonia" for the following: **Activity intolerance** related to fatigue, p. 6.

E. Patient–Family Teaching and Discharge Planning

Provide patient and SOs with verbal and written information for the following:

1. Administration of medications (especially warfarin), including dose, schedule, rationale, precautions, and potential side effects.

2. Necessity for limiting and pacing activities.

3. Need for follow-up appointments with MD and obtaining PT results at scheduled intervals.

4. Planning home activities to minimize potential for injury/bleeding.

5. Wearing a Medic-Alert bracelet or carrying an identification card if patient is on long-term anticoagulant therapy.

V. Hemothorax

Hemothorax is an accumulation of blood in the pleural space caused by an injury to the chest wall and/or lungs. Mediastinal shift and lung collapse can occur, depending on the amount of accumulated blood. A hemothorax usually is present after a penetrating chest wound and it can occur after thoracic surgery, with anticoagulant therapy, or after the insertion of a central venous catheter.

A. Assessment

If the hemothorax is very small, the patient may be asymptomatic. The presence or degree of the following will vary, depending on the severity of the hemothorax.

Signs and symptoms: Chest pain, dyspnea, anxiety, cyanosis, restlessness.

Physical exam: Tachypnea, tachycardia, and shock if blood loss is significant. The affected side will show decreased or absent thoracic movement, dullness with percussion, and decreased or absent breath sounds with auscultation.

B. Diagnostic Tests

1. <u>Chest x-ray</u>: Will show presence of fluid in the pleural space and confirm the presence of a mediastinal shift, if present.

2. <u>ABG values</u>: May confirm the presence of respiratory acidosis as evidenced by decreased pH, increased $Paco_2$, and hypoxemia as indicated by a decreased Pao_2.

3. <u>CBC</u>: May reveal a decrease in hemoglobin, proportionate to the amount of blood loss.

4. <u>Pulmonary function study</u>: Will show a reduced vital capacity.

C. Medical Management and Surgical Interventions

1. **Thoracocentesis:** To remove blood from the pleural space.

2. **Insertion of a chest tube** with connection to **underwater seal drainage:** To drain accumulated blood and assess for further bleeding.

3. **Analgesics:** For pain management.

4. **IV replacement of fluids and blood products:** If there is significant blood loss.

5. **Thoracotomy:** To locate and control the bleeding if blood loss exceeds 200 mL/h over 2 hours.

D. Nursing Diagnoses and Interventions

Potential alteration in respiratory function related to blockage or dislodging of chest tube

Desired outcome: Patient does not exhibit signs of respiratory dysfunction.

1. Assess respiratory status by inspecting, palpating, and auscultating anterior, lateral, and posterior lung fields and by monitoring VS q2h or more frequently, as indicated by patient's condition. After thoracocentesis, monitor VS q15min during the first hour or longer until patient becomes stable.

2. Ensure patency and closed seal of chest tube drainage system by avoiding kinks in tubing, securely taping connection sites, and monitoring fluid level in collection chamber and water movement in water seal chamber. Until the lung re-expands and the patient no longer requires chest drainage, there will be fluctuations (tidaling) in the water seal chamber with inspiration and expiration. Monitor the amount of blood in the collection chamber. Amounts >100 mL/h are considered excessive and should be reported to MD immediately.

3. Unless it is contraindicated, milk or strip the drainage tubing q2–4h or per hospital protocol to help maintain patency of the tubes for drainage.

4. **Do not clamp chest tube unless directed by MD** when changing drainage system or if the chest tube becomes disconnected from drainage system. To prevent a tension hemothorax or pneumothorax, clamp the tube for no longer than a minute or two or place the end of the tube in a small bottle of sterile water held below the level of the chest.

5. Keep a sterile petrolatum (Vaseline) gauze pad at the bedside in case the chest tube becomes dislodged from the patient's body. If this occurs, remove the dressing and press the gauze pad over the insertion site.

See "Pneumothorax" for the following: **Impaired gas exchange,** p. 3, and **Alteration in comfort,** p. 4.

E. Patient–Family Teaching and Discharge Planning

Provide patient and SOs with verbal and written information for the following:

1. Medications, including name, purpose, dosage, schedule, precautions, and potential side effects.
2. Importance of medical follow-up; confirm date and time of next appointment if it is known.
3. Avoiding physical exertion until approved by MD.
4. Indications of respiratory and wound infections and the importance of seeking prompt attention if they occur.

VI. Atelectasis

Atelectasis is a collapse of all or part of the lung, and it is most commonly seen immediately after major abdominal or thoracic surgery. It can be either an acute or chronic condition, and it occurs more frequently in patients with COPD. In the postoperative period it can be precipitated by the effects of anesthesia, sedation, and decreased mobility on pulmonary function. Other potential causes include mucous plugs, foreign objects in the lung, aneurysm, pleural effusion, and bronchogenic carcinoma. Atelectasis can lead to respiratory infection.

A. Assessment

The clinical picture is determined by the site of collapse and rate of development. It can include all or some of the following:

Signs and symptoms: Dyspnea, fever, cyanosis, weakness.

Physical exam: Decreased thoracic movement, absent or decreased breath sounds, bronchial breath sounds in the presence of consolidation, and dullness over affected area with percussion.

History of: Recent surgery of long duration, incision high on abdomen or thorax, lung disease, smoking, obesity, immobility.

B. Diagnostic Test

Chest x-ray: Will reveal higher density in the affected area, and may show decreased lung size.

C. Medical Management

1. **Chest percussion and postural drainage (chest physiotherapy):** To remove secretions if mucous plugs are the cause of the condition.
2. **Deep breathing and coughing exercises.**
3. **Hyperinflation therapy**: To expand partially collapsed lung areas.
4. **Analgesics:** To facilitate coughing for patients who are guarding because of pain.
5. **Bronchoscopy.**
6. **Oxygen therapy:** As needed.

D. Nursing Diagnoses and Interventions

Potential alteration in respiratory function related to prolonged inactivity and/or omission of deep breathing (for all patients on bed rest and/or at risk for atelectasis)

Desired outcome: Patient demonstrates deep breathing at frequent intervals and effective coughing (if needed) and does not exhibit signs of respiratory dysfunction.

1. Teach the patient to deep breathe q1–2h to facilitate expansion of the lung, and to cough to clear the secretions (if needed).
2. Instruct patient in use of incentive spirometer or other hyperinflation device to assist with deep breathing. Ensure that the patient inhales slowly and deeply and holds the breath at the end of inspiration. Encourage the use of

the hyperinflation device q1–2h, followed by coughing, if needed, to raise secretions.

3. If coughing is ineffective to raise secretions, suction may be necessary to stimulate the cough reflex and promote secretion clearance.

4. When appropriate, instruct the patient in the use of a pillow or folded arms to splint the incision during coughing.

5. If prescribed and needed, perform chest physiotherapy to assist in clearance of secretions.

6. Assess respiratory status by auscultating anterior and posterior lung fields as needed and with each therapy.

7. In nonrestricted patients, encourage fluid intake of at least 2–3 L/day to loosen secretions.

8. Encourage ambulation, or reposition patient on bed rest by turning q2h, to promote effective airway clearance.

9. When bronchodilators such as metaproterenol sulfate and albuterol are used, stay with patient during treatment and assess for significant irregularities or elevation in heart rate.

Alteration in comfort: Pain related to surgical incision or disease process

Desired outcome: Patient relates a reduction in discomfort and does not exhibit signs of uncontrolled pain.

1. Assess patient for pain level and effectiveness of pain management.

2. Administer analgesics one half-hour before coughing and deep breathing or chest physiotherapy to reduce pain and enhance compliance.

3. Instruct patient to assume Fowler's position and use splinting technique for comfort during coughing and deep breathing.

4. Assist patient with repositioning and ambulation as necessary.

E. Patient–Family Teaching and Discharge Planning

Provide patient and SOs with verbal and written information for the following:

1. Medications, including name, purpose, dosage, route, schedule, precautions, and potential side effects.

2. Use of hyperinflation device.

3. Importance of walking to tolerance and changing positions while in bed to promote optimal lung expansion.

4. Notifying MD if signs of increased lung collapse (eg, dyspnea and cyanosis) or respiratory infection (eg, SOB, increased sputum or coughing, altered color of sputum) occur.

5. Importance of medical follow-up; confirm time and date of next appointment if known.

6. Precipitating factors for development of atelectasis: mucous plug (in patients with COPD); smoking; and inactivity, especially for patients with COPD or bronchogenic carcinoma.

VII. Pleural Effusion

A pleural effusion is an accumulation of fluid in the pleural space. It is caused by a number of inflammatory, circulatory, or neoplastic diseases, such as congestive heart failure, ascites, pneumonia, or pulmonary embolism. *Transudate effusion* is usually caused by congestive heart failure or cirrhosis. *Exudate effusion* is caused by infection or a tumor.

A. Assessment

Clinical indications of pleural effusion are related to the underlying disease. Dyspnea is present when there is a large effusion; with a small effusion, the patient may be asymptomatic.

Signs and symptoms: Pleuritic pain, diaphoresis, cough.

Physical exam: Fever. Over the affected lung area there will be decreased breath sounds with auscultation, dullness with percussion, and decrease in tactile fremitus with palpation. With a large effusion, the trachea might deviate away from the affected side.

B. Diagnostic Tests

1. <u>Chest x-ray:</u> Will show evidence of effusion if there is >300 mL of fluid present in the pleural space. The costophrenic angle will be obliterated.

2. <u>Thoracocentesis:</u> Allows removal and examination of fluid from pleural space to provide the definitive diagnosis and determine the type of effusion.

3. <u>Pleural biopsy:</u> Determines the cause of effusion. Tissue is removed by biopsy needle and sent to pathology for examination.

C. Medical Management

1. **Multiple thoracocenteses** or **insertion of chest tube attached to a closed drainage system:** To remove fluid if the effusion is large. Fluid should not be drained too quickly.

2. **Tetracycline** or **nitrogen mustard instillation via chest tube:** To sclerose the area if a tumor is causing the effusion. **Note:** During the instillation, the patient is repositioned to disperse the medication. The MD will designate position and length of time it is to be maintained.

3. **Oxygen therapy:** As needed.

4. **Other medical treatment:** Performed as determined by the underlying condition.

D. Nursing Diagnoses and Interventions

Alteration in respiratory function related to decreased lung expansion secondary to fluid accumulation in the pleural space

Desired outcomes: Patient complies with the therapeutic regimen and does not exhibit signs of respiratory dysfunction. If appropriate, the patient can demonstrate apical expansion breathing exercises.

1. Assess respiratory status q2–4h by auscultating anterior and posterior lung fields for breath sounds and monitoring VS, including respiratory rate and depth. Report significant findings to MD.

2. If present, ensure that chest tube drainage system is patent and draining well. (See guidelines for closed chest drainage system with hemothorax, p. 11.) Monitor amount of drainage q4h or more frequently, as necessary.

3. Provide prescribed oxygen therapy as indicated. Instruct patient to notify staff if SOB occurs.

4. Provide hyperinflation therapy (eg, incentive spirometry) at frequent intervals.

5. For patients with gross pleural effusion, provide the following instructions for apical expansion breathing exercises: Sit upright, if possible; position the fingers just below the clavicles; inhale and attempt to push the upper chest wall against the pressure of the fingers; hold the breath for a few moments; and exhale passively. Explain that this exercise, when done at frequent inter-

vals, will help re-expand the involved lung tissue, minimize flattening of the upper chest, and help mobilize secretions.

See "Pneumonia" for the following: **Activity intolerance**, p. 6.

E. Patient–Family Teaching and Discharge Planning

Provide patient and SOs with verbal and written information for the following:

1. Importance of not smoking.
2. Signs of respiratory distress and importance of notifying MD should they develop.
3. Use of at-home equipment such as oxygen, hand-held nebulizer, incentive spirometer.
4. Need for pacing activities and providing for frequent rest periods.

▶ Section Two   **Acute Respiratory Failure**

Acute respiratory failure (ARF) develops when the lungs are unable to exchange oxygen and carbon dioxide adequately. The diagnosis is determined by ABG values, which will show a decreased Pao_2 (<50 mm Hg), possibly an increase in $Paco_2$, and a decreased pII when breathing room air. Conditions that can lead to ARF include central nervous system depression from barbiturate ingestion; head injury; intracranial hemorrhage; neuromuscular diseases such as Guillain-Barré syndrome and multiple sclerosis; flail chest; and respiratory conditions such as emphysema, pulmonary emboli, chronic bronchitis, asthma, pneumonia, and pleural effusion. If ARF is not treated in a timely manner, coma, cardiac failure, and death can ensue.

A. Assessment

The clinical picture can vary, depending on the underlying condition.

Signs and symptoms: *Hypoxemia* causing disorientation, restlessness, agitation, hypertension, and dysrhythmias; *hypercapnia* causing somnolence, confusion, and hypotension; headache; diaphoresis.

Physical exam: Changes in the rate and depth of respirations, including tachypnea; presence of crackles (rales), rhonchi, and diminished breath sounds with auscultation; increased work of breathing as evidenced by use of accessory (sternocleidomastoid) muscles.

B. Diagnostic Tests

1. <u>ABG values:</u> The most important diagnostic tool. Typically, patient will have a decreased Pao_2, possibly an increase in $Paco_2$, and a decreased pH while breathing room air.
2. <u>EKG:</u> May reveal either atrial or ventricular dysrhythmias.
3. <u>Chest x-ray:</u> May reveal the extent of ARF as well as the precipitating underlying condition.
4. <u>WBC count:</u> If elevated, will show evidence of infection.

C. Medical Management

1. **Humidified oxygen therapy:** As determined by ABG values. Optimally, the Pao_2 is maintained at 55 mm Hg or above, $Paco_2$ at 35–45 mm Hg, and pH at

7.3–7.5. If oxygen therapy does not reverse the hypoxemia and hyper-capnia, intubation and mechanical ventilation might be necessary. The $Paco_2$ and pH levels are especially important in the management of patients with COPD. A venturi mask (high-flow system) provides a consistent oxygen concentration that is not dependent on the breathing pattern, and therefore is commonly used in low concentrations (24–28%) for patients with COPD.

2. **IV aminophylline:** To treat bronchospasms. It is regulated according to aminophylline blood levels. Therapeutic range = 10–20 mg/mL.

3. **IPPB with bronchodilators (isoproterenol, isoetharine):** q2–4h to minimize co_2 retention.

4. **Chest physiotherapy:** To assist patient with expectoration of secretions.

5. **Steroids** (IV or PO), such as prednisone 1 mg/kg daily: To help relieve symptoms.

6. **Coughing and deep breathing**: If coughing is ineffective, suctioning may be necessary to stimulate the cough reflex.

7. **Hydration:** Via IV fluids.

8. **Antibiotics:** If infection is present.

9. **Additional treatment:** Determined by the underlying condition.

D. Nursing Diagnoses and Interventions

Impaired gas exchange related to chronic tissue hypoxia secondary to disease process

Desired outcome: Patient demonstrates VS and ABG values within acceptable limits.

1. Assess and document respiratory status at least q2h by auscultating anterior, lateral, and posterior lung fields for presence of adventitious breath sounds, including crackles (rales) and rhonchi, monitoring respiratory rate and depth, and observing for dyspnea and cyanosis. Monitor VS and LOC as well. Report significant findings to MD.

2. Watch for >45 mm Hg of $Paco_2$, which is indicative of carbon dioxide retention (hypercapnia), and for a drop in Pao_2, which occurs with hypoxemia. If elevation in $Paco_2$ and a decrease in Pao_2 continue, intubation with mechanical ventilation probably will be necessary. Report significant ABG values to MD immediately so that appropriate therapy can be initiated.

3. Administer prescribed oxygen therapy. For patients with COPD, maintain venturi mask at prescribed low concentrations or deliver low-flow oxygen device at 1–3 L/min, or as prescribed.

4. Enhance air exchange by having patient assume high Fowler's position and turn from side to side q2h.

5. Encourage ambulation if patient's condition permits.

6. Administer bronchodilator therapy as prescribed and monitor for side effects of the treatment, including fast or irregular heart beat.

7. Ensure patency of IV device for aminophylline infusion. Check the site and drip rate at least q1–2h. Be alert to signs of toxicity, such as tachycardia, dysrhythmias, and decreasing BP.

8. Observe for presence of circumoral cyanosis, which is a late sign of decreased oxygenation.

9. Keep a manual resuscitator at the bedside.

Sleep pattern disturbance related to awakening secondary to dyspnea and treatment schedule

Desired outcome: Patient relates the attainment of adequate rest.

1. Anticipate interrupted sleep pattern because of breathing problems and treatment schedules; encourage patient to sleep between care activities.
2. Schedule care activities in a flexible manner, whenever possible, to allow periods of uninterrupted sleep.
3. Keep patient's environment calm and quiet; limit the number of visitors.

Ineffective airway clearance related to ineffective coughing

Desired outcome: Patient demonstrates the ability to clear the airway.

1. If bronchodilator therapy has been prescribed, administer chest physiotherapy as directed to assist patient with airway clearance.
2. Evaluate efficacy of chest physiotherapy and bronchodilator therapy by ausculating anterior and posterior lung fields for presence of adventitious breath sounds.
3. Instruct patient in effective coughing technique: Sit upright with upper body flexed slightly forward; take two deep breaths and exhale passively; then take a deep breath, hold it, and cough forcefully. **Note:** To avoid small-airway collapse, patients with COPD should cough twice sharply from the mid-inspiratory point rather than after a deep breath.
4. If patient is unable to cough up secretions, perform tracheal suctioning to stimulate the cough reflex and enhance airway clearance.

Potential fluid volume deficit related to decreased intake secondary to fatigue and/or prescribed limitations

Desired outcome: Patient does not exhibit signs of dehydration.

1. Monitor I&O and weight daily.
2. Assess skin turgor, mucous membranes, and VS as indicators of hydration status.
3. Give oral fluids, and administer IV fluids as prescribed. **Note:** Depending on underlying condition, fluids may be limited to prevent further compromise to cardiac and respiratory system.

See "Appendix One" for nursing diagnoses and interventions for the care of patients with life-disrupting illnesses, p. 544.

E. Patient–Family Teaching and Discharge Planning

ARF is an acute condition that is symptomatically treated during the patient's hospitalization. Discharge planning and patient–family teaching should be directed to the underlying condition and treatment for that condition. See sections of this book that describe the content pertaining to the precipitating condition.

▶ Section Three   **Chronic Obstructive Pulmonary Disease**

Chronic obstructive pulmonary disease (COPD) is any chronic respiratory condition that obstructs the flow of air to or from the bronchioles. Causative factors include aging, smoking, allergens, and environmental and occupational pollutants. COPD also is referred to as chronic obstructive lung disease (COLD).

I. Asthma

Asthma is a disorder in which there is obstruction of airflow in the bronchioles and smaller bronchi, producing bronchospasm, mucosal edema, and excessive mucus production. It can occur in any age group, and its symptoms are intermittent and usually alleviated with treatment. *Extrinsic asthma* is precipitated by environmental allergens, including pollens, dust, feathers, animal dander, and foods. *Intrinsic asthma* is believed to be caused by an infection in the upper or lower respiratory tract and occurs more frequently in individuals over age 35.

A. Assessment

Signs and symptoms: Dyspnea with a prolonged expiratory phase, productive cough with thick sputum.

Physical exam: Wheezing that is often audible without a stethoscope, high-pitched wheezes and a prolonged expiratory phase heard with auscultation, use of accessory muscles for respirations, flared nostrils, retraction of intercostal spaces, neck vein distention, and tachycardia.

▶ **Note:** If symptoms are not treated, the condition can progress to *status asthmaticus*, a state in which there is almost no air exchange; if it is not reversed, death will ensue.

B. Diagnostic Tests

1. <u>ABG values:</u> To assess the severity of the asthma attack. Respiratory acidosis (decreased pH, increased $Paco_2$) usually is present. Serial ABG values reflect the effectiveness of the treatment.

2. <u>Chest x-ray:</u> May reveal hyperinflation of the lungs during an attack; may also rule out conditions such as pneumonitis that can produce similar symptoms.

3. <u>WBC and sputum specimen analysis:</u> To determine the presence of infection.

4. <u>Skin testing:</u> To identify the allergen that produced the attack.

5. <u>Pulmonary function testing:</u> To evaluate the degree of obstruction. Will reveal a decreased vital capacity, increased residual volume, and a decreased forced expiratory volume.

6. <u>EKG:</u> To reveal the degree of tachycardia and right heart strain and the presence of cardiac disease.

C. Medical Management

For acute episode:

1. **Pharmacotherapy:** Parenteral or inhalant epinephrine, bronchodilators, and corticosteroids. Antibiotics are given if there is evidence of infection. **Caution:** Unless the patient is intubated, sedatives are contraindicated because they diminish respirations.

2. **Oxygen therapy** (based on ABG results): Low-flow, typically 1–3 L/min via nasal cannula or high-flow via venturi mask.

3. **Serial ABG values:** To evaluate patient's condition and the effectiveness of treatment.

4. **IV catheter insertion:** For hydration and delivery of IV medications.

5. **Chest physiotherapy:** To enhance secretion expectoration if necessary. This treatment is used with caution, however, because it can exacerbate symptoms.

For continued therapy:

1. **Aminophylline:** Dosage determined by blood levels of aminophylline. Blood specimen is drawn 2 hours after oral dose of medication to check for peak level. It is desirable to reach a therapeutic level in which patient is symptom free. Therapeutic range = 10–20 mg/mL.

2. **Identification of stressors that precipitate or exacerbate asthmatic attacks.**
3. **Nebulized bronchodilators and/or steroids.**

D. Nursing Diagnoses and Interventions

Impaired gas exchange related to chronic tissue hypoxia secondary to obstructive process in the bronchioles and bronchi

Desired outcome: Patient demonstrates VS and ABG values within acceptable limits.

1. Assess VS and auscultate anterior, lateral, and posterior lung fields for breath sounds q1–2h or more frequently as necessary. Report to MD any significant changes in VS and respiratory pattern, such as increasing dyspnea or tachycardia.
2. Observe for presence of cyanosis (circumoral, nailbed, mucous membrane, and underside of tongue) as a late sign of hypoxemia.
3. Review ABG results, noting changes in pH, $Paco_2$, and Pao_2. Respiratory acidosis is most often seen during an acute asthma attack in which the pH is below normal and the $Paco_2$ is increased. Any increase in acidosis signals a worsening condition. Notify MD of significant findings.
4. Maintain low concentrations of high-flow oxygen via a venturi mask or low-flow oxygen at 1–3 L/min, or as prescribed.
5. Enhance air exchange by assisting patient into high Fowler's position.
6. Administer bronchodilator therapy if prescribed. Monitor for the presence of tachycardia/dysrhythmias.

Ineffective airway clearance related to excessive mucus production and ineffective coughing

Desired outcome: Patient demonstrates appropriate coughing technique and the ability to raise secretions.

1. Administer percussion and postural drainage, as prescribed, to assist with clearing of airways.
2. Instruct COPD patient in the "double cough" technique: Sit upright with the upper body flexed forward slightly; take 2–3 breaths and exhale passively; inhale again, but only to the midinspiratory point; then exhale by coughing quickly two or three times. This technique prevents small airway collapse, which can occur with one forceful cough.
3. Auscultate anterior, lateral, and posterior lung fields to evaluate breath sounds q2–4h and after coughing.

Alteration in nutrition: Less than body requirements related to decreased intake secondary to fatigue and anorexia

Desired outcome: Patient does not exhibit signs of malnutrition or weight loss.

1. Monitor I&O and record food intake daily; weigh patient at least weekly.
2. Encourage intake of foods high in protein and carbohydrates. Provide small, frequent meals to minimize fatigue and enhance patient's compliance with eating.
3. When necessary, involve dietician in meal planning.
4. Minimize the potential for distention by avoiding gas-producing foods and carbonated beverages.
5. Provide oral care at frequent intervals to enhance appetite.

Anxiety related to perceived threat to biologic integrity secondary to sensation of suffocation

Desired outcomes: Patient does not exhibit ineffective coping mechanisms. Patient relates the presence of psychologic comfort.

1. Keep patient and SOs well informed of activities, therapy, and procedures in which patient will participate. Involve patient in decisions about care activities.

2. Remain with patient during acute episodes. Answer questions and provide care in a calm, reassuring manner.

3. Facilitate transition to home care by initiating discharge planning early in patient's hospital stay.

4. Encourage patient to establish realistic goals for return to wellness.

See "Acute Respiratory Failure" for the following: **Sleep pattern disturbance**, p. 16. See "Pneumoconioses" for the following: **Potential for infection** (recurring URIs), p. 26

E. Patient–Family Teaching and Discharge Planning

Provide patient and SOs with verbal and written information for the following:

1. Medications to be taken at home, including name, schedule, dosage, purpose, route, precautions, and potential side effects. Caution patient about overmedicating in an attempt to relieve symptoms. For example, overmedication of any of the bronchodilators can increase the heart rate and cause nausea, vomiting, and abdominal pain.

2. Use of at-home therapy, including hand-held nebulizers for administering bronchodilators and steroids. Counsel patient on the need to taper the dosage of steroids gradually rather than abruptly. Advise steroid-dependent asthmatics about the need for additional steroids in the event of a serious injury or surgery.

3. Signs and symptoms that necessitate medical intervention, including increased dyspnea unrelieved by prescribed dosage of medication, increased lethargy, increased sputum production (an indicator of infection), or an interruption of the sleep pattern related to dyspnea.

4. Avoiding exposure to infectious individuals, particularly those with URIs.

5. Importance of pacing activities to tolerance and allowing for intermittent rest periods.

6. Introduction to local American Lung Association activities and pulmonary rehabilitation programs.

7. Potential need for change in environment such as the elimination of certain foods, pets, feather pillows, dust.

8. Availability of emergency phone numbers, including that of MD.

9. Maintenance of diet high in protein and carbohydrates.

10. Identification and alleviation of emotional stressors by using visualization and biofeedback, as appropriate.

11. Importance of follow-up appointments with MD.

II. Chronic Bronchitis

Chronic bronchitis is the most common respiratory disease. It occurs in individuals who have smoked cigarettes for a long period of time and/or lived in areas of severe air pollution. The extent of the disease is dependent on the number of cigarettes smoked, the length of time smoking has occurred, and/or the length of time spent living in the polluted air.

Lung changes that occur with this disease include inflammation, loss of ciliary action, hypertrophy of mucosal glands, hyperinflation of the alveoli, and edema of bronchial mucosae, all of which result in an increase of mucus production. When this occurs, mucous plugs develop in the stretched alveoli, causing obstruction of the bronchioles. As the disease progresses, there is further destruction of the lung tissue, causing inadequate ventilation and perfusion. Recurrent URIs are common in these patients, especially during the winter. As the disease progresses, acute episodes increase in severity and length. Respiratory failure and cardiac problems (right ventricular failure due to pulmonary hypertension) can develop. Centrilobular emphysema is common.

A. Assessment

Chronic indicators: Morning cough, production of clear and copious sputum, anorexia, cyanosis, edema.

Acute indicators: Fever, dyspnea, thick and tenacious sputum.

Physical exam: Use of accessory muscles for respiration; digital clubbing; prolonged expiratory phase, rhonchi, and wheezes heard with auscultation; dullness over areas of consolidation elicited with percussion; decreased thoracic expansion with palpation. Dependent edema will be present if there is right ventricular failure.

B. Diagnostic Tests

1. ABG values: Reveal hypoxemia and hypercapnia (in most cases) in which Pao_2 is below normal and $Paco_2$ is elevated. The severity of the respiratory acidosis is directly related to the severity of the condition.

2. Sputum culture: May reveal the presence of infection.

3. Chest x-ray: Will reveal a normal A–P diameter, nearly normal diaphragm position, and increased peripheral lung markings.

4. Pulmonary function tests: Will show a reduced vital capacity, increased residual volume (trapping of air), and a decreased expiratory reserve volume.

5. CBC: Will reveal an increased WBC count in the presence of bacterial infection, and an elevated hematocrit in the presence of hypoxemia.

C. Medical Management

1. **Bronchodilator therapy**: Oral, IV, and/or inhalant to relieve bronchospasm.

2. **Oxygen therapy:** To treat hypoxemia. With severe hypoxemia, exhaustion, and/or acidosis, patient might require intubation and ventilator support.

3. **Antibiotics:** If bacterial infection is present.

4. **Chest physiotherapy:** To assist in removal of secretions.

5. **Adequate fluid intake:** By oral and/or IV routes to maintain hydration.

6. **Diuretics** and **salt restriction:** In the presence of cardiac complications.

7. **Corticosteroids:** To decrease inflammation and improve air exchange.

8. **Restrict smoking.**

D. Nursing Diagnoses and Interventions

Impaired gas exchange related to chronic tissue hypoxia secondary to bronchiole obstruction

Desired outcome: Patient exhibits VS and ABG values within acceptable range.

1. Assess VS and auscultate anterior, lateral, and posterior lung fields for breath sounds q1–2h or more frequently as necessary. Report to MD any significant changes, including dyspnea and tachycardia.

2. Assist patient into high Fowler's position, and turn patient from side to side q2h to enhance aeration.

3. Maintain low-flow oxygen at 1–3 L/min, or as prescribed.

4. Review ABG values, noting changes in pH, $Paco_2$, Pao_2, and HCO_3. With chronic bronchitis the pH is typically low-normal (because of the compensatory action of the kidneys), $Paco_2$ is increased, and HCO_3 is increased (because the kidneys excrete more hydrogen ions with compensation).

5. Observe for presence of cyanosis (underside of tongue, mucous membrane, and circumoral) as a late indicator of decreased oxygenation. Also be alert to somnolence, which can signal increased hypoxemia and hypercapnia.

6. Administer bronchodilator therapy as prescribed. Remain with patient to monitor for side effects of therapy, which can include tachycardia and dysrhythmias.

Potential alterations in fluid volume: *Excess* related to retention secondary to decreased cardiac output; *deficit* related to decreased intake or fluid restriction

Desired outcome: Patient does not exhibit signs of dehydration or overhydration.

1. Monitor I&O, assess skin turgor and mucous membranes, and weigh patient daily to assess hydration.

2. In the nonrestricted patient, encourage fluid intake of at least 2–3 L/day to ensure adequate hydration and help keep secretions thin to promote their expectoration.

3. As the disease progresses, cardiac complications are likely and fluid restriction becomes necessary. The assessment of the patient's level of hydration and response to fluids is essential. Be especially alert to neck vein distention, VS changes, increased dyspnea, and crackles (rales). **Note:** Be aware that fluid restriction will also thicken the secretions and complicate the condition if the patient is unable to expectorate.

See "Acute Respiratory Failure" for the following: **Sleep pattern disturbance**, p. 16. See "Asthma" for the following: **Ineffective airway clearance**, p. 19, **Alteration in nutrition**, p. 19, and **Anxiety**, pp. 19–20. See "Pneumoconioses" for the following: **Potential for infection** (recurring URIs), p. 26. See "Appendix One" for nursing diagnoses and interventions for the care of patients with life-disrupting illnesses, p. 544.

E. Patient–Family Teaching and Discharge Planning

Provide patient and SOs with verbal and written information for the following:

1. Medications, including drug name, dosage, purpose, schedule, route, precautions, and potential side effects. Caution patient about overmedicating in an attempt to relieve symptoms.

2. Indications of changes in condition that warrant medical attention: changes in color, consistency, and amount of sputum; increased dyspnea; fever and chills; increased cough; decreased activity tolerance; and/or feeling of tightness in chest.

3. Use of at-home oxygen therapy, including indications for use, precautions (eg, warning not to increase flow rate above that prescribed), and community resources for oxygen replacement when necessary.

4. Importance of avoiding infectious individuals, especially those with URIs; the availability of flu and pneumococcal vaccine.

5. Pacing activities to tolerance and allowing for intermittent rest periods.

6. Diet planning, including list of foods high in protein and carbohydrates and discussing the need for adequate hydration.

7. Introduction to local American Lung Association activities and pulmonary rehabilitation programs.

8. Referral to dietician if weight reduction or sodium restriction is necessary.

III. Emphysema

Pulmonary emphysema is characterized by the destruction of pulmonary elastic tissue, reduction of elastic recoil of the lungs, and the formation of cystic areas in the lungs that diminish air exchange. There is enlargement of the air passages distal to the terminal bronchioles and airway collapse on expiration, reducing expiratory airflow. There are three types of emphysema.

Centrilobular: The most common type, frequently associated with chronic bronchitis. The destruction is limited to the bronchioles, and it is found in the upper lung fields. It can progress to panlobular emphysema.

Panlobular: Caused by a deficiency of alpha-antitrypsin and considered to be an inherited disease. There is uniform destruction of alveoli, usually in the lower lung fields.

Paraseptal: Caused by conditions that produce scarring or fibrosis of lung tissue. The alveolar sac is involved.

Emphysema is a progressive disease, and affected individuals can become totally disabled by using all available energy for breathing. In later stages, pulmonary hypertension develops, leading to cor pulmonale, which produces cardiac as well as respiratory problems.

A. Assessment

Chronic indicators: Nonproductive cough (unless patient also has chronic bronchitis), dyspnea on exertion.

Acute indicators: Increased dyspnea and coughing, fever, peripheral edema (indicative of cardiac involvement), fatigue.

Physical exam: Weight loss with muscle wasting producing an emaciated look, increased A–P chest diameter, pursed lip breathing, hypertrophy of accessory (sternocleidomastoid) muscles of respiration, hyperresonance elicited over affected lung fields with percussion, decreased breath sounds and a prolonged expiratory phase heard with auscultation, decreased fremitus over affected lung fields, and decrease in thoracic excursion with palpation. Digital clubbing appears in later stages of the disease.

B. Diagnostic Tests

1. <u>Chest x-ray:</u> Will show hyperinflation, an increased A–P diameter, a lowered and flattened diaphragm, and a small cardiac silhouette.

2. <u>ABG values:</u> May reveal a slight decrease in Pao_2. As the disease progresses, Pao_2 will continue to decrease (hypoxemia), and the $Paco_2$ will increase because of hypoventilation and CO_2 retention.

3. <u>Pulmonary function studies:</u> Will show an increased total lung capacity, increased residual volume, and decreased forced expiratory volume. The vital capacity will be normal or slightly decreased.

4. <u>CBC:</u> Will reveal an increased hemoglobin later in the disease phase secondary to increased hypoxemia.

5. <u>EKG:</u> May reveal atrial and ventricular dysrhythmias. Most patients will have an atrial dysrhythmia secondary to atrial dilation and right ventricular hypertrophy caused by pulmonary hypertension.

6. <u>Sputum culture:</u> May reveal presence of a respiratory infection.

C. Medical Management

1. **Oxygen therapy:** As determined by ABG results.

2. **Bronchodilator therapy.**

3. **Antibiotics:** If there is evidence of infection.
4. **Fluids:** For maintenance of hydration.
5. **Corticosteroids:** To improve airflow.
6. **Restrict smoking.**

D. Nursing Diagnoses and Interventions

Impaired gas exchange related to decreased lung capacity and trapping of CO_2 secondary to pulmonary tissue destruction and/or cystic tissue formation

Desired outcomes: Patient exhibits VS and ABG values within acceptable limits. Patient can demonstrate technique for pursed lip breathing.

1. Assess patient's VS and respiratory status q2–4h by auscultating anterior, lateral, and posterior lung fields. Report any significant changes in VS or respiratory status to MD.

2. Teach patient the following procedure for pursed lip breathing to enhance air exchange: Sit upright with hands on the thighs; inhale normally through the nose, with the mouth closed; exhale slowly through the mouth, with the lips pursed in a whistling position. The exhalation should be twice as long as the inhalation and the patient should make a whistling sound when exhaling.

3. Administer bronchodilator therapy as prescribed. Remain with the patient and monitor for side effects of the therapy, including dysrhythmias and tachycardia.

4. Administer oxygen as prescribed. **Caution:** Be aware that higher flow can depress respiratory drive in hypoxic patients.

5. Monitor ABG values, which will reveal the extent of the disease. The Pao_2 shows the level of hypoxemia and the $Paco_2$ will show hyper/hypoventilation. The $Paco_2$ will increase with hypoventilation and trapping of CO_2. Patients with chronic alveolar hypoventilation will have chronic compensated respiratory acidosis in which the pH is low-normal and the HCO_3 is increased because of renal compensation.

See "Acute Respiratory Failure" for the following: **Sleep pattern disturbance,** p. 16. See "Asthma" for the following: **Alteration in nutrition,** p. 19, and **Anxiety,** pp. 19–20. See "Chronic Bronchitis" for the following: **Fluid volume deficit or fluid volume excess,** p. 22. See "Pneumoconioses" for the following: **Potential for infection** (recurring URIs), p. 26. See "Appendix One" for nursing diagnoses and interventions for the care of patients with life-disrupting illnesses, p. 544.

E. Patient–Family Teaching and Discharge Planning

Provide patient and SOs with verbal and written information for the following:

1. Medications, including drug name, dosage, schedule, purpose, route, precautions, and potential side effects.

2. Signs and symptoms that necessitate medical attention: increased dyspnea; fatigue; increased coughing; changes in the amount, color, and consistency of sputum; swelling in ankles and legs; fever; and sudden weight gain.

3. Use of oxygen, including instructions for when to use it, importance of not increasing prescribed flow rate, precautions, and community resources for oxygen replacement when necessary.

4. Avoiding infectious individuals, especially those with URIs.

5. Increasing and pacing activities to tolerance.

6. Follow-up visits with MD; confirm date and time of next appointment.

7. Local American Lung Association activities and pulmonary rehabilitation programs.

▶ Section Four   **Restrictive Respiratory Disorders**

I. Pneumoconioses

The pneumoconioses include a number of disorders that are occupational in origin. They are characterized by permanent retention of inhaled particles, which results in inflammation and fibrosis. Because these particles remain in the lung tissue for the life of the individual, damage to lung tissue is ongoing.

Asbestosis: Develops from exposure to asbestos fibers in occupations such as mining of asbestos, construction, and paint production. It also can occur in family members who are exposed to the asbestos fibers on the clothing of the asbestos worker. Inhalation of these fibers causes lung tissue fibrosis, usually in the lower lobes. In turn, the fibrosis decreases lung volume and elasticity of the tissues, which ultimately leads to pulmonary failure. When exposed to asbestos fiber, cigarette smokers and individuals with COPD are at a greater risk of getting this disease.

Silicosis: Occurs in individuals who inhale dust from quartz rock containing silica. This may occur during mining, tunneling in rock, or sandblasting. The inhaled particles adhere to the lung tissue and produce fibrotic nodules. Long-term exposure to silica dust is necessary before there is evidence of lung tissue changes. Many individuals who have silicosis also develop tuberculosis (TB). Cigarette smokers and individuals with COPD have a greater risk of developing this disease.

Coal miner's pneumoconiosis (black lung): Occurs in individuals who work in coal mines and inhale coal dust. The minute dust particles are retained in the lung tissue, resulting in fibrosis, usually in the upper lobes. Although continued exposure to coal dust causes the disease to advance, the disease can be nonprogressive if there has been limited exposure.

A. Assessment

Usually, no symptoms appear until the disease is in an advanced stage.

Chronic indicators: Cough—either dry or productive, depending on the progression; sputum production—green, yellow, or black in color with black lung; wheezes with asbestosis.

Acute indicators: Dyspnea on exertion, chest pain, cyanosis, tachypnea, recurrent URIs, and potential hemoptysis with silicosis. With asbestosis, signs and symptoms of right ventricular heart failure, including neck vein distention and peripheral edema, can develop.

B. Diagnostic Tests

1. Chest x-ray: Reveals the presence of diffuse infiltrates in the lower lobes with asbestosis, and nodules throughout the lungs with cavitations in the advanced stages of silicosis and black lung.
2. ABG values: Will reveal decreased Pao_2 and increased $Paco_2$ in advanced disease.
3. Sputum culture: Will show presence of fibers with asbestosis and black lung.
4. Pulmonary function tests: Will show decreases in vital capacity and pulmonary compliance in advanced disease.
5. CBC with differential: Will show presence of inflammation and/or infection.

C. Medical Management

Management is directed toward symptoms and complications. There is no one specific treatment for these disorders.

1. **Oxygen therapy:** If need is determined by ABG results.
2. **Antibiotic therapy:** If infection is present.
3. **Bronchodilator therapy with hand-held nebulizer:** To open the airways and aid in loosening secretions.
4. **Corticosteroids:** To slow the inflammatory process.
5. **Maintenance of adequate fluid intake**: Either oral or IV.
6. **Chest physiotherapy:** To aid in expectoration of sputum.
7. **Digoxin and diuretics:** To treat cardiac complications of asbestosis in advanced disease.
8. **Antituberculosis medications:** For silicosis if TB is also present.

D. Nursing Diagnoses and Interventions

Impaired gas exchange related to decreased lung capacity secondary to ongoing lung tissue destruction

Desired outcomes: Patient exhibits VS and ABG values within an acceptable range. Patient can demonstrate technique for diaphragmatic breathing.

1. Assess and document VS and patient's respiratory status q4h or more frequently, as necessary; report any increase in respiratory distress to MD.
2. Review ABG results, noting changes in Pao_2 and $Paco_2$. Respiratory distress is evidenced by a decrease in Pao_2. $Paco_2$ will increase with hypoventilation and decrease with hyperventilation, indicating a significant change in respiratory status. ABG values should be correlated with physical assessment data to provide the total clinical picture.
3. Administer oxygen therapy as prescribed.
4. Anticipate care activities that may increase work of breathing and adjust activities accordingly.
5. Instruct patient in technique for diaphragmatic breathing: Assume a supine position, and place the hands over the abdomen while breathing in and out through the nose and consciously attempting to push the abdomen outward. If done correctly, the hands should rise and fall with each breath. Teach patient to use this breathing technique diligently until it no longer requires a conscious effort.

Potential for infection (recurring URIs) related to vulnerability secondary to ongoing lung tissue inflammation and destruction

Desired outcome: Patient demonstrates effective coughing and does not exhibit signs of URI.

1. Measure patient's temperature q2–4h, and report elevation to MD.
2. Monitor CBC results, especially WBCs for elevation.
3. Assist patient with coughing productively by administering prescribed chest physiotherapy.
4. Administer prescribed antibiotics.
5. Instruct patient in effective coughing technique: Sit with the upper body flexed slightly forward; take 2–3 breaths with passive exhalation; take a deep breath and hold it briefly; then cough forcefully. Explain that taking a drink of water before coughing may enhance the mobilization of secretions.

See "Asthma" for the following: **Alteration in nutrition:** Less than body requirements, p. 19. See "Appendix One" for nursing diagnoses and interventions for the care of patients with life-disrupting illnesses, p. 544.

E. Patient—Family Teaching and Discharge Planning

Provide patient and SOs with verbal and written information for the following:

1. Breathing and coughing positions that facilitate expectoration of secretions and diminish work of breathing.
2. Importance of limiting exposure to individuals known to have infections, especially URIs.
3. Medications, including the drug name, dosage, schedule, route, purpose, precautions, and potential side effects.
4. Signs and symptoms that necessitate medical attention: increased dyspnea and coughing; increased heart and respiratory rates; and changes in amount, consistency, and color of sputum.
5. Importance of pacing activities and providing frequent rest periods.
6. A diet high in protein and carbohydrates and an intake of fluids of at least 2–3 L/day in nonrestricted patients. As appropriate, involve dietician to give patient and SOs dietary instructions.

II. Tuberculosis

Tuberculosis (TB) is caused by the acid-fast organism *Mycobacterium tuberculosis*, which causes the formation of tubercles on the lungs and then spreads through the lymphatic system into other body organs. The infection is spread via airborne droplets projected by sneezing or coughing.

Not everyone exposed to the organism contracts the disease, and it can lie dormant for years before symptoms develop. Typically, the primary lesion develops 6 weeks after the initial infection. When the immune response occurs, the organism circulating in the bloodstream becomes trapped in organs such as the kidney. Individuals most prone to contract TB are those who are malnourished, alcoholic, have uncontrolled diabetes, or live in crowded conditions.

A. Assessment

Patient can be asymptomatic during the early stages of the disease.

Signs and symptoms: Malaise, low-grade fever, fatigue, weight loss, cough, night sweats, hemoptysis.

Physical exam: Dullness with percussion over the affected lung fields; crackles (rales) or wheezes with auscultation.

B. Diagnostic Tests

Results can mimic those for pneumonia, lung abscess, or bronchogenic carcinoma.

1. Chest x-ray: Will show node enlargement and presence of calcification. The upper lung fields are usually affected and cavitation might be present. In the early stages, patchy cavities are noted; in advanced stages calcium deposits in lymph nodes and lungs (coin lesions) are present.
2. Tuberculin skin test with purified protein derivative (PPD): Test is positive if it reveals 10 mm or more of induration around the site within 24–72 hours.
3. Sputum smear and culture: Will show presence of *M tuberculosis*. It should be obtained in the early morning and sent immediately to the lab. Three to five specimens are needed for accurate indentification.

4. <u>Gastric culture:</u> Will show presence of *M tuberculosis* if the patient swallows sputum. It should be obtained in the morning after patient has been NPO for 8 hours.

5. <u>Lymph node biopsy:</u> Performed when lymph nodes are enlarged and might show the presence of *M tuberculosis*.

C. Medical Management

1. **Bedrest:** If there is fever, hemoptysis, and/or cough.

2. **Isolation:** During contagious period.

3. **Antitubercular pharmacotherapy:** The following are used in combination: Isoniazid, ethambutol hydrochloride, rifampin, and streptomycin sulfate. **Note:** When isoniazid is used, close monitoring of SGOT and SGPT is necessary to evaluate hepatic integrity. Hepatic complications can be fatal in the elderly.

4. **Corticosteroids:** Sometimes given if there is evidence of TB in organs other than the lungs.

D. Nursing Diagnoses and Interventions

Alteration in nutrition: Less than body requirements related to decreased intake secondary to fatigue and anorexia

Desired outcome: Patient does not exhibit signs of malnutrition or weight loss.

1. Monitor and record I&O and weight daily.

2. Request dietician's assistance in planning meals that are high in protein and carbohydrates; offer small, frequent meals and between-meal snacks.

3. Request dietician's evaluation of patient's nutrition status with the use of anthropometric measurements of body size and proportions, including height, weight, triceps skinfold measurement, and mid-arm circumference to evaluate the patient's fat and protein reserves. For the total clinical picture, correlate these results with lab values, including albumin, creatinine, and transferrin, and the total leukocyte count. For more information, see "Providing Nutritional Therapy," pp. 512–519 in Chapter 11, "Metabolic Disorders."

Ineffective breathing pattern related to hyperpnea secondary to infectious process

Desired outcome: Patient exhibits a respiratory rate and depth within acceptable range.

1. Monitor VS and assess patient's respiratory status q2–4h.

2. Observe for circumoral cyanosis, use of accessory muscles for breathing, dyspnea, and tachycardia.

3. Encourage patient to take slow, deep breaths.

4. Report any significant change in VS or respiratory pattern to MD.

Activity intolerance related to fatigue secondary to infectious process

Desired outcome: Patient relates the attainment of adequate rest.

1. Provide frequent rest periods between care activities.

2. Advise patient to perform activities to tolerance.

3. Reassure patient that normal activity tolerance will return with wellness.

4. Involve patient in decision making regarding care activities and need for rest periods.

Potential for infection (for other patients and staff members) related to susceptibility secondary to communicable nature of the disease

Desired outcome: Other patients and staff members do not exhibit signs of infection.

1. Until patient is no longer communicable, maintain tuberculosis isolation (AFB isolation) according to the following 1983 guidelines from Centers for Disease Control:

   □ Provide private room with special ventilation; keep door closed; patients infected with same organism can share a room.

   □ Use mask if patient is coughing and does not cover mouth reliably.

   □ Wear gown, if needed, to prevent gross contamination of clothing. (Gloves are not necessary.)

   □ Wash hands after touching patient or potentially contaminated articles.

   □ Articles used in patient care should be cleaned and disinfected or discarded, although they are rarely involved in the transmission of TB.

2. Instruct patient to cough or sneeze into tissues and discard them into specially designated bag.

3. Instruct patient and SOs regarding isolation precautions.

4. Consult with hospital's infection control nurse for additional information.

5. Reinforce need for the patient to adhere to medication routine, both in the hospital and at home.

See "Appendix One" for nursing diagnoses and interventions for the care of patients with life-disrupting illnesses, p. 544.

E. Patient–Family Teaching and Discharge Planning

Provide patient and SOs with verbal and written information for the following:

1. Medications, including drug name, dosage, purpose, schedule, precautions, and potential side effects.

2. Importance of follow-up appointments with MD; confirm time and date of next appointment if it is known. Explain the need for tuberculin skin tests for SOs.

3. Recognizing causative factors for TB and altering lifestyle and/or home environment as necessary, such as minimizing the number of individuals in patient's residence, providing for nutritious meals, and encouraging patient's attendance at programs such as Alcoholics Anonymous, if appropriate.

4. Method of transmission of TB and potential for recurrence if medical treatment is not followed.

5. Referral to public health nurse, if appropriate.

6. Pacing activities to tolerance and providing for frequent rest periods.

7. Checking with MD before taking additional medications that can exacerbate the disease. For example, the use of corticosteriods can precipitate the rupture of a tubercle.

III. Pulmonary Fibrosis

The causes of pulmonary fibrosis are unknown, but it is theorized that it is a reaction to the inhalation of noxious gases or exposure to radiation. It is seen in patients with silicosis, tuberculosis, and collagen diseases. The fibrotic process is a continuous one and does not abate even when the causative agent is no longer present. The fibrosis primarily affects the alveoli and causes an increase in the bronchial diameter in relationship to lung volume. Often the patient has a viral illness at the time of initial diagnosis. Work of breathing is increased because of decreased lung compliance, and affected individuals adopt a rapid, shallow breathing pattern because it requires the least amount of energy. Cardiac complications can occur as a result of the pulmonary hypertension.

A. Assessment

Chronic indicators: Dyspnea, cyanosis, digital clubbing.

Acute indicators: Increased dyspnea, tachycardia, dysrhythmias.

Physical exam: Dullness with percussion over affected lung fields; decreased breath sounds with auscultation.

B. Diagnostic Tests

1. <u>Lung biopsy:</u> To rule out other respiratory disorders such as infection of the lung tissue and determine prognosis.
2. <u>CBC:</u> Will show elevated WBCs in the presence of infection.
3. <u>Pulmonary function testing:</u> Assesses extent of lung damage.
4. <u>ABG values:</u> Help evaluate the level of hypoxemia and hypercapnia.
5. <u>Chest x-ray:</u> Reveals the extent of fibrosis.

C. Medical Management

Management is directed toward reversing or halting disease progression.

1. **Corticosteroids:** To decrease inflammation and fibrosis.
2. **Chest physiotherapy:** To assist with removal of secretions.
3. **Antibiotics:** If infection is present.
4. **Oxygen therapy:** To correct hypoxemia.

D. Nursing Diagnoses and Interventions

Alteration in nutrition: Less than body requirements related to decreased intake secondary to fatigue and anorexia

Desired outcome: Patient does not exhibit signs of malnutrition or weight loss.

1. Monitor I&O and weight daily.
2. If necessary, request dietician assistance with meal planning.
3. Offer small, frequent meals to encourage adequate nutrition.
4. Provide encouragement during mealtimes to promote eating.

Ineffective breathing patterns related to hyperpnea secondary to decreased lung compliance

Desired outcome: Patient exhibits a respiratory rate and depth within acceptable range.

1. Review ABG values and report them to MD. Watch for a decrease in Pao_2, which would indicate worsening hypoxemia, and an increase in $Paco_2$, which is indicative of hypoventilation (CO_2 retention). Assess VS and respiratory status q4h or more frequently, as necessary. Monitor for indicators of increasing respiratory distress, including dyspnea, cyanosis, and tachycardia.
2. Reinforce the importance of taking slow, deep breaths.
3. Minimize activity level in the presence of increased work of breathing.
4. Admininster prescribed oxygen as indicated.

   See "Pneumoconioses" for the following: **Potential for infection** (recurring URIs), p. 26. See "Appendix One" for nursing diagnoses and interventions for the care of patients with life-disrupting illnesses, p. 544.

E. Patient–Family Teaching and Discharge Planning

Provide patient and SOs with verbal and written information for the following:

1. Importance of pacing activities to tolerance and avoiding strenuous exercises that would increase cardiac and respiratory symptoms.

2. Medications, including drug name, dosage, purpose, schedule, precautions, and potential side effects. It is likely that patient will take corticosteroids while at home. Provide instructions to ensure patient takes correct amount, especially for period during which the medication is tapered.

3. Limiting exposure to persons known to have infections such as colds or the flu. Teach patient the signs of URI that require treatment (eg, changes in the amount, consistency, and color of sputum; SOB; and/or fever).

4. If possible, limiting exposure to geographic areas known to have air pollution.

5. Use of oxygen and the necessary precautions if it is prescribed for at-home therapy.

▶ Section Five **Bronchogenic Carcinoma**

The occurrence of bronchogenic carcinoma is closely related to smoking—the number of cigarettes smoked and years the individual has smoked. The disease is rare in nonsmokers, although some industries produce carcinogens that cause lung cancer. Prognosis is poor when the diagnosis is made in advanced disease. The rate of tumor growth varies, depending on the type of cancer (squamous cell, oat cell, adenocarcinoma); the cure rate is 8–10%. Often the tumor is found in the larger bronchi of the right lung. The tumor creates areas of decreased perfusion, which causes ventilation problems. Because of lung tissue obstruction, secondary diseases can occur, including pneumonia, pleural effusion, and pneumothorax. Metastasis most likely occurs in the brain, long bones, cervical lymph nodes, liver, and kidney.

A. Assessment

Chronic indicators: Nonproductive cough, hemoptysis, wheezing, digital clubbing, hoarseness, anorexia, dyspnea.

Acute indicators: Increasing dyspnea, productive cough, chest pain, headache, nausea and vomiting, anorexia, malaise, disorientation, pain in bones, unexplained weight loss.

Physical exam: Decreased breath sounds, crackles (rales), and rhonchi heard with auscultation; dullness elicited over the affected lung field with percussion.

B. Diagnostic Tests

1. Sputum cytology: May reveal the presence of cancerous cells. The specimen should be obtained first thing in the morning after the patient has coughed deeply.

2. Chest x-ray: Reveals the presence of solitary nodules and possibly pleural effusion, atelectasis, and lymph node enlargement.

3. Pulmonary function testing: Measures vital capacity, inspiratory capacity, expiratory reserve volume, total lung capacity, tidal volume, functional residual volume, minute volume, forced vital capacity, and lung compliance. The test results will be normal unless there is a blockage of the major airways.

4. Needle aspiration biopsy: Uses fluoroscopy to remove a sample of lung tissue for pathologic examination.

5. Thoracocentesis: Allows examination of the pleural fluid to detect the presence of cancer cells.

6. Bronchoscopy: Determines whether tumor can be removed surgically.

7. <u>Lymph node biopsy in neck and axillary area:</u> Reveals metastasis, if present.
8. <u>CT scan:</u> To show presence of malignancy in other organs.
9. <u>EKG:</u> Determines cardiac status, including presence of dysrhythmias, ischemia, and enlargement of the heart chambers.
10. <u>ABG values:</u> To determine disease progression and need for oxygen therapy.

C. Medical Management and Surgical Interventions

1. **Chemotherapy medications** (used in combination for treatment): lomustine, cyclophosphamide, methotrexate, doxorubicin, dacarbazine, and vinblastine.

2. **Antiemetics:** Given before chemotherapy and during course of treatment to minimize nausea and vomiting.

3. **Analgesics:** For pain.

4. **Oxygen therapy:** If determined by ABG results and patient's condition.

5. **Radiation therapy:** To reduce tumor size.

6. **Thoracotomy:** To excise tumor or determine its presence. Pneumonectomy wedge resections also are done, depending on the size and location of the tumor. If lymph nodes are involved, they too are removed.

D. Nursing Diagnoses and Interventions

Alteration in repiratory function related to decreased lung capacity secondary to thoracotomy

Desired outcomes: Patient does not exhibit signs of respiratory dysfunction. Patient can demonstrate apical expansion exercises.

1. Assess patient's VS and respiratory patterns q2–4h, or as indicated.

2. Instruct patient in apical expansion exercises: Sit upright; position fingers under the clavicles and apply moderate pressure; inhale while attempting to expand the upper chest wall against the pressure of the fingers; maintain the expansion for a few moments; then exhale quietly and passively. This exercise helps re-expand the remaining lung tissue, mobilize secretions, and prevent flattening of the upper chest wall.

See "Appendix One" for nursing diagnoses and interventions for the care of preoperative and postoperative patients, pp. 528–532, care of the patient on prolonged bed rest, pp. 533–537, and care of patients with cancer and other life-disrupting illnesses, pp. 544–551.

E. Patient–Family Teaching and Discharge Planning

Provide patient and SOs with verbal and written information for the following:

1. Medications, including drug name, dosage, schedule, precautions, and potential side effects.

2. Equipment that will be used at home such as an oxygen system and a bedside commode.

3. Referral to public health or visiting nurse, if necessary.

4. American Cancer Society pamphlets and programs.

5. Need for follow-up care with MD; confirm date and time of next appointment if it is known.

6. Signs and symptoms of respiratory complications that may necessitate medical attention: increased dyspnea, cyanosis, and agitation. In addition, if sur-

gery was performed, teach patient the indicators of wound infection (eg, persistent redness, local warmth, purulent discharge, swelling, pain, and fever).

7. Hospice care if there is a facility nearby.

▶ Selected References

Baum G, et al: *Textbook of Pulmonary Disease*, 3rd ed. Little, Brown, 1983.

Bordow RA, Stool EW, Moser KM (editors): *Manual of Clinical Problems in Pulmonary Medicine*. Little, Brown, 1979.

Byrne C, et al: *Laboratory Tests: Implications for Nursing Care*, 2nd ed. Addison-Wesley, 1986.

Carpenito LJ: *Handbook of Nursing Diagnosis*. Lippincott, 1984.

Carpenito LJ: *Nursing Diagnosis: Application to Clinical Practice*. Lippincott, 1983.

Centers for Disease Control 1981–84: Guidelines for Isolation Precautions. In: *Guidelines for Prevention and Control of Nosocomial Infections*. US Department of Health and Human Services.

Emanuelson K, et al: *Acute Respiratory Care*. Wiley, 1981.

Henshaw HC, et al: *Diseases of the Chest*. Saunders, 1980.

Hughes J: Post-operative pulmonary care: Past, present, and future. *Critical Care Quarterly* 1983; 6:67–71.

Krupp M, et al: *Current Medical Diagnosis and Treatment*. Lange, 1983.

Morrison ML (editor): *Respiratory Intensive Care Nursing*, 2nd ed. Little, Brown, 1979.

Moser K, et al: *Better Living and Breathing: A Manual for Patients*. Mosby, 1980.

Nursing Clinical Library: *Respiratory Disorders*. Springhouse, 1984.

Saxton D, et al: *The Addison-Wesley Manual of Nursing Practice*. Addison-Wesley, 1983.

Spearman C, et al: *Egan's Fundamentals of Respiratory Therapy*, 4th ed. Mosby, 1982.

Swearingen PL: *The Addison-Wesley Photo-Atlas of Nursing Procedures*. Addison-Wesley, 1984.

Thompson P, et al: Compliance challenges in a black lung clinic. *Nurs Clin North Amer* 1982; 17:513–521.

Traver GA (editor): *Respiratory Nursing: The Science and the Art*. Wiley, 1982.

Wade J: *Comprehensive Respiratory Care: Physiology and Technique*, 3rd ed. Mosby, 1982.

West JB: *Pulmonary Pathophysiology: The Essentials*. Williams & Wilkins, 1978.

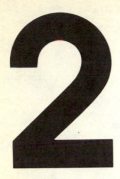
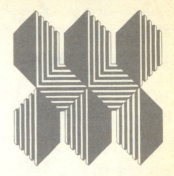

Cardiovascular Disorders

► Section One   **Degenerative Cardiovascular Disorders**

I. Pulmonary Hypertension

As blood passes through the pulmonary vasculature, it exchanges carbon dioxide and particulate matter for oxygen. Normally the pulmonary vascular bed offers little resistance to blood flow, but when resistance occurs, pulmonary hypertension results. Possible causes include increased pulmonary blood flow from a ventricular or atrial shunt, left ventricular failure, chronic hypoxia related to COPD, pulmonary embolus, pulmonary stenosis, or any physiologic occurrence that increases pulmonary vascular resistance or constriction of the vessels in the pulmonary tree.

A. Assessment

Acute indicators: Exertional dyspnea, syncope, and precordial chest pain, all of which result from low cardiac output or hypoxia. Cough and palpitations also can occur.

Chronic indicators: Signs of right and/or left ventricular failure.

□ *Right ventricular failure:* Peripheral edema; increased venous pressure and pulsations; liver engorgement.

□ *Left ventricular failure:* Dyspnea; SOB, particularly on exertion; decreased BP; oliguria; and orthopnea.

Physical exam: Cyanosis from decreased cardiac output and subsequent systemic vasoconstriction, systolic murmur caused by tricuspid regurgitation or pulmonary stenosis, diastolic murmur due to pulmonary valvular incompetence.

B. Diagnostic Tests

1. <u>Hematologic tests such as CBC and electrolytes:</u> Usually normal, although polycythemia can occur in the presence of hypoxemia due to compensation.

2. <u>Liver function tests:</u> May be abnormal if venous congestion is significant. Examples include increased SGOT, SGPT, and bilirubin.

3. <u>EKG:</u> Will show evidence of right atrial enlargement and right ventricular enlargement secondary to the increased pressure needed to force blood through the hypertensive pulmonary vascular bed.

4. <u>Chest x-ray:</u> Will show enlargement of the pulmonary artery and right atrium and ventricle.

5. <u>Pulmonary function test:</u> Results are usually normal, although some individuals will have increased residual volume and reduced maximum voluntary ventilation.

6. <u>ABG analysis:</u> May show low $Paco_2$ and high pH, which occur with hyperventilation.

7. <u>Echocardiography:</u> Often valuable for showing increased right ventricular dimension, thickened right ventricular wall, and possible tricuspid or pulmonary valve dysfunction.

8. <u>Cardiac catheterization with angiography:</u> Necessary to confirm pulmonary hypertension. Pulmonary vascular resistance will be very high, and pulmonary artery and right ventricular pressures can approach or equal systemic arterial pressures. (See "Cardiac Catheterization," pp. 72–75, for further detail.)

C. Medical Management and Surgical Interventions

1. **Oxygen:** Usually 2–5 L/min by nasal cannula. If hypoxia is severe, oxygen is administered by mask.

2. **Diet:** Low in sodium if signs of heart failure are present.

3. **Pharmacotherapy**

   □ *Diuretics:* If indicators of right and/or left heart failure are present.

   □ *Anticoagulants (warfarin sodium):* Although prophylactic use is controversial, it may be administered if pulmonary emboli are present.

   □ *Vasodilators and calcium antagonists:* To decrease cardiac workload.

4. **Treat causative factor if possible:** For example, by surgically closing arteriovenous shunts or replacing defective valves.

5. **Heart–lung transplantation:** For advanced pulmonary vascular disease.

D. Nursing Diagnoses and Interventions

Impaired gas exchange related to altered oxygen transport secondary to pulmonary capillary constriction and restricted blood flow

Desired outcome: Patient's VS, ABG values, and respiratory status are within acceptable limits.

1. Auscultate lung fields q4–8h to assess lung sounds. Note the presence of adventitious sounds, which can occur with fluid extravasation.

2. Monitor ABG results for evidence of hyperventilation: low $Paco_2$ and high pH.

3. Observe for and document presence of cyanosis, which can occur with decreased gas exchange.

4. Teach patient to take slow, deep breaths to enhance gas exchange.

5. Assist patient into Fowler's position, if possible, to decrease work of breathing.

6. Administer prescribed low-flow oxygen as indicated.

Activity intolerance related to fatigue and weakness secondary to right and left ventricular failure

Desired outcome: Patient progresses to his or her highest level of mobility with decreasing evidence of cardiac intolerance.

1. Observe for and document any changes in VS. Monitor systemic BP at least q4h. Report drops >10–20 mm Hg, which can signal decompensation of the cardiac muscle. Also be alert to other signs of left ventricular failure, including dyspnea, SOB, and crackles (rales).

2. Measure and document I&O and weight, reporting any steady gains or losses. Be alert to other signs of right ventricular failure, including peripheral edema, both pedal and sacral; ascites; distended neck veins; and increased CVP.

3. Administer diuretics, vasodilators, and calcium channel blockers as prescribed.

4. Provide periods of undisturbed rest; limit visitors as appropriate.

5. Keep frequently used items within patient's reach so that exertion can be avoided as much as possible.

6. Assist patient with ROM exercises at frequent intervals. To help prevent complications of immobility, plan progressive ambulation and exercise based on patient's tolerance and prescribed activity restrictions. For examples, see **Potential impairment of physical mobility** related to inactivity, p. 535, in "Appendix One."

Knowledge deficit: Disease process and treatment

Desired outcome: Patient can verbalize knowledge of the disease, its treatment, and measures that promote wellness.

1. Assess the patient's level of knowledge of the disease process and its treatment.

2. Discuss the purposes of the medications: to ease the workload of the heart (vasodilators), "relax" the heart (calcium antagonists), and prevent fluid accumulation (diuretics).

3. Support the patient in dealing with the concept of having a chronic disease.

4. If the etiology of pulmonary hypertension is known, reinforce explanations of the disease process, treatment, and the need for changing lifestyle, if appropriate.

5. Explain the value of relaxation techniques, including tapes, soothing music, meditation, and biofeedback.

6. If the patient smokes, explain that smoking increases the workload of the heart by causing vasoconstriction. Provide materials that explain the benefits of quitting smoking, such as the pamphlets prepared by the American Heart Association.

7. Confer with MD regarding the type of exercise program that will benefit the patient; provide patient teaching as indicated.

8. If appropriate, involve the dietitian to assist patient with planning meals that are low in sodium.

See "Heart Failure" for the following: **Fluid volume excess**: Edema (due to decreased cardiac output), p. 49, **Knowledge deficit**: Precautions and negative side effects of diuretic therapy, p. 49, and **Knowledge deficit**: Precautions and negative side effects of vasodilators, p. 50.

E. Patient–Family Teaching and Discharge Planning

Provide patient and SOs with verbal and written information for the following:

1. Indicators that necessitate medical attention: decreased exercise tolerance, increasing SOB or dyspnea, swelling of ankles and legs, steady weight gain.

2. Medications, including drug name, purpose, dosage, schedule, precautions, and potential side effects.

3. See additional interventions under **Knowledge deficit**, pp. 37–38.

II. Cardiomyopathy

Cardiomyopathy is a disorder of the heart muscle. It is unique among cardiovascular diseases because it is not caused by ischemic, valvular, hypertensive, or congenital disorders. Cardiomyopathy is categorized into the following types:

Dilated cardiomyopathy: Characterized by hypertrophy of all four of the heart chambers, especially the ventricles. Contractile dysfunction is usually the first sign, followed by congestive heart failure. There is progressive deterioration of cardiac muscle function caused by toxic, metabolic, or infectious agents. The mortality rate is high, and although a minority of patients improve, most die within 4 years of onset of the symptoms.

Hypertrophic cardiomyopathy: Characterized by an abnormally stiff left ventricle during diastole, which restricts ventricular filling. This causes increased left atrial, left ventricular, and pulmonary pressures resulting in dyspnea. Cardiac function can remain normal for varying periods of time before decompensation occurs. Symptoms include increased diastolic BP, decreased cardiac output, pulmonary hypertension, and right ventricular failure. Although it is theorized that hypertrophic cardiomyopathy has a strong hereditary link, the etiology is unknown. Possible causes include increased circulating catecholamines, subendocardial ischemia, or abnormal conduction patterns that lead to abnormal ventricular contraction.

Restrictive cardiomyopathy: Least common in Western countries, it is characterized by restrictive ventricular filling caused by fibrosis, infiltration, hypertrophy, and cardiac stiffness.

A. Assessment

Signs and symptoms: Dyspnea is usually the symptom that brings the patient to the physician. Decreased exercise tolerance, fatigue, weakness, syncope, peripheral edema, palpitations, right or left ventricular failure, and peripheral or pulmonary emboli also can occur.

Physical exam: Presence of S3 or S4 heart sounds and valve murmurs, increased venous pressure and pulsations, crackles (rales), decreased BP, and increased heart and respiratory rates related to decreased cardiac output. In addition, hepatomegaly and mild to severe cardiomegaly may be present.

B. Diagnostic Tests

1. <u>Chest x-ray:</u> To detect cardiac enlargement, particularly of the ventricles and left atrium. Pulmonary hypertension also may be seen.

2. <u>EKG results:</u> Determined by the extent and location of myocardial involvement. EKG changes indicative of cardiomyopathy include left ventricular hypertrophy, conduction defects, nonspecific ST segment changes, and Q waves that resemble those found with infarction.

3. <u>Echocardiography:</u> Will identify thickened ventricular walls and chamber dilation or restriction, depending on the type of cardiomyopathy. Poor contractility also may be seen if myocardial muscle deterioration has progressed.

4. <u>Cardiac catheterization:</u> Does not confirm cardiomyopathy, but it can be valuable for ruling out other disorders such as ischemic heart disease. Findings may include decreased cardiac output, decreased ventricular movement, increased filling pressures, and valvular regurgitation. For detail, see "Cardiac Catheterization," pp. 72–75.

5. <u>Endomyocardial biopsy:</u> Sometimes necessary to identify the type of pathologic agent; can be done during cardiac catheterization procedure.

C. Medical Management and Surgical Interventions

Medical management is aimed toward support, maintenance of normal function for as long as possible, and delaying disease progression.

1. **Control symptoms of heart failure:** See "Heart Failure," pp. 47–48.

2. **Limit or restrict activity.**

3. **Prohibit alcohol intake:** Alcohol can worsen myopathy.

4. **Pharmacotherapy**

    □ *Antiarrhythmic agents:* To control dysrhythmias.

    □ *Beta blockers:* To decrease outflow obstruction during exercise.

    □ *Calcium antagonists:* To produce arterial vasodilation and decrease cardiac workload.

    □ *Anticoagulants (warfarin sodium):* To prevent embolus formation.

5. **Surgical replacement of valves:** See "Cardiac Surgery," pp. 75–76.

D. Nursing Diagnoses and Interventions

Activity intolerance related to weakness and fatigue secondary to decrease in cardiac muscle contractility

Desired outcome: Patient progresses to his or her highest level of mobililty with decreasing evidence of cardiac intolerance.

1. Monitor BP and VS q4h, and report changes such as irregular heart rate, heart rate >110/min, or decreasing BP.

2. Observe for and report signs of acute decreased cardiac output, including oliguria, decreasing BP, decreased mentation, and dizziness.

3. Assess integrity of peripheral perfusion by monitoring peripheral pulses and

urine output. Report changes such as decreased amplitude of pulses and decreased urinary output.

4. In the presence of acute decreased cardiac output, ensure that the patient's needs are met so that activity can be avoided, for example, by keeping water at the bedside and urinal or commode nearby, maintaining a quiet environment, and limiting visitors as appropriate.

5. Plan nursing care to allow for periods of undisturbed rest.

6. Administer medications as prescribed.

7. To help prevent complications of immobility, assist patient with passive and some active or assistive ROM and other exercises, depending on patient's tolerance and prescribed limitations. For discussion of a progressive in-bed exercise program, see **Potential impairment of physical mobility** related to inactivity, p. 535, in "Appendix One."

Potential alteration in tissue perfusion: Cardiopulmonary and peripheral related to impaired circulation secondary to embolus formation

Desired outcome: Patient's VS and other physical findings are within acceptable limits.

1. Observe for and report indicators of pulmonary emboli, eg, sudden onset of chest pain, dyspnea, SOB, and hemoptysis.

2. Observe for and report indicators of peripheral emboli, eg, decreased peripheral pulses and calf pain or tenderness.

3. In the *absence* of decreased peripheral pulses and calf pain or tenderness, assess for a positive Homan's sign by flexing the knee 30° and dorsiflexing the foot. Pain elicited in the calf signifies a positive Homan's sign, which occurs in the presence of deep-vein thrombosis. Report significant findings to MD.

▶ **Note:** For patients who are *a*symptomatic of embolization, see interventions for prevention of this disorder in "Caring for Patients on Prolonged Bed Rest," p. 533, in "Appendix One."

See "Pulmonary Embolism" in Chapter 1 (Respiratory Disorders) for the following: **Potential for injury** (bleeding with anticoagulant therapy), p. 9. See "Pulmonary Hypertension" for the following: **Activity intolerance**, p. 37. See "Coronary Artery Disease" for the following: **Knowledge deficit**: Precautions and negative side effects of beta blockers, p. 43. See "Heart Failure" for the following: **Knowledge deficit**: Precautions and negative side effects of diuretic therapy, p. 49, **Fluid volume excess**: Edema, p. 49, and **Knowledge deficit**: Precautions and negative side effects of vasodilators, p. 50. See "Appendix One" for nursing diagnoses and interventions for the care of patients on prolonged bed rest, pp. 533–537, and for the care of patients with life-disrupting illnesses, pp. 544–546.

E. Patient–Family Teaching and Discharge Planning

Provide patient and SOs with verbal and written information for the following:

1. Medications, including drug name, purpose, dosage, schedule, precautions, and potential side effects.

2. Signs and symptoms that necessitate immediate medical attention: dyspnea, decreased exercise tolerance, alterations in pulse rate/rhythm, loss of consciousness (caused by dysrhythmia or decreased cardiac output), and steady weight gain (caused by heart failure).

3. Reinforcement that cardiomyopathy is a chronic disease requiring lifetime treatment.

4. Importance of abstaining from alcohol, which increases cardiac muscle deterioration.
5. Need for physical support from family and outside agencies as disease progresses.
6. Availability of community and/or medical support such as American Heart Association.

III. Coronary Artery Disease

The coronary arteries are the vessels that supply the myocardial muscle with oxygen and nutrients necessary for optimal function. Atherosclerotic lesions within these arteries are a major cause of obstruction and subsequent ischemia, which ultimately can lead to myocardial infarction. The most common symptom of coronary artery disease (CAD) is angina, a result of decreasing blood flow and decreased oxygen supply through narrowed or obstructed arteries (ischemia). Often, CAD is diagnosed only after the patient presents with angina or myocardial infarction.

A. Assessment

Chronic indicators: Stable or progressively worsening angina that occurs when myocardial demand for oxygen is more than the supply, such as during exercise. The pain is usually described as pressure or a crushing or burning substernal pain that radiates down one or both arms. It also can be felt in the neck, cheeks, and teeth. Usually, it is relieved with discontinuation of exercise and/or administration of nitroglycerine.

Acute indicators: CAD is considered unstable (acute) when angina becomes more frequent and is unrelieved by nitroglycerine and rest, when it occurs during sleep or rest, or when it occurs with progressively lower levels of exercise.

Risk factors: Increasing age, male gender, family history, smoking, diet high in sodium and cholesterol, hypertension, obesity, abnormal glucose tolerance, "type A" behavior, sedentary and/or stressful lifestyle.

B. Diagnostic Tests

1. Chest x-ray: Usually normal unless heart failure is present.
2. EKG: Usually normal unless a myocardial infarction has occurred or the individual is experiencing angina at the time of the EKG.
3. Treadmill exercise test: To determine the amount of exercise that causes angina as well as the degree of ischemia and EKG changes produced. Significant findings can include 1 mm or more ST segment depression or elevation and ventricular ectopic beats.
4. Thallium treadmill test: A type of radionuclide imaging. When injected, the thallium produces "cold spot" images of ischemic areas or scarring in conjunction with treadmill exercise. A follow-up rest imaging is performed to compare resting and exercise (stress) usage.
5. Holter monitoring: A 24-hour EKG monitoring that can show activity-induced ST segment changes or ischemia-induced dysrhythmias.
6. Magnetic resonance (MR) imaging: Allows visualization of one or more planes at a given time.
7. Coronary arteriography via cardiac catheterization: Provides the ultimate diagnosis of CAD. Arterial lesions (plaque) are located and the amount of occlusion is determined. At this time, feasibility for coronary artery bypass grafting (CABG) or angioplasty is determined. For details, see "Cardiac Surgery," pp. 75–76.

C. Medical Management and Surgical Interventions

1. **Management of risk factors:** Eliminating tobacco, reducing BP, reducing serum lipids, controlling weight and stress, and initiating an exercise program.

2. **Oxygen by nasal cannula**: During angina attacks.
3. **Pharmacotherapy**

   □ *Sublingual nitroglycerine:* During angina to increase microcirculation, perfusion to the myocardium, and venodilation.

   □ *Beta blockers:* To decrease oxygen demand of the myocardium.

   □ *Calcium antagonists:* To reduce oxygen demands.

   □ *Long-acting nitrates or topical nitroglycerine:* For anginal prophylaxis.

4. **Diet:** Low in cholesterol, sodium, calories, and/or triglycerides, as appropriate.

D. Nursing Diagnoses and Interventions

Alteration in comfort: Angina related to decreased oxygen supply to the myocardium

Desired outcome: Patient relates a decrease in discomfort and does not exhibit signs of uncontrolled pain.

1. Emphasize to patient the importance of immediately reporting to staff any manifestations of angina.
2. Keep sublingual nitroglycerine within reach of patient, and explain that it is to be administered as soon as angina begins, repeating q5 min × 3 if necessary.
3. Assess the location, character, and severity of the pain. Record the severity on a subjective 1–10 scale. Also record the number of nitroglycerine tablets needed to relieve each episode and the factor or event that precipitated the pain.
4. Stay with patient and provide reassurance during periods of angina. If indicated, request that visitors leave the room.
5. Monitor for presence of headache and hypotension after administration of nitroglycerine. Keep patient recumbent during angina as well as during nitroglycerine administration.
6. Avoid activities and factors that are known to cause stress for the patient and may precipitate angina.
7. Discuss the value of relaxation techniques, including tapes, soothing music, biofeedback, meditation, or yoga.

Activity intolerance related to weakness and fatigue secondary to tissue ischemia (myocardial infarction)

Desired outcome: Patient progresses to his or her highest level of mobility with decreasing evidence of cardiac intolerance.

1. Observe for and report the following: increasing frequency of angina, angina that occurs at rest, angina that is unrelieved by nitroglycerine, or decreased exercise tolerance without angina.
2. Assist patient with recognizing and limiting activities that increase oxygen demands, such as exercise and anxiety.
3. Maintain oxygen as prescribed for angina attacks.
4. Have patient perform ROM exercises, depending on tolerance and prescribed activity limitations. Because cardiac intolerance to activity can be further aggravated by prolonged bed rest, consult with MD regarding in-bed exercises and activities that can be performed by the patient as the condition improves. Examples are found in **Potential impairment of physical mobility** related to inactivity, pp. 535–536, in "Appendix One."

Alterations in nutrition: More than body requirements related to excessive intake of calories, sodium, and/or fats

Desired outcome: Patient demonstrates knowledge of and compliance with the dietary regimen.

1. If patient is over the ideal body weight (see Table 11–2, p. 518), explain that a low-calorie diet is necessary.
2. Teach patient how to decrease dietary intake of saturated (animal) fats and increase intake of polyunsaturated (vegetable oil) fats.
3. Teach patient to limit dietary intake of cholesterol to <300 mg/day.
4. Teach patient to limit dietary intake of refined/processed sugar.
5. Teach patient to limit dietary intake of sodium chloride to <4 g/day (mild restriction).
6. Encourage intake of fresh fruits, natural carbohydrates, fish, poultry, legumes, fresh vegetables, and grains for a healthy, balanced diet.

Knowledge deficit: Precautions and negative side effects of nitrates

Desired outcome: Patient can verbalize understanding of the precautions and side effects of the prescribed medication.

1. Instruct patient to report to MD or staff the presence of a headache associated with nitroglycerine, in which case the MD may alter the dosage.
2. Teach patient to assume a recumbent position if a headache occurs. Explain that the vasodilation effect of the drug causes a decrease in BP, which can result in orthostatic hypotension and headache.

Knowledge deficit: Precautions and negative side effects of beta blockers

Desired outcome: Patient can verbalize understanding of the precautions and side effects of beta blockers.

1. Instruct patient to be alert to depression, fatigue, dizziness, erythematous rash, respiratory distress, and sexual dysfunction, which can occur as side effects of beta blockers. Explain the importance of notifying MD promptly should they occur.
2. Explain that weight gain and peripheral and sacral edema can occur as negative side effects of beta blockers. Teach patient how to assess for edema and the importance of reporting signs and symptoms promptly should they occur.
3. Explain that BP and pulse rate are assessed prior to administration of beta blockers because the drug can cause hypotension and excessive slowing of the heart.
4. Caution patient about skipping or abruptly stopping beta blockers, which can result in rebound angina or even myocardial infarction.

E. Patient–Family Teaching and Discharge Planning

Provide patient and SOs with verbal and written information for the following:

1. Medications, including drug name, dosage, purpose, schedule, precautions, and potential side effects. Discuss the potential for headache and dizziness after nitroglycerine administration. Caution patient about using nitroglycerine more frequently than prescribed and notifying MD if 3 tablets do not relieve angina.
2. Importance of reducing intake of caffeine, which causes vasoconstriction and increases the heart rate.
3. Dietary changes: low saturated fat, low salt, low cholesterol; the need for weight loss if appropriate.
4. Prescribed exercise program and importance of maintaining a regular exercise schedule. Remind patient of the need to measure pulse, stop if pain occurs, and stay within prescribed exercise limits.

5. Indicators that necessitate medical attention: progression to unstable angina, loss of consciousness, decreased exercise tolerance, unrelieved pain, angina that is unrelieved by nitroglycerine, increasing frequency of angina, and need to increase the number of nitroglycerine tablets to relieve angina.

6. Elimination of smoking; refer patient to a "stop smoking" program, as appropriate.

7. Importance of involvement and support of SOs in patient's lifestyle changes.

8. Importance of getting BP checked at regular intervals (at least once a month if the patient is hypertensive).

9. Avoiding strenuous activity for at least an hour after meals to avoid excessive oxygen demands.

IV. Myocardial Infarction

Ischemic heart disease accounts for approximately one-third of all deaths in the United States, and of patients with ischemic heart disease, half die because of myocardial infarction (MI). Most MIs are caused by critical narrowing of the coronary arteries due to atherosclerosis (see "Coronary Artery Disease," pp. 41–44). Occlusion also can be caused by thrombus formation or coronary artery spasm. When ischemia is prolonged and unrelieved, irreversible damage (infarction) occurs. MI can occur in various areas of the heart, depending on the location of the coronary artery occlusion and distribution of blood supply.

A. Assessment

Signs and symptoms: Chest pain, substernal pressure and/or burning, pain that radiates to the jaw and arm. Weakness, diaphoresis, nausea, vomiting, and acute anxiety also can occur. The heart rate can be abnormally slow (bradycardia) or rapid (tachycardia).

Physical exam: Possible minor hypotension, increasing respiratory rate, and crackles (rales) if ventricular failure occurs. Temperature elevations to 39.4C (104F) can occur secondary to the inflammatory process. Intensity of S1 and S2 heart sounds may be decreased if papillary muscle rupture has occurred. S3 and S4 sounds may be present if heart failure has occurred.

History of: Sudden onset of intense chest pain that is unrelieved by nitroglycerine.

B. Diagnostic Tests

1. Serum enzymes: Will reveal myocardial muscle damage. The following enzyme levels will increase: creatinine phosphokinase (CPK), the MB isoenzyme, serum glutamic oxaloacetic transaminase (SGOT), and lactic dehydrogenase (LDH).

2. Serial EKGs: For comparison to the baseline. Lead changes identify the area of infarct.

3. Chest x-ray: Usually reveals cardiomegaly and signs of left ventricular failure.

4. Radioisotope studies (using pyrophosphate and technetium): May help localize area of infarct. Ventricular function may be assessed via gated blood pool studies with isotopes.

5. Echocardiography: Detects abnormalities of left ventricular wall motion, which usually correspond to the EKG site of infarction.

6. Magnetic resonance (MR) studies: Allow volumetric measurements of the ventricle through visualization of one or more planes.

7. Hemodynamic monitoring in the CCU: Measures cardiac output and pulmonary artery pressures, which are usually reflective of infarction.

8. Angiography: Determines areas of stenosis or occlusion and suitability for coronary artery bypass grafting.

9. <u>ABG studies:</u> May reveal hypoxemia (decreased Pao_2) and hyperventilation (decreased $Paco_2$).

10. <u>CBC:</u> May reveal leukocytosis secondary to the inflammatory process.

11. <u>Erythrocyte sedimentation rate (ESR):</u> Increases in the presence of an inflammatory process.

C. Medical Management and Surgical Interventions

1. **Relieve acute pain:** Usually with IV morphine sulfate in small increments (2 mg) until relief is obtained.

2. **Oxygen:** Usually 2–4 L/min by nasal cannula or mask for 2–3 days. Hypoxia is common and adds stress to the compromised myocardium.

3. **Bed rest with commode privileges.**

4. **Treat dysrhythmias:** Antiarrhythmic agents (eg, lidocaine) for ventricular premature beats; atropine for bradycardias.

5. **Manage fluid imbalance:** Oral or IV fluids for dehydration; diuretics for fluid overload.

6. **Treat ventricular failure**: See "Heart Failure," p. 48.

7. **Limit infarct size by decreasing cardiac workload:** Rest, beta blockade, controlled exercise program, risk-factor management.

8. **Medical reperfusion:** Streptokinase for thrombus resolution and percutaneous transluminal coronary angioplasty for removal of plaque (see "Cardiac Catheterization," p. 73).

9. **Surgical reperfusion**: Coronary artery bypass graft (see "Cardiac Surgery," pp. 75–76).

10. **Transfer to CCU:** For close monitoring, if needed.

D. Nursing Diagnoses and Interventions

Alteration in comfort: Pain related to ischemia and infarction of myocardial tissue

Desired outcome: Patient relates control of discomfort and does not exhibit signs of uncontrolled pain.

1. Assess location, character, and intensity of pain.

2. Administer prescribed pain medications (usually morphine sulfate) and document quality of relief obtained and the time interval from administration to expressed relief.

3. Provide reassurance during episodes of pain; stay with patient if possible.

4. Observe for and report side effects of pain medications, such as hypotension, slowed respiratory rate, and difficulty with urination.

5. Administer oxygen as prescribed, usually 2–4 L/min.

Fluid volume excess: Edema related to retention secondary to decreased cardiac output

Desired outcome: Patient is able to control thirst and does not exhibit signs of fluid overload.

1. Record I&O, and report imbalances.

2. Observe for and report any indicators of fluid accumulation in the lungs such as dyspnea, crackles (rales), and SOB.

3. Be alert to and report decreasing urine output (particularly <30 mL/h) and increasing specific gravity (>1.030).

4. Assess for peripheral (sacral, pedal) edema.

5. Maintain IV infusion as prescribed. Usually, fluids are limited to prevent failure and circulatory overload.

6. If fluids are limited, help control thirst by offering ice chips or Popsicles, if they are allowed; record the amount of intake. Teach patient and SOs the importance of fluid limitation.

Activity intolerance related to fatigue and weakness secondary to decreased strength of cardiac contraction

Desired outcome: Patient progresses to his or her highest level of mobility with decreasing evidence of cardiac intolerance.

1. Observe for and report any symptoms of decreased cardiac output and/or cardiac failure, such as decreasing BP, cold extremities, oliguria, decreased peripheral pulses, and increased heart rate.
2. Monitor I&O, and be alert to urinary output <30 mL/h. Auscultate lung fields q2h for presence of crackles (rales), which can occur with fluid retention and cardiac failure.
3. Palpate peripheral pulses at frequent intervals. Be alert to irregularities and decreased amplitude, which can signal cardiac failure.
4. Administer oxygen and medications as prescribed.
5. During acute periods of decreased cardiac output and as prescribed, support patient in maintaining bed rest by keeping personal articles within reach, providing a calm and quiet atmosphere, and limiting visitors to ensure periods of undisturbed rest.
6. Assist patient to commode if bathroom privileges are allowed.
7. Assist patient with passive and/or assistive ROM exercises, as determined by tolerance and activity limitations. Consult with MD regarding the type and amount of in-bed exercises the patient can perform as the condition improves. Examples of in-bed exercises can be found in the nursing diagnosis **Potential impairment of physical mobility** related to inactivity, p. 535, in "Appendix One."
8. As appropriate, teach patient self-measurement of pulse rate for gauging exercise tolerance.

Impaired gas exchange related to tissue hypoxia secondary to fluid accumulation in the lungs

Desired outcome: Patient demonstrates ABG values and VS within acceptable limits.

1. Auscultate lung fields q2h for presence of crackles (rales), which occur with fluid accumulation.
2. Assess ABG levels, and be alert to evidence of hypoxemia (decreased Pao_2) or hyperventilation (decreased $Paco_2$).
3. Monitor for sudden changes in respiratory pattern (increased dyspnea or slowed rate), which can occur with an extension of the infarction and should be reported immediately.
4. Administer oxygen as prescribed. Deliver oxygen with humidity to help prevent its drying effects on oral and nasal mucosa.
5. Monitor BP. In the absence of marked hypotension, place patient in semi-Fowler's position to ease dyspnea.
6. Administer prescribed analgesics (usually morphine sulfate) or antianxiety agents (usually diazepam) to relax patient, decrease cardiac workload, and ease respiratory effort.

Sleep pattern disturbance related to awakening for VS assessment or medication administration

Desired outcome: Patient relates the attainment of adequate rest.

1. Plan care activities so that they do not interfere with patient's rest.
2. Provide periods of at least 1½ hours for undisturbed sleep.

3. Administer mild sedatives, if prescribed, to facilitate sleep.
4. Involve SOs in the care plan; coordinate visiting times.
5. If necessary, limit visitors so that patient can attain rest/sleep.
6. Question patient about interventions used at home that promote sleep.

See "Appendix One" for nursing diagnoses and interventions for the care of patients on prolonged bed rest, pp. 533–537, and for the care of patients with life-disrupting illnesses, pp. 544–546.

E. Patient–Family Teaching and Discharge Planning

Provide patient and SOs with verbal and written information for the following :

1. Process of myocardial infarction and extent of the patient's injury.
2. Indicators that necessitate immediate medical attention: unrelieved pain, decreased activity tolerance, sudden onset of SOB, weight gain.
3. Medications, including drug name, purpose, dosage, schedule, precautions, and potential side effects.
4. Exercise program specific to patient's condition.
5. Importance of avoiding overexertion and getting rest when tired.
6. Resumption of sexual activity as directed, usually after 4–8 weeks, but will vary with each patient.
7. Diet regimen as prescribed.
8. Elimination of smoking; refer patient to programs that specialize in this process.
9. Phone number and/or address for American Heart Association, local heart rehabilitation programs, family physician, and primary nurse.
10. Referral to stress management programs, if appropriate.

V. Heart Failure

Heart (cardiac) failure is the state in which the heart is unable to pump blood at a rate sufficient to meet metabolic requirements of the tissues. Heart failure can occur as a result of myocardial or cardiac muscle damage such as after large infarcts, or when an adequate cardiac muscle is stressed or forced to work harder over a period of time. When the heart is unable to pump sufficient blood to meet metabolic demands, it relies on three main compensatory mechanisms:

□ *Increasing cardiac fluid* to increase fiber length and subsequently increase force of contraction (Frank-Starling law). The fluid that fills the ventricles before systole is termed "preload," and it is a critical factor in patients with cardiac failure. It is important to have enough volume to stretch the fibers, but not so much of a stretch that decreased contractility and decreased cardiac output occur.

□ *Increasing catecholamine discharge* (epinephrine and norepinephrine) to increase contractility. This causes systemic vasoconstriction, which, in turn, increases workload of the heart by increasing resistance. This is called "afterload."

□ *Myocardial hypertrophy* to increase the mass of working contractile tissue. The hypertrophy will be either right sided, left sided, or both, depending on the cause of failure. Conditions that can result in primary right-sided heart failure include right ventricular MI, COPD, left-to-right shunts, and pulmonary valve stenosis. Primary left-sided heart failure is caused by conditions such as left ventricular MI, aortic valve stenosis, mitral regurgitation, and hypertension. Over time, left-sided failure can result in the involvement of both sides of the heart.

A. Assessment

Signs and symptoms: Orthopnea, fatigue, weakness, nocturia, cardiac cachexia (anorexia), and confusion, which can occur late in the disease course. In addition, decreased right ventricular output can cause increased central venous pressure (CVP), distended neck veins, and peripheral edema; and decreased left ventricular output can cause dyspnea and SOB, as well as other indicators of pulmonary edema.

Physical exam: Decreased BP, dysrhythmias, tachycardia, tachypnea, increased venous pulsations and pressure, crackles (rales), pitting edema, ascites, galloping heart sounds, and pulsus alternans (alternating strong and weak heart beats). Hepatomegaly may occur in the presence of right-sided heart failure.

History of: Noncompliance with medication or diet regimen, sleeping on extra pillows to enhance respirations, decreased exercise tolerance, or increasing SOB.

B. Diagnostic Tests

1. <u>Chest x-ray:</u> Will show the presence of cardiomegaly and engorged pulmonary vasculature.

2. <u>Serum electrolytes:</u> May reveal hyponatremia (dilutional); hyperkalemia if glomerular filtration is decreased; or hypokalemia, which can result from some diuretics.

3. <u>Serum enzymes:</u> May reveal an elevated SGOT with hepatic congestion and decreased liver function.

4. <u>Serum bilirubin:</u> May reveal hyperbilirubinemia in the presence of liver dysfunction.

5. <u>Circulation time:</u> Sodium dehydrocholate is given IV, and the time is measured until the patient begins to experience a bitter taste in the mouth. In the presence of heart failure, the time is often increased at rest, but in mild cases it may be normal at rest and increase with exercise or hepatic compression.

6. <u>CBC:</u> May reveal a decreased hemoglobin and hematocrit in the presence of anemia.

C. Medical Management and Surgical Interventions

1. **Treat underlying cause:** Surgically repair abnormalities such as valvular lesions or treat conditions such as hypertension or endocarditis.

2. **Treat precipitating factors:** Such as infection or dysrhythmias.

3. **Physical and emotional rest.**

4. **Low-sodium diet:** In less severe disease states, this may mean elimination of table salt only.

5. **Weight control:** If appropriate.

6. **Pharmacotherapy**

   □ *Diuretics:* To control fluid accumulation and reduce blood volume.

   □ *Digitalis:* To increase strength of cardiac contraction.

   □ *Vasodilators:* To decrease cardiac workload by decreasing sympathetic nervous system vasoconstriction. Although there is some controversy about when to initiate vasodilator therapy, it is believed that it is appropriate when patients are symptomatic with light activity or when they are being treated with digitalis. This provides a combination of increased contractility (digitalis) and decreased afterload (vasodilator). The administration of IV vasodilators such as sodium nitroprusside and nitroglycerine necessitates the patient's transfer to the CCU.

   □ *Inotropic drugs:* Administered during acute exacerbation to increase BP and the strength of contractions. Administration of inotropic drugs also necessitates the patient's transfer to the CCU for close monitoring of vasoactive effects.

D. Nursing Diagnoses and Interventions

Activity intolerance related to weakness and fatigue secondary to decreased strength of cardiac contraction

Desired outcome: Patient progressives to his or her highest level of activity with decreasing evidence of cardiac intolerance.

1. Monitor VS q2h or as necessary, and report decreasing BP, increasing heart rate, or increasing respiratory rate, which can occur with worsening failure related to sympathetic nervous system discharge and fluid retention.

2. Administer vasodilators and other cardiac drugs as prescribed.

3. If symptoms worsen, discuss the need for activity limitations with patient. Assist patient with ADLs to prevent SOB and plan nursing care and limit visitors to allow for periods of undisturbed rest

4. Discuss ways to decrease activities at home, such as not climbing stairs.

5. If appropriate, refer patient to an OT to learn how to conserve energy so that ADLs can be performed with a minimum of exertion.

6. Assist patient with passive and/or assistive ROM exercises, depending on tolerance and prescribed activity limitations. Because cardiac intolerance to activity can be further aggravated by prolonged bed rest, consult with MD regarding the type and amount of in-bed exercises that can be initiated as the patient's condition improves. For details, see **Potential impairment of physical mobility** related to inactivity, p. 535, in "Appendix One."

Fluid volume excess: Edema related to retention secondary to decreased cardiac output

Desired outcome: Patient does not exhibit signs of fluid overload.

1. Auscultate lung fields at least q shift; report presence of crackles (rales), which occur with fluid volume excess.

2. Monitor and document I&O at least q shift. Report imbalances, including urinary output <30 mL/h, which can occur with decreased renal bloodflow.

3. Monitor weight daily, and report unusual gains. Be alert to the presence of pitting edema.

4. Auscultate heart sounds; be alert to S3 gallop, an early sign of heart failure.

5. Administer diuretics as prescribed. Observe for indicators of decreased effective circulating volume such as hypotension, decreased CVP, and tachycardia.

6. If appropriate, teach patient the importance of decreasing intake of sodium (or table salt).

7. If fluids are limited, help relieve patient's thirst by offering ice chips or Popsicles. Record the amount of intake on the I&O record.

Knowledge deficit: Precautions and negative side effects of diuretic therapy

Desired outcome: Patient can verbalize knowledge of the precautions and negative side effects of diuretic therapy.

1. Depending on type of diuretic used, teach patient to report signs and symptoms of the following:

   □ *Hypokalemia:* Anorexia, irregular pulse, nausea, apathy, muscle cramps.

   □ *Hyperkalemia:* Muscle weakness, hyporeflexia, and irregular heart rate, which can occur with potassium-sparing diuretics.

   □ *Hyponatremia:* Fatigue, weakness, edema.

2. For patients on long-term diuretic therapy, explain the importance of follow-up monitoring of blood levels of sodium and potassium.

3. As appropriate, instruct patient to use care when rising from a sitting or recumbent position to prevent injury from orthostatic hypotension.

Knowledge deficit: Precautions and negative side effects of digitalis therapy

Desired outcome: Patient can verbalize understanding of the precautions and negative side effects associated with digitalis therapy.

1. Teach patient the technique and importance of assessing pulse rate before taking digitalis. Explain that he or she should obtain pulse rate parameters from MD, but that digitalis is usually withheld when it is <60 beats/min if the usual heart rate before digitalis administration is greater.

2. Explain that serum potassium levels are monitored routinely because low potassium levels can potentiate digitalis toxicity.

3. Explain that the apical heart rate and peripheral pulses are assessed for irregularity, which is a sign of digitalis toxicity.

4. Teach patient to be alert to other indicators of digitalis toxicity, including nausea, vomiting, anorexia, diarrhea, blurred vision, and mental confusion. Explain the importance of reporting signs and symptoms promptly to MD or staff should they occur.

Knowledge deficit: Precautions and negative side effects of vasodilators

Desired outcome: Patient can verbalize knowledge of the precautions and negative side effects associated with vasodilators.

1. Explain that a headache can occur after administration of a vasodilator and that lying down will help alleviate the pain.

2. Teach the importance of assessment of weight gain and for signs of peripheral or sacral edema, any of which can occur as side effects of vasodilator therapy.

3. Instruct patient to alert MD to negative side effects of this therapy.

See "Coronary Artery Disease" for the following: **Alterations in nutrition:** More than body requirements of sodium, calories, and/or fats, p. 42, and **Knowledge deficit:** Precautions and negative side effects of beta blockers, p. 43. See "Myocardial Infarction" for the following: **Sleep pattern disturbance**, p. 46, and **Impaired gas exchange**, p. 46. See "Appendix One" for nursing diagnoses and interventions for the care of patients on prolonged bed rest, pp. 533–537, and for the care of patients with life-disrupting illnesses, pp. 544–546.

E. Patient–Family Teaching and Discharge Planning

Provide patient and SOs with verbal and written information for the following:

1. Medications, including drug name, purpose, dosage, schedule, precautions, and potential side effects. Stress the importance of taking medications regularly and *not* stopping them without MD consultation. Teach patient and SOs how to measure pulse rate for digitalis therapy.

2. Diet: Advise patient that sodium restriction may be lessened as cardiac function improves. Assist patient with diet planning or refer to a nutrition specialist if major dietary changes are necessary.

3. Signs and symptoms that necessitate medical attention: irregular pulse, bradycardia, unusual SOB, increased orthopnea, decreased exercise tolerance, and unusual or steady weight gain.

4. Importance of quitting smoking, which causes vasoconstriction and increases cardiac workload. As appropriate, refer patient to programs that specialize in quitting smoking.

5. Importance of limiting exertional activities at home (eg, minimizing bending and lifting and/or avoiding stair climbing).

6. Emergency telephone numbers to call if needed.

7. Importance of follow-up care; confirm date and time of next medical appointment.

▶ Section Two   **Inflammatory Heart Disorders**

The disorders described in this section are inflammations or infections involving mainly the heart muscle and linings: pericardium, myocardium, and endocardium. The inflammation can be acute or chronic, and prognosis usually depends on extent of the involvement, structures involved, and secondary disorders that occur.

I. Pericarditis

Pericarditis is an inflammation of the stiff, fibrous sac (pericardium) that surrounds, supports, and protects the heart. The pericardium is composed of a fibrous outer layer and a serous inner layer. The inflammatory condition produces friction between the layers during cardiac movement. Acute pericarditis causes exudate production and formation of chronic fibrinous adhesions. Pericarditis occurs in a vast number of medical disorders. The most common causes are viral or bacterial infections, uremia, acute myocardial infarction, neoplastic diseases, and trauma.

A. Assessment

Chronic indicators: Elevated systemic venous pressure (CVP) and signs secondary to systemic venous congestion, including edema, ascites, and hepatic congestion. If fibrous constriction is severe, symptoms of left-sided heart failure may appear, such as dyspnea, cough, and orthopnea.

Acute indicators: Chest pain localized to the retrosternal and left precordial regions, or pain that mimics acute abdominal pain or ischemic pain. Unlike ischemic pain, however, it is often increased with deep inspirations, movement, or lying down and eased by sitting up and leaning forward. Other indicators include dyspnea, if the increased pericardial fluid is severe enough to cause constriction of the bronchi, and fever.

Physical exam: Characteristic pericardial friction rub (a scratching, grating, high-pitched sound) heard on auscultation.

B. Diagnostic Tests

1. <u>Serial EKGs:</u> Typically show widespread ST elevation in most leads, unlike localized ischemic ST segment elevation.
2. <u>CBC:</u> Often shows presence of increased WBCs (leukocytosis).
3. <u>ESR:</u> Increases in the presence of inflammation.
4. <u>Cardiac enzymes:</u> Probably will be normal, although the MB fraction of CPK may increase with epicardial inflammation.
5. <u>Echocardiogram:</u> Reveals increase in pericardial fluid, which occurs with infection or irritation.

C. Medical Management and Surgical Interventions

1. **Treat underlying disorder.**
2. **Bed rest:** Until pain and fever are relieved.
3. **Pharmacotherapy**
   - □ *Nonsteroidal anti-inflammatory agents.*
   - □ *Corticosteroids:* For example, prednisone 60–80 mg qd in divided doses for 5–7 days and tapered thereafter, if symptoms are unrelieved by nonsteroidal anti-inflammatory agents.
   - □ *Antibiotics:* Given only in the presence of purulent pericarditis.
4. **Emergency pericardiocentesis:** If cardiac tamponade (accumulation of fluid that restricts ventricular filling and reduces cardiac output) develops.

This procedure involves needle aspiration of the fluid in the pericardial sac to relieve pressure and allow for normal cardiac muscle contraction. Usually it is done under local anesthetic in the ICU, operating room, or cardiac catheterization lab.

5. **Partial or total pericardectomy:** To allow normal cardiac movement and function if pericarditis is recurrent and has produced scar tissue and constriction. This procedure involves the removal of part (pericardial "window") or all of the pericardium to prevent constriction by scar tissue, exudate, or bleeding.

D. Nursing Diagnoses and Interventions

Activity intolerance related to weakness and dyspnea secondary to inflammation of the cardiac muscle and restriction of contraction

Desired outcome: Patient progresses to his or her highest level of mobility with decreasing evidence of cardiac intolerance.

1. Ensure that patient maintains bed rest during febrile period and understands the rationale.

2. Anticipate patient's needs by placing personal articles within easy reach.

3. Advise patient about the importance of frequent periods of rest during convalescence.

4. Monitor VS for changes that are indicative of cardiac or pulmonary decompensation, such as decreasing BP and increasing heart and respiratory rates.

5. Be alert to signs of cardiac tamponade, including narrowed pulse pressure, rapid pulse, hypotension, dyspnea, distended neck veins, and distant or decreased heart sounds. Report positive findings to MD and prepare for emergency pericardiocentesis.

6. Assist patient with turning at least q2h, and provide passive ROM exercises at frequent intervals to help prevent complications of immobility. As the patient's condition improves, consult with MD regarding in-bed exercises that require more cardiac tolerance. Examples are found with the nursing diagnosis **Potential impairment of physical mobility** related to inactivity, p. 535, in "Appendix One."

Potential alteration in tissue perfusion: Peripheral, cardiopulmonary, and cerebral related to impaired circulation secondary to dysfunctional cardiac muscle

Desired outcome: Patient's mentation and VS are within acceptable limits.

1. Observe for and report increasing restlessness or anxiety and changes in mentation, which can occur with decreased cerebral perfusion.

2. Palpate peripheral pulses at least q2–4h to assess peripheral perfusion.

3. Assess for pulsus paradoxus (decrease in pulse volume and systolic BP > 10 mm Hg during inspiration), which is produced by pericardial restriction and subsequent decreased ventricular filling. The assessment is performed as follows:

   □ Ask the patient to take a deeper-than-usual breath, and palpate the peripheral pulse. Be alert to decreased amplitude or strength.

   □ Tell the patient to breathe normally, and inflate the BP cuff.

   □ Ask the patient to take another deeper-than-usual breath, and slowly deflate the cuff. Note and record the systolic reading during the inspiration phase.

   □ Tell the patient to breathe normally again. Continue deflating the cuff, and record the point at which systolic sounds are heard with normal respirations. The difference in millimeters of mercury is the measurement of the pulsus paradoxus.

4. Instruct patient to perform foot and leg exercises q4h to enhance venous circulation.

5. If patient exhibits signs of decreased cerebral perfusion, reorient and institute safety precautions as necessary.

Alteration in comfort: Chest (pericardial) pain related to friction rub

Desired outcome: Patient relates a reduction in discomfort and does not exhibit signs of uncontrolled pain.

1. Assess and document character, intensity, and duration of pain. Administer pain medications as prescribed, and document their effectiveness. Advise patient to notify staff as soon as pain occurs so that the medication can be administered early.

2. Use the following interventions to enhance the effectiveness of the medication: Support the patient in a side-lying position with pillows, and/or place the patient in Fowler's position; provide emotional support; and control environmental stimuli by limiting visitors, dimming the lights, and providing a quiet environment.

3. Administer oxygen as prescribed, typically 2–3 L/min by nasal cannula.

Ineffective breathing pattern related to guarding secondary to pericardial pain

Desired outcome: Patient demonstrates a respiratory rate and depth within acceptable limits.

1. Assess breath sounds and respirations at least q4h. Report the presence of rhonchi or areas of diminished breath sounds.

2. Assess the breathing effort for adequate depth at least q2h, and teach the patient to breathe deeply. Teach the use of an incentive spirometer.

3. Place the patient in semi-Fowler's or high Fowler's position to ease the pressure on the heart, which will help decrease the effort of breathing.

See "Appendix One" for nursing diagnoses and interventions for the care of patients on prolonged bed rest, pp. 533–537.

E. Patient–Family Teaching and Discharge Planning

Provide patient and SOs with verbal and written information for the following:

1. Importance of frequent rest periods during convalescence.

2. Importance of prompt treatment if symptoms of pericarditis recur.

3. Procedure for measuring temperature, which can be an indicator of recurring inflammation.

4. Importance of avoiding individuals with URI and promptly seeking medical attention if flu or cold symptoms occur.

5. Medications, including drug name, purpose, dosage, schedule, precautions, and potential side effects.

In addition,

6. Explain that feelings of wellness do not necessarily mean that the inflammation has completely resolved.

II. Myocarditis

Myocarditis is an inflammation of the myocardium (middle layer of the heart walls, composed of cardiac muscle), and is often caused by a virus, bacterium, or protozoon. Clinical consequences range from focal inflammation with spontaneous recovery to more severe processes such as acute congestive cardiomyopathy and chronic dilated cardiomyopathy. The condition can be acute or chronic.

A. Assessment

Chronic indicators: Signs of congestive heart failure may appear, including distended neck veins, pulmonary congestion, dyspnea, and tachycardia.

Acute indicators: Fatigue, dyspnea, palpitations, continuous precordial discomfort, fever.

Physical exam: Cardiomegaly with diffuse point of maximal impulse (PMI), soft heart sounds, heart murmur of tricuspid or mitral regurgitation, S3 and S4 heart sounds.

History of: URI or GI complaints.

B. Diagnostic Tests

1. <u>EKG:</u> Changes are usually transient and involve the ST segment and T wave or intraventricular conduction defects.

2. <u>Chest x-ray:</u> Heart varies in size from normal to enlarged, depending on extent of involvement and subsequent muscle damage.

3. <u>Radionuclide scans:</u> May identify areas of the myocardium that are necrotic or akinetic.

4. <u>Cardiac enzymes:</u> To assess for elevated CPK or CPK isoenzyme.

5. <u>Cultures and sensitivities by blood studies or muscle biopsy:</u> To identify causative organism.

C. Medical Management and Surgical Interventions

1. **Oxygenation and bed rest:** Hypoxia and exercise contribute to muscle damage. Usually, oxygen is administered by nasal cannula at 2–3 L/min.

2. **Pharmacotherapy**

   □ *Antibiotics:* Type is determined by the causative organism.

   □ *Diuretics and digitalization:* To treat congestive heart failure. Close observance for digitalis toxicity is important because these patients are particularly sensitive to digitalis.

   □ *Anti-arrhythmic agents:* For prompt treatment of dysrhythmias. Drugs with negative inotropic action (such as propranolol), which further decrease the strength of contraction, should be avoided because of the weakness of the already compromised myocardial muscle.

   □ *Steroids:* Controversial with this disorder, and are used mostly for patients with acute viral myocarditis.

D. Nursing Diagnoses and Interventions

Activity intolerance related to weakness and fatigue secondary to dysfunction of myocardial muscle

Desired outcome: Patient progresses to his or her highest level of mobility with decreasing evidence of cardiac intolerance.

1. Observe for and immediately report signs of congestive heart failure, including dyspnea, distended neck veins, and crackles (rales).

2. Be alert to steady weight gains, which can occur with heart failure. Monitor I&O and report imbalances.

3. Administer and maintain oxygen as prescribed.

4. Ensure that the patient maintains bed rest during the febrile period; advise patient about the importance of frequent periods of rest during the convalescent period.

5. Anticipate patient's needs by placing personal items within reach.

6. Assist patient with turning q2h, and provide assistance with ROM exercises at frequent intervals to help prevent complications of immobility. As the patient's condition improves, consult with MD regarding progressive in-bed exercises that require increasing cardiac tolerance. These are discussed with the nursing diagnosis **Potential impairment of physical mobility** related to inactivity, p. 535, in "Appendix One."

See "Heart Failure" for the following: **Knowledge deficit**: Precautions and negative side effects of digitalis therapy, p. 49. See "Pericarditis" for the following: **Alteration in comfort**: Chest (pericardial) pain related to friction rub, p. 53. See "Infective Endocarditis" for the following: **Knowledge deficit**: Disease process and therapeutic regimen, p. 56. See "Osteomyelitis" in Chapter 8 for the following: **Knowledge deficit**: Adverse side effects from prolonged use of potent antibiotics, p. 387. See "Appendix One" for nursing diagnoses and interventions for the care of patients on prolonged bed rest, pp. 533–537.

E. Patient–Family Teaching and Discharge Planning

Provide patient and SOs with verbal and written information for the following:

1. Indicators of recurring inflammation and/or heart failure. The signs of heart failure, which must be reported *stat*, include steady weight gain, decreased exercise tolerance, fatigue, dyspnea, and SOB.

2. Medications to be taken at home, including drug name, purpose, dosage, schedule, precautions, and potential side effects.

3. Importance of helping to fight infection with a well-balanced diet that includes vegetables, fruits, and protein. Advise patients with congestive heart failure not to add salt to their food.

4. Importance of immunization and vaccination as preventive measures.

5. Technique for measuring body temperature and importance of regular measurement to detect elevations, which can signal recurring infection. Suggest that the patient measure body temperature at least once a week if asymptomatic, and more frequently if symptoms of colds and flu, fatigue, or weakness occur.

6. Notifying MD if URI or viral infections occur, because they can precipitate myocarditis.

7. Importance of regular follow-up; confirm date and time of next medical appointment.

III. Infective Endocarditis

Inflammation of the inner lining of the atria, ventricles, and covering of the heart valves is called endocarditis. This infection involves the left side of the heart more frequently than the right side and is characterized by vegetations (fibrous network of platelets, blood cells, and pathogenic organisms), which are found most frequently on the mitral and aortic valves. Vegetations on the valves can prevent adequate closure and/or adherence of the valve flaps, resulting in stenosis. When the vegetations affect the chamber lining, muscle fibers eventually undergo degenerative changes, and the patient becomes at risk for emboli because parts of the vegetations can break off. In addition, there is a tendency for fibrin and platelets to deposit on the vegetations and these may embolize as well. Endocarditis is usually classified as acute or subacute.

A. Assessment

Chronic indicators: Murmurs (sign of valvular involvement) and dyspnea, distended neck veins, peripheral edema, pulmonary congestion, splenomegaly, and activity intolerance (signs of congestive heart failure).

Acute indicators: Temperature elevation, malaise, anorexia, weight loss, tachycardia, and pallor.

History of: URI, flu, or other infectious process.

B. Diagnostic Tests

1. <u>Blood cultures:</u> To identify causative organism.

2. <u>ESR:</u> Usually elevated.

3. <u>WBC count:</u> May be normal in subacute forms and can range from 15,000–20,000 in acute disease.

4. <u>Two-dimensional echocardiography:</u> May be used to detect intracardiac complications such as valvular disorders or wall motion abnormalities. This test uses sound waves (or echoes), which allow visualization of the cardiac wall and valvular movement.

C. Medical Management and Surgical Interventions

1. **Specific antibiotic therapy:** Will depend on the causative organism and its susceptibility or sensitivity to drugs. In the subacute form of the disorder, it is satisfactory to wait until the organism is identified, but with acute endocarditis, broad-spectrum antibiotic therapy is instituted immediately after blood cultures are drawn and then adjusted if necessary after organism identification. Intermittent IV antibiotics are given q4–6h. The duration of therapy is usually 4–6 weeks.

2. **Bed rest.**

3. **Well-balanced diet:** To maintain resistance to infection.

4. **Surgical repair or valve replacement:** Performed when congestive heart failure does not respond to medical management; when an infection does not respond to antimicrobial therapy within 1 week; when repeated episodes of embolization occur, especially when vascular occlusions are found in the eyes, brain, coronary arteries, and kidneys; when repeated infections occur (eg, relapse after 3 months); and when fungal endocarditis is found. (See discussion of mitral valve replacement in "Mitral Stenosis," p. 58.)

D. Nursing Diagnoses and Interventions

Knowledge deficit: Disease process and therapeutic regimen

Desired outcome: Patient can verbalize understanding of the disease process and measures that are taken to prevent bacteremia.

1. Assess patient's level of knowledge about the disease and therapy.

2. As indicated, explain the disease process and the need for prolonged antibiotic therapy.

3. Because of the increased risk for bacteremia, discuss the need for antibiotic prophylaxis before dental procedures and all major and minor surgical procedures and early treatment of common infections (eg, UTI, URI, and wound infection).

4. Teach patient the early indicators of infection, eg, low-grade fever and malaise, and the importance of reporting indicators to MD promptly. Teach patient how to measure body temperature and the importance of monitoring temperature weekly if asymptomatic and more frequently if weakness, fatigue, or symptoms of cold or a flu occur.

See "Pulmonary Embolism" in Chapter 1 for the following: **Potential for injury** (bleeding with anticoagulation therapy), p. 9. See "Cardiomyopathy" for the following: **Potential alteration in tissue perfusion** (embolization), p. 40. See "Pericarditis" for the following: **Activity intolerance**, p. 52. See "Osteomyelitis" in Chapter 8 for the following: **Knowledge deficit**: Adverse side effects from prolonged use of potent antibiotics, pp. 387–389. See "Appendix One" for nursing diagnoses and interventions for the care of patients on prolonged bed rest, pp. 533–537.

E. Patient–Family Teaching and Discharge Planning

Provide patient and SOs with verbal and written information for the following:

1. Need for prolonged antibiotic therapy, including prophylaxis before dental and surgical procedures.

2. Other medications to be taken at home, including drug name, purpose, dosage, schedule, precautions, and potential side effects. **Note:** The patient may be required to self-administer IV antibiotics at home to decrease the length of hospital stay; teach the technique if indicated.

3. Importance of medical follow-up to check valve function; confirm date and time of next medical appointment.

4. Signs and symptoms of URI and other infections that can precipitate recurrence of endocardial infection, and/or indicators of recurrence of endocarditis and the importance of getting prompt medical attention if they occur.

5. Importance of reporting signs of increasing cardiac failure *stat*. These include steady weight gain, decreased exercise tolerance, fatigue, and dyspnea.

6. Importance of regular temperature measurement, eg, weekly if asymptomatic and more frequently if weakness, fatigue, or symptoms of a cold or flu occur.

▶ Section Three **Valvular Heart Disorders**

I. Mitral Stenosis

The most common cause of mitral valve stenosis is rheumatic heart disease, although it also can be caused by a virus or malignancy. In the diseased mitral valve the orifice becomes narrowed either by calcification or thickening of the valve leaflets. Because the mitral valve is located between the left atrium and ventricle, stenosis results in decreased ventricular filling and increased left atrial and pulmonary pressures. As the severity of the stenosis increases, maintenance of cardiac output becomes more difficult. In addition, high pulmonary pressures cause fluid extravasation into the alveoli, which results in pulmonary edema.

Patients with valvular disorders are predisposed to endocarditis (see "Infective Endocarditis," pp. 55–57). Bacteria in the bloodstream have a tendency to lodge in the malfunctioning valves because of calcium deposits and/or turbulent blood flow, so special care should be taken whenever a systemic infection is present or the patient is undergoing major or minor surgical procedures such as dental work.

A. Assessment

Chronic indicators: Decreased exercise tolerance secondary to decreased cardiac output; increased pulmonary artery pressures.

Acute indicators: Dyspnea is usually the first symptom of worsening stenosis. Orthopnea, hemoptysis, thromboembolism, and chest pain with subsequent right ventricular failure may occur with elevated pulmonary pressure. In some patients, chest pain occurs secondary to decreased oxygen perfusion.

Physical exam: Decreased arterial pulse volume, as determined by palpation or Doppler; elevated venous pulsations; low-pitched diastolic murmur; elevated CVP; and hepatomegaly. Left ventricular impulse may be displaced by an enlarged right ventricle. Normally, it is best heard over the mitral area, fifth intercostal space, mid-clavicular line.

B. Diagnostic Tests

1. <u>Chest x-ray:</u> May reveal an enlarged left atrium and right ventricle.

2. <u>Echocardiography:</u> Can readily diagnose mitral stenosis by poor valve leaflet separation and thickened leaflets; also may demonstrate pulmonary hypertension.

3. <u>EKG:</u> Although not useful for a definitive diagnosis, it will demonstrate characteristic changes associated with left atrial and right ventricular enlargement.

4. <u>Cardiac catheterization:</u> To determine extent of the stenosis (see "Cardiac Catheterization," pp. 72–75).

C. Medical Management and Surgical Interventions

1. **Restrict physically strenuous activities.**

2. **Antibiotic prophylaxis for endocarditis:** Before and after invasive procedures, including dental work (see "Infective Endocarditis," p. 56).

3. **Pharmacotherapy**

   □ *Oral diuretics:* To reduce pulmonary artery pressures and relieve dyspnea.

   □ *Digitalis glycosides:* To increase the strength of contraction for patients with ventricular failure.

   □ *Oral anticoagulants (warfarin sodium):* May be prescribed to prevent thromboemboli.

4. **Mitral commissurotomy:** To relieve stenosis by incising the valve and removing calcifications. This procedure involves a heart–lung bypass. Usually the chest is entered through the left fifth intercostal space. The left atrial appendage is incised and a dilator is inserted and guided through the mitral orifice.

5. **Mitral valve replacement:** For patients who continue to be symptomatic after a commissurotomy. Using a midline sternotomy incision, a prosthetic mitral valve is inserted while the patient is on a heart–lung bypass machine. Usually the patient remains in ICU for 48 hours after the procedure.

D. Nursing Diagnoses and Interventions

Activity intolerance related to fatigue and weakness secondary to decreased left ventricular filling

Desired outcome: Patient progresses to his or her highest level of mobility with decreasing evidence of cardiac intolerance.

1. Monitor VS at frequent intervals, and report significant (10 mm Hg or greater) decrease in BP to MD. Assess for orthostatic changes in BP, which occur when the patient moves from a supine to standing position.

2. Assess peripheral pulses, capillary refill, and temperature and color of the extremities as indicators of adequate cardiac output.

3. Provide rest periods at frequent intervals, especially between care activities.

4. Confer with MD regarding in-bed exercises that can be incorporated as the patient's condition improves. Examples are found in "Appendix One," **Potential impairment of physical mobility** related to inactivity, p. 535. Increase

ambulation progressively and to the patient's tolerance; be alert to indicators of activity intolerance, including SOB, dyspnea, and fatigue.

Fluid volume excess: Edema related to retention secondary to right-sided heart failure

Desired outcome: Patient does not exhibit signs of overhydration.

1. Observe for and report the following indicators of right-sided heart failure: increasing CVP, peripheral edema, dyspnea, hepatic enlargement on palpation, and jugular vein distention.

2. Monitor I&O and administer fluids only as prescribed to ensure that patient maintains adequate volume without overload. Weigh patient daily and report significant I&O imbalance.

3. If fluids are limited, offer ice chips and Popsicles to help patient control thirst. Record the amount of intake.

4. Administer cardiac glycosides as prescribed to increase the strength of contraction.

5. Administer diuretics as prescribed to decrease volume load.

Knowledge deficit: Potential for development of endocarditis

Desired outcome: Patient can verbalize knowledge of the potential for endocarditis, indicators of the disorder, and measures that prevent it.

1. Assess patient's knowledge of the disease process and potential for endocarditis. As indicated, explain how endocarditis affects the heart and its valves and why individuals with valvular disorders are predisposed toward developing this disorder.

2. Discuss the importance of antibiotic prophylaxis before and after any major or minor surgical procedures.

3. Teach patient the following indicators of endocarditis: temperature increases, malaise, anorexia, tachycardia, and pallor. Explain the importance of reporting the symptoms early.

4. Teach patient the indicators of frequently encountered infections (eg, URI, UTI, wound), and stress the importance of reporting them to MD promptly should they occur.

Potential for infection (with concomitant endocarditis) related to increased susceptibility secondary to valvular disorder

Desired outcome: Patient does not exhibit signs of infection.

1. Ensure good handwashing before patient contact, and maintain aseptic technique for all invasive procedures.

2. Monitor temperature q4h and report significant increases to MD.

3. Be alert to rising heart rate, which can signal the presence of an infection.

4. Administer prescribed antibiotics on time.

5. Maintain adequate hydration, as prescribed, through oral and prescribed IV fluids. **Caution:** Notify MD and limit fluids if any signs of heart failure and/or fluid overload occur.

See "Pulmonary Embolism" in Chapter 1 for the following: **Potential for injury** (bleeding with anticoagulant therapy), p. 9. See "Heart Failure" for the following: **Knowledge deficit** (side effects of diuretics), p. 49, and **Knowledge deficit** (side effects of digitalis), p. 49. As appropriate, see nursing diagnoses and interventions in "Cardiac Catheterization," p. 73–74, and "Cardiac Surgery," p. 75–76.

E. Patient–Family Teaching and Discharge Planning

Provide patient and SOs with verbal and written information for the following:

1. Medications, including drug name, purpose, dosage, schedule, precautions, and potential side effects
2. Gradually increasing exercise, avoiding heavy lifting (>5 lb), incorporating rest periods.
3. Name and phone number of a resource person (eg, MD, primary nurse) should questions arise after hospital discharge.
4. Referral to cardiac rehabilitation program if appropriate.
5. Resumption of sexual activity as directed by MD.
6. Indicators that necessitate immediate medical attention: decreased exercise tolerance, signs of infection, SOB, bleeding.
7. Importance of consulting MD before using OTC medications, especially aspirin products, which can prevent platelet aggregation.
8. Importance of follow-up care; confirm date and time of next medical appointment.

II. Mitral Regurgitation and Mitral Valve Prolapse

Abnormalities of the mitral valve cause mitral regurgitation (MR). The most common cause of MR is mitral valve prolapse (MVP) syndrome, which can be caused by a variety of clinical conditions that result in a "floppy" or incompetent mitral valve, including heredity, papillary muscle dysfunction, cardiomyopathy, or inflammatory heart disorders. The significant effects of MR and MVP occur during ventricular systole. Normally, the mitral valve is closed during ventricular systole, but with MR the valves allow approximately half of the ventricular volume back into the left atrium rather than forcing it forward into the aorta. MR is often associated with coronary artery disease and myocardial infarction.

A. Assessment

Chronic indicators: A majority of patients with MVP remain asymptomatic, although weakness and low exercise tolerance secondary to low cardiac output may be present. Anxiety and patient complaints of intermittent palpitations and chest discomfort also can occur.

Acute indicators: Fatigue, exhaustion, dyspnea, palpitations, and signs of pulmonary edema.

Physical exam: Holosystolic murmur heard at the apex, radiating toward the axilla; possible presence of S3 heart sounds; characteristic ejection click.

B. Diagnostic Tests

1. <u>EKG:</u> Will show left atrial enlargement, possibly with atrial fibrillation.
2. <u>Chest x-ray:</u> Will demonstrate cardiomegaly with left ventricular and left atrial enlargement.
3. <u>Echocardiography:</u> Provides a definitive diagnosis and reveals severity of the disorder.
4. <u>Radioisotope imaging:</u> Often useful in follow-up; progressive increases in end-systolic or end-diastolic volumes can indicate a worsening condition.
5. <u>Angiography and ventriculogram:</u> Will show decreased contraction and dilation.

C. Medical Management and Surgical Interventions

1. **Endocarditis prophylaxis with antibiotics**: Initiated before major or minor surgical procedures.

2. **Pharmacotherapy**

□ *Beta blockade:* To decrease cardiac workload and prevent chest pain and irregularities in rhythm.

□ *Digitalis:* To increase strength of contraction.

□ *Vasodilators:* To decrease afterload and increase cardiac output.

□ *Diuretics:* To control fluid accumulation.

□ *Anticoagulants (heparin or warfarin):* To prevent embolization.

3. **Diet:** Low in sodium.

4. **Mitral valve replacement:** If necessary. (See "Mitral Stenosis," p. 58.)

D. Nursing Diagnoses and Interventions

Activity intolerance related to fatigue and weakness secondary to decreased cardiac output with valvular regurgitation

Desired outcome: Patient progresses to his or her highest level of mobility with decreasing evidence of cardiac intolerance.

1. Provide frequent rest periods, especially between care activities.
2. As necessary, assist patient with ADLs to avoid shortness of breath.
3. Discuss ways to decrease energy output at home.
4. Progressively increase ambulation to patient's tolerance. Be alert to dyspnea, fatigue, and SOB with activity. Modify or restrict activities, as indicated.

See "Pulmonary Embolism" in Chapter 1 for the following: **Potential for injury** (bleeding with anticoagulant therapy), p. 9. See "Coronary Artery Disease" for the following: **Knowledge deficit:** Precautions and negative side effects of beta blockers, p. 43. See "Heart Failure" for the following: **Fluid volume excess:** Edema (due to decreased cardiac output), p. 49, **Knowledge deficit:** Precautions and negative side effects of diuretic therapy, p. 49, **Knowledge deficit:** Precautions and negative side effects of digitalis therapy, p. 49, and **Knowledge deficit:** Precautions and negative side effects of vasodilators, p. 50. See "Mitral Stenosis" for the following: **Knowledge deficit:** Potential for development of endocarditis, p. 59, and **Potential for infection** (with concomitant endocarditis), p. 59. As appropriate, see nursing diagnoses and interventions in "Cardiac Catheterization," pp. 73–74. See "Cardiac Surgery," pp. 75–76, for all nursing diagnoses and interventions related to postsurgical care.

E. Patient–Family Teaching and Discharge Planning

See "Heart Failure," p. 50, and "Cardiac Surgery," p. 76.

III. Aortic Stenosis

Aortic stenosis is a condition that obstructs outflow from the left ventricle. It is either congenital or acquired and it results from adhesions and fusion of the valve cusps. Usually, normal left ventricular output can be maintained by compensatory left ventricular hypertrophy, but eventually progressive stenosis causes signs of low cardiac output such as cool extremities, fluid accumulation, decreased urinary output, and cardiac failure.

A. Assessment

Signs and symptoms: Often, patients are asymptomatic until around age 60, when angina, orthostatic hypotention, syncope with exertion, orthopnea, signs of pulmonary edema, and cardiac failure are seen. Signs of left ventricular failure also may be present, including dyspnea and SOB.

Physical exam: Decreased systolic BP, decreased pulse pressure (the difference between the systolic and diastolic pressures), increased left ventricular impulse (palpable at 5th intercostal space, midclavicular line, as a "lift" of the chest wall during ventricular systole), and systolic ejection murmur (best heard at the apex of the heart, 2nd intercostal space).

B. Diagnostic Tests

1. <u>EKG:</u> Will show presence of left ventricular hypertrophy.

2. <u>Chest x-ray:</u> May reveal aortic valve calcification.

3. <u>Cardiac catheterization with angiography:</u> Demonstrates the degree of thickness of the stenotic valve.

4. <u>Echocardiography:</u> Allows visualization of the narrowed valve opening. Two-dimensional echocardiography can be helpful in determining severity of the stenosis.

C. Medical Management and Surgical Interventions

1. **Antibiotics:** A prophylaxis against endocarditis.

2. **Treatment of congestive heart failure:** If present. See "Medical Management and Surgical Interventions" in "Heart Failure," p. 48.

3. **Aortic valve replacement:** Appropriate for patients with left ventricular dysfunction and symptoms of decreased cardiac output and functional disability. Aortic valve replacement is performed using heart–lung bypass, and the patient is in ICU for 2–3 days postoperatively. **Note:** Artificial mechanical valves, as well as those obtained from animals, may be used. Patients with artificial valves are maintained on lifetime anticoagulant therapy.

D. Nursing Diagnoses and Interventions

See "Mitral Stenosis" for the following: **Knowledge deficit** (potential for endocarditis), p. 59, and **Potential for infection** (endocarditis), p. 59. See "Pulmonary Embolism" in Chapter 1 for the following: **Potential for injury** (bleeding with anticoagulant therapy), p. 9. See "Heart Failure" for the following: **Fluid volume excess:** Edema, p. 49, **Knowledge deficit** (side effects of vasodilator therapy), p. 50, **Knowledge deficit** (side effects of digitalis therapy), p. 49, and **Knowledge deficit** (side effects of diuretic therapy), p. 49. See "Coronary Artery Disease" for the following: **Knowledge deficit** (side effects of beta blockers), p. 43. As appropriate, see nursing diagnoses and interventions in "Cardiac Catheterization," pp. 73–74, and "Cardiac Surgery," pp. 75–76.

E. Patient–Family Teaching and Discharge Planning

See "Heart Failure," p. 50, and "Cardiac Surgery," p. 76.

IV. Aortic Regurgitation

Many disorders can cause aortic valve regurgitation, but the most common is rheumatic fever. The cusps of the valve become fibrotic and retract, preventing valve closure during diastole. Incompetence of this valve allows backward flow, which results in a large ventricular volume. If the condition develops slowly the patient remains asymptomatic longer because the left ventricle hypertrophies to accommodate a larger volume.

A. Assessment

Signs and symptoms: With slowly developing regurgitation, the patient can remain asymptomatic for years. When the heart begins to fail, signs associated with left ventricular failure develop, including dyspnea, orthopnea, decreasing BP, changes in mentation, peripheral vasoconstriction, and pulmonary edema.

Physical exam: Decreased aortic pulse pressure (the difference between systolic and diastolic pressures), low diastolic BP, low-pitched diastolic murmur located in the second intercostal space to the right of the sternum, tachycardia, crackles (rales), and increased pulmonary arterial pressures.

B. Diagnostic Tests

1. <u>EKG:</u> Will demonstrate left axis deviation and left ventricular conduction defects with chronic aortic regurgitation. With acute regurgitation, nonspecific ST segment changes or left ventricular hypertrophy will be seen.
2. <u>Chest x-ray:</u> Results depend on the severity and duration of the disorder, but it eventually demonstrates cardiac enlargement.
3. <u>Cardiac catheterization with angiography:</u> Useful in determining severity of the regurgitation
4. <u>Echocardiography:</u> May identify the cause of regurgitation by revealing damaged cusps or vegetations caused by endocarditis.

C. Medical Management and Surgical Interventions

1. **Pharmacotherapy**
   - □ *Cardiac glycosides (digitalis):* To maintain ventricular function.
   - □ *Vasodilators:* To decrease afterload.
2. **Treatment of heart failure:** See "Heart Failure," p. 48.
3. **Surgical interventions:** Heart failure is not uncommon in patients with aortic regurgitation, even with aggressive medical treatment. Therefore, aortic valve replacement is usually recommended. Indications for this surgery include chronic aortic regurgitation that has become symptomatic and ventricular dysfunction during exercise.

D. Nursing Diagnoses and Interventions

See "Pulmonary Embolism" in Chapter 1 for the following: **Potential for injury** (bleeding with anticoagulant therapy), p. 9. See "Coronary Artery Disease" for the following: **Knowledge deficit** (side effects of beta blockers), p. 43. See "Heart Failure" for the following: **Fluid volume excess:** Edema, p. 49, **Knowledge deficit** (side effects of digitalis therapy), p. 49, **Knowledge deficit** (side effects of diuretic therapy), p. 49, and **Knowledge deficit** (side effects of vasodilator therapy), p. 50. See "Mitral Stenosis" for the following: **Knowledge deficit** (potential for endocarditis), p. 59, and **Potential for infection** (endocarditis), p. 59. As appropriate, see nursing diagnoses and interventions in "Cardiac Catheterization," pp. 73–74, and "Cardiac Surgery," pp. 75–76.

E. Patient–Family Teaching and Discharge Planning

See "Heart Failure," p. 50, and "Cardiac Surgery," p. 76.

▶ Section Four   **Cardiovascular Conditions Secondary to Other Disease Processes**

I. Cardiac and Noncardiac Shock (Circulatory Failure)

A shock state exists when tissue perfusion decreases to the point of cellular metabolic dysfunction. Shock is classified according to the causative event.

Hematogenic (hemorrhagic or hypovolemic) shock: Occurs when blood volume is insufficient to meet metabolic needs of the tissues, eg, with severe hemorrhage.

Cardiogenic shock: Occurs when cardiac failure results in decreased tissue perfusion, such as in myocardial infarction.

Neurogenic shock: Result of a neurologic event (eg, head injury) that causes massive vasodilation and decreased perfusion pressures.

Anaphylactic shock: A severe systemic response to an allergen (foreign protein), resulting in massive vasodilation, decreased perfusion, decreased venous return, and subsequent decreased cardiac output.

Septic shock: Occurs when bacterial toxins cause an overwhelming systemic infection.

A prolonged shock state from any cause can result in death, so early recognition and intervention are essential.

A. Assessment

Early signs and symptoms: Cool, pale, and clammy skin; dry and pale mucous membranes; restlessness; hyperventilation; anxiety; nausea; thirst; weakness.

Physical exam: Rapid heart rate; decreased systolic BP and increased diastolic BP secondary to catecholamine (sympathetic) response.

Late signs and symptoms: Decreased urinary output, hypothermia, drowsiness, diaphoresis, confusion, and lethargy, all of which can progress to a comatose state.

Physical exam: Irregular heart rate; continually decreasing BP, usually with systolic pressure palpable at 60 mm Hg or less; rapid and possibly irregular respiratory rate.

B. Diagnostic Tests

Diagnosis is usually based on the presenting symptoms and clinical signs.

1. <u>ABG values:</u> Will reveal metabolic acidosis caused by anaerobic metabolism.
2. <u>Serial measurement of urinary output:</u> Less than 30 mL/h is indicative of decreased perfusion and decreased renal function.

For septic shock:

3. <u>Serial creatinine and BUN levels:</u> To assess for potential renal complications and dysfunction.
4. <u>Serum electrolyte levels:</u> Identify renal complications and dysfunctions as evidenced by hyperkalemia and hypernatremia.
5. <u>Blood culture:</u> To identify the causative organism.
6. <u>WBC and ESR:</u> Elevated in the presence of infection.

For hematogenic shock:

7. <u>CBC:</u> Hematocrit and hemoglobin will be decreased.

For anaphylactic shock:

8. <u>WBC count:</u> Will reveal increased eosinophils.

C. Medical Management

Interventions are determined by clinical presentation and severity of the shock state. Patients are transferred to ICU to assess severity of the shock state and closely monitor status.

For cardiogenic shock:

1. **Vascular support**: Intra-aortic balloon counterpulsation is used to augment perfusion pressures.

2. **Optimize blood volume**: Either with volume expanders such as dextran or with diuretics if fluid overload is the problem.

3. **Pharmacotherapy**

   □ *Sympathomimetics:* For example, dopamine infusion at low doses (2–5 μg/kg/min) to increase renal perfusion and decrease systemic vasocontriction. Moderate doses (5–8 μg/kg/min) help strengthen cardiac contraction.

   □ *Vasodilators:* To increase peripheral perfusion and reduce afterload vasoconstriction.

   □ *Osmotic diuretics:* To increase renal blood flow.

4. **Oxygen support**: As needed, to maintain adequate ventilation.

For anaphylactic shock:

1. **Pharmacotherapy**

   □ *Epinephrine (0.5 mL, 1:1000 in 10-mL saline):* To promote vasoconstriction and decrease the allergic response by counteracting vasodilation caused by histamine release.

   □ *Bronchodilators:* To relieve bronchospasm.

   □ *Antihistamines:* To prevent relapse.

   □ *Hydrocortisone:* For its anti-inflammatory effects.

2. **Oxygen and airway support**: As needed.

For hemorrhagic shock:

1. **Control hemorrhage.**

2. **Fresh whole blood:** To increase oxygen delivery at the tissue level when >2 L of blood have been lost.

3. **Albumin or dextran:** Sometimes used to increase vascular volume.

4. **Ringer's solution:** Often used as an isotonic solution to replace electrolytes and ions lost with bleeding in hemorrhagic shock.

D. Nursing Diagnoses and Interventions

Alteration in tissue perfusion: Peripheral, cardiopulmonary, cerebral, and renal related to impaired circulation secondary to decreased circulating blood volume

Desired outcome: Patient's VS, mentation, and physical findings are within acceptable limits.

1. Assess and document peripheral pulses. Report significant findings such as coolness and pallor of the extremities, decreased amplitude of pulses, and delayed capillary refill.

2. Monitor BP at frequent intervals; be alert to readings >20 mm Hg below patient's normal or to other indicators of hypotension, such as dizziness, altered mentation, or decreased urinary output.

3. If hypotension is present, place patient in a supine position to promote venous return. Remember that BP must be at least 80/60 mm Hg for adequate coronary and renal artery perfusion.

4. Monitor CVP (if line is inserted) to determine adequacy of venous return and blood volume; 4–10 cm H_2O are usually considered adequate levels. Values near zero can indicate hypovolemia, especially when associated with decreased urinary output, vasoconstriction, and increased heart rate, which are found with hypovolemia.

5. Observe for indicators of decreased cerebral perfusion such as restlessness, confusion, and decreased LOC. If positive indicators are present, protect patient from injury by raising side rails and placing bed in its lowest position. Reorient patient as indicated.

6. Monitor for indicators of decreased coronary artery perfusion such as chest pain and an irregular heart rate.

7. Monitor urinary output hourly. Notify MD if it is <30 mL/h in the presence of adequate intake. Check weight daily for evidence of gain.

8. Monitor lab results for elevated BUN and creatinine; report increases.

9. Monitor serum electrolyte values for evidence of imbalances, particularly sodium and potassium. Be alert to signs of hyperkalemia such as increased serum levels, muscle weakness, hyporeflexia, and irregular heart rate. Also monitor for signs of hypernatremia such as increased serum levels, fluid retention, and edema.

10. Administer fluids as prescribed to increase vascular volume. The type and amount of fluid will depend on the type of shock and the patient's clinical situation.

   □ *Cardiogenic shock:* Fluids probably will be limited to prevent overload, yet dehydration must be avoided to ensure support of vascular space and cardiac muscle.

   □ *Hypovolemic shock:* The amount lost is replaced. As much as 1000 mL/h of Ringer's solution may be administered if volume loss is severe. Most often, this includes blood replacement.

   □ *Septic shock:* Ringer's solution, plasma, and blood are administered.

Impaired gas exchange related to tissue hypoxia secondary to decreased circulating blood volume

Desired outcome: Patient exhibits ABG values and VS within acceptable limits.

1. Monitor respirations q30 min; note and report presence of tachypnea and/or dyspnea.

2. Teach patient to breathe slowly and deeply to promote oxygenation.

3. Ensure that the patient has a patent airway; suction secretions as needed to assist with gas exchange.

4. Administer oxygen as prescribed.

5. Monitor ABG results. Be alert to and report presence of hypoxemia (decreased Pao_2), hypercapnia (increased $Paco_2$), and acidosis (decreased pH, increased $Paco_2$).

6. Report significant findings to MD.

See "Appendix One" for nursing diagnoses and interventions for the care of patients with life-disrupting illnesses, pp. 544–546.

E. Patient–Family Teaching and Discharge Planning

For interventions, see discussion with patient's primary diagnosis.

II. Cardiac Arrest

▶ **Note:** This section is intended as an overview only. In the event of a cardiac arrest, the reader should refer to cardiac arrest procedures established by the institution.

Cardiac arrest occurs when the heart stops beating, or when the contraction is ineffective (such as in ventricular tachycardia or ventricular fibrillation) in maintaining cardiac output. Many conditions can precipitate cardiac arrest, including myocardial infarction, heart failure, shock state, severe electrolyte disturbances, drowning, electrocution, drug overdose, and hypoxia. Often, the events that precipitate cardiac arrest occur in a vicious cycle. For example, a cardiac rhythm disturbance leads to decreased cardiac output, which leads to decreased tissue perfusion, which results in hypoxia, which leads to more rhythm disturbances, and the cycle goes on. Management of the pre-arrest stage is directed toward breaking this cycle and correcting the condition to prevent cardiac arrest. To help prevent an arrest from occurring, accurate and prompt nursing assessment is crucial. However, an arrest can occur without prior warning. This is an emergency situation, which requires *immediate* medical intervention.

A. Assessment

Signs and symptoms: Loss of consciousness—inability to be aroused by shaking and shouting.

Physical exam: Absence of carotid pulse; loss of audible or palpable BP; and usually, absence of respirations.

B. Medical Management

1. **Management of pre-arrest phase:** Includes treatment for shock, oxygen therapy or airway support, transfer to ICU, antiarrhythmic drugs, and pain relief.

2. **Basic life support:** Cardiopulmonary resuscitation (CPR) to provide maintenance of cardiac pumping action and ventilation until normal cardiac rhythm is restored.

3. **Ventilation:** To prevent hypoxia and subsequent anaerobic metabolism. The method depends on the patient's clinical presentation. Mouth-to-mouth breathing, oxygen mask with 100% oxygen if the patient is breathing, oral or nasal airways, endotracheal intubation, and manual ventilation may be used.

4. **Closed chest compressions:** An adjunct to circulation. If done properly, cardiac compression can provide 25–30% of the normal cardiac output.

5. **Establish IV access line:** In arrest situations, it is often difficult to establish a peripheral IV line because of vascular collapse or constriction. In addition, with decreased peripheral perfusion, absorption of drugs can be variable. The MD may instead insert a central venous catheter into the femoral, jugular, or subclavian vein.

6. **Treat cardiac rhythm abnormalities:** Lidocaine to suppress ventricular ectopic beats; atropine for bradycardias; defibrillation and/or epinephrine to combat ventricular fibrillation.

7. **Restore effective ventilation and circulation and a stable cardiac rhythm before transfer to ICU.**

C. Nursing Diagnoses and Interventions

Alterations in cardiac output: Decreased: Impaired oxygen transport secondary to cardiac arrest

Desired outcome: Patient's VS, ABG values, and physical findings are within acceptable limits.

1. Ensure adequate oxygenation by hyperextending the neck of stuporous patients and providing oxygen support as prescribed.

2. Maintain or establish an IV line. Typically, dextrose 5% in water (D_5W) is run at a rapid rate unless otherwise prescribed.

3. Assess and document BP at frequent intervals (q5–15 min) and report drops in pressure to MD immediately.

4. Assess and document heart rate; report irregularities or apical/radial deficit.

5. Administer antiarrythmic agents such as quinidine and procainamide and inotropic drugs such as digitalis glycosides or dopamine hydrochloride as prescribed.

6. Observe ventilatory status and be alert to indicators of hypoxia or inadequate ventilation such as changes in rhythm, adventitious lung sounds, or breath sounds that are not equal in both lungs. Be alert to ABG results that signal hypoxemia, hypercapnia, or acidosis, such as low pH (<7.35), low Pao_2 (<80 mm Hg), and high $Paco_2$ (>45 mm Hg). Report significant findings.

7. Monitor peripheral perfusion (femoral pulses). Be alert to and report decreasing amplitude of pulse pressures.

See "Appendix One" for nursing diagnoses and interventions for the care of patients with life-disrupting illnesses, pp. 544–546.

D. Patient–Family Teaching and Discharge Planning

See discussion under patient's primary diagnosis.

III. Pulmonary Edema

Acute pulmonary edema is an emergency situation in which hydrostatic pressure in the pulmonary vessels is greater than the vascular oncotic pressure that holds fluid in the vessels. As a result, fluid moves into the alveoli. When the alveoli contain fluid, their ability to participate in gas exchange is reduced and hypoxia can occur. The most common cause or precipitating factor in acute pulmonary edema is acute left ventricular failure, or an acute exacerbation of congestive heart failure. Other causes include hypertension, volume overload, or nervous system disorders such as head trauma and grand mal seizures, which result in sympathetic nervous system hyperactivity and produce shifts in blood volume to the pulmonary system to increase pulmonary capillary pressure. Pulmonary edema can develop suddenly, or it can develop slowly over a period of hours or days.

A. Assessment

Signs and symptoms: Anxiety, restlessness, frothy and blood-tinged sputum, orthopnea, extreme dyspnea. The patient exhibits "air hunger" and may thrash about and describe a sensation of drowning.

Physical exam: Crackles (rales), tachycardia, tachypnea, engorged neck veins.

History of: Recent myocardial infarction or "heart problems" in the past; hypertension; fluid overload, often from IV fluids.

B. Diagnostic Tests

1. <u>ABG values:</u> Will reveal hypoxemia.
2. <u>Chest x-ray:</u> Will delineate interstitial fluid and may reveal an increased heart size.

C. Medical Management

1. **Transfer to ICU.**
2. **Oxygen:** High flow either by non-rebreathing mask or endotracheal intubation and mechanical ventilation.
3. **High Fowler's position:** To decrease venous return.
4. **Morphine sulfate:** In small increments (2–4 mg IV slowly) to decrease anxiety, work of breathing, and sympathetic vasoconstriction. **Note:** Morphine is avoided when pulmonary edema is associated with bronchial asthma, COPD, or CO_2 retention.
5. **Diuretics:** Usually injected over a 2-minute period.
6. **Rotating tourniquets:** Occasionally used to decrease venous return. Wide, soft rubber tubing or BP cuffs are applied in a rotating system to three of the four extremities and inflated to approximately 10 mm Hg below diastolic pressure. This allows arterial flow but impedes venous return from the ex-

tremity. Every 15 minutes the tourniquets are rotated so that each extremity is relieved of a tourniquet one out of every four rotations.

7. Other pharmacotherapy

□ *Vasodilators such as nitroprusside:* May be used to reduce systemic and venous pressures. Nitroglycerine (0.3–0.6 mg sublingual) also may be given for venodilation and to decrease preload.

□ *Digitalis:* To decrease ventricular rate and strengthen contractions for patients who are not already using the drug.

□ *Theophylline:* If bronchospasms further complicate the pulmonary edema.

D. Nursing Diagnoses and Interventions

Fear related to life-threatening situation

Desired outcome: Patient relates psychologic comfort and does not exhibit signs of uncontrolled anxiety or fear.

1. Provide the opportunity for patient and SOs to express feelings and fears. Be reassuring and supportive.
2. Help make the patient as comfortable as possible with prompt pain relief and positioning, typically high Fowler's.
3. Keep the environment as calm and quiet as possible.
4. Explain all treatment modalities, especially those that may be uncomfortable, eg, oxygen face mask and rotating tourniquets.
5. Remain with patient if at all possible, providing emotional support both for the patient and SOs.

Alteration in tissue perfusion: Cardiopulmonary, peripheral, and cerebral related to impaired circulation secondary to decreased cardiac output

Desired outcome: Patient's VS, mentation, and physical findings are within acceptable limits.

1. Monitor BP q15min, or more frequently if unstable. Be alert to decreases >20 mm Hg or changes such as dizziness and decreased mentation.
2. Check pulse rate q15–30min. Monitor for irregularities, increased heart rate, or skipped beats, which can signal decompensation and decreased function.
3. Monitor for indicators of peripheral vasoconstriction such as cool extremities, pallor, and diaphoresis. Evaluate capillary refill; pink color should return within 1–3 seconds after applying pressure to the nail beds.
4. Monitor for indicators of decreased cerebral perfusion such as restlessness, anxiety, confusion, lethargy, stupor, and coma. Institute safety precautions accordingly.
5. Administer digitalis as prescribed.
6. Administer vasodilators as prescribed, and monitor the effects closely. Be alert to problems such as hypotension and irregular heart beats.
7. Implement measures for decreasing venous return and increasing peripheral perfusion such as placing patient in high Fowler's position.

Impaired gas exchange related to tissue hypoxia secondary to fluid accumulation in the alveoli

Desired outcome: Patient exhibits VS, ABG values, and physical findings within acceptable limits.

1. Auscultate lung fields for breath sounds; be alert to the presence of crackles (rales), which signal alveolar fluid congestion.
2. Assist patient into high Fowler's position to decrease work of breathing and enhance gas exchange.

3. Teach patient to take slow, deep breaths to increase oxygenation.

4. Administer oxgyen as prescribed. If ABGs are drawn, monitor the results for the presence of hypoxemia (decreased Pao_2) and hypercapnia (increased $Paco_2$).

5. Be alert to signs of increasing respiratory distress: increased respiratory rate, gasping for air, cyanosis, or rapid heart rate.

6. Administer diuretics as prescribed. Monitor potassium levels because of the potential for hypokalemia in patients taking certain diuretics.

7. As indicated, have emergency equipment (eg, airway and manual resuscitator) available and functional.

Fluid volume excess: Edema related to retention secondary to decreased cardiac output

Desired outcome: Patient does not exhibit signs of fluid overload.

1. Closely monitor I&O, including insensible losses from diaphoresis and respirations.

2. Record weight daily, and report steady gains.

3. Assess for edema (interstitial fluids), especially in dependent areas such as the ankles and sacrum.

4. Assess the respiratory system for indicators of fluid extravasation such as crackles (rales) or pink-tinged, frothy sputum.

5. Monitor IV rate of flow to prevent volume overload. Use a commercial infusion controller, if possible.

6. Unless contraindicated, provide ice chips and/or Popsicles to help patient control thirst. Record the amount on the I&O record.

7. Administer diuretics as prescribed, and record patient's response.

See "Coronary Artery Disease" for the following: **Knowledge deficit** (side effects of nitrates), p. 43. See "Heart Failure" for the following: **Knowledge deficit** (negative side effects of digitalis therapy), p. 49, **Knowledge deficit** (negative side effects of diuretic therapy), p. 49, and **Knowledge deficit** (negative side effects of vasodilator therapy), p. 50. See "Appendix One" for nursing diagnoses and interventions that relate to the care of patients with life-disrupting illnesses, pp. 544–546.

E. Patient–Family Teaching and Discharge Planning

See the primary diagnosis.

▶ Section Five   **Special Cardiac Procedures**

I. Pacemakers

A mechanical pacemaker delivers an electrical impulse to the heart to stimulate contraction when the heart's natural pacemakers fail to maintain normal rhythm. Patients for whom pacemakers are indicated have a history of syncopal episodes, dizziness, intolerance to exercise, blacking out, or an episode of cardiac arrest. When patients suffer from temporary or transient rhythm disturbances such as severe bradycardia or a conduction block, a temporary pacemaker can be inserted. Temporary pacemakers are seen most often in ICUs and on an emergency basis. The lead wire is inserted through a peripheral vein into the right side of the heart, where it lodges in the tissue to deliver the electrical impulse.

Some patients who have had temporary pacemakers inserted are observed for the possibility of permanent pacing. Permanent pacemakers are indicated for patients with a complete or incomplete conduction block that recurs or is not transient. Stokes-Adams syncope (an intermittent heart block), symptomatic bradycardia, and uncontrollable tachydysrhythmias also are indications for permanent pacing. The pacemaker is implanted subcutaneously under local anesthesia, and it is completely internal.

The increasing complexity of pacemakers has led to the development of a three-letter code for universal language by the International Council on Heart Disease. The first letter represents the chamber that is paced: ventricle (V), atrium (A), both (D). The second letter is the chamber that is sensed: ventricle (V), atrium (A), both (D), or none (O). The third letter is the mode of response: inhibited by ventricular activity (I), triggered by ventricular activity (T), both mechanisms (D), or neither, in that it works continuously (O).

Types of pacemakers include:

Asynchronous or fixed rate: Discharges an impulse to the ventricle at a prescribed rate, without a sensing mechanism. Asynchronous or fixed-rate pacemakers can be VOO, AOO, or DOO.

Ventricular demand: Senses intrinsic cardiac function and discharges only when the ventricle fails to do so (at the prescribed rate). This type of pacemaker is coded VVI or VVT.

Synchronous: Senses the activity in the atrium and stimulates the ventricle. This type of pacemaker is coded VAT.

Sequential: Senses the activity in the atrium and ventricle and stimulates both sequentially if no intrinsic activity occurs. This type of pacemaker is coded DVI, VDD, or DDD.

Temporary pacemakers are often inserted in ICU, where the patient can be closely monitored. Permanent pacemakers are implanted in the operating room, after which the patient is transferred to the telemetry unit for 24–48 hours of close monitoring. After implantation, physical activity, especially arm movement, is restricted for approximately 48 hours to allow the lead and pacemaker to affix and imbed. The MD may put the patient's affected arm and shoulder in a sling or other immobilizer to restrict movement.

A. Nursing Diagnoses and Interventions

Knowledge deficit: Pacemaker insertion procedure and pacemaker function

Desired outcome: Patient can verbalize knowledge of the insertion procedure and function of the pacemaker.

1. Assess patient's knowledge of the insertion procedure and function of the pacemaker. As appropriate, describe the procedure and explain that the pacemaker stimulates the patient's own heart to beat when the heart becomes lazy or slows down.

2. Begin a teaching program specific to the patient's rhythm disorder and type of pacemaker inserted, including normal function of the heart, patient's disorder of rhythm that requires a pacemaker, and how the patient's pacemaker works.

3. Reinforce explanation by MD of the length of time of the procedure, use of local anesthetic, and postprocedure care.

Potential alteration in tissue perfusion: Peripheral and cardiopulmonary related to impaired circulation secondary to pacemaker malfunction

Desired outcome: Patient's VS and physical findings are within acceptable limits.

1. Monitor perfusion by assessing BP at frequent intervals.

2. Assess rate and regularity of apical and radial pulses. At minimum, it should be the rate established for the pacemaker.

3. Assess for apical/radial deficit, which if present indicates that the heart is mechanically contracting but there is no perfusion.

4. Be alert to pulse irregularity, which can signal pacemaker malfunction or decreasing patient response.

5. Ensure that patient maintains strict bed rest for 48 hours postoperatively to prevent pacemaker dislodgement.

6. Maintain patient's arm in a sling or other immobilizer to prevent pacemaker dislodgement caused by arm movement.

7. Alert MD to significant findings.

Alteration in comfort: Pain related to pacemaker insertion

Desired outcome: Patient relates a reduction in discomfort and does not exhibit signs of uncontrolled pain.

1. Assess for pain, and medicate as prescribed.

2. Assist patient with positioning for comfort, using pillows for support as needed.

3. Adjust the sling or shoulder support to avoid incisional pressure and pressure areas.

See "Appendix One" for nursing diagnoses and interventions for the care of preoperative and postoperative patients, pp. 528–532.

B. Patient–Family Teaching and Discharge Planning

Provide patient and SOs with verbal and written information for the following:

1. Activity restrictions as directed by MD, such as heavy lifting, and instructions about the amount and type of exercise allowed. Resumption of sexual activity probably will not be affected, but depends on patient's underlying condition.

2. Technique for measuring radial pulse.

3. Signs and symptoms that necessitate medical attention, such as decreasing pulse rate, irregular pulse, dizziness, passing out, and signs of infection.

4. Necessity of follow-up care, usually at pacemaker clinic; confirm date of next appointment.

5. Medications, including drug name, purpose, dosage, schedule, precautions, and potential side effects.

6. Importance of using caution around strong magnetic fields, which can alter the function of the pacemaker. **Note:** Strong magnetic fields such as microwave ovens can convert some pacemakers to a fixed-rate mode. Once the patient moves away from the magnetic field, the pacemaker will return to normal programmed function. Generally, this is not a problem for the newer pacemakers.

7. Expected life of the pacemaker battery, which is approximate and can vary from 5–10 years, depending on the type of battery.

II. Cardiac Catheterization

Cardiac catheterization is an invasive diagnostic procedure used to assess the extent of coronary artery disease or valvular heart disease. It involves the insertion of a radiopaque catheter through a peripheral vessel into the heart. Subsequently, pressure measurements are made and the amount of cardiac output is determined to diagnose valvular stenosis and resistance to blood flow. Then dye is injected so that the heart structures, including ventricular chambers, coronary arteries, great vessels, and valves, can be visualized with fluoroscopy.

Associated procedures may include *His bundle EKG* to assess conduction system abnormalities and ectopic (irregular) beats. If indicated, *transvenous intracardiac pacing wires* also may be inserted to assess conduction defects and determine the exact location of the disorder. Another procedure performed in the cardiac catheterization laboratory is the *intracoronary injection of streptokinase*, a therapeutic measure used to dissolve a clot or thrombus that is occluding a coronary artery. This procedure restores circulation to the myocardial muscle distal to the occlusion.

Patients are sedated before cardiac catheterization and given a local anesthetic so that they can be awake to alert the MD to any chest pain and cooperate with position changes. Usually, cardiac catheterization is an elective, scheduled procedure, but it also might be performed in emergency situations.

Percutaneous transluminal coronary angioplasty (PTCA): A treatment similar to cardiac catheterization that offers an alternative to cardiac surgery for some patients with coronary artery occlusions and disease. After basic procedures (eg, coronary artery visualization) are performed, a balloon catheter is inserted until it is positioned at the point of stenosis. The balloon is then inflated in increments of pressure to compress the plaque and allow distal perfusion.

A. Nursing Diagnoses and Interventions

Knowledge deficit: Catheterization procedure and postcatheterization regimen

Desired outcome: Patient can verbalize knowledge of the catheterization procedure and postcatheterization regimen.

1. Assess patient's knowledge of the catheterization procedure. As appropriate, reinforce MD's explanation of the procedure, and answer any questions or concerns the patient and SOs have. If possible, arrange for an orientation visit to the catheterization laboratory before the procedure.

2. Before the cardiac catheterization, have the patient practice techniques (eg, Valsalva maneuver, coughing, and deep breathing) that will be used during the catheterization.

3. Explain that after the procedure, bed rest will be required, and that VS, circulation, and the insertion site will be checked at frequent intervals to ensure integrity. In addition, explain that sandbags may be used over the insertion site, and that flexing of the insertion site (arm or groin) is contraindicated to prevent bleeding.

4. Stress the importance of reporting signs and symptoms of hemorrhage, hematoma formation, or embolization promptly.

Potential alteration in tissue perfusion: Peripheral, cardiopulmonary, and cerebral related to impaired circulation secondary to the catheterization procedure

Desired outcome: Patient's VS and physical findings are within acceptable limits.

1. Monitor BP q15min until stable on three successive checks, q2h for the next 12 hours, and q4h thereafter. If the systolic pressure drops 20 mm Hg below previous readings, lower the head of the bed and notify MD. **Note:** If the insertion site was the antecubital space, measure BP on the unaffected arm.

2. Be alert to and report indicators of decreased perfusion, including cool extremities, cyanosis, decreased LOC, decreased urinary output, and SOB.

3. Monitor patient's heart rate, and notify MD if dysrhythmias occur. If the patient is not on a cardiac monitor, auscultate apical and radial pulses with every BP check, and report irregularities or apical/radial discrepancies.

Potential fluid volume deficit related to loss secondary to hemorrhage/hematoma formation after arterial puncture

Desired outcome: Patient does not exhibit signs of excessive bleeding and/or hypovolemia.

1. Be alert to indicators of shock or hemorrhage such as a decrease in BP or increase in pulse rate.
2. Inspect dressing on the groin or antecubital space for presence of frank bleeding or hematoma formation (fluctuating swelling).
3. If bleeding occurs, maintain pressure at the insertion site as prescribed. Typically, this is done with a pressure dressing or a 2½–5 pound sandbag.
4. Monitor peripheral perfusion and be alert to decreased amplitude or absence of distal pulses, delayed capillary refill, coolness of the extremities, and pallor, which can signal embolization or hemorrhagic shock.
5. To minimize the risk of bleeding, caution patient about flexing the elbow or hip for 6–8 hours, or as prescribed.

Potential alteration in tissue perfusion: Peripheral related to impaired circulation secondary to embolization

Desired outcome: Patient's VS and physical findings are within acceptable limits.

1. Assess peripheral perfusion by palpating peripheral pulses q15min for 30 minutes, then q30min for 1 hour, then qh for 2 hours, or per protocol.
2. Monitor for and report any indicators of arterial embolization in the involved limb, such as faintness or absence of pulse, coolness of extremity, mottling, decreased capillary refill, cyanosis, and complaints of numbness, tingling, and/or pain at the insertion site. Instruct patient to report any of these signs or symptoms promptly.
3. If there is *no* evidence of an embolus or thrombus formation, instruct patient to move fingers or toes and rotate wrist or ankle to promote circulation.
4. Ensure that patient maintains bed rest for 4–6 hours, or as prescribed.

Potential alteration in tissue perfusion: Renal related to impaired circulation secondary to decreased cardiac output or reaction to contrast dye

Desired outcome: Patient's VS and physical findings are within acceptable limits.

1. Because contrast dye for cardiac catheterization may cause osmotic diuresis, monitor for indicators of dehydration such as poor skin turgor, dry mucous membranes, and high urine specific gravity.
2. Monitor I&O. Notify MD if urinary output is <30 mL/h in the presence of an adequate intake.
3. If urinary output is insufficient in spite of adequate intake, restrict fluids. Be alert to and report indicators of fluid overload such as crackles (rales) on auscultation of lung fields, distended neck veins, and SOB. Notify MD of significant findings.
4. If patient does not exhibit signs of cardiac or renal failure, encourage daily intake of 2–3 L of fluids, or as prescribed, to flush the contrast dye out of the system.

See "Coronary Artery Disease" for the following: **Alteration in comfort** (angina), p. 42, **Knowledge deficit** (negative side effects of nitrates), p. 43, and **Knowledge deficit** (negative side effects of beta blockers), p. 43.

B. Patient–Family Teaching and Discharge Planning

Provide patient and SOs with verbal and written information for the following:

1. Use of nitroglycerine, including purpose, dosage, schedule, precautions, and potential side effects such as headache and dizziness. Caution patient to avoid using nitroglycerine more frequently than prescribed and to notify MD if three tablets do not relieve pain.

2. Use of calcium antagonists, beta blockers, antiarrhythmic agents, and antihypertensive agents, including the drug name, purpose, dosage, schedule, precautions, and potential side effects. Advise patient about the importance of taking the medications regularly and not discontinuing them without MD approval.

3. Signs and symptoms necessitating immediate medical attention, including chest pain unrelieved by nitroglycerine, decreased exercise tolerance, increasing SOB, and loss of consciousness.

4. Activity and dietary limitations as prescribed.

5. Importance of follow-up with MD; confirm date and time of next appointment.

III. Cardiac Surgery

Cardiac surgery is performed to correct a variety of heart disorders. For example, coronary artery bypass grafting (CABG) is a technique used to treat blocked coronary arteries; a portion of the saphenous vein or internal mammary artery is used to shunt blood around the blocked portions of arteries to maintain flow to the heart muscle. Valve replacement, another type of cardiac surgery, is performed for patients with valvular stenosis or valvular incompetence of the mitral, tricuspid, pulmonary, or aortic valve. Cardiac surgery is also performed to correct heart defects that are either acquired or congenital, such as ventricular aneurysm, ventricular or atrial septal defects, transposition of great vessels, and tetralogy of Fallot.

Unless an emergency occurs, patients are usually admitted to the hospital the day before surgery. Most institutions that perform cardiac surgery have special units called transitional care, special care, or step-down units where preoperative cardiac patients are admitted. After surgery, most patients are in an ICU for 24–72 hours and then transferred to a medical–surgical unit. However, this is highly variable and depends on the patient's postoperative course and need for close cardiac monitoring.

A. Nursing Diagnoses and Interventions

Knowledge deficit: Diagnosis, surgical procedure, preoperative routine, and postoperative course

Desired outcome: Patient can verbalize knowledge of the diagnosis, surgical procedure, and the preoperative and postoperative regimen.

1. Assess patient's level of knowledge pertaining to the diagnosis and surgical procedure, and provide information where necessary. Encourage questions, and allow time for verbalization of concerns and fears.

2. If appropriate for the patient, provide orientation to the ICU and equipment that will be used postoperatively.

3. Provide instructions for deep breathing and coughing in the preoperative teaching.

4. Reassure patient that postoperative discomfort will be relieved with medication.

5. Advise patient that in the immediate postoperative period, speaking will be impossible because of the presence of an endotracheal tube, which will assist with breathing. Also explain that a chest tube(s) will be present. Teach patient how he or she will move, deep breathe, and cough with a chest tube in place. (Refer to Chapter 1, p. 11 for care considerations for patients with chest tubes.)

Activity intolerance related to weakness secondary to cardiac surgery

Desired outcome: Patient progresses to his or her highest level of mobility with decreasing evidence of cardiac intolerance.

1. Monitor VS at frequent intervals, and be alert to indicators of cardiac failure, including hypotension, tachycardia, crackles (rales), tachypnea, and decreased peripheral pulses. Notify MD of significant findings.

2. To help minimize myocardial oxygen consumption, ensure that the patient has frequent rest periods.

3. Assess perfusion to the brain by checking patient's orientation to time and place.

4. As prescribed, administer medications that decrease myocardial oxygen consumption, such as beta blockers or calcium antagonists.

5. Assist patient with ROM and other exercises, depending on tolerance and prescribed activity limitations. Consult with MD regarding patient's readiness to participate in exercises that require increased cardiac tolerance. For a discussion of in-bed exercises that may be used, see **Potential impairment of physical mobility** related to inactivity, p. 535, in "Appendix One."

See "Pulmonary Embolism" in Chapter 1 for the following: **Potential for injury** (bleeding with anticoagulant therapy), p. 9. See "Coronary Artery Disease" for the following: **Alteration in nutrition** (more than body requirements of sodium, calories, and fat), p. 42. See "Atherosclerotic Arterial Occlusive Disease" for the following: **Potential alteration in tissue perfusion:** Renal, p. 80. See "Appendix One" for the following: **Alteration in tissue perfusion** (peripheral), p. 533, and for nursing diagnoses and interventions for the care of preoperative and postoperative patients, pp. 528–532.

B. Patient–Family Teaching and Discharge Planning

Provide patient and SOs with verbal and written information for the following:

1. Medications, including drug name, dosage, schedule, purpose, precautions, and potential side effects.

2. Untoward symptoms requiring medical attention for patients taking warfarin, such as bleeding from the nose, hemoptysis, hematuria, melena, and excessive bruising. In addition, stress the following: Take warfarin at the same time every day; notify MD if *any* signs of bleeding occur; keep appointments for PT checks; avoid OTC medications unless approved by MD; wear a Medic-Alert bracelet or card; avoid constrictive or restrictive clothing; and use soft-bristled toothbrushes and electric razors.

3. Maintenance of low-sodium, low-fat, low-cholesterol diet.

4. Importance of pacing activities at home and allowing frequent rest periods.

5. Technique for assessing radial pulse, temperature, and weight, if these indicators require monitoring at home, and reporting significant changes to MD.

6. Introduction to local American Heart Association activities.

7. Telephone number of nurse available to discuss concerns and questions or clarify instructions that are unclear.

8. Importance of follow-up visits with MD; confirm date and time of next appointment.

9. Signs and symptoms that necessitate immediate medical attention: chest pain, dyspnea, SOB, weight gain, and decrease in exercise tolerance.

10. Activity restrictions, eg, lifting (> 5 lb), pushing, and pulling for at least 6 weeks; prescribed exercise program; and resumption of sexual activity, work, and driving a car, as directed.

11. Care of the incision site; importance of assessing for signs of infection such as drainage, fever, persistent redness, and local warmth and tenderness.

▶ Section Six   **Disorders of the Peripheral Vascular System**

I. Atherosclerotic Arterial Occlusive Disease

Arteriosclerosis is a normal aging process of changes occurring in the arteries, including thickening of the walls, loss of elasticity, increase in calcium deposits, and usually, an increase in external diameter and a decrease in internal diameter. In contrast, *atherosclerosis* refers to a pathologic process of focal changes in the arteries, usually involving the accumulation of lipids, carbohydrates, calcium, blood components, and fibrous tissue. Although the two processes differ, they usually occur simultaneously.

The process of atherosclerotic disease results in narrowing of the arterial lumen, which limits blood flow. Thrombosis or aneurysm can occur, depending on the reaction of the tissue that is supplied by the atherosclerotic vessels. Arterial occlusion and insufficiency are usually found in the lower extremities in patients over age 50. *Thromboangiitis obliterans* (Buerger's disease) is an arterial occlusive disease that differs from atherosclerosis in that there is recurrent arterial inflammation. The cause is unknown, but the risk factors appear to be the same as those for atherosclerosis. It usually occurs in individuals 20–35 years of age and begins in the small arteries. *Raynaud's disease* is another type of impairment that tends to affect younger individuals and women. It is characterized by vasospasm of small arteries and arterioles in the extremities, particularly associated with an oversensitivity to the sympathetic nervous system effects of cold. The cause of Raynaud's disease is unknown.

A. Assessment

Signs and symptoms: Severe, cramping pain (called intermittent claudication) that follows exercise and is usually relieved by rest. It is indicative of ischemia secondary to decreased blood flow. The patient also can have delayed healing, collapsed veins, and decreased sensory or motor function.

Physical exam: Decreased pulse amplitude, decreased or absent peripheral pulses, decreased hair distribution, and bluish discoloration of the extremities and areas of decreased circulation. The skin may appear shiny and the nails thickened. Capillary filling will be >3 seconds (with normal circulation, capillary filling occurs in <3 seconds).

Risk factors: Hypertension, cigarette smoking, diabetes mellitus, family history of atherosclerotic disease, and hyperlipoproteinemia. Use of beta blocker drugs can exacerbate patient's symptoms because of their peripheral vasoconstricting effect.

B. Diagnostic Tests

1. <u>Angiography of peripheral vasculature:</u> Will locate obstruction and reveal extent of vascular lesions. This invasive study is usually done only if surgery is planned.
2. <u>Doppler flow studies:</u> Uses an electronic stethoscope to determine the amount of blood flow in arteries in which palpable pulses are difficult to obtain.
3. <u>Digital subtraction angiography:</u> Uses computerized tomography to visualize arteries radiologically and determine presence and extent of occlusion.
4. <u>Exercise testing:</u> To determine the amount of exercise that precipitates ischemia and claudication.
5. <u>Oscillometry:</u> Uses a BP cuff connected to a manometer to locate occlusive sites, as evidenced by decreased pressure readings.

C. Medical Management and Surgical Interventions

1. **Regular lower extremity exercise program:** To increase circulation. This can include a walking program or Buerger-Allen exercises. Activity may be con-

traindicated for some patients with severe disease, who may instead require bed rest to decrease oxygen demands.

2. **Restriction of cigarette smoking:** To prevent increased vasoconstriction and severity of the circulation deficit.

3. **Control of hyperlipidemia and cholesterol levels:** To help prevent progression of atherosclerosis. This is accomplished through low-fat, low-cholesterol diets or the controversial antilipemic drugs, which may be used if diet control is ineffective. Examples of these drugs include clofibrate and cholestyramine.

4. **Control of hypertension:** Administration of agents such as thiazide diuretics.

5. **Provide warmth, eg, with warm towels or heating pads:** To promote arterial flow. **Caution:** Care must be taken not to apply extreme heat because the patient's sensitivity to temperature is often decreased and burns can result.

6. **Pharmacotherapy**
   □ *Mild analgesics:* For relief of pain.
   □ *Antiplatelet agents such as aspirin and dipyridamole:* May be used to help prevent platelet adherence and thromboembolism. The use of anticoagulants such as warfarin to prevent thrombus formation is controversial.

   □ *Pentoxyphylline:* To increase flexibility of erythrocytes, which enhances their movement through the microcirculation, and to prevent aggregation of RBCs and platelets.

7. **Surgical management:** For patients who are severely limited by the occlusion and for whom the occlusion is fairly localized.

   □ *Endarterectomy:* Removal of the atheromatous obstruction via an arterial incision.

   □ *Bypass vascular grafting:* Removal or bypass of the obstructed segment by suturing a graft proximally and distally to the obstruction.

   □ *Sympathectomy:* Relief of arterial vasoconstriction to help improve circulation. Nerves that stimulate vasoconstriction (sympathetic) are incised and ligated to decease constriction and relax the vessels.

   □ *Percutaneous transluminal angioplasty:* May be used to treat focal arterial obstruction. A balloon-tipped catheter is inserted through the vein or artery to the area of the occlusion. The balloon is gradually inflated to ablate the obstruction.

   □ *Amputation:* See discussion, p. 405, in Chapter 8.

D. Nursing Diagnoses and Interventions

Knowledge deficit: Interventions that increase peripheral circulation

Desired outcome: Patient can verbalize understanding of measures that increase circulation.

1. Teach patient to elevate HOB to increase circulation to the lower extremities. Explain that this can be accomplished at home by raising the HOB on 6-inch blocks.

2. Explain to patient that walking and ROM exercises to the hip, knee, and ankle promote collateral circulation.

3. Discuss an exercise program with MD, and describe the routine to the patient. Often, this includes walking to the patient's tolerance (without pain).

4. If prescribed, teach the patient Buerger-Allen exercises:
   □ Teach patient to lie flat in bed with the legs elevated above the level of the heart for 2–3 minutes.
   □ Have the patient sit on the edge of the bed for 2–3 minutes with the legs relaxed and dependent.

□ In the same position, instruct patient to flex, extend, invert, and evert the feet, holding each position for 30 seconds.

□ Finally, have the patient lie flat, with the legs at heart level, and covered with a warm blanket for approximately 5 minutes.

5. Teach patient to assess peripheral pulses, warmth, color, hair distribution, and capillary filling. To check for capillary filling, teach the patient to press on a nail bed until blanching occurs and release the pressure. Explain that with normal capillary filling, color (pink) returns in 1–3 seconds.

▶ **Note:** Bed rest without exercise may be prescribed to decrease oxygen demand in acute, severe cases.

Alteration in comfort: Chronic pain related to ischemia secondary to atherosclerotic obstructions

Desired outcome: Patient relates a reduction in discomfort and does not exhibit signs of uncontrolled pain.

1. Assess for the presence of pain, and administer pain medications as prescribed.

2. Teach patient to rest and stop exercising before claudication (severe, cramping pain) occurs.

3. Because the pain may be chronic and continuous, explore alternate methods of pain relief such as visualization, guided imagery, biofeedback, meditation, and relaxation exercises or tapes.

4. Institute measures to increase circulation to ischemic extremities, such as Buerger-Allen exercises and walking.

Knowledge deficit: Potential for infection and impaired skin integrity due to decreased arterial circulation

Desired outcome: Patient can verbalize knowledge of the potential for infection and impaired skin integrity as well as measures to prevent these problems.

1. Teach patient how to assess for signs of infection or problems with skin integrity and to report significant findings to MD.

2. Caution patient about the increased potential for easily traumatizing the skin, for example, from bumping the lower extremities.

3. Stress the importance of wearing shoes or slippers that fit properly.

4. Instruct patient to cut toenails straight across to prevent ingrown toenails.

5. Advise patient to cover corns or calluses with pads to prevent further injury.

6. Encourage patient to keep the feet clean and dry, using mild soap and warm water for cleansing, and applying a mild lotion to prevent dryness.

7. Advise patient not to scratch or rub the skin on the feet as this can result in abrasions that easily can become infected.

8. Suggest that patient keep the feet warm with loose-fitting socks and warm soaks. Caution the patient to check the temperature of warm soaks and bath water carefully to protect the skin from burns.

Potential alteration in tissue perfusion: Peripheral related to impaired circulation secondary to graft occlusion

Desired outcome: Patient's VS and physical findings are within acceptable limits.

1. Assess peripheral pulses on patient's return from surgery and q2h thereafter. Also monitor BP, another indicator of perfusion pressure; report to MD a significant increase or decrease (>15–20 mm Hg, or as directed).

2. If necessary, use the Doppler ultrasonic probe to check pulses, holding the probe to the skin at a 45° angle to the blood vessel. In the presence of blood flow, wavelike "whooshing" sounds will be heard. Record the rate and character of the sounds as well as the frequency and intensity.

3. To prevent pressure on the tissue, keep sheets and blankets off the legs and feet with an overbed cradle.

4. For the first 48–72 hours after surgery (or as directed), prevent acute hip flexion, which can occlude blood flow for patient with a femoral graft.

Potential alteration in tissue perfusion: Renal related to impaired circulation secondary to decreased blood supply during surgery

Desired outcome: Patient's VS and physical findings are within acceptable limits.

▶ **Note:** During many vascular surgical procedures, the aorta is clamped temporarily to facilitate endarterectomy and grafting. Although all body systems are affected to a degree, the renal system is especially sensitive to the lack of blood flow.

1. Monitor I&O. Report output <30 mL/h.

2. Monitor results of renal function tests. Be alert to increases in serum creatinine and BUN, which occur with decreasing renal function.

3. Monitor for signs of fluid retention, eg, distended neck veins, crackles (rales), and peripheral edema.

4. In the absence of acute cardiac or renal failure, encourage adequate fluid intake (2–3 L/day) to help maintain adequate renal blood flow and promote fluid balance.

See "Appendix One" for nursing diagnoses and interventions for the care of preoperative and postoperative patients, pp. 528–532.

E. Patient–Family Teaching and Discharge Planning

Provide patient and SOs with·verbal and written information for the following:

1. "Stop Smoking" programs, if appropriate.

2. Importance of avoiding factors and activities that cause vasoconstriction, eg, tight clothing and crossing the legs at the knee.

3. Exercise program as prescribed by MD; importance of rest periods if claudication occurs.

4. Skin care.

5. Measures that optimize arterial blood flow.

6. Medications, including drug name, rationale, dosage, schedule, precautions, and potential side effects.

II. Aneurysms: Abdominal, Thoracic, and Femoral

An aneurysm is a localized outpouching sac that is formed at a weak point in an arterial wall. The most common cause of aneurysm is atherosclerosis, although vessel wall trauma, congenital defect, and infection are other causes. Loss of vessel wall elasticity and atherosclerotic deposits cause the vessel to weaken, resulting in gradual dilation. Unless this condition is recognized and surgically treated, rupture and exsanguination can occur. Although aneurysms can develop in any vessel, peripheral vessel aneurysms are most commonly found in the abdominal aorta, thoracic aorta, and femoral arteries. *Dissecting aneurysms* occur in aortic vessels that have atherosclerotic lesions and develop intimal tears, allowing bleeding into the layers of the vessel, which causes weakening and hematoma formation.

Until the aneurysm reaches sufficient size to press on adjacent organs, the individual may be asymptomatic. Complications include rupture and bleeding, exsanguination, and embolization. Most individuals with aneurysms are hypertensive.

A. Assessment

Chronic indicators

☐ *Abdominal aneurysm:* Patient describes sensation of "heart beat" in the abdomen. Chronic abdominal pain in the middle or lower abdomen also may be present.

☐ *Thoracic aneurysm:* Patient may be asymptomatic for years. Pressure from the aneurysm on adjacent structures can result in dull pain in the upper back, dyspnea, cough, dysphagia, and hoarseness.

☐ *Femoral aneurysm:* Signs of decreased distal arterial blood flow. See the indicators discussed with "Atherosclerotic Arterial Occlusive Disease," p. 77.

Acute rupture indicators: Sudden onset of severe pain, often described as tearing or ripping; pallor; diaphoresis; back pain; and sudden loss of consciousness.

Physical exam: Decreased BP and pulses, tachycardia, cyanosis, and cool and clammy skin. Patient may have pulsating abdominal mass or systolic bruit over the abdomen (abdominal aneurysm) or a diastolic murmur (thoracic aneurysm).

B. Diagnostic Tests

1. <u>Chest x-ray:</u> May reveal the outline of an aneurysm, especially if there is calcification.

2. <u>Aortography:</u> Uses contrast dye to locate the lesion and identify its size as well as the condition of the proximal and distal vessels.

3. <u>Sonogram:</u> May assist in diagnosis when x-ray and physical exam are inconclusive. The sound waves may help determine the size, shape, and location of the aneurysm.

4. <u>Digital subtraction angiography:</u> To confirm diagnosis via computerized tomography, which visualizes the arteries radiographically.

5. <u>EKG:</u> May help differentiate the pain of thoracic aneurysm from that of myocardial infarction.

C. Medical Management and Surgical Interventions

1. **Decrease BP:** Using antihypertensive agents such as atenolol or hydralazine.

2. **Decrease aortic pulsatile flow:** Using medications that decrease myocardial contractility, such as propranolol.

3. **Analgesics:** For pain relief.

4. **Surgical interventions:** Indicated if the aneurysm is larger than 4 cm in diameter, peripheral embolization has occurred, there is rupture (a surgical emergency), or a stable aneurysm suddenly becomes tender or causes severe pain. The procedure involves resection of the aneurysm and restoration of vascular flow with a vascular graft or a graft prosthesis made of Teflon or dacron.

D. Nursing Diagnoses and Interventions

Knowledge deficit: Potential for aneurysmal rupture (if surgery is not immediately planned)

Desired outcomes: Patient and SOs can verbalize knowledge of the potential for aneurysm rupture, the symptoms of rupture, and the importance of seeking immediate medical attention should symptoms occur.

1. Assess patient's knowledge of the potential for rupture, and intervene accordingly. Teach patient and SOs the symptoms of rupture.

2. Emphasize the importance of seeking immediate medical attention should

any signs and symptoms of rupture occur. Provide numbers of emergency services in the area.

3. Encourage questions, and answer them clearly.

Knowledge deficit: Surgical procedure and postoperative regimen

Desired outcome: Patient can verbalize knowledge of the surgical procedure and postoperative regimen and does not exhibit signs of harmful anxiety.

1. Assess patient's knowledge of the surgical procedure and postoperative period and intervene accordingly.
2. Explain the postoperative regimen. If appropriate, this should include a tour of the ICU or a description of the unit. Also alert the patient to the potential for postoperative intubation, presence of chest tube, and cardiac monitoring. Teach deep-breathing and coughing exercises.
3. Provide time for patient and SOs to verbalize fears and anxieties and ask questions.

Potential fluid volume deficit related to loss secondary to postsurgical bleeding/hemorrhage

Desired outcome: Patient does not exhibit signs of excessive bleeding and/or hypovolemia.

1. After the patient has been transferred from the ICU, monitor BP and peripheral pulses q30min during the first hour; then q2h or as necessary.
2. Check the operative site for the presence of frank bleeding.
3. Assess apical and peripheral pulses, and report the presence of tachycardia or a decreased amplitude of peripheral pulses, which can occur with bleeding.
4. Monitor abdomen for increasing girth.
5. Be alert to patient complaints of low back pain, which in addition to signs of hypovolemic shock, may signal retroperitoneal hemorrhage.
6. Monitor LOC as a measure of cerebral perfusion; report changes.
7. Instruct patient to alert staff promptly to untoward signs and symptoms.
8. Notify MD immediately of significant findings.

Potential alteration in tissue perfusion: Peripheral related to impaired circulation secondary to postoperative embolization

Desired outcome: Patient's VS and physical findings are within acceptable limits.

1. Assess peripheral pulses at least qh, and report decreases in amplitude or absence of a pulse.
2. Report any changes in color, capillary refill, or temperature of the extremities.
3. Maintain patient on bed rest until otherwise directed.
4. Keep patient flat to maintain graft patency and ensure healing with decreased risk of embolization.
5. Instruct patient to report untoward signs and symptoms promptly to staff.

See "Appendix One" for nursing diagnoses and interventions for the care of preoperative and postoperative patients, pp. 528–532.

E. Patient–Family Teaching and Discharge Planning

Provide patient and SOs with verbal and written information for the following:

1. Importance of regular medical follow-up to ensure graft patency and prompt identification of the development of a new aneurysm.

2. Prevention of recurrence of aneurysm by avoiding factors that accelerate atherosclerosis, such as cigarette smoking, obesity, and hypertension.

3. Necessity of a regularly scheduled exercise program that alternates exercise with rest.

4. Indicators of wound infection and thrombus or embolus formation, and the need to report them promptly to MD should they occur.

5. Medications, including drug name, purpose, dosage, schedule, precautions, and potential side effects.

6. Telephone number of nurse available to discuss concerns and questions or clarify instructions that are unclear.

7. Importance of follow-up visits with MD; confirm date and time of next appointment.

III. Arterial Embolism

An embolus is a fragment of a thrombus, globule of fat, clump of tissue, fragment of an atherosclerotic lesion, bacteria, or a bubble of air that moves in the circulation, lodges in a vessel, and ultimately obstructs flow.

Emboli can be venous (see "Venous Thrombosis/Thrombophlebitis," pp. 84–87) or arterial. An arterial embolism most commonly arises from thrombi that develop in the chambers of the heart secondary to valvular heart disease, atrial fibrillation (a dysrhythmia with ineffective atrial contraction), myocardial infarction, congestive or chronic cardiac failure, or vascular injury or disease. Emboli also can arise from atherosclerotic plaque lesions in any vessel. The clinical course following embolism depends on the size of the embolus, the vessel(s) affected, degree of obstruction, and distal tissue involved.

A. Assessment

Signs and symptoms: Sudden onset of severe pain and a gradual decrease in sensory and motor functioning; presence of tingling, numbness, blanching, coolness, and cyanosis. If the coronary arteries are involved, the patient may present with signs of decreased cardiac function, angina pectoris, or myocardial infarction.

Physical exam: Possible presence of a darkened extremity; diminished or absent pulse(s). Necrosis or gangrene can occur if there is total occlusion and absence of collateral flow.

History of: Vascular injury, infection, valvular heart disease, cardiac dysrhythmias.

B. Diagnostic Tests

1. Ultrasonic Doppler flow studies: Will reveal decreased or absent arterial blood flow distal to the embolus.

2. Angiography: Provides visualization of the embolus in the arterial tree and collateral circulation.

C. Medical Management and Surgical Interventions

1. **Bed rest:** To prevent further embolization.

2. **Anticoagulation with heparin via continuous IV drip:** To prevent further embolization.

3. **Thrombolytic drugs such as streptokinase:** To speed up the process of clot lysis.

4. **Analgesics:** To relieve pain caused by distal vasospasm and ischemia.

5. **Embolectomy:** Surgical removal of the embolus.

D. Nursing Diagnoses and Interventions

Potential alteration in tissue perfusion: Peripheral related to impaired circulation secondary to embolization (preoperative period)

Desired outcome: Patient's physical findings are within acceptable limits.

1. Maintain patient on bed rest to prevent further embolization.

2. Monitor peripheral circulation. Keep extremities warm (room temperature). Advise patient to avoid chilling by wearing socks and/or slippers.

3. Protect extremities from trauma. Provide an overbed cradle to keep sheets and blankets off tissue that has decreased circulation.

4. If prescribed, keep the lower extremities slightly dependent (but not >45°) to promote circulation.

5. Teach patient signs and symptoms of embolization, which necessitate immediate medical attention.

See "Pulmonary Embolism" in Chapter 1 for the following: **Potential for injury** (bleeding secondary to anticoagulant therapy), p. 9. See "Appendix One" for nursing diagnoses and interventions for the care of preoperative and postoperative patients, pp. 528–532.

E. Patient–Family Teaching and Discharge Planning

Provide patient and SOs with verbal and written information for the following:

1. Prescribed exercise plan to prevent stasis of blood.

2. Signs and symptoms that necessitate immediate medical attention: extremity pain, coolness, pallor, and cyanosis.

3. Indicators of wound infection, if surgery was performed.

4. Oral anticoagulant therapy: need for regular medical checkups and immediate reporting of epistaxis, ecchymosis, hemoptysis, melena, or hematuria; administration at the same time every day; not changing regular dietary habits (eg, becoming a vegetarian) without first consulting MD or nurse; importance of consulting with MD before taking any OTC medications, especially aspirin products, which affect platelet aggregation and potentiate the anticoagulant effect of warfarin.

5. Other medications, including drug name, purpose, dosage, schedule, precautions, and potential side effects.

IV. Venous Thrombosis/Thrombophlebitis

Although venous thrombosis and thrombophlebitis are different disorders, clinically they are referred to as a single entity, and the terms are used interchangeably to refer to the development of a venous thrombus or thrombi, with associated inflammation. Disturbances in the venous system can have a variety of causes and precipitating factors, including stasis of blood, hemoconcentration, venous trauma, inflammation, or altered coagulation. Venous stasis can occur with heart failure, shock states, immobility from prolonged bed rest, or as a side effect of anesthesia. Vessel trauma can result from chemical irritation caused by IV solutions or direct trauma. Altered coagulation states are usually related to liver disease or withdrawal from anticoagulants. Venous thrombosis and thrombophlebitis most often occur in the lower extremities, and the most serious complication is embolization.

A. Assessment

Signs and symptoms: Pain, edema, tenderness, erythema, local warmth, and prominence of superficial veins. Sometimes the first sign is a pulmonary embolus (see "Pulmonary Embolism," p. 8).

Physical exam: A knot or bump occasionally can be felt on palpation. **Caution:** Because of the risk of embolization, never test for a positive Homan's sign in the presence of clinical indicators of venous thrombosis or thrombophlebitis.

Risk factors: Prolonged bed rest and immobility, leg trauma, recent surgery, use of oral contraceptives, obesity.

B. Diagnostic Tests

1. <u>Contrast phlebography (venography):</u> Although an expensive, time-consuming test, it is very precise in its visualization of the venous system and therefore is diagnostic of the disorder. A contrast dye is injected into the venous system that is to be studied, allowing visualization of the veins by showing filling or absence of filling.

2. <u>Doppler ultrasound:</u> Identifies changes in blood flow secondary to presence of a thrombus.

3. <u>I-fibrinogen injection test:</u> Useful screening device for early detection of thrombosis because the isotope identifies clots that are forming.

C. Medical Management and Surgical Interventions

1. **Prevention:** Involves identifying patients at risk, increasing fluid intake to at least 2–3 L/day, promoting leg exercises to prevent stasis, and prescribing elastic stockings and early ambulation.

2. **Therapeutic anticoagulation:** Prevents development of a pulmonary embolus. Heparin is used during the acute phase, and long-term warfarin therapy is used after the acute phase.

3. **Thrombolytic therapy:** Instituted in some medical centers to lyse and digest the clot. Streptokinase or urokinase may be used.

4. **Bed rest:** During the acute phase.

5. **Analgesics for pain:** Usually acetaminophen.

6. **Anti-inflammatory agents** such as corticosteroids: To reduce inflammation.

7. **Exercise regimen:** Walking or leg exercises after the acute phase.

8. **Warm moist packs:** To reduce discomfort and pain.

9. **Thrombectomy:** Necessary when the danger of pulmonary embolism is extreme, the patient cannot tolerate anticoagulation, or extremity damage from the absence of venous drainage is imminent.

D. Nursing Diagnoses and Interventions

Potential alteration in tissue perfusion: Peripheral and pulmonary related to impaired circulation secondary to embolization

Desired outcome: Patient's VS and physical findings are within acceptable limits.

1. Be alert to and promptly report early indicators of thrombus formation: pain, edema, erythema, and local warmth.

2. Monitor for and immediately report signs of pulmonary embolus: sudden onset of chest pain, dyspnea, tachypnea, increased heart rate, hemoptysis, and diaphoresis. Should they occur, prompt medical attention is crucial.

3. Administer anticoagulants as prescribed. Double-check drip rates and dosages with a colleague.

Alteration in comfort: Pain related to inflammatory process secondary to thrombus formation

Desired outcome: Patient relates a reduction in discomfort and does not exhibit signs of uncontrolled pain.

1. Monitor patient for the presence of pain, and administer analgesics as prescribed.

2. Ensure that the patient maintains bed rest during the acute phase to minimize painful engorgement and the potential for embolization.

3. If prescribed, apply warm, moist packs. Be sure that the packs are warm (but not extremely so) and not allowed to cool. If appropriate, use a Kock-Mason dressing (warm towel covered by plastic wrap and a K-pad) to provide continuous moist heat.

4. To enhance venous drainage and reduce engorgement, keep the legs elevated above heart level (but not >45°).

Alteration in tissue perfusion: Peripheral related to impaired circulation secondary to venous engorgement

Desired outcome: Patient's physical findings are within acceptable limits.

1. Elevate patient's legs above heart level (not >45°) to promote venous drainage.

2. As prescribed for patients without evidence of thrombus formation, apply antiembolic hose, which compress superficial veins to increase blood flow to the deeper veins. Remove the stockings for approximately 15 minutes q8h. Inspect the skin for evidence of irritation.

3. Encourage patient to perform ankle circling and active or assisted ROM exercises on the lower extremities to prevent venous stasis. Perform passive ROM if patient is unable to do this. **Caution:** If there are any signs of acute thrombus formation such as calf hardness or tenderness, the exercises are contraindicated because of the risk of embolization. Notify MD.

4. Encourage deep breathing, which creates increased negative pressure in the lungs and thorax to assist in the emptying of large veins.

5. Arterial circulation usually will not be impaired unless there is arterial disease or severe edema compressing arterial flow. Assess pulses regularly, however, to confirm the presence of good arterial flow.

Potential impairment of skin integrity related to vulnerability secondary to venous stasis and rupture of small veins

Desired outcome: Patient can verbalize knowledge of measures that prevent further tissue breakdown and participates in a program that promotes healing.

1. Protect the extremities from trauma. If indicated, use a bed cradle to keep bedding off compromised tissues.

2. Keep the skin clean and dry.

3. If patient is wearing antiembolic hose, ensure that they do not cause pressure areas.

4. At frequent intervals, assess the extremities for redness or breakdown. Teach patient signs and symptoms that necessitate prompt attention.

5. Report significant findings to MD.

See "Pulmonary Embolism" in Chapter 1 for the following: **Potential for injury** (bleeding with anticoagulant therapy), p. 9.

E. Patient–Family Teaching and Discharge Planning

Provide patient and SOs with verbal and written information for the following:

1. Exercise program as prescribed by MD. Usually, walking is the best exercise.

2. Avoiding restrictive clothing, eg, tight socks, stockings, and pants.

3. Avoiding prolonged periods of standing still.

4. If possible, elevating legs above heart level when sitting.

5. Weight reduction program, if appropriate. Provide consultation with a nutritional therapist, if indicated.

6. Keeping extremities and feet clean and dry; being alert to early signs of venous stasis ulcers, such as redness and skin breakdown.

7. Importance of avoiding trauma to the extremities.

8. Wearing antiembolic hose, if prescribed. The hose must fit properly and should be snug over the feet and progressively less snug as they reach the knee or thigh. Stress the importance of avoiding wrinkles in the hose.

9. Signs and symptoms that require medical attention: persistent redness, swelling, tenderness, decreased pulses, and ulcerations on the extremity.

In addition,

10. If the patient is discharged from the hospital on warfarin therapy, provide information about the following:

   □ As directed, seeing MD for scheduled PT checks.

   □ Taking warfarin at same time each day; do not skip days unless directed to by MD.

   □ Wearing a Medic-Alert bracelet.

   □ Avoiding alcohol consumption and changes in diet (eg, changing to a vegetarian diet), both of which can alter the body's response to warfarin.

   □ Informing other physicians and dentists when making appointments with them that warfarin is being taken.

   □ Being alert to indicators that necessitate immediate medical attention: hematuria, melena, epistaxis, ecchymosis, hemoptysis, dizziness, and weakness.

   □ Avoiding taking OTC medications (eg, aspirin, which potentiates the anticoagulant effect of warfarin) without consulting MD or nurse.

V. Varicose Veins

Varicose veins are enlarged, tortuous, and dilated, and they occur as a result of incompetent valves or increased venous pressure. As the vessels dilate, they lose their elasticity and become less functional. This can result in venous stasis and subsequent thrombosis formation. Varicose veins are most often found in the lower extremities.

A. Assessment

Signs and symptoms: If only the superficial veins are involved, the patient can be asymptomatic except for the appearance of dilated veins. Increases in venous pressure can cause swelling, pain, leg fatigue, and muscle aches and cramps. As the condition progresses, discomfort increases and ulcerations can develop.

Physical exam: Increased firmness of calf muscles, redness, and swelling; tenderness elicited at the affected site.

Risk factors: Pregnancy, prolonged periods of standing, familial history of varicose veins, obesity, lack of exercise.

B. Diagnostic Tests

1. <u>Brodie-Trendelenburg test:</u> Demonstrates the presence of backward flow through incompetent venous valves. While the patient is supine, the leg is elevated to empty the venous system. A tourniquet is then applied to occlude the superficial veins and the patient is asked to stand. If the communicating valves are incompetent, blood will flow superficially and engorge the superficial veins. This test determines the appropriate treatment.

2. <u>Doppler flow studies:</u> Detect backward blood flow through incompetent valves.

3. <u>Phlebography:</u> Allows visualization of veins via injection of contrast medium to reveal dilatations, incompetent valves, and thrombi.

C. Medical Management and Surgical Interventions

1. **Prevention through health teaching**.

2. **Support hose or antiembolic hose:** To compress the superficial veins, decrease engorgement, and shunt venous flow to the deeper, stronger veins.

3. **Weight reduction program:** If obesity is a contributing factor.

4. **Walking or leg-exercise program:** To prevent venous stasis.

5. **Vein ligation and stripping:** When pain from the varicose veins is severe and/or the risk of thrombus formation increases. Usually this involves ligation of the saphenous vein at the groin, where the saphenous and femoral veins meet. Another small incision is made at the ankle, and a wire is passed into the vein, "stripping" it as it passes. For tortuous veins, multiple incisions may be required.

D. Nursing Diagnoses and Interventions

Alteration in comfort: Pain related to preoperative venous engorgement and/or surgical procedure

Desired outcome: Patient relates a reduction in discomfort and does not exhibit signs of uncontrolled pain.

1. Monitor patient for the presence of pain, and administer analgesics as prescribed.

2. To prevent increased venous pressure and promote venous drainage, encourage patient to keep the legs elevated above the level of the heart.

3. Maintain elastic wraps and antiembolic hose for support and venous drainage.

4. To promote circulation and prevent venous stasis, initiate postoperative leg exercises and ambulation as soon after surgery as possible (as directed by MD). To minimize discomfort, advise patient not to sit with the legs dependent or to stand still for prolonged periods.

See "Venous Thrombosis/Thrombophlebitis" for the following: **Alteration in tissue perfusion:** Peripheral (venous engorgement), p. 86, and **Potential impairment of skin integrity**, p. 86. See "Appendix One" for nursing diagnoses and interventions for the care of preoperative and postoperative patients, pp. 528–532.

E. Patient–Family Teaching and Discharge Planning

Provide patient and SOs with verbal and written information for the following:

1. Medications, including drug name, purpose, dosage, schedule, precautions, and potential side effects.

2. Importance of preventive measures, including the following: Wear support hose, elevate legs when possible, avoid prolonged periods of sitting and standing still, initiate a walking or exercise program, change positions at frequent intervals, and start a weight reduction program, if appropriate.

3. Necessity of frequent rest periods for at least the first 6 weeks after surgery.

4. Importance of regular medical follow-up.

5. Avoiding constricting clothing or knee-high stockings, which can obstruct venous flow.

▶ Selected References

Braunwald E (editor): *Heart Disease: A Textbook of Cardiovascular Disease*, vols 1 and 2. Saunders, 1984.

Brunner LS, Suddarth DS: *Textbook of Medical-Surgical Nursing*, 5th ed. Lippincott, 1984.

Cantwell JD: Exercise and coronary heart disease: Role in primary prevention. *Heart Lung* 1984; 13:6−13.

Carpenito LJ: *Nursing Diagnosis: Application to Clinical Practice*. Lippincott, 1983.

Gershan JA, Juricka JK: PTCA: Implications for nursing. *Focus on Critical Care* August 1984; 11:28−35.

Goldberger E: *Textbook of Clinical Cardiology*. Mosby, 1982.

Gurevich I, Mineola MA: Infectious complications after open heart surgery. *Heart Lung* 1984; 13:472−481.

Guyton AC: *Textbook of Medical Physiology*, 6th ed. Saunders, 1981.

Holloway N: *Nursing the Critically Ill Adult: Applying Nursing Diagnosis*, 2nd ed. Addison-Wesley, 1984.

Johanson BC, et al: *Standards for Critical Care*. Mosby, 1981.

Johnson GP, Johanson BC: Beta blockers. *AJN* July 1983; 83:1034−1043.

Jones DA, Dunbar CF, Jirovec MM: *Medical-Surgical Nursing: A Conceptual Approach*, 2nd ed. McGraw-Hill, 1982.

Mathewson M: Prolapsed mitral valve syndrome. *AJN* August 1980; 80:1431−1433.

Michaelson CR (editor): *Congestive Heart Failure*. Mosby, 1983.

Mitman L: Pulmonary hypertension. *Nursing 82* Feb 1982; 12:61.

Newton KM: Coronary artery disease risk factors. In: *Cardiovascular Critical Care Nursing*. Wood SL (editor). Churchill-Livingston, 1983.

Partridge S: The nurse's role in percutaneous transluminal coronary angioplasty. *Heart Lung* Nov-Dec 1982; 11:505−511.

Pinneo R: Living with coronary artery disease: The nurse's role. *Nurs Clin North Am* 1984; 19:459−468.

Saxton DF, et al: *The Addison-Wesley Manual of Nursing Practice*. Addison-Wesley, 1983.

Slusarczyk SM, Hicks FD: Helping your patient to live with a permanent pacemaker. *Nursing 83* April 1983; 13:58−63.

Urrows S: Fluid and electrolyte balance in the patient with a myocardial infarction. *Nurs Clin North Am* 1980; 15:603−615.

3

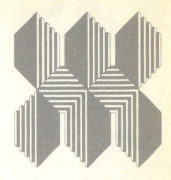

Renal–Urinary Disorders

▶ Section One   **Renal Disorders**

I. Glomerulonephritis

Glomerulonephritis (GN) is the name of a group of diseases that damage the renal glomeruli. When the glomerulus is injured, protein and RBCs are allowed to enter the renal tubule and be excreted in the urine. GN can be acute or chronic. Most individuals with acute GN recover completely within 1–2 years, but renal damage continues to progress for those with chronic GN. Chronic GN is the most common cause of chronic renal failure. Most forms of GN are the result of immunological processes.

See "Acute Renal Failure," p. 106, and "Chronic Renal Failure," p. 111, as appropriate.

A. Assessment

Indicators can range from subtle to blatant, depending on the patient's level of renal function.

Acute indicators: Hematuria, proteinuria, oliguria, dull bilateral flank pain, headache, low-grade fever.

Chronic indicators: Fatigue, lethargy, anorexia, nausea, nocturia.

Physical exam: Presence of edema (peripheral, periorbital, sacral), crackles (rales), elevated BP.

History of: Recent URI or other infection; systemic lupus erythematosus or other autoimmune disease; bloody urine.

B. Diagnostic Tests

1. <u>Urinalysis and 24-hour urinary protein excretion:</u> Red cell casts and protein excretion >3.5 g/day are common with GN.

2. <u>BUN and serum creatinine:</u> Will increase in the presence of decreased renal function.

3. <u>Plasma complement, antinuclear antibody titer, antistreptolysin O titer, throat and blood cultures, hepatitis B antigen, and immunoelectrophoresis of the serum and urine:</u> Optional tests to determine cause of GN.

4. <u>Renal biopsy:</u> Indicated when tissue diagnosis is needed to direct therapy or provide prognostic data. Usually a percutaneous (closed) renal biopsy is performed. Postbiopsy care includes keeping the patient supine with a rolled towel under the biopsy site for 12 hours and frequent monitoring of VS (q15min initially). **Note:** Two possible complications are bleeding and infection. Severe pain, hypotension, persistant gross hematuria, or fever should be reported to MD immediately.

C. Medical Management

1. **Bed rest:** For patients with acute GN.

2. **Decrease level of antigen availability:** When possible (eg, treat infections with antibiotics).

3. **Pharmacotherapy**

   □ *Corticosteroids and cytotoxic agents:* To suppress the immune system and reduce antibody formation.

   □ *Anticoagulants:* To reduce non-immunological mediators of glomerular damage.

Table 3-1 Diuretics

Generic Name	Common Brand Names	Usual Dosage/24 hours
acetazolamide	Diamox	250–375 mg (qod)
*amiloride HCl	Midamor	5–10 mg
chlorothiazide sodium	Diuril	250–1000 mg
chlorthalidone	Hygroton	25–100 mg
ethacrynic acid	Edecrin	25–200 mg
furosemide	Lasix	20–160 mg
hydrochlorothiazide	Esidrix	25–100 mg
metolazone	Zaroxolyn, Diulo	2.5–10 mg
*spironolactone	Aldactone	25–200 mg
*triamterene	Dyrenium	50–300 mg

*Although most diuretics can cause hypokalemia, these diuretics might cause hyperkalemia. For this reason they are often used in combination with thiazide diuretics.

> ☐ *Diuretics:* To remove excess fluid (see Table 3-1).
>
> ☐ *Antihypertensives:* To control BP.

4. **Plasmapheresis:** To remove immune complexes or antiglomerular basement antibodies.

5. **Diet:** Restricted sodium and fluids if edema or hypertension is present. A high-carbohydrate diet is encouraged to maintain nutrition and prevent tissue catabolism. If renal function is markedly decreased, protein and potassium may be limited to prevent hyperkalemia and retention of excess nitrogenous wastes.

6. **Peritoneal dialysis or hemodialysis:** To maintain homeostasis or prevent uremic complications if renal function is markedly decreased (see "Renal Dialysis," p. 116).

D. Nursing Diagnoses and Interventions

Activity intolerance related to lost endurance secondary to prolonged bed rest and weakness secondary to renal dysfunction

Desired outcomes: Patient maintains bed rest until BUN, BP, and protein excretion are normal or near normal. Patient demonstrates ability to assume normal activity levels after enforced bed rest.

1. During the period of enforced bed rest, assist patient with ADLs as necessary. For patients with acute GN, bed rest usually lasts 10 days–2 weeks.

2. Provide bed exercises within the prescribed activity limitations. Establish a progressive activity regimen that will allow patient to return to normal activities without complications. For more information, see "Appendix One," p. 535, **Potential impairment of physical mobility** related to inactivity secondary to prolonged bed rest.

3. Before patient resumes activities, ensure that BUN and BP are normal and urine protein excretion is near normal. Notify MD if elevations occur after patient resumes activities.

Fluid volume excess: Edema related to retention secondary to decreased renal function

Desired outcomes: Patient does not exhibit signs of overhydration. Patient states that thirst is controlled, can list foods that are high in sodium, and plans a 3-day menu that excludes foods high in sodium.

1. Monitor I&O closely. Notify MD of sudden changes in output.

2. Monitor weight daily. Report unusual or steady gains or losses.

3. Observe for indicators of fluid overload: edema, hypertension, crackles (rales), tachycardia, lethargy, distended neck veins, SOB, and increased CVP. **Note:** Not all patients with edema are fluid-overloaded. Edema also can occur because of decreased serum albumin secondary to urinary losses.

4. Offer ice chips or Popsicles to minimize thirst in the fluid-restricted patient; be sure to record the amount on the intake record. Frequent mouth care also may help minimize thirst.

5. Provide patient with data regarding foods high in sodium, which should be avoided. Examples include foods made with soy sauce and monosodium glutamate (MSG), bacon, salted nuts, potato chips, corn chips, and commercial luncheon meats. In addition, many over-the-counter (OTC) preparations are also high in sodium, eg, mouthwashes and antacids. Advise patient to read all labels carefully.

Knowledge deficit: Signs and symptoms of fluid and electrolyte imbalance (caused by decreased renal function and/or diuretic therapy)

Desired outcome: Patient can verbalize knowledge of the signs and symptoms of fluid and electrolyte imbalance and the importance of reporting them promptly to MD or staff should they occur.

1. Alert patient and SOs to the following signs and symptoms of fluid and electrolyte imbalance:

   □ *Hypokalemia:* Abdominal cramps, lethargy, dysrhythmias.

   □ *Hyperkalemia:* Muscle cramps and weakness.

   □ *Hypocalcemia:* Neuromuscular irritability such as twitching.

   □ *Hyperphosphatemia:* Excessive itching.

   □ *Uremia:* Confusion, lethary, restlessness.

2. Instruct patient to report the above signs and symptoms to MD or staff promptly should they occur.

Knowledge deficit: Negative side effects of corticosteroids and cytotoxic agents

Desired outcome: Patient can verbalize knowledge of the negative side effects of corticosteroids and cytotoxic agents and the importance of reporting them promptly to staff or MD should they occur.

1. Corticosteroids and cytotoxic agents are potent medications with potentially serious side effects. For the patient on corticosteroids, alert him or her to the potential for the following: infection, increasing BP, mental changes, hyperglycemia, and/or GI bleeding.

2. For the patient on cytotoxic agents, alert him or her to the potential for the following: infection and cystitis, bleeding, and abnormal hair loss.

3. Stress the importance of notifying MD or staff promptly should any of the above occur.

Potential for infection related to increased susceptibility secondary to corticosteroid therapy, immobility, invasive procedures, and impaired skin integrity

Desired outcome: Patient does not exhibit signs of infection.

1. Because the respiratory system is a common site for infection in the immunocompromised patient, be alert to indications of infection such as increased body temperature, adventitious breath sounds, and increased, thickened, or yellow airway secretions. If secretions are noted, encourage coughing at frequent intervals. **Note:** Uremic and elderly individuals tend to run subnormal temperatures, so even slight fevers can be significant.

2. Use meticulous, sterile technique when performing invasive procedures or manipulating urinary catheters, IV lines, or venous catheters.

3. Provide oral hygiene and skin care at frequent intervals. Edema, bed rest, and uremia all increase the potential for skin breakdown, which further increases the risk of infection.

See "Pulmonary Embolism" in Chapter 1 for the following: **Potential for injury** related to increased risk of bleeding secondary to anticoagulant therapy, p. 9. See "Appendix One" for nursing diagnoses and interventions for the care of patients on prolonged bed rest, pp. 533–537.

E. Patient–Family Teaching and Discharge Planning

Provide patient and SOs with verbal and written information for the following:

1. Medications, including drug name, purpose, dosage, schedule, precautions, and potential side effects.

2. Diet, including fact sheet listing foods that should be avoided or limited. If patient has been directed to limit potassium, see Table 3-2, p. 96. Inform patient that diet and fluid restrictions may be altered as renal function changes.

3. Indicators that require medical attention: irregular pulse, fever, unusual SOB or edema, sudden change in urine output, or unusual weakness.

4. Techniques for measuring temperature and pulse and recording I&O.

5. Necessity for continued medical evaluation; confirm date and time of next MD appointment, if known.

6. Importance of adjusting and gradually increasing activities to avoid fatigue.

7. Necessity of avoiding infections and seeking treatment promptly should they occur. Teach the signs and symptoms of URI, otitis media, UTI, and impetigo.

In addition:

8. Coordinate family and social service support for the patient who must continue bed rest at home. Consider such factors as meals, housework, child care, and transportation.

II. Nephrotic Syndrome

Nephrotic syndrome (NS) is a complex of symptoms that can occur with any disease that causes glomerular damage and consequent increased glomerular permeability to protein. The hallmarks of NS are increased urinary excretion of protein, decreased serum albumin, increased serum lipids, and edema. The two main causes of NS are glomerulonephritis and diabetic nephropathy, and its course and prognosis depend on the status of the disease that caused it. In adults, NS usually progresses to chronic renal failure.

See "Glomerulonephritis," p. 92, and "Chronic Renal Failure," p. 111, as appropriate.

A. Assessment

Signs and symptoms: Anorexia, nausea, diarrhea, lethargy, fatigue. Patient also may have ascites, pleural effusion, decreased urinary output, and weight gain.

Physical exam: Pallor; edema (periorbital, abdominal, sacral, dependent); and either hypertension or hypotension, depending on the primary renal disease and effective circulating volume.

History of: Glomerulonephritis or diabetes mellitus.

Table 3-2 Foods Relatively High in Potassium

apricots	nuts
bananas	oranges
cantaloupe	potatoes
carrots	pumpkin
cauliflower	salt substitute
chocolate	spinach
dried beans, peas	Swiss chard
dried fruits such as raisins, prunes	sweet potatoes
grapefruit	tomatoes
mushrooms	

B. Diagnostic Tests

1. <u>24-hour protein excretion:</u> To diagnose the syndrome. NS is defined as the urinary excretion of >3.5 g/day of protein. Protein loss can be >10 g/day.

2. <u>Urinalysis:</u> Will show sediment-containing casts, oval fat bodies, and RBCs.

▶ **Note:** All urine samples should be sent to the lab immediately after they are obtained, or refrigerated if this is not possible. Urine left at room temperature has greater potential for bacterial growth, turbidity, and alkalinity, any of which can distort the results.

---

3. <u>Serum tests:</u> Will show low albumin, elevated cholesterol and triglycerides, and low total calcium. BUN and creatinine may be elevated. Additional lab tests might be performed, depending on the suspected cause of NS.

4. <u>Renal biopsy:</u> Often necessary to determine the cause, direct the therapy, and indicate the prognosis of NS. See "Glomerulonephritis," p. 92, for further discussion.

C. Medical Management

1. **Bed rest.**

2. **Diet:** Low in sodium, rich in high biological value protein (1.5 g/kg body weight/day), with adequate caloric intake. Liberal protein intake is required to provide necessary amino acids for albumin synthesis.

3. **Pharmacotherapy** may include the following:

   □ *Diuretics:* Used cautiously to reduce edema (see Table 3-1, p. 93).

   □ *Antibiotics:* To treat infection.

   □ *Corticosteroids, anticoagulants, or cytotoxic agents:* To treat glomerulonephritis. See "Glomerulonephritis," p. 92.

   □ *Antihypertensive agents:* To treat hypertension.

D. Nursing Diagnoses and Interventions

Potential alterations in fluid volume: *Deficit* related to vascular dehydration secondary to pharmacotherapy; *Excess* related to retention secondary to decreased serum albumin and renal retention of sodium and water

Desired outcomes: Patient does not exhibit signs of dehydration or overhydration. Patient can verbalize knowledge of foods high in sodium and the rationale for avoiding them.

1. Monitor I&O closely; document q shift.

2. Monitor weight daily. Report unusual or steady gains or losses.

3. Observe for and document changes in hydration and VS after administration of diuretics, antihypertensives, or osmotic agents.

4. Limit sodium intake as prescribed. Instruct patient about foods that are high in sodium (see "Glomerulonephritis," **Fluid volume excess**, pp. 93–94).

5. Measure abdominal girth q shift in patients with ascites.

6. Auscultate lung fields q shift for evidence of pleural effusion (bronchial or decreased breath sounds), and be alert to signs of respiratory distress. Notify MD of significant changes.

7. Observe for indicators of decreased effective circulating volume (eg, hypotension, tachycardia, and decreased CVP), which can occur as a result of sodium restriction and the administration of diuretics or certain antihypertensives.

Alteration in nutrition: Less than body requirements related to decreased intake secondary to anorexia and increased need secondary to urinary losses of protein

Desired outcomes: Patient maintains a diet high in protein, does not exhibit signs of weight loss or malnutrition, and can verbalize knowledge of foods high in protein.

1. Provide prescribed high-protein diet in small, frequent feedings.

2. Teach patient about foods high in protein (eg, meat, poultry, fish, cheeses, nuts, lentils, and eggs).

3. Develop diet plan with dietitian, patient, and SOs, adjusting it to patient preference.

4. Encourage SOs to bring in patient's favorite high-protein foods as allowed.

5. Record calorie intake and weigh patient daily.

Potential for infection related to vulnerability secondary to treatment with immunosuppressive agents, prolonged immobility, invasive procedures, and disease process

Desired outcomes: Patient does not exhibit signs of infection. Patient can verbalize knowledge of the indicators of infection and the importance of seeking medical attention promptly should they occur.

▶ **Note:** NS causes an increased susceptibility to infection, which is believed to be caused by the loss of serum-immune globulins in the urine. The risk of infection is further increased if the patient is being treated with immunosuppressive agents.

---

1. Minimize the risk of exposing patient to individuals with infections by providing a private room, if possible.

2. For other interventions, see the same nursing diagnosis in "Glomerulonephritis," p. 94.

See "Glomerulonephritis" for the following: **Activity intolerance**, p. 93, **Knowledge deficit**: Signs and symptoms of fluid and electrolyte imbalance, p. 94, and **Knowledge deficit**: Negative side effects of corticosteroids and cytotoxic agents, p. 94. See "Pulmonary Embolism" in Chapter 1 for the following: **Potential for injury** related to increased risk of bleeding secondary to anticoagulant therapy, p. 9. See "Appendix One" for nursing diagnoses and interventions for the care of patients on prolonged bed rest, pp. 533–537.

E. Patient–Family Teaching and Discharge Planning

Provide patient and SOs with verbal and written information for the following:

1. Medications, including drug name, purpose, dosage, schedule, precautions, and potential side effects.
2. Diet: Advise patient and SOs that diet and fluid restrictions may be altered as renal function changes. Provide lists of advocated and restricted foods.
3. Signs and symptoms that require medical attention: irregular pulse, fever, unusual SOB or edema, sudden change in urinary output, or unusual weakness.
4. Need for continued medical evaluation; confirm time and date for the next MD appointment, if known.
5. Importance of avoiding infections and seeking treatment promptly should signs and symptoms appear. Teach the indicators of URI, otitis media, impetigo, and UTI.
6. Importance of skin care, especially that over edematous areas.

In addition:

7. Coordinate family and social service support for the patient who must continue bed rest at home. Consider such factors as meals, housework, child care, and transportation.

III. Acute Pyelonephritis

Acute pyelonephritis is an infection of the renal parenchyma and pelvis, which usually occurs secondary to an ascending UTI. UTIs typically result from anatomic or functional obstruction to urine flow, eg, from prostatic hypertrophy or renal calculi, or instrumentation such as catheterization or cystoscopy. Hematogenous infection also can occur in acute pyelonephritis when bacteria reach the kidney via the bloodstream.

The incidence of acute pyelonephritis increases with advancing age. In the absence of anatomical obstruction or instrumentation, acute pyelonephritis is almost exclusively a disease of females. The infecting organism is usually a type of fecal flora such as *Escherichia*, *Klebsiella*, or *Enterobacter*. Recurrent infections are common; chronic renal failure is a rare complication.

A. Assessment

Signs and symptoms: Fever, chills, flank pain, nausea, vomiting, malaise, frequency and urgency of urination, dysuria, cloudy and foul-smelling urine. **Note:** These indicators can be nonspecific, especially in the elderly.

Physical exam: Tender, enlarged kidneys; abdominal rigidity; and costovertebral tenderness.

History of: UTI and/or obstruction; recent urologic procedure.

B. Diagnostic Tests

Unless an anatomic or pre-existing renal disease is present, renal function should remain normal.

1. Urine culture: Should be positive for the causative organism. **Note:** Asymptomatic bacteriuria is common in the elderly.
2. Urinalysis: Will reveal presence of WBCs, WBC casts, RBCs, and bacteria.

▶ **Note:** All urine samples should be sent to the lab immediately after they are obtained, or refrigerated if this is not possible. Urine left at room temperature has greater potential for bacterial growth, turbidity, and alkalinity, any of which can distort the test results.

3. Blood culture: Positive for the causative organism in hematogenous infection. It is obtained in patients who appear septic or are hypotensive.
4. IVP or retrograde pyelogram: May be performed if there are recurrent episodes or if obstruction is suspected.

C. Medical Management and Surgical Interventions

1. **Bed rest.**
2. **Pharmacotherapy**
   - □ *Antibiotics:* For the infection; initially parenteral, then oral.
   - □ *ASA or acetaminophen:* To control the fever and treat the discomfort.
3. **Surgical intervention:** May be necessary if an obstruction is present.

D. Nursing Diagnoses and Interventions

Alteration in comfort: Dysuria related to infection

Desired outcome: Patient relates relief from discomfort and does not exhibit signs of uncontrolled pain.

1. Monitor patient for the presence of dysuria. As appropriate, administer the prescribed analgesics, and document their effectiveness.
2. If it is not contraindicated, increase the patient's fluid intake to help relieve dysuria.
3. Notify MD of unrelieved or increasing flank pain.
4. As appropriate, assist patient with repositioning if it is effective in relieving discomfort.
5. Use nonpharmacologic interventions when possible, eg, relaxation techniques, guided imagery, and distraction.

Potential for infection (or its recurrence) related to increased susceptibility secondary to disease process

Desired outcomes: Patient exhibits absence or reduction of fever and other indicators of infection. Patient can verbalize knowledge of the signs and symptoms of infection and the importance of reporting them promptly should they occur.

1. Monitor patient's temperature at least q4h. Report temperature spikes to MD. Monitor for the presence of flank or labial pain, foul-smelling and/or cloudy urine, and frequency and urgency of urination. Teach these indicators to the patient and stress the importance of reporting them promptly to MD or staff should they occur.
2. Monitor BP and pulse at least q4h. The presence of hypotension and tachycardia can be indicative of sepsis and bacteremic shock.
3. Administer prescribed antibiotics as scheduled. Draw prescribed antibiotic serum levels at correct times to ensure reliable results. **Note:** Most antibiotics are measured at peak (30–60 minutes after infusion) and trough (30–60 minutes before the next dose) levels.
4. Use urinary catheters only when mandatory. Use meticulous, sterile technique when inserting and irrigating. Provide perineal care at least every shift. For indwelling catheters, maintain unobstructed flow, and always keep the urinary collection container below the level of the patient's bladder to prevent reflux of urine. **Note:** Intermittent catheterization carries less of a risk of UTI than indwelling catheterization.

5. Offer cranberry, plum, or prune juices, which leave an acid ash in the urine and inhibit bacteriuria.

6. Teach female patients the importance of wiping the perineal area from front to back to minimize the risk of introducing fecal flora into the urinary tract.

7. Treat fever with prescribed antipyretics and tepid baths as needed.

Alteration in nutrition: Less than body requirements related to decreased intake secondary to nausea and/or anorexia

Desired outcome: Patient does not exhibit signs of malnutrition or weight loss.

1. Provide nauseated or anorexic patient with frequent, small meals and carbonated beverages.

2. Treat nausea and vomiting with prescribed medications.

3. Record accurate calorie intake, and weigh patient daily.

4. Alert MD to inadequate nutritional intake.

Fluid volume deficit related to decreased intake secondary to anorexia and abnormal loss secondary to vomiting and diaphoresis

Desired outcomes: Patient does not exhibit signs of dehydration. Patient verbalizes knowledge of the importance of a fluid intake of at least 2–3 L/day.

1. Maintain adequate fluid intake to avoid dehydration. An intake of at least 2–3 L/day is usually indicated; however, the appropriate amount depends on the patient's output, which includes NG, fecal, urinary, and insensible losses. Obtain parameters for the desired amount of fluid intake/restriction from MD. Teach nonrestricted patients the importance of maintaining a fluid intake of at least 2–3 L/day.

2. Monitor I&O and daily weights as indicators of hydration status.

3. Report indicators of dehydration: poor skin turgor, thirst, dry mucous membranes, tachycardia, or orthostatic hypotension.

4. Instruct patient in fluid intake goals as well as other interventions in which he or she may participate to enhance wellness.

E. Patient–Family Teaching and Discharge Planning

Provide patient and SOs with verbal and written information for the following:

1. Medications, including drug name, purpose, dosage, schedule, precautions, and potential side effects.

2. Importance of taking medications for prescribed length of time, even if feeling well.

3. Necessity of reporting the following indicators of UTI to MD: urgency, frequency, dysuria, flank pain, cloudy or foul-smelling urine, and fever.

4. Importance of perineal hygiene for female patients and the necessity of wiping from front to back.

5. Importance of emptying the bladder at least q3–4h and once during the night to help prevent UTI caused by residual urine.

6. Necessity of maintaining a fluid intake of at least 2–3 L/day and drinking fruit juices (cranberry, plum, prune) that leave an acid ash in the urine.

7. Importance of continued medical follow-up because of the high incidence of recurrence.

IV. Renal Calculi

The kidneys excrete several substances that singly or in combination are highly insoluble. Normally, these substances are excreted with minimal crystal formation; but diet, medications, metabolic abnormalities, systemic disease, or infection can increase the tendency for crystals to form and stones to develop. Altered urine pH and concentration also can be important factors in stone formation.

Stones can lodge and cause obstruction or be passed in the urine. Giant staghorn calculi occasionally develop and fill the entire renal pelvis. The most common types of stones are made of calcium, struvite, cystine, and uric acid. Renal calculi are often recurrent and a common medical problem. Complications include infection and hydronephrosis.

A. Assessment

Signs and symptoms: The primary symptom is pain, with the location and severity depending on the area in which the stone has lodged. Vague back pain occurs when the stone lodges in the calyces or pelvis. Renal colic (severe flank pain radiating to the groin) is typical when the stone has lodged at the junction of the pelvis and ureter. Other indicators are hematuria, nausea, vomiting, syncope, and fever.

Physical exam: Diaphoresis, pallor, and obvious distress.

History of: Previous stone formation, UTI, or urinary tract obstruction; diet high in calcium, purine, or oxalate.

B. Diagnostic Tests

See "Ureteral Calculi," p. 122.

C. Medical Management and Surgical Interventions

1. See "Ureteral Calculi," p. 123.
2. **Surgical interventions:** Indications for surgery include complete obstruction; persistent infection; severe, uncontrollable pain; renal pelvic calculus that is too large to pass spontaneously.

   □ *Pyelolithotomy* (incision into the renal pelvis).

   □ *Nephrolithotomy* (incision into the renal parenchyma).

   □ *Nephrectomy* (removal of the kidney if it is severely damaged).

   □ *Nephrolithotripsy* (breaking up the stone with sound waves; see "Ureteral Calculi," p. 123, for further information).

D. Nursing Diagnoses and Interventions for the Surgical Patient

Potential fluid volume deficit related to abnormal loss secondary to postoperative bleeding or postobstructive diuresis

Desired outcome: Patient does not exhibit signs of hypovolemia or excessive bleeding.

1. Monitor I&O, daily weight, and skin turgor as indicators of hydration status.
2. Observe for signs of hemorrhage. Urine is usually dark red or pink for approximately 48 hours postoperatively in the patient who has had a pyelolithotomy or nephrolithotomy. Urine should not be bright red or contain clots. **Note:** The postnephrectomy patient should have clear urine. Alert MD to inappropriate hematuria.
3. Monitor BP and pulse for signs of hidden bleeding, eg, hypotension and rapid pulse rate.
4. Check dressings and sheets under the dressing q4h for evidence of bleeding from the incision.

Potential impairment of skin integrity related to irritation secondary to wound drainage

Desired outcome: Patient does not exhibit signs of impaired skin integrity at the wound site.

1. After a pyelolithotomy, there can be drainage of urine from the incision for several days to 2 weeks. Apply an ostomy pouch with a skin barrier to collect drainage and protect the skin.

2. Closely monitor skin integrity, especially in elderly patients who are at increased risk for skin breakdown.

3. Ensure that the drainage tube remains in its proper position; notify MD immediately if it dislodges, as it can be difficult to reinsert after 30 minutes.

See "Appendix One" for nursing diagnoses and interventions for the care of preoperative and postoperative patients, pp. 528–532.

E. Patient–Family Teaching and Discharge Planning

Provide patients and SOs with verbal and written information for the following:

1. Medications, including drug name, purpose, dosage, schedule, precautions, and potential side effects.

2. When appropriate, a diet that prevents recurrence of stones. Provide lists of foods that should be limited or avoided, including those that are high in calcium (eg, dairy products), purine (eg, meats, fish, poultry), and oxalate (eg, beets, figs, nuts, spinach, black tea, chocolate). Encourage a daily fluid intake of at least 3 L/day in nonrestricted patients. A high fluid intake is especially important in preventing recurrent stones in patients with cystinuria.

3. Need for continued use of medications and medical follow-up because of the high rate of recurrence.

4. Requirements for maintaining alterations in urinary pH to prohibit stone precipitation and the necessity of urine pH testing.

5. Importance of seeking prompt medical treatment for signs and symptoms of UTI (eg, fever, flank or labial pain, cloudy and/or foul-smelling urine) or obstruction (eg, anuria, oliguria, and pain that is dull and aching or sharp and sudden).

6. Care of drains or catheters if patient is discharged with them.

7. Care of the surgical incision and indicators of wound infection, which necessitate medical attention: persistent redness, swelling, pain, local warmth, and purulent drainage.

8. Postoperative activity precautions: Avoid heavy lifting (>5 lb) for the first 6 weeks, be alert to fatigue, get maximum amounts of rest, and gradually increase activities to tolerance.

V. Hydronephrosis

Hydronephrosis is the dilatation of the renal pelvis and calyces secondary to the obstruction of urinary flow. It results from any condition or abnormality that causes urinary tract obstruction. If the obstruction is not corrected, the affected kidney eventually atrophies and fails. Obstruction in the urethra or bladder willl affect both kidneys, while obstruction in a single ureter or kidney will affect only the involved kidney.

Dramatic postobstructive diuresis can occur as a result of measures to relieve kidney obstruction. Inappropriate loss of sodium and water can in turn lead to volume depletion.

A. Assessment

Indicators are determined by the level, severity, and duration of obstruction.

Kidney/ureteral obstruction: Flank pain and abdominal tenderness, renal colic, gross hematuria, paralytic ileus.

Bladder neck/urethral obstruction: Frequency, hesitancy, dribbling, incontinence, nocturia, signs and symptoms of renal insufficiency, suprapubic pain, anuria.

Physical exam: Enlarged kidney(s) and distended bladder if bladder neck obstruction is present; crackles (rales) and possibly hypertension and edema if patient is fluid overloaded.

History of: UTI or obstruction.

B. Diagnostic Tests

1. <u>BUN and serum creatinine:</u> To determine level of renal function.

2. <u>Urinalysis:</u> To determine the presence of stone formation or infection.

3. <u>Renal ultrasound:</u> Noninvasive technique that uses high-frequency sound waves to assess renal size, contour, and structural changes. Because it does not rely on dye uptake, it can be used to evaluate poorly functioning kidneys.

4. <u>Abdominal x-ray, IVP, and/or retrograde pyelogram:</u> To identify cause of obstruction.

C. Medical Management and Surgical Interventions

Management of hydronephrosis depends on the cause and duration of the urinary tract obstruction. Major causes of obstruction in the pelvis and ureter are calculi (see "Renal Calculi," p. 100) and neoplasms. Major causes of obstruction in the bladder and urethra are neoplasm (see "Cancer of the Bladder," p. 128), neurogenic bladder (see "Neurogenic Bladder," p. 139), and prostatic hypertrophy (see "Benign Prostatic Hypertrophy," p. 447). Also see "Urinary Tract Obstruction," p. 126, for a general discussion of urinary tract obstruction. See "Acute Renal Failure," p. 106, and "Chronic Renal Failure," p. 111, as appropriate.

Management of hydronephrosis might include the insertion of a nephrostomy tube into the renal pelvis to drain urine and relieve pressure. It is inserted percutaneously under local anesthesia or in an open surgical procedure.

D. Nursing Diagnoses and Interventions

Potential for injury related to risk of complications secondary to insertion/presence of nephrostomy tube

Desired outcomes: Patient does not exhibit signs of infection or excessive bleeding. Signs of perforation or tube malfunction are promptly detected and treated, resulting in absence of injury to the patient.

1. Maintain sterile technique when providing dressing changes and nephrostomy tube care.

2. Observe for and report indicators of infection such as fever, pain, purulent drainage, and tachycardia. Document changes in color, odor, or clarity of urine. Infection is common with hydronephrosis.

3. Do not change, clamp, or irrigate the nephrostomy tube unless specifically prescribed by MD. **Caution:** Because of the tiny renal pelvis, never insert more than 5 mL at one time into the tube unless a larger amount has been specifically prescribed by the MD.

4. Keep the urine collection container and tubing in a dependent position. Avoid kinks in the tubing.

5. Report gross hematuria (urine that is bright red, possibly with clots). Transient hematuria can be expected for 24–48 hours after tube insertion.

6. Notify MD of leakage around the catheter, which can occur with blockage, as well as a sudden decrease in urine output, which can signal a dislodged catheter.

7. Report a sudden onset of or increase in pain, which can indicate perforation of a body organ by the catheter.

8. Keep the tube securely taped to the patient's flank with elastic tape. If the tube becomes accidently dislodged, cover the site with a sterile dressing; notify MD immediately.

▶ **Note:** Before removing the nephrostomy tube, the MD may request that it be clamped for several hours at a time to evaluate patient tolerance. While the tube is clamped, monitor the patient for the following indications of ureteral obstruction: flank pain, diminished urinary output, and fever.

Fluid volume deficit related to abnormal loss secondary to postobstructive diuresis

Desired outcome: Patient does not exhibit signs of dehydration.

1. Monitor I&O. Initially, output should exceed intake.

2. Monitor weight daily. Alert MD to steady weight loss.

3. Observe for and report indicators of volume depletion, including postural hypotension, tachycardia, poor skin turgor, elevated hematocrit, and decreased CVP.

4. As prescribed, encourage fluids in nonrestricted patients who are dehydrated.

See "Glomerulonephritis" for the following: **Knowledge deficit**: Signs and symptoms of fluid and electrolyte imbalance, p. 94.

E. Patient–Family Teaching and Discharge Planning

Provide patient and SOs with verbal and written information for the following:

1. Medications, including drug name, purpose, dosage, schedule, precautions, and potential side effects.

2. Care of the nephrostomy catheter, if discharged with one; procedure to follow should the catheter become dislodged.

3. Frequency of and procedure for dressing changes. Patient and/or SOs should demonstrate safe dressing-change technique before hospital discharge.

4. Need for continued medical follow-up; confirm date and time of next MD appointment, if known.

5. Signs and symptoms that necessitate medical attention: fever, cloudy or foul-smelling urine, flank or labial pain, increased catheter drainage, and drainage around the catheter site.

VI. Renal Artery Stenosis

Stenosis of the renal artery or one of its main branches is usually the result of congenital fibromuscular hyperplasia or arteriosclerotic changes. A reduction in the lumen of the renal artery causes a decrease in blood flow to the affected kidney, which in turn stimulates the renin–angiotensin system, causing systemic hypertension. The elevation in blood pressure is usually proportional to the degree of ischemia in the affected kidney. If the hypertension is left untreated, the nonischemic kidney will develop arteriolar hyperplasia. When both kidneys are involved, renal failure can occur.

A. Assessment

Signs and symptoms: Headache, nose bleeds, tinnitus.

Physical exam: Auscultation of a bruit in the mid-epigastric area. BP can be severely elevated.

B. Diagnostic Studies

1. <u>IVP</u>: Visualizes kidneys via excretion of idodine-containing contrast medium; will demonstrate an ischemic kidney.

2. <u>Renal arteriography</u>: Injection of contrast medium into the renal arteries to visualize renal vasculature. The arteriogram can be false positive in the older adult. Complications include allergic reaction to the contrast medium, contrast medium-induced acute renal failure, hemorrhage, embolus, and infection.

3. <u>Radioisotope renogram</u>: Will demonstrate a delayed transit time of the radioisotope through the affected kidney.

4. <u>Renal vein renin levels</u>: Will show a difference between the two kidneys in unilateral disease. The renin level from the ischemic kidney should be 1.5 times that of the nonischemic kidney.

5. <u>BUN and serum creatinine</u>: To determine the level of renal function.

C. Medical Management and Surgical Interventions

Renovascular hypertension can be treated either medically or surgically. Patients over age 55 or those with diabetes mellitus or diffuse arteriosclerotic vascular disease may be considered poor surgical risks. Type and duration of the disease are additional factors that can contribute to the decision to treat patients medically.

Surgical interventions include the following

1. *Percutaneous transluminal angioplasty:* Performed if the patient is a suitable candidate and the necessary equipment and personnel are available. Angioplasty involves the insertion of a balloon-tipped catheter to dilate the narrowed vessel. It can be performed under local anesthesia and requires minimal hospitalization.

2. *Resection or bypass of the lesion:* Performed for those patients who are unsuitable candidates for angioplasty, or when angioplasty is unavailable.

D. Nursing Diagnoses and Interventions

Knowledge deficit: Technique for measuring BP and the rationale for frequent assessments after angioplasty

Desired outcomes: Patient verbalizes knowledge of the potential complications of angioplasty and the importance of frequent VS checks, and demonstrates BP measurement technique prior to hospital discharge.

1. Explain the rationale for measuring BP under the same conditions each day: sitting, standing, lying down. Teach the technique for measuring BP to the patient and SOs.

2. Explain the rationale for measuring VS q15 min immediately after angioplasty. Teach patient and SOs the importance of monitoring the integrity of the pulses distal to the angioplasty site.

3. Alert patient and SOs to the potential for bleeding and hematoma formation at the angioplasty site, as well as symptoms of hidden bleeding, including hypotension and tachycardia. Explain that if a hematoma is noted, it will be circled with ink and the time will be noted to detect further bleeding.

See "Glomerulonephritis" for the following: **Knowledge deficit**: Signs and symptoms of fluid and electrolyte imbalance, p. 94. See "Appendix One" for nursing diagnoses and interventions for the care of preoperative and postoperative patients, pp. 528–532.

E. Patient–Family Teaching and Discharge Planning

Provide patients and SOs with verbal and written information for the following:

1. Medications, including drug name, purpose, dosage, schedule, precautions, and potential side effects.
2. Diet: low in sodium. Include lists of foods high in potassium if patient is taking diuretics that cause hypokalemia (see Table 3-2, p. 96). Provide sample menus, and have the patient demonstrate understanding of the diet by planning meals for 3 days.
3. Technique for measuring BP. Patient and/or SOs should demonstrate proficiency before discharge.
4. Care of incision or angioplasty site. Teach patient the indicators of wound infection and the importance of reporting them promptly to the MD.
5. Need for continued medical follow-up to evaluate effectiveness of the treatment.

▶ Section Two **Renal Failure**

I. Acute Renal Failure

Acute renal failure (ARF) is a sudden decrease in renal function that may or may not be accompanied by oliguria. The kidney loses its ability to maintain biochemical homeostasis, causing dramatic alterations in fluid and electrolyte and acid–base balance. Although the renal damage is usually reversible, ARF has a high mortality rate.

The most common cause of ARF is acute tubular necrosis (ATN), which is usually caused by ischemia or nephrotoxins (antibiotics, heavy metals, or radiographic contrast media). ATN also can occur after transfusion reactions, septic abortions, or crushing injuries. The clinical course of ATN can be divided into the following three phases: oliguric (lasting approximately 7–21 days); diuretic (7–14 days); and recovery (3–12 months). Causes of ARF other than ATN include acute poststreptococcal glomerulonephritis, malignant hypertension, and hepatorenal syndrome. The mortality rate of ARF varies greatly with etiology, the patient's age, and other medical problems. The overall mortality rate for ATN is 40–60%.

A decrease in renal function secondary to decreased renal perfusion, but without kidney damage, is called pre-renal failure. A reduction in urine output because of obstruction of urine flow is called post-renal failure. Prolonged pre-renal or post-renal problems can lead to kidney damage and ARF, so early detection and correction of these problems are critical.

A. Assessment

Electrolyte disturbance: Muscle weakness, dysrhythmias, pruritis.

Fluid volume excess: Oliguria, pitting edema, hypertension, pulmonary edema.

Metabolic acidosis: Kussmaul respirations (hyperventilation), lethargy, headache.

Uremia: Altered mental state, anorexia, nausea, diarrhea, pale and sallow skin, purpura, decreased resistance to infection, anemia, fatigue.

▶ **Note:** Uremia adversely affects all body systems.

Physical exam: Pallor and edema (peripheral, periorbital, sacral); crackles (rales) and elevated BP in patient who has fluid overload.

History of: Exposure to nephrotoxic substances, recent blood transfusion, prolonged hypotensive episodes or decreased renal perfusion, abortion, or a recent URI.

B. Diagnostic Tests

1. **BUN and serum creatinine:** Assess the progression and management of ARF. Although both BUN and creatinine will increase as renal function decreases, creatinine is a better indicator of renal function because it is not affected by diet, hydration, or tissue catabolism.

2. **Creatinine clearance:** Measures the kidney's ability to clear the blood of creatinine and approximates the glomerular filtration rate. It will decrease as renal function decreases. Creatinine clearance is normally decreased in the elderly. **Note:** Failure to collect all urine during the period of study can invalidate the test.

3. **Urinalysis:** Can provide information about the cause and location of renal disease as reflected by abnormal urinary sediment (casts and cellular debris).

4. **Urinary osmolality and urinary sodium:** To rule out renal perfusion problems (pre-renal). In ATN the kidney loses the ability to adjust urine concentration and conserve sodium.

▶ **Note:** All urine samples should be sent to the lab immediately after collection, or refrigerated if this is not possible. Urine left at room temperature has greater potential for bacterial growth, turbidity, and alkalinity, any of which can distort the reading.

---

5. **Renal ultrasound:** Provides information about renal anatomy and pelvic structures, evaluates renal masses, and detects obstruction and hydronephrosis.

6. **Renal scan:** Provides information about the perfusion and function of the kidneys.

C. Medical Management

The goal is to remove the precipitating cause, maintain homeostatic balance, and prevent complications until the kidneys are able to resume function. Initially, a trial of fluid and diuretics may be used to rule out pre-renal problems.

1. **Restrict fluids:** Replace losses plus 400 mL/24h. **Note:** Insensible fluid losses are only partially replaced to offset the water formed during the metabolism of protein, carbohydrates, and fats.

2. **Packed cells:** For active bleeding or if anemia is poorly tolerated.

3. **Pharmacotherapy**

   □ *Diuretics:* In non-oliguric ARF for fluid removal (see Table 3-1, p. 93).

   □ *Antihypertensives:* To control BP.

   □ *Aluminum hydroxide antacids:* Bind phosphorus to control hyperphosphatemia.

   □ *Cation exchange resins (Kayexalate):* To control hyperkalemia (see "Fluid and Electrolyte Disturbances," p. 503, for additional treatment).

   □ *Calcium or vitamin D supplements:* For hypocalcemic patients.

   □ *Sodium bicarbonate:* To treat acidosis. It is used cautiously in hypocalcemic or fluid-overloaded patients.

   □ *Vitamins B and C:* To replace losses if patient is on dialysis.

Table 3-3 Drug Usage in Renal Failure

Drugs that are handled primarily by the kidney have an increased effect in patients with renal failure. Usually they require modification of dosage and/or frequency. Some of these medications are:

Antibiotics
*carbenicillin
*cefazolin
*gentamicin
*kanamycin
*tobramycin
 vancomycin

Sedatives
*phenobarbital

Hypoglycemic Agents
 insulin

Antiarrhythmics
 digoxin
*procainamide

Drugs that usually do not require dosage modification include:

Antibiotics
*chloramphenicol
 clindamycin
 dicloxacillin
 erythromycin
 nafcillin sodium

Antihypertensive Agents
 hydralazine
 clonidine HCl
 prazosin HCl
 minoxidil
*methyldopa

Sedatives
 diazepam
 chlordiazepoxide HCl

Diuretics
 murosemide
 Metolazone

Hypoglycemic Agent
 tolbutamide

Anti-inflammatory
 indomethacin

Narcotics
 codeine
 morphine

Anti-arrhythmic Agents
 propranolol
*quinidine gluconate

*Dialyzable drugs, which might require extra dosage after dialysis.

▶ **Note:** Medications that are excreted primarily by the kidneys require modification of dosage and/or frequency. Dialyzable medications may need to be increased, or held and given after dialysis (see Table 3-3).

4. **Diet:** High carbohydrate, low protein, low potassium, and low sodium. Sodium is limited to prevent thirst and fluid retention. Potassium is limited because of the kidney's inability to excrete excess potassium. Protein is limited to minimize retention of nitrogenous wastes. **Note:** Because of the loss of potassium during the diuretic phase, potassium might need to be increased during this time (see Table 3-2, p. 96).

5. **TPN:** May be necessary for patients unable to maintain adequate oral/enteral intake.

6. **Peritoneal dialysis or hemodialysis:** Administered if the above therapy is inadequate for maintaining homeostasis or preventing complications (see "Renal Dialysis," p. 116).

D. Nursing Diagnoses and Interventions

Fluid volume excess: Edema related to fluid retention secondary to renal dysfunction: Oliguric phase

Desired outcome: Patient adheres to prescribed fluid restriction and does not exhibit signs of fluid volume overload.

1. Closely monitor and document I&O.
2. Monitor weight daily. A steady weight gain reflects excessive fluid volume.

3. Observe for indicators of fluid overload, including edema, hypertension, crackles (rales), tachycardia, distended neck veins, SOB, and increased CVP.

4. Carefully adhere to prescribed fluid restriction. Provide oral hygiene at frequent intervals, and offer ice chips or Popsicles to minimize thirst. Hard candies also may be given to decrease thirst. Spread allotted fluids evenly over a 24-hour period, and record the amount given. Instruct patient and SOs about the need for fluid restriction.

▶ **Note:** Patients nourished via TPN are at increased risk for fluid overload because of the necessary fluid volume.

Fluid volume deficit related to abnormal loss secondary to excessive urinary output: Diuretic phase

Desired outcome: Patient does not exhibit signs of dehydration.

1. Closely monitor and document I&O.

2. Monitor weight daily. A weight loss greater than 0.5 kg/day may reflect excessive volume loss.

3. Observe for indicators of volume depletion, including poor skin turgor, hypotension, tachycardia, and decreased CVP.

4. As prescribed, encourage fluids in the dehydrated patient.

5. Report significant findings to MD.

Activity intolerance related to fatigue and weakness secondary to uremia and anemia

Desired outcome: Patient verbalizes decreases in weakness and fatigue and exhibits signs of improving endurance.

1. Hematocrit will decrease and stabilize at around 20–25%. Usually, patients are not transfused unless their hematocrit drops below 20–25% or their anemia is poorly tolerated. Notify MD of increased weakness, fatigue, dyspnea, chest pain, or a further decrease in hematocrit. **Note:** Muscle weakness can be an indicator of dangerous hyperkalemia and should be reported immediately.

2. Assist with ADLs as necessary; encourage independence to patient's tolerance.

3. Establish a progressive activity regimen within patient's activity limitations that will help patient to return to normal activities without complications. For more information see **Potential impairment of physical mobility** related to inactivity secondary to prolonged bed rest, p. 535, in "Appendix One."

Potential for injury related to sensorimotor and mentation alterations secondary to uremia, electrolyte imbalance, and metabolic acidosis

Desired outcomes: Patient does not exhibit signs of injury, is oriented to time, place, and person, and can verbalize knowledge of the signs and symptoms of electrolyte imbalance and metabolic acidosis and the importance of reporting them promptly should they occur.

1. Avoid giving patient foods high in potassium (see Table 3-2, p. 96).

2. Minimize tissue catabolism by controlling fevers, maintaining adequate nutritional intake (especially protein and calories), and preventing infections.

3. Assess for and alert patient to indicators of the following:

   □ *Hypokalemia (may occur during the diuretic phase):* Abdominal cramps, lethargy, and dysrhythmias. See "Fluid and Electrolyte Disturbances," p. 505, for treatment.

□ *Hyperkalemia:* Muscle cramps, dysrhythmias, muscle weakness, peaked T waves on EKG. **Note:** A normal serum potassium is necessary for normal cardiac function. Hyperkalemia is a common and potentially fatal complication of ARF during the oliguric phase. See "Fluid and Electrolyte Disturbances," p. 503, for treatment.

□ *Hypocalcemia:* Neuromuscular irritability and positive Trousseau and Chvostek signs.

□ *Hyperphosphatemia:* Excessive itching.

□ *Uremia:* Confusion, lethargy; restlessness.

□ *Metabolic acidosis:* Rapid, deep respirations; confusion.

4. Prepare patient for the possibility of altered taste and smell.

5. Patients with renal failure tend to have increased magnesium levels because of decreased urinary excretion of dietary magnesium, and thus magnesium-containing medications should be avoided. For example, patients using magnesium-containing antacids are typically switched to aluminum hydroxide preparations.

6. Administer aluminum hydroxide antacids as prescribed. Experiment with different brands or try capsules for patients who refuse certain liquid antacids.

7. Assure patient and SOs that irritability, restlessness, and altered thinking are temporary. Facilitate orientation through calendars, radios, familiar objects, and frequent reorientation.

8. Ensure safety measures (eg, padded side rails, airway, tongue blade) for patients who are confused or severely hypocalcemic. For patients who exhibit signs of hyperkalemia, have emergency supplies (eg, manual resuscitator bag, crash cart, and emergency drug tray) available.

Potential for infection related to increased susceptibility secondary to uremia

Desired outcome: Patient does not exhibit signs of infection.

▶ **Note:** One of the primary causes of death in ARF is sepsis.

1. Monitor temperature and secretions for indicators of infection. Even minor increases in temperature can be significant because uremia masks the febrile response and inhibits the body's ability to fight infection.

2. Use meticulous, aseptic technique when changing dressings or manipulating venous catheters, IV lines, or indwelling catheters.

3. Avoid the use of indwelling urinary catheters since they are a common source of infection. When it is indicated, use intermittent catheterization instead.

4. Provide oral hygiene and skin care at frequent intervals. Use emollients and gentle soap to avoid drying and cracking of skin, which can lead to breakdown and infection.

Alteration in bowel elimination: Constipation related to negative side effects of drugs (eg, phosphate binders), restrictions of fresh fruit and fluids, and prolonged bed rest

Desired outcomes: Patient relates that bowel movements are within normal pattern. Patient can verbalize knowledge of foods and activities that promote bowel movements.

1. Monitor and record the quality and number of bowel movements.

2. Provide prescribed stool softeners and bulk-building supplements as necessary.

3. Suggest alternate dietary sources of fiber, such as unsalted popcorn or un-processed bran.

4. Encourage exercise and activity as appropriate.

5. Provide Fleets, oil-retention, or tap-water enemas as prescribed *only* if the above measures fail. Avoid use of large-volume water enemas because excess fluid can be absorbed from the GI tract.

E. Patient–Family Teaching and Discharge Planning

Provide patient and SOs with verbal and written information for the following:

1. Medications, including drug name, purpose, dosage, schedule, precautions, and potential side effects

2. Diet: Include fact sheet that lists foods to restrict.

3. Care and observation of the dialysis access if the patient is being discharged with one (see "Renal Dialysis," pp. 116–122).

4. Importance of continued medical follow-up of renal function.

5. Instructions regarding the signs and symptoms of potential complications. These should include indicators of infection, electrolyte imbalance, fluid overload or deficit, and bleeding (especially from the GI tract for patients who are uremic).

In addition:

6. If the patient requires dialysis after discharge, coordinate discharge planning with dialysis unit staff. Arrange visit to dialysis unit if possible.

II. Chronic Renal Failure

Chronic renal failure (CRF) is a slowly progressive, irreversible loss of kidney function, which can develop over months to years. Eventually it may progress to end-stage renal disease (ESRD). The patient with ESRD requires dialysis or a kidney transplant to sustain life. Prior to ESRD, the patient can lead a relatively normal life with CRF, managed by diet and medications. This period can last from days to years, depending on the cause of renal failure and the patient's level of renal function at the time of diagnosis.

There are many causes of CRF. Some of the most common include glomerulo-nephritis, diabetes mellitus, polycystic kidney disease, and hypertension. In some patients, the etiology of CRF is unknown.

A. Assessment

Fluid volume abnormalities: Crackles (rales), hypertension, edema, oliguria, or anuria.

Electrolyte disturbances: Muscle weakness, dysrhythmias, pruritis, tetany.

Uremia—retention of metabolic wastes: Weakness, malaise, anorexia, dry and dis-colored skin, peripheral neuropathy, irritability, clouded thinking, ammonia odor to breath. **Note:** Uremia adversely affects all body systems.

Metabolic acidosis: Rapid respirations, lethargy, headache.

Potential acute complications

□ *Congestive heart failure:* Crackles, dyspnea, orthopnea.

□ *Pericarditis:* Chest pain, SOB.

□ *Cardiac tamponade:* Hypotension, distant heart sounds, pulsus paradoxus (exag-gerated inspiratory drop in systolic BP).

Physical exam: Pallor, dry and discolored skin, edema (peripheral, periorbital, sac-ral). With fluid overload, crackles and elevated BP may be present.

History of: Glomerulonephritis, diabetes mellitus, polycystic kidney disease, hypertension, systemic lupus erythematosus, chronic pyelonephritis, or analgesic abuse, especially the combination of phenacetin and aspirin.

B. Diagnostic Tests

1. <u>BUN and serum creatinine:</u> Both will be elevated. **Note:** Nonrenal problems such as dehydration or GI bleeding also can cause the BUN to increase, but there will not be a corresponding increase in creatinine.

2. <u>Creatinine clearance:</u> Measures the kidney's ability to clear the blood of creatinine and approximates the glomerular filtration rate. Creatinine clearance will decrease as renal function decreases. Dialysis is usually begun when the creatinine clearance is less than 10 mL/min. Creatinine clearance is normally decreased in the elderly. **Note:** Failure to collect all urine specimens during the period of study will invalidate the test.

3. <u>Urinalysis:</u> Can provide information about the cause and location of renal disease as reflected by abnormal urinary sediment. **Note:** For accurate assessment of urinary sediment, the specimen should be sent to the lab and examined within one hour of voiding.

4. <u>X-ray of the kidneys, ureters, and bladder (KUB):</u> Documents the presence of two kidneys, changes in size or shape, and some forms of obstruction.

5. <u>IVP, renal ultrasound, renal biopsy, renal scan (using radionuclides), and CT scan:</u> Additional tests for determining the cause of renal insufficiency. Once the patient has reached ESRD, these tests are not performed.

6. <u>Serum chemistries, chest and hand x-rays, and nerve conduction velocity test:</u> To assess for development and progression of uremia and its complications.

C. Medical Management and Surgical Interventions

Prior to ESRD, medical management is aimed at slowing the progression of CRF. Once the patient reaches ESRD, management is aimed at avoiding complications, alleviating uremic symptoms, and providing dialysis or renal transplantation.

1. **Diet:** Carbohydrates are increased in protein-restricted patients to ensure adequate caloric intake and prevent catabolism. Depending on existing renal function, sodium is limited to prevent thirst and fluid retention, potassium is limited because of the kidney's inability to excrete excess potassium, and protein is limited to minimize retention of nitrogenous wastes.

2. **Pharmacotherapy**
   □ *Aluminum hydroxide antacids:* Bind phosphorus to control hyperphosphatemia.

   □ *Antihypertensives:* To control BP.

   □ *Multivitamins and folic acid:* For patients with dietary restrictions or who are on dialysis (water-soluble vitamins are lost during dialysis).

   □ *Anabolic steroids, parenteral iron, or ferrous sulfate:* To treat anemia.

   □ *Diphenhydramine:* To treat itching.

   □ *Sodium bicarbonate:* To treat acidosis.

   □ *Vitamin D preparations:* To treat hypocalcemia.

   □ *Deferoxamine:* To treat iron or aluminum toxicity (experimental use).

   ▶ **Note:** Medications that are excreted primarily by the kidney require modification of dosage and/or frequency. Dialyzable medications may need to be increased, or held and given postdialysis (see Table 3-3, p. 108).

3. **Packed cells:** To treat severe or symptomatic anemia.

4. **Maintain homeostasis and prevent complications** by avoiding the following: volume depletion, hypotension, use of radiopaque contrast medium, and nephrotoxic substances. Pregnancy is contraindicated.

5. **Renal transplant or dialysis:** If the above therapies are inadequate.

D. Nursing Diagnoses and Interventions

Activity intolerance related to fatigue and weakness secondary to anemia and uremia

Desired outcomes: Patient verbalizes decreases in weakness and fatigue and exhibits evidence of improving endurance.

1. Anemia is usually proportional to the degree of azotemia. Hematocrit can be as low as 20% or less, but usually stabilizes at around 20–25%. Typically, these patients are not transfused unless hematocrit drops below 20% or anemia is poorly tolerated. Notify MD of increased weakness, fatigue, dyspnea, chest pain, or further decreases in hematocrit. **Note:** Anemia is better tolerated in the uremic than in the nonuremic patient.

   □ Provide and encourage optimal nutrition.

   □ Administer anabolic steroids (eg, nandrolene) if prescribed. Prepare female patients for side effects, including increasing facial hair, deepening voice, and menstrual irregularities.

   □ Coordinate lab studies to minimize blood drawing.

   □ Observe for and report evidence of occult blood and blood loss.

   □ Report symptomatic anemia: weakness, SOB, chest pain.

   □ Do not administer ferrous sulfate at the same time as aluminum hydroxide antacids. The two medications should be given at least 1 hour apart to maximize absorption of the ferrous sulfate.

   □ Administer parenteral iron if prescribed. Anaphylaxis is a possible complication.

2. Assist patient with identifying activities that cause increased fatigue and adjusting those activities accordingly.

3. Assist the patient with ADLs while encouraging maximum independence to the patient's tolerance.

4. Establish with the patient realistic, progressive exercises and activity goals that are designed to increase endurance. Ensure that they are within the patient's prescribed limitations. Examples are found in "Appendix One," **Potential impairment of physical mobility** related to inactivity secondary to prolonged bed rest, p. 535.

Impairment of skin integrity related to pruritus secondary to uremia

Desired outcome: Patient states that pruritus is controlled and can verbalize knowledge of the cause, preventive factors, and treatment.

1. Pruritus is common in uremic patients, causing frequent, intense scratching. Pruritus often decreases with a reduction in BUN and improved phosphorus control. Encourage the use of phosphate binders and the reduction of dietary phosphorus (see p. 235) if elevated phosphorus is a problem. Give phosphate binders with meals for maximum effects. If necessary, administer antihistamines as prescribed. Keep patient's fingernails short.

2. Because uremia retards wound healing, instruct the patient to monitor scratches for evidence of infection and seek early medical attention should signs and symptoms of infection appear.

3. Uremic skin is often dry and scaly because of reduction in oil gland activity. Encourage the use of skin emollients. Patients should avoid hard soaps and

excessive bathing. Advise patient to bathe every other day and use bath oils as needed if dry skin is a problem.

4. Clotting abnormalities and capillary fragility place the uremic patient at increased risk for bruising. Advise patient and SOs that this can occur.

Knowledge deficit: Need for frequent BP checks and compliance with antihypertensive therapy and the potential for change in insulin requirements for diabetics

Desired outcomes: Patient can verbalize knowledge of the importance of frequent BP checks and compliance with antihypertensive therapy. Diabetic patient can verbalize knowledge of the potential for change in insulin requirements.

▶ **Note:** Patients with CRF may experience hypertension because of fluid overload, excess renin secretion, and/or arteriosclerotic disease.

---

1. Teach patient the importance of getting BP checked at frequent intervals and complying with the prescribed antihypertensive therapy.

2. Teach diabetic patients that insulin requirements often decrease as renal function decreases. Instruct diabetic patients to be alert to indicators of hypoglycemia, including confusion, diaphoresis, and hypotension.

Potential for injury related to sensorimotor and mentation alterations secondary to electrolyte and acid–base imbalances and uremia

Desired outcomes: Patient does not exhibit signs of injury and can verbalize orientation to time, place, and person. Patient can relate knowledge of the importance of avoiding foods and products that contain potassium.

1. Hyperkalemia is a common complication of CRF. Avoid salt substitutes (KCl) and "light" salts (contain KCl) and potassium-containing medications such as potassium penicillin G. (For a list of foods that are high in potassium, see Table 3-2, p. 96.)

2. If the patient requires multiple blood transfusions, observe for indicators of hyperkalemia, because old banked blood may contain as much as 30 mEq/L of potassium. Use fresh-packed cells when possible.

3. For other interventions, see the same nursing diagnosis in "Acute Renal Failure," p. 109.

See "Acute Renal Failure" for the following: **Potential for infection**, p. 110, **Alteration in bowel elimination:** Constipation, p. 110, and **Fluid volume excess** (oliguric phase), p. 108. See "Appendix One," pp. 544–546, for appropriate nursing diagnoses and interventions for the care of patients with life-disrupting illnesses.

E. Patient–Family Teaching and Discharge Planning

Provide patient and SOs with verbal and written information for the following:

1. Medications, including drug name, purpose, dosage, schedule, precautions, and potential side effects.

2. Diet. Include fact sheet listing foods that are to be restricted or limited. Inform patient that diet and fluid restrictions may be altered as renal function decreases. Provide sample menus and have the patient demonstrate understanding by preparing 3-day menus that incorporate dietary restrictions.

3. Care and observation of dialysis access if the patient has one (see "Renal Dialysis," pp. 116–122).

4. Signs and symptoms that necessitate medical attention: irregular pulse, fever,

unusual SOB or edema, sudden change in urine output, and unusual muscle weakness.

5. Need for continued medical follow-up; confirm date and time of next MD appointment.

6. Importance of avoiding infections and seeking treatment promptly should one develop. Instruct the patient in the indicators of frequently encountered infections, eg, URI, UTI, impetigo, otitis media.

In addition:

7. For the patient with or approaching ESRD, provide data concerning the various treatment options and support groups. The local chapter of the National Kidney Foundation can be helpful in identifying support groups and organizations in the area. Patient and SOs should meet with the renal dietitian and social worker before discharge.

8. Coordinate discharge planning and teaching with the dialysis unit or facility. If possible, have patient visit dialysis unit before discharge.

> ▶ Section Three   **Care of the Renal Transplant Patient**

Annually, approximately 5000–6000 patients with end-stage renal disease (ESRD) receive renal transplants. Although patients receive transplants at major medical centers and are cared for postoperatively in specialized units, they may be admitted to any hospital for treatment of a rejection episode, medication complication, or unrelated illness. The majority of the transplanted kidneys come from cadavers, although living family members might also donate. Unless the graft is donated from an identical twin, transplant success depends on the suppression of graft rejection. This is accomplished by carefully matching donors to recipients through tissue typing before transplantation and immunosuppression after transplantation. Rejection is the major complication of renal transplant.

A. Immunosuppression

1. Necessary for the life of the graft.

2. Puts the patient at increased risk for infection and development of malignancy in the long term.

3. Usual immunosuppressive medications

   □ *Azathioprine (Imuran):* Side effects include decreased WBC and platelet counts.

   □ *Prednisone:* Side effects include muscle wasting, aseptic necrosis of bone, cataracts, bleeding, sodium retention, altered carbohydrate metabolism, mood and behavior changes, and Cushingoid changes.

4. New medication: *Cyclosporine*—a potent immunosuppressive. Side effects include nephrotoxicity, hepatotoxicity, hirsutism, tremors, gum hyperplasia, hypertension, infection, malignancy. Route is either PO or IV. If IV, administer slowly over 2–4-hour period and monitor for anaphylaxis. If route is PO, use a glass container; mix with orange juice or chocolate milk to make it more palatable. Do not allow solution to stand.

B. Rejection

1. *Acute:* 1 week–4 months after surgery; potentially reversible; treated with increased immunosuppression.

2. *Chronic:* Months to years after transplant; irreversible; managed conservatively with diet and antihypertensives until dialysis is required.

3. *Indicators of rejection:* Oliguria, tenderness over kidney (located in iliac fossa), sudden weight gain, fever, malaise, hypertension, and increased BUN and serum creatinine.

C. Nursing Diagnoses and Interventions

Potential for infection related to increased susceptibility secondary to invasive procedures, exposure to infected individuals, and immunosuppression

Desired outcomes: Patient does not exhibit signs of infection. Patient can verbalize knowledge of the indicators of infection and the importance of reporting them promptly to MD or staff.

1. Observe for indicators of infection, such as fever and unexplained tachycardia. Instruct the patient to be alert to signs and symptoms of commonly encountered infections and the importance of reporting them promptly.

2. Teach patient to avoid exposure to individuals known to have infections.

3. Use aseptic technique with all invasive procedures and dressing changes.

Knowledge deficit: Signs and symptoms of rejection, negative side effects of immunosuppressive agents, and importance of protecting the fistula

Desired outcome: Patient can verbalize knowledge of the signs and symptoms of rejection, the side effects of immunosuppressive therapy, and the importance of protecting the hemodialysis vascular access.

1. Explain the importance of renal function monitoring: I&O, daily weight, and BUN and serum creatinine values.

2. Alert patient to the signs and symptoms of rejection and the importance of reporting them promptly should they occur.

3. Explain that significant decreases in white cell and platelet counts can be a side effect of immunosuppressive agents, and therefore serial monitoring is essential.

4. Explain that GI bleeding is a potential side effect of immunosuppressive agents. Alert patient to the signs and symptoms and the importance of reporting them promptly should they occur.

5. If the patient has a patent fistula (hemodialysis vascular access), explain that it must be handled with care because the patient will need it if a return to dialysis is indicated. Explain that taking blood pressures, drawing blood, and starting IVs is contraindicated in the fistula arm; therefore, patient should warn others about these contraindications. For additional information see the discussion that follows in "Renal Dialysis."

▶ Section Four   **Renal Dialysis**

▶ **Note:** This section does not include care of the patient during dialysis; rather, it provides essential background data, including nursing therapeutics for the care of patients undergoing dialysis.

Peritoneal dialysis and hemodialysis are lifesaving procedures used to treat severely decreased or absent renal function. Dialysis can be either temporary, until the kidneys are able to resume adequate function, or permanent. Dialysis is defined as the selective movement of water and solutes from one fluid compartment to another across a semipermeable membrane. The two fluid compartments are the patient's blood and the dialysate (electrolyte and glucose solution). With hemodialysis, the semipermeable membrane is an artificial one; with peritoneal dialysis, the peritoneum serves as a natural dialysis membrane.

Indications for dialysis: Acute renal failure or acute episodes of chronic renal failure that cannot be managed by diet, medications, and fluid restriction; ESRD; drug overdose; hyperkalemia; fluid overload; or metabolic acidosis.

Functions of dialysis: Correction of electrolyte abnormalities; removal of fluid and metabolic wastes; correction of acid–base abnormalities. **Note:** Dialysis does not compensate completely for the lack of functioning kidneys. Medications and dietary and fluid restrictions are often necessary to supplement dialysis.

Peritoneal dialysis: Slow; does not require heparinization; can be performed by trained floor nurses; requires a minimum of equipment.

Hemodialysis: Fast; requires heparinization, specially trained staff, expensive and complex equipment; patient must have adequate vasculature for access.

I. Care of the Peritoneal Dialysis Patient

Peritoneal dialysis utilizes the peritoneum as the dialysis membrane. Dialysate is instilled into the peritoneal cavity via a special catheter, and movement of solutes and fluid occurs between the patient's capillary blood and the dialysate. At set intervals the peritoneal cavity is drained and new dialysate is instilled.

A. Components of Peritoneal Dialysis

1. *Catheter:* Silastic tube that is either implanted as a surgical procedure for chronic patients or inserted at the bedside for acute dialysis.

2. *Dialysate:* Sterile electrolyte solution similar in composition to normal plasma. The electrolyte composition of the dialysate can be adjusted according to individual need. The most commonly adjusted electrolyte is potassium. Glucose is added to the dialysate in varying concentrations to remove excess body fluid via osmosis. **Note:** Some glucose crosses the peritoneal membrane and enters the patient's blood. Diabetic patients may require additional insulin. Observe for and report indicators of hyperglycemia, eg, complaints of thirst or changes in sensorium.

B. Types of Peritoneal Dialysis

1. Intermittent peritoneal dialysis (IPD): The patient is dialyzed for 8–10-hour periods, 4–5 times per week. A predetermined amount of dialysate (usually 2 L) is instilled for a set length of time (usually 20–30 min). It is then allowed to drain by gravity, and the process is repeated. IPD can be performed manually with individual bottles and bags, or mechanically using a proportioning machine or cycler. The patient is restricted to a chair or bed. Peritoneal dialysis also can be performed as an acute, temporary procedure. Continuous hourly exchanges are performed for 48–72 hours. This type of dialysis usually requires a critical care setting. The patient is restricted to bed.

2. Continuous ambulatory peritoneal dialysis (CAPD): The patient attaches a specialized bag of dialysate to the peritoneal catheter; allows the dialysate to drain in; clamps the catheter, leaving the bag attached; and goes about his or her daily routine. After 4 hours (8 hours at night) the clamp is opened and the dialysate is allowed to drain out. Using aseptic technique, the patient attaches a new bag of dialysate and the process is repeated. Dialysis exchanges are done continuously, 7 days a week. CAPD is used primarily for ESRD.

3. Continuous cycling peritoneal dialysis (CCPD): This is a combination of IPD and CAPD. A cycler performs three dialysate exchanges at night. In the

morning a fourth exchange is instilled and left in the peritoneal cavity for the entire day. At the end of the day, the fourth exchange is allowed to drain out and the process is repeated. The patient is ambulatory by day and restricted to bed at night.

C. Nursing Diagnoses and Interventions

Potential for infection related to increased vulnerability secondary to direct access of the catheter to the peritoneum

Desired outcomes: Patient does not exhibit signs of infection. Patient can verbalize understanding of the signs and symptoms of infection and demonstrates sterile technique for bag, tubing, and dressing changes.

1. The most common complication of peritoneal dialysis is peritonitis. Observe for and report indications of peritonitis, including fever, abdominal pain, cloudy outflow, nausea, and malaise. **Caution:** It is essential that sterile technique be used when connecting and disconnecting the catheter from the dialysis system.

2. The dialysate must remain sterile because it is instilled directly into the body. Maintain sterile technique when adding medications to the dialysate.

3. Follow agency policy for dressing the catheter exit site.

4. Observe for and report redness, drainage, or tenderness at exit site. Culture any exudate and report the results to the MD.

5. Report to MD if dialysate leaks around the catheter exit site. This can indicate an obstruction or the need for another purse-string suture around the catheter site. Continued leakage at the site can lead to peritonitis.

6. Instruct the patient in the above interventions and observations if peritoneal dialysis will be used after discharge.

Potential alterations in fluid volume: *Excess* related to fluid retention or inadequate exchange secondary to catheter problems and/or peritonitis; *Deficit* related to abnormal loss secondary to hypertonicity of the dialysate

Desired outcome: Patient does not exhibit signs of dehydration, fluid overload, or retained dialysate.

1. Fluid retention can occur because of catheter complications that prevent adequate outflow, or a severely scarred peritoneum that prevents adequate exchange. Observe for and report indicators of fluid overload, such as hypertension, tachycardia, distended neck veins, or increased CVP. Also be alert to incomplete dialysate returns. Accurate measurement and recording of outflow is critical.

2. Outflow problems can occur because of the following:

   ☐ *Full colon:* Use stool softeners, high-fiber diet, or enemas if necessary.

   ☐ *Catheter occlusion by fibrin (usually occurs soon after insertion):* Obtain order to irrigate with heparinized saline.

   ☐ *Catheter obstruction by omentum:* Turn patient from side to side, elevate HOB, or apply firm pressure to the abdomen.

   ▶ **Note:** Notify MD for unresolved outflow problems.

3. Monitor I&O and weight daily. A steady weight gain is indicative of fluid retention.

4. Respiratory distress can occur because of compression of the diaphragm by the dialysate. If this occurs, elevate the HOB, drain the dialysate, and notify MD.

5. Bloody outflow may appear with initial exchanges. Report gross bloody outflow.

6. Coordinate lab studies to limit blood drawing, since patients with renal failure are anemic due to alteration in erythropoietin, causing decreased RBC production and longevity.

7. Volume depletion can occur with excessive use of hypertonic dialysate. Observe for and report indicators of volume depletion, including poor skin turgor, hypotension, tachycardia, and decreased CVP.

Alteration in nutrition: Less than body requirements related to increased need secondary to protein loss in the dialysate

Desired outcome: Patient does not exhibit signs of malnutrition and can verbalize knowledge of the prescribed dietary regimen.

1. Protein crosses the peritoneum and a significant amount is lost in the dialysate. An increased intake of protein is necessary to prevent excessive tissue catabolism. Protein loss increases with peritonitis. Ensure adequate dietary intake of protein: 1.2–1.5 g/kg body weight daily.

2. Peritoneal dialysis patients typically have fewer dietary restrictions than those on hemodialysis. Ensure that a dietary evaluation and teaching program is performed when the patient changes from one type of dialysis to the other.

3. Provide a list of restricted and encouraged foods, with menus that illustrate their integration into the daily diet. Ensure understanding by having the patient plan a 3-day menu that incorporates the appropriate foods and restrictions.

Potential for injury related to sensorimotor and mentation alterations secondary to uremia and serum electrolyte imbalance

Desired outcomes: Patient does not exhibit signs of injury and can verbalize orientation to person, place, and time and knowledge of the signs and symptoms of uremia and serum electrolyte imbalance.

1. Instruct patient and staff to observe for and report indications of the following:

   □ *Increased uremia:* Confusion, lethargy, and restlessness. Monitor BUN and serum creatinine values, which can signal the need for increased diaylsis.

   □ *Hyperkalemia:* Muscle cramps and muscle weakness. Monitor serum potassium values.

   □ *Hypokalemia (secondary to dialysis):* Abdominal cramps, lethargy, and dysrhythmias. Monitor serum potassium values. **Note:** Alert MD to the development of an irregular pulse, because it can be indicative of dangerous hypokalemia. This is especially important for patients on digitalis, as hypokalemia potentiates digitalis toxicity.

2. Promptly report abnormal lab values to the MD. The dialysate or length of dialysis time may require adjustment to compensate for the abnormal lab values.

3. For other interventions, see the same nursing diagnosis in "Acute Renal Failure," p. 109.

II. Care of the Hemodialysis Patient

During hemodialysis, a portion of the patient's blood is removed via a special vascular access, heparinized, pumped through an artificial kidney (dialyzer), and then returned to the patient's circulation. Hemodialysis is either a temporary, acute procedure performed as needed, or it is performed chronically three times a week for 3–6 hours each treatment.

A. Components of Hemodialysis

1. *Artificial kidney* (dialyzer): Composed of a blood compartment and dialysate compartment, separated by a semipermeable membrane that allows the diffusion of solutes and the filtration of water. Protein and bacteria do not cross the artificial membrane.

2. *Dialysate:* An electrolyte solution similar in composition to normal plasma. Each of the constituents may be varied according to patient need. The most commonly altered component is potassium. Glucose may be added to prevent sudden drops in serum osmolality and serum glucose during dialysis.

3. *Vascular access:* Necessary to provide a blood flow rate of 200–300 mL/min for an effective dialysis.

B. Nursing Diagnoses and Interventions

Potential alterations in fluid volume: *Excess* related to fluid retention secondary to renal failure; *Deficit* related to excessive fluid removal secondary to dialysis

Desired outcomes: Patient does not exhibit signs of overhydration or dehydration. Patient can verbalize understanding of the signs and symptoms of overhydration and dehydration.

1. Monitor I&O and daily weight as indicators of fluid status. A steady weight gain is indicative of retained fluid. The patient's weight is an important guideline for determining the quantity of fluid that needs to be removed during dialysis. Weigh patient at the same time each day, using the same scale, and wearing the same amount of clothing (or with same items on the bed if using a bed scale) .

2. Instruct patient and staff to observe for and report indications of fluid overload: edema, hypertension, crackles (rales), tachycardia, distended neck veins, SOB, and increased CVP.

3. After dialysis observe for and report indicators of volume depletion, including hypotension, decreased CVP, and tachycardia. Describe the signs and symptoms to the patient and explain the importance of reporting them promptly should they occur. **Note:** Because of autonomic neuropathy, the uremic patient may not develop a compensatory tachycardia when hypovolemic.

▶ **Note:** Antihypertensive medications are usually held before and during dialysis to help prevent hypotension during dialysis. Clarify medication prescriptions with the MD.

Potential for injury related to increased risk of bleeding secondary to heparinization with dialysis

Desired outcome: Patient does not exhibit signs of excessive bleeding.

1. Observe for bleeding (gums, needle sites, incisions) postdialysis. Alert patient to the potential for bleeding from these areas.

2. To prevent hematoma formation, do not give IM injection for at least 1 hour postdialysis.

3. GI bleeding is common in patients with renal failure, especially after heparinization. Guaiac all stools for evidence of bleeding. Report findings.

Potential for injury related to risk of complications secondary to the creation of the vascular access for hemodialysis

Desired outcomes: Patient does not exhibit signs of injury from vascular access complications. If complications occur, they are detected and reported promptly, resulting in immediate treatment and absence of injury to the patient.

1. Monitor the vascular access as follows: Assess for patency, auscultate for bruit, and palpate for thrill. Report severe or unrelieved pain, and observe for and report numbness, tingling, and swelling of the extremity distal to the access, any of which can signal inadequate blood supply. Expect postoperative swelling along the fistula, and elevate the extremity.

2. Notify MD if the extremity distal to vascular access becomes cool, has decreased capillary refill, or is discolored, as these problems can occur with vascular insufficiency.

3. Follow the three principles of nursing care common to all types of vascular access: Prevent bleeding, prevent clotting, and prevent infection. Explain the monitoring and care procedures to the patient. Remember that the vascular access is the patient's lifeline. Monitor it closely and handle it with care. Vascular accesses include the following:

Shunt: An external, temporary connection between an artery and a vein.

□ *Prevent bleeding:* Keep shunt securely wrapped with gauze, exposing a portion of the loop to allow evaluation of patency. Tape shunt connection. Do not puncture tubing. Never cut dressings off. Keep bulldog or other smooth rubber-shod clamps at the bedside in case the shunt becomes disconnected. If shunt is pulled out, apply firm pressure at site and call MD stat. If necessary, apply tourniquet above the site.

□ *Prevent clotting:* Do not kink tubing. Do not take BP, start IVs, or draw lab work from shunt arm. Document patency at least q shift. Blood within shunt tubing should be warm and bright red. Palpate for thrill and auscultate for bruit above venous cannula exit site. Observe for and immediately report indications of clotting: dark or separated blood within the shunt, shunt cool to the touch, absence of thrill and bruit.

□ *Prevent infection:* Use aseptic technique with dressing changes. Observe for and report indications of infection: redness, swelling, local warmth, exudate, and tenderness at the exit site. Culture any drainage.

Subclavian or femoral lines: External, temporary catheters inserted into a large vein.

□ *Prevent bleeding:* Anchor catheter securely since it might not be sutured in. Tape all connections. Keep clamps at bedside in case line becomes disconnected. If the line is removed or accidentally pulled out, apply firm pressure to site for at least 10 min.

▶ **Note:** An air embolus can occur if a subclavian line accidently becomes disconnected. If this occurs, immediately clamp the line. Then turn the patient into a left side-lying position to help prevent the air from blocking the pulmonary artery, and lower the head of the bed into Trendelenburg's position to increase intrathoracic pressure. This will decrease the flow of inspiratory air into the vein. Notify MD.

□ *Prevent clotting:* Keep line patent by priming with heparin or by constant infusion with a heparinized solution. Follow protocol or obtain specific order from MD. Attach a label to all lines that are primed with heparin to alert other personnel.

□ *Prevent infection:* Perform aseptic dressing changes according to agency protocol. Observe for and report indications of infection, including redness, local warmth, exudate, swelling, and tenderness at exit site. Report and culture any drainage.

Fistula: Internal, permanent connection between an artery and a vein, or the insertion of an internal graft that is joined to an artery and vein. Grafts can be straight or U-shaped. They are located in the arm or thigh.

□ *Prevent bleeding:* Inspect needle puncture sites postdialysis for bleeding. Should it occur, apply just enough pressure over the site to stop it. Release the pressure and check for bleeding q5–10 min.

□ *Prevent clotting:* Do not take BP, start IV, or draw blood in the fistula arm. Avoid tight clothing, jewelry, name bands, or restraint on fistula extremity. Palpate for thrill and auscultate for bruit at least q shift and after hypotensive episodes. Notify MD stat if bruit or thrill is absent.

□ *Prevent infection:* Observe for and report indications of infection: redness, local warmth, swelling, exudate, and unusual tenderness. Culture and report any drainage.

See "Care of the Peritoneal Dialysis Patient" for the following: **Potential for injury** (sensorimotor and mentation alterations), p. 119.

► Section Five   **Disorders of the Urinary Tract**

I. Ureteral Calculi

Ureteral calculi are a common urologic condition. Although the cause of stones is unknown in 50% of reported cases, it is believed that they originate in the kidney and are passed through the kidney to the ureter; 90% of all stones pass from the ureter into the bladder and out of the urinary system spontaneously.

See "Renal Calculi," p. 100, for related information.

A. Assessment

Signs and symptoms: Pain that is sharp, sudden, and intense or dull and aching. Pain can be intermittent as the stone moves along the ureter, subsiding when it enters the bladder. Nausea, vomiting, diarrhea, abdominal pain, and paralytic ileus can occur. Patient may experience frequency, void in small amounts, and have hematuria.

Physical exam: Pallor and diaphoresis may be noted; chills and fever may be present in the acute stage. There can be absence of bowel sounds secondary to ileus, and the abdomen may be distended and tympanic.

History of: Sedentary lifestyle, residence in geographic area in which water supply is high in stone-forming minerals, vitamin A deficiency, vitamin D excess, hereditary cystinuria.

B. Diagnostic Tests

1. <u>Serum tests:</u> To assess calcium, phosphorus, and uric acid levels.

2. <u>Serum and urine creatinine tests:</u> To evaluate renal function. Abnormalities are reflected by high serum creatinine and low urine creatinine.

3. <u>Urinalysis:</u> To test urine pH and specific gravity and for presence of RBCs, WBCs, crystals, and casts.

4. <u>Urine culture:</u> To assess for infection.

5. <u>24-hour urine collection:</u> To test for high levels of uric acid, cystine, oxalate, calcium, phosphorus, or creatinine.

► **Note:** All urine samples should be sent to the lab immediately after they are obtained, or refrigerated if this is not possible. Urine left at room temperature has greater potential for bacterial growth, turbidity, and alkaline pH, any of which can distort the reading.

6. **Kidney, ureter, bladder (KUB) x-ray:** To outline gross structural changes in the kidneys and urinary system. Typically, calcification is seen. Serial radiography monitors progressive movement of the stone.

7. **IVP/excretory urogram:** To outline radiopaque stones within the ureters.

8. **CT scan with or without injection of contrast medium:** To delineate cysts, tumors, calculi, and other masses; ureteral dilation; and bladder distention.

C. Medical Management and Surgical Interventions

1. Pharmacotherapy during the acute stage

☐ *Narcotic and antispasmodic agents:* To relieve pain and ureteral spasms.

☐ *Antiemetics:* For nausea and vomiting.

☐ *Antibiotics:* For infection.

2. Prophylactic pharmacotherapy

☐ *For uric acid stones:* Allopurinol, sodium bicarbonate, potassium or sodium citrate, or citric acid is given to reduce uric acid production or alkalinize the urine.

☐ *For calcium stones:* Ascorbic acid, ammonium chloride, potassium acid phosphate, sodium and potassium phosphates, or hydrochlorothiazide is given to acidify the urine, produce solubility, or reduce urinary calcium.

☐ *For cystine stones:* Penicillamine is given to lower cystine levels in the urine.

3. IV therapy: For patients who are dehydrated.

4. Increase fluid intake: To help flush stone from ureter to the bladder and out through the system.

5. Diet: Specific to patient's stone type. (See **Knowledge deficit**: Diet and its relationship to stone formation, p. 125, for detail.)

6. Endoscopic removal of calculi via cystoscope: A basketing catheter is placed beyond the stone and rotated in a downward movement to capture and remove the stone.

7. Ureteral catheters (stents): Positioned above the stone to promote ureteral dilation, allowing the calculus to pass. These catheters also can be used for intermittent or continuous irrigation with an acidic solution to combat alkalinity. They may be placed temporarily after removal of the stone to allow for healing and promote patency of the ureter in the presence of edema.

8. Ureterolithotomy: Removal of calculi that are unable to pass through the ureter. The ureter is surgically incised and the stone is manually removed.

9. Percutaneous ultrasonic lithotripsy (PUL): Used when the stone is easily accessible such as in the renal pelvis, calyx, or upper ureter. A small tube is placed through a nephrostomy tract against the stone. An ultrasonic probe is passed through this tube, allowing ultrasound waves to shatter the stone. Fragments are removed by suction or irrigation.

10. Extracorporeal shock wave lithotripsy (ESWL): The patient is anesthetized (epidural or general) and placed in a water bath. The affected area is positioned under an electric shock generator, which shatters the calculi. Usually, 500-1500 shock waves over a 30–60 second period are adequate to break the calculi into fine particles. The fragments are passed in the patient's urine within a few days.

D. Nursing Diagnoses and Interventions

Alteration in comfort: Acute pain related to calculus or surgical procedure to remove it

Desired outcome: Patient expresses a reduction in discomfort and does not exhibit signs of uncontrolled pain.

1. Assess and document quality, location, intensity, and duration of the pain. Notify MD of sudden onset of pain.

2. Notify MD of a sudden cessation of pain, which can signal the passage of the stone. (Strain all urine for solid matter and send it to the laboratory for analysis.)

3. Medicate patient with prescribed analgesics, narcotics, and antispasmodics; evaluate and document the response.

4. Provide warm blankets, heating pad to affected area, or warm baths to increase regional circulation and relax tense muscles.

5. Provide back rubs. These are especially helpful for postoperative patients who were in the lithotomy position during surgery.

Alteration in pattern of urinary elimination: Dysuria, urgency, or frequency related to the presence of a ureteral calculus

Desired outcomes: Patient relates the return of normal voiding pattern. Patient can verbalize knowledge of the importance of a 2–3 L/day fluid intake and demonstrates self-recording of I&O and self-straining of urine.

1. Determine and document patient's normal voiding pattern.

2. Monitor the quality and color of the urine. Optimally it is straw colored, clear, and has a characteristic urine odor. Dark urine is often indicative of dehydration, and blood-tinged urine can result from the rupture of ureteral capillaries as the calculus passes through the ureter.

3. In patients for whom fluids are not restricted, encourage a fluid intake of at least 2–3 L/day to help flush calculus through ureter into the bladder and out through the system.

4. Record accurate I&O; teach patient how to self-record I&O.

5. Strain all urine for evidence of solid matter; teach patient the procedure.

6. Send any solid matter to the laboratory for analysis.

Potential alteration in pattern of urinary elimination related to obstruction or positional problems of the ureteral catheter

Desired outcome: Patient does not exhibit alterations in urinary elimination caused by obstruction or positional problems of the ureteral catheter.

1. Occasionally, patients return from surgery with a ureteral catheter. If patient has more than one, label one "right" and the other "left"; keep all drainage records separate.

2. Monitor output from ureteral catheter. Amount will vary with each patient and depend on catheter dimension. If drainage is scanty or absent, milk the catheter and tubing gently to try to dislodge obstruction. If this fails, notify MD.

3. **Caution:** Never irrigate this catheter without specific MD prescription. If irrigation is prescribed, use gentle pressure and aseptic technique. Always aspirate with sterile syringe prior to instillation to prevent ureteral damage from overdistention. Use another sterile syringe to insert amounts no greater than 3 mL per instillation.

4. Typically, patient will require bed rest if ureteral catheter is indwelling. Explain to patient that semi-Fowler's and side-lying positions are acceptable. Fowler's position should be avoided, however, because sutures are seldom used and gravity can cause catheter to move into the bladder.

5. Ureteral catheters are often attached to the urethral catheter after placement in the ureters. Carefully monitor the urethral catheter for movement, and ensure that it is securely attached to the patient.

▶ **Note:** After the ureteral catheters have been removed (usually simultaneously with the urethral catheter), monitor for indicators of ureteral obstruction, including flank pain, nausea, and vomiting.

Potential impairment of skin integrity related to irritation secondary to postoperative wound drainage

Desired outcome: Patient does not exhibit signs of impaired skin integrity at the wound site.

1. Monitor incisional dressings frequently during the first 24 hours and change or reinforce as needed. Excoriation can result from prolonged contact of urine with the skin.

2. Note and document odor, consistency, and color of drainage. Immediately after surgery, drainage may be red.

3. To facilitate frequent dressing changes, use Montgomery straps rather than tape to secure dressing.

4. If drainage is copious after drain removal, apply wound draingage or ostomy pouch with a skin barrier over the incision. Use a pouch with an anti-reflux valve to prevent contamination from reflux.

Knowledge deficit: Diet and its relationship to stone formation

Desired outcomes: Patient can verbalize knowledge of foods to limit and demonstrates this knowledge by planning a 3-day menu that excludes or limits these foods from the diet.

1. Assess patient's knowledge of diet and its relationship to stone formation.

2. As appropriate, provide the following information:

   □ *For uric acid stones:* Limit intake of foods high in purines, such as lean meat, legumes, whole grains.

   □ *For calcium stones:* Limit intake of foods high in calcium, such as milk, cheese, green leafy vegetables, yogurt.

   □ *For oxalate stones:* Limit intake of foods high in oxalate, such as chocolate, caffeine-containing drinks, beets, spinach. Explain that vitamin C supplements should be avoided because as much as half is converted to oxalic acid.

3. Have the patient demonstrate knowledge of the dietary restrictions by planning a 3-day menu that excludes or limits the appropriate foods.

See "Appendix One" for nursing diagnoses and interventions for the care of preoperative and postoperative patients, pp. 528–532.

E. Patient–Family Teaching and Discharge Planning

Provide patient and SOs with verbal and written information for the following:

1. Medications, including drug name, purpose, dosage, schedule, precautions, and potential side effects.

2. Indicators of UTI and/or recurrent calculi, which necessitate medical attention: chills, fever, hematuria, flank pain, cloudy and/or foul-smelling urine.

3. Care of incision, including cleansing and dressing. Teach patient signs and symptoms of infection, including redness, swelling, local warmth, tenderness, and purulent drainage.

4. Care of drains or catheters if patient is discharged with them.

5. Importance of daily fluid intake of at least 2–3 L/day in nonrestricted patients.

6. Dietary changes as specified by MD.

7. Activity precautions as directed for patient who has had surgery: Avoid lifting heavy objects (>5 lbs) for the first 6 weeks, be alert to fatigue, get maximum rest, increase activities gradually to tolerance.

8. Use of nitrazine paper to assess pH of urine. Desired pH will be determined by type of stone formation to which the patient is prone. Instructions for use are on nitrazine paper container.

II. Urinary Tract Obstruction

Urinary tract obstruction is usually the result of blockage from pelvic tumors, calculi, and urethral strictures. Additional causes include neoplasms, benign prostatic hypertrophy, ureteral or urethral trauma, inflammation of the urinary tract, and pelvic or colonic surgery in which ureteral damage has occurred. The obstruction acts like a dam, causing urine to collect and pool. Muscles in the area contract to push urine around the obstruction, and dilation of the structures behind the obstruction begins to occur. Hydrostatic pressure increases, and filtration and concentration processes within the urinary system are compromised. Obstructions can occur anywhere along the urinary tract, but the most common sites are the ureteropelvic and ureterovesical junctions, bladder neck, and urethral meatus. Obstructions in the upper urinary tract can lead to bilateral involvement of the ureters and kidneys as well as of the bladder.

A. Assessment

Signs and symptoms: Anuria, pain that is sharp and intense or dull and aching, nausea, vomiting, local abdominal tenderness, hesitancy, straining to start a stream, dribbling, oliguria, and nocturia.

Physical exam: Bladder distention, mass in flank area, and "kettle drum" sound over bladder with percussion.

History of: Recent fever (possibly caused by the obstruction); hypertensive episodes (caused by increased hormone production from the body's attempt to increase renal blood flow).

B. Diagnostic Tests

1. Serum elecrolytes, BUN, and creatinine: To assess renal function.

2. Hemoglobin and hematocrit: To assess for systemic bleeding and/or anemia, which may be related to decreased renal secretion of erythropoietin.

3. Urinalysis, urine culture, IVP, and KUB radiology: See "Ureteral Calculi," p. 122, for discussion of these tests.

C. Medical Management and Surgical Interventions

1. **Catheterization:** To establish drainage of urine.

2. **Pharmacotherapy**
   - □ *Narcotics:* For pain relief.
   - □ *Antispasmodics:* For relief of spasms.
   - □ *Antibiotics:* For bacterial infection.
   - □ *Corticosteroids:* For reduction of local swelling.

3. **IV therapy:** For acutely ill, dehydrated patients.

4. **Serial urine and serum tests:** For ongoing analysis of electrolytes and osmolality.

5. **Cystoscopy:** To determine degree of bladder outlet obstruction.

6. **Establish drainage:** Via catheters or drains (ureteral, urethral, or suprapubic) above point of obstruction.

7. **Surgical removal of obstruction or dilation of strictures.**

D. Nursing Diagnoses and Interventions

Potential fluid volume deficit related to excessive urinary loss and/or hemorrhage secondary to rapid bladder decompression during catheterization procedure

Desired outcome: Patient does not exhibit signs of dehydration or excessive bleeding during or after catheterization procedure.

1. Do not allow rapid emptying of the bladder; clamp the catheter if drainage exceeds 800–1000 mL within the first 5 minutes after catheterization. **Caution:** Rapid decompression can lead to hemorrhage, acute fluid and electrolyte imbalance, and shock.

2. Follow MD directions for slow decompression of the bladder.

3. Monitor VS for signs of hypotension: decreasing BP, changes in LOC, tachycardia, tachypnea, thready pulse.

4. Record accurate output; notify MD if output exceeds 200 mL/hour because this can occur with postobstruction diuresis, potentially resulting in a serious electrolyte imbalance.

5. Observe for and report indicators of the following:

   □ *Hypokalemia:* Abdominal cramps, lethargy, dysrhythmias.

   □ *Hyperkalemia:* Diarrhea, colic, irritability, nausea, muscle cramps, weakness, irregular apical or radial pulses.

   □ *Hypocalcemia:* Muscle weakness and cramps, complaints of tingling in fingers, positive Trousseau and Chvostek signs.

   □ *Hyperphosphatemia:* Excessive itching.

6. Monitor mentation, noting signs of disorientation, which can occur with electrolyte imbalance.

7. Weigh patient daily using the same scale and at the same time of day, eg, before breakfast. Weight fluctuations of 2–4 lb (0.9–1.8 kg) normally occur in a diuresing patient.

Alteration in comfort: Pain related to bladder spasms

Desired outcome: Patient expresses a reduction in discomfort and does not exhibit signs of uncontrolled pain.

1. Assess for and document patient complaints of pain in the suprapubic or urethral area; reassure patient that spasms are normal with obstruction.

2. Medicate with antispasmodics or analgesics as prescribed.

3. Teach patient the procedure for slow, diaphragmatic breathing.

4. If the patient is losing urine around the catheter and has a distended bladder (with or without bladder spasms), check the catheter and drainage tubing for evidence of obstruction. Inspect for kinks and obstructions in drainage tubing, compress and roll catheter gently between fingers to assess for gritty matter within catheter, milk drainage tubing to release obstructions, and/or instruct patient to turn from side to side. Obtain prescription for catheter irrigation if these measures fail to relieve the obstruction.

5. In nonrestricted patients, encourage intake of at least 2–3 L/day of fluids to help reduce frequency of spasms.

6. Instruct patient in the use of nonpharmacologic methods of pain relief such as guided imagery, relaxation techniques, and/or distraction.

See "Ureteral Calculi" for the following: **Potential impairment of skin integrity** (from wound drainage), p. 125. See "Appendix One" for nursing diagnoses and interventions for the care of preoperative and postoperative patients, pp. 528–532.

E. Patient–Family Teaching and Discharge Planning

Provide patient and SOs with verbal and written information for the following:

1. Medications, including drug name, dosage, purpose, schedule, precautions, and potential side effects.

2. Indicators that signal recurrent obstruction and require prompt medical attention: pain, fever, decreased urinary output.

3. Necessity of limiting activites during postoperative period.

4. Care of drains or catheters if patient is discharged with them; care of the surgical incision.

5. Indicators of *wound infection*: persistent redness, local warmth and tenderness, drainage, swelling; and *URI*: dysuria, flank or suprapubic pain, cloudy or foul-smelling urine, chills, and/or fever.

III. Cancer of the Bladder

Cancer of the bladder is the second most common form of urinary system cancer. Causes are not clearly understood, but industrial exposure to certain chemicals such as b-naphthylamine is believed to be a factor, as is smoking and the consumption of large amounts of coffee and saccharin.

Bladder cancer often begins in the bladder lumen, but the bladder neck and ureteral orifices also can be involved. Cellular proliferation can occur throughout the transitional epithelium that lines the kidneys, ureters, and mucosa of the bladder. Metastasis can appear in the lymph nodes and spread to the bones, liver, and lungs.

A. Assessment

Signs and symptoms: Dysuria, painless hematuria, burning with urination. Depending on tumor size, the patient may experience suprapubic pain. If the tumor causes urinary obstruction, see "Urinary Tract Obstruction," p. 126, for further data.

Physical exam: Presence of a mass, which may be palpated by using both hands on the abdomen in an effort to feel the outline of the tumor.

B. Diagnostic Tests

1. Urinalysis, urine culture, IVP: See "Ureteral Calculi," p. 122, for a discussion of these tests.

2. Urine cytology: To assess for abnormal cells.

3. WBC, Hgb, and Hct: To check for presence of infection, bleeding, and anemia.

4. Alkaline phosphatase test: To assess for metastasis to the bones.

5. Biopsy in conjunction with cystoscopy: A cystoscope is inserted through the urethra and into the bladder to visualize the structures. If abnormalities are seen, a section of the tissue is removed for biopsy. Because the procedure is very uncomfortable under a local anesthetic, general anesthesia is usually used.

6. Cystogram (cystography): To outline tumors that are present in the bladder. A radiopaque medium is introduced into the bladder via a urethral catheter. X-rays are taken both before and after urination.

C. Medical Management and Surgical Interventions

1. **Grading and staging the disease:** To formulate a prognosis and guide treatment. The degree of grading and staging is determined by the extent of metastasis and tissue involvement: the greater the metastasis, the higher the grade and stage.

2. **Chemotherapy:** Methotrexate, doxorubicin, fluorouracil, cyclophospha-mide, mitomycin C, and cisplatin may be used. Intravesical chemotherapy, which is used for superficial bladder cancers, involves instillation of medica-tion into the bladder via an indwelling catheter.

3. **Palliative radiation therapy:** Used primarily in the late stages for pain relief, but it also can be used early in treatment.

4. **Radon seeds:** May be implanted around the base of the tumor in an attempt to eradicate the bladder tumor and prevent regrowth. Typically, this is done after a transurethral resection (TUR) and fulguration of the bladder tumor. Severe cystitis is likely to occur from the irradiation.

5. **Supervoltage radiation therapy:** Often used in conjunction with surgery or chemotherapy to shrink very large tumors or for pain relief if the cancer has metastasized widely.

6. **Pharmacotherapy**

   □ *Analgesics and narcotics:* For pain relief.

   □ *Antibiotics:* For therapy-induced infections.

7. **TUR and fulguration:** Removal of the tumor with electrocautery via cysto-scope and resectoscope.

8. **Segmental resection:** Performed if the dome of the bladder is involved. The top half of the bladder is removed via an abdominal incision.

9. **Urinary diversion:** See p. 131 for discussion.

D. Nursing Diagnoses and Interventions

Potential alterations in fluid volume: *Excess* related to retention secondary to irriga-tion; *Deficit* related to loss secondary to postsurgical hemorrhage (after TUR or seg-mental resection)

Desired outcomes: Patient does not exhibit signs of dehydration or fluid overload. Hemorrhage and electrolyte imbalance are detected and reported promptly.

1. Monitor and record VS and I&O; record color and consistency of catheter drainage at least q8h. Drainage may be dark red after surgery, but it should lighten to pink or blood-tinged within 24 hours. **Note:** Patients with a TUR may have clots passing through the drainage tubing. Continuous bladder irri-gation (CBI) is often used to flush bloody drainage from the bladder to pre-vent clot formation, which can occlude the urethral catheter.

2. Be alert to hypotension and rapid pulse rate, and watch for bright-red, thick drainage or drainage that does not lighten after irrigation, either of which can signal arterial bleeding within the operative area and necessitate immedi-ate surgical intervention.

3. Monitor TUR patient's postoperative mental status, being alert to changes in mentation such as confusion, which can denote a change in electrolyte bal-ance and necessitate medical attention. Water intoxification and hypona-tremia can occur because of the high volumes of irrigation fluid that are used with a TUR.

Potential for infection related to vulnerability secondary to presence of suprapubic catheter and opening of a closed drainage system

Desired outcome: Patient does not exhibit signs of infection.

1. Using aseptic technique, cleanse the area surrounding the suprapubic cathe-ter with an antimicrobial solution such as povidone-iodine. Apply sterile 4×4 gauze pad(s) over the catheter exit site and tape securely. Change the dress-ing as soon as it becomes wet, and use a pectin wafer skin barrier to protect the insertion site if indicated. **Note:** If a trocar system is used, clean around

the plastic cover and keep the area dry. Tape the plastic edges securely to the skin to prevent accidental removal.

2. Wash hands *before* and *after* manipulating the catheter, and use aseptic technique when opening the closed drainage system, changing dressings, and irrigating the catheter.

3. Irrigate catheter *only* if there is an obstruction and by MD prescription.

4. Protect the catheter by keeping it securely taped to the patient's lateral abdomen.

5. If the catheter is accidentally pulled out of the insertion site, immediately cover the site with a sterile 4×4 and notify MD.

6. To keep urine dilute to help prevent UTI, encourage a fluid intake of at least 2–3 L/day in nonrestricted patients.

7. Keep the drainage collection container below the level of the patient's bladder to prevent infection from reflux of urine.

Potential alteration in pattern of urinary elimination related to obstruction of suprapubic catheter or anuria/dysuria secondary to removal of catheter

Desired outcomes: Patient's urinary output is appropriate for the amount of intake. Patient denies discomfort before and after removal of the suprapubic catheter.

1. Keep drainage from suprapubic catheter separate from that of other catheters and drains.

2. Prevent external obstruction of the catheter, assessing frequently for patency. Irrigate *only* if internally obstructed and with MD order.

3. Before removal of suprapubic catheter, MD may request a 3–4 hour clamping routine to assess patient's ability to void normally. After patient has voided, unclamp the catheter and measure the residual urine that flows into the drainage collection container. Once the residual urine is <100 mL after each of two successive voidings, notify MD. Usually the catheter can be removed at that time.

4. After removal of the catheter, evaluate patient's ability to void by recording the time and amount during the first 24 hours. Patients with segmental resections will void frequently and in small amounts at first because the bladder capacity is approximately 60 mL. Explain to the patient the bladder will expand to 200–400 mL within a few months.

5. If patient cannot void 8–12 hours after catheter removal and experiences abdominal pain or has a distended bladder, notify MD for intervention.

6. If patient experiences burning with urination, encourage an increased intake of fluids and apply heat over the bladder area with a warm blanket, heating pad, or sitz bath, any of which will increase circulation to the area and relax the muscles.

See "Urinary Tract Obstruction" for the following: **Alteration in comfort**: Pain related to bladder spasms, p. 127. See "Appendix One" for nursing diagnoses and interventions for the care of preoperative and postoperative patients, pp. 528–532; and the care of patients with cancer and other life-disrupting illnesses, pp. 544–551.

E. Patient–Family Teaching and Discharge Planning

See discussion in "Urinary Tract Obstruction," p. 128.

▶ Section Six **Urinary Diversions**

A. Surgical Interventions

Cystectomy is the complete removal of the bladder and is a radical treatment for bladder neoplasm. After a cystectomy, the urine produced by the kidneys must be channeled by a urinary diversion, of which there are three types.

Ureterosigmoidostomy: The ureters are resected from the bladder and implanted into the sigmoid colon, allowing the urine to pass with the feces through the rectum. With this procedure there is no stoma, and consequently, no external appliance is required.

Ileal conduit: This is the most frequently performed diversion. A 15–20 cm section of the ileum is resected from the intestine to form a passageway for the urine. The proximal end is closed and the distal end is brought out through the abdomen, forming a stoma. The ureters are resected from the bladder and anastomosed to the ileal segment. After anastomosis, the intestine continues to function normally.

Cutaneous ureterostomy: The ureters are resected from the bladder and brought out through the surface of the abdomen either separately, or with one attached to the other inside the body, resulting in only one abdominal stoma. Typically, the stoma is flush with the abdomen rather than protruding.

▶ **Note:** For a discussion of bladder cancer, see p. 128.

B. Nursing Diagnoses and Interventions

Alteration in bowel elimination related to disruption of normal function secondary to ureterosigmoidostomy

Desired outcomes: Patient with ureterosigmoidostomy can demonstrate procedure for insertion of rectal tube and verbalize knowledge of foods that may result in incontinence of urine and/or feces.

1. Auscultate patient's abdomen for bowel sounds and assess for distention q8h, measure abdominal girth daily, and document findings. Bowel sounds should reappear within 48–72 hours of surgery. Notify MD of significant findings.

2. After ureterosigmoidostomy, the patient will have a rectal tube.

    □ Monitor output from tube. Expect to see drainage that is fecal and/or blood–tinged. A lack of output can signal an obstruction of the tube; notify MD accordingly.

    □ Irrigate the rectal tube *only* with MD prescription, with no more than 20–30 mL normal saline. Use gentle pressure to avoid damaging the ureteral attachment to the sigmoid colon.

    □ Usually during the first four postoperative days, only the surgeon removes and replaces the rectal tube. After this period of time, if the patient needs to have a bowel movement and the rectal tube is still in place, remove the tube cautiously and replace it after the patient has finished. **Caution:** Never insert the tube more than 10 cm (4 inches) into the rectum because the anastomosis is usually 15–20 cm from the anus.

    □ Before the patient's discharge from the hospital, teach the technique for rectal tube insertion for drainage of urine during the night.

    □ Inform the patient that gas-forming foods such as beans or cabbage should be avoided because the resulting flatulence can cause incontinence of urine and/or feces.

□ Inform the patient that stools will be soft and diarrhea-like because of urine in the colon.

Potential for injury related to alterations in mentation and/or motor function secondary to reabsorption of electrolytes through the urinary diversion (ureterosigmoidostomy) or loss of sodium and potassium (ileal conduit)

Desired outcome: Patient does not exhibit signs of injury caused by mentation or motor dysfunction.

1. For patients with ureterosigmoidostomies, electrolytes are easily reabsorbed or passed to the urine from the urinary diversion. The longer the contact of urine with the mucosa, the greater are the risks for electrolyte imbalance. For these patients, assess for the following:

    □ *Hyperchloremic acidosis:* Nausea, vomiting, irregular pulse, muscle weakness, tachypnea, lethargy, diarrhea.

    □ *Reabsorption dehydration:* Thirst, headache, increased urinary outpt.

    □ *Hypokalemia:* Irregular pulse, anorexia, lethargy, confusion, flaccid paralysis.

    □ *Metabolic acidosis:* Apathy, disorientation, weakness, Kussmaul's respirations.

2. For patients with ureterosigmoidostomies whose rectal tubes and ureteral catheters have been removed, encourage rectal evacuation at least q4h to minimize the absorption of urinary electrolytes through the colonic mucosa.

3. For patients with ileal conduits, assess for indicators of hypokalemia and hyponatremia, including changes in LOC (from sleepy to combative), muscle tone (convulsions to flaccidity), and changes in heart rate.

4. If patient is confused or exhibits signs of motor dysfunction, keep the bed in the lowest position and raise the siderails. Notify MD of significant findings.

5. Encourage oral intake as directed, and assess for the need for IV management. MD may prescribe IV fluids with potassium supplements.

6. If patient is hypokalemic and allowed to eat, encourage foods high in potassium, such as bananas, cantaloupes, and apricots. See Table 3-2, p. 96, for a list of foods that are high in potassium.

7. Encourage patient to ambulate by the 2nd or 3rd day after surgery. Mobility will help prevent urinary stasis, which increases the risk of electrolyte problems.

Potential for infection related to vulnerability secondary to invasive procedures, reflux of feces into the urinary tract, and contact of pouch with the suture line

Desired outcome: Patient does not exhibit signs of infection.

1. To help prevent contamination and cross-contamination, wash your hands before and after caring for the patient.

2. Patients with cystectomies may have an indwelling urethral catheter to drain serosanguinous fluid from the peritoneal cavity. **Caution:** Do not irrigate this catheter because irrigation can result in peritonitis.

3. Monitor the patient's temperature q4h during the first 24–48 hours after surgery. Notify MD of fever spikes. **Caution:** Do not measure the temperature rectally for a patient with a ureterosigmoidostomy, as this can damage the anastomosis site.

4. Inspect the dressing q4h during the first 24–48 hours after surgery. Assess for the presence of stool or purulent drainage on the dressing; notify MD if these are noted. Change the dressing when it becomes wet, using sterile technique. Use extra care to prevent disruption of the drains.

5. Note the condition of the incision. Be alert to indicators of infection, including redness, tenderness, local warmth, puffiness, and purulent drainage.

6. Monitor and record the character of the urine at least q8h. Mucous particles are normal in the urine of patients with ileal conduits and ureterosigmoid-ostomies because of the nature of the bowel segment used. Cloudy urine, however, is abnormal and can signal an infection. The urine should be yellow or pink–tinged during the first 24 hours after surgery. Assess for other indicators of UTI, including flank pain, chills, and fever. The patient with a ureterosigmoidostomy is especially susceptible to UTI because of the increased risk of reflux of feces into the urinary tract.

7. Note the position of the stoma to the incision. If they are close together, apply the pouch first to avoid the overlap of the pouch with the suture line. If necessary, cut the pouch down on one side, or place it at an angle to avoid contact with drainage, which may loosen the adhesive.

8. Encourage a fluid intake of at least 2–3 L/day as this helps flush urine through the urinary tract, preventing stasis. Encourage the patient to drink cranberry, prune, or plum juices, which leave an acid ash in the urine and lower the pH to help prevent infection.

Potential fluid volume deficit related to abnormal blood loss secondary to surgical procedure

Desired outcome: Patient does not exhibit signs of excessive bleeding or hypovolemia.

1. Note the amount and character of the drainage at least q4h. Initially it will be reddish in color, with only small amounts of urine. Serosanguinous drainage should continue for 3–4 days.

2. Be alert to the presence of gross hematuria, along with decreasing BP, tachycardia, and tachypnea, which can signal hemorrhage.

3. Report significant findings to the MD.

Potential impairment of skin integrity: Stoma and peristomal area related to erythema, improper appliance, or sensitivity to appliance material

Desired outcomes: Patient does not exhibit signs of peristomal or stomal irritation or breakdown. Patient can verbalize knowledge of factors that may injure the skin or stoma and can demonstrate the technique for pouch change and skin care before hospital discharge.

1. Patch-test the patient's skin for a 24-hour period, at least 24 hours before ostomy surgery to assess for allergies to the different tapes that might be used on the postoperative appliance. If redness, swelling, itching, weeping, or other indicators of tape allergy occur, document the type of tape that caused the reaction and note on the cover of the chart "Allergic to _____ tape."

2. Patients with urinary diversions, except for those with ureterosigmoid-ostomies, will have a pouch when they return from surgery. For the first 24 hours, remove the pouch from the faceplate at least q shift and inspect the stoma and peristomal skin. The color of the stoma should be pink or red–tinged. A stoma that is very pale or dark with a purple cast can signal impaired circulation and should be reported to the MD immediately. Also assess the degree of swelling, if present, and inform the patient that the stoma will shrink considerably over the first 6–8 weeks, and less significantly over the next year. Evaluate the height of the stoma and plan care accordingly. The stoma formed by a cutaneous ureterostomy is usually flush and more challenging to pouch.

3. Assess the integrity of the peristomal skin and question the patient about the presence of itching or burning. If leakage of urine has occurred, the skin will be inflamed and it will itch and burn. In the absence of leakage, the patient can wear the same postoperative pouch for 3–4 days.

4. Assess for inflamed hair follicles (folliculitis) or a reaction to the tape. Report the presence of a rash to the MD, since this often occurs with a yeast infection and will require topical medication.

5. When changing the pouch, measure the stoma with a measuring guide and ensure that the opening of the skin barrier is cut to the exact size of the stoma to protect the peristomal skin. The pouch opening should be ⅛ inch larger than the stoma to provide an adhesive seal with the skin barrier.

6. Wash the peristomal skin with water and a non-oily soap such as Ivory. An oily soap will prevent adequate adherence of the pouch. Dry the skin thoroughly before applying the skin barrier and pouch.

7. When changing the pouch, instruct the patient to hold a gauze pad on (but not in) the stoma to absorb the urine and protect the skin.

8. After applying the pouch, connect it to the bedside drainage system if the patient is on bed rest. When the patient is no longer on bed rest, empty the pouch by opening the spigot at the bottom of the pouch and draining the urine into the patient's measuring container. Do not allow the pouch to become too full as this could break the seal of the appliance with the patient's skin. Instruct the patient accordingly.

9. If the peristomal skin becomes irritated, expose it to air 20–30 min/day and dry it with a hair dryer on a "cool" setting. Instruct the patient to hold a gauze or tampon wick on the stoma to absorb the urine.

10. Change the incisional dressing as often as it becomes wet, using sterile technique.

11. Patients with ureterosigmoidostomies will require frequent inspections of the perianal area and careful skin care to prevent skin breakdown caused by the drainage of urine and feces.

Alteration in the pattern of urinary elimination related to postoperative use of catheters, stents, and/or rectal tube

Desired outcomes: Patient's urinary output is within acceptable limits. Patients with ureterosigmoidostomies can demonstrate self-insertion of the rectal tube for rectal evacuation and can verbalize knowledge of the rationale for not advancing the tube farther than 10 cm into the rectum.

1. Check for the presence of stents or ureteral catheters that protrude from the stoma into the pouch and label them "right" or "left" as appropriate. These stents maintain the patency of the ureters and assist in the healing of the anastomosis by keeping it urine-free. The MD will remove them around the fifth postoperative day. After removal, assess for indicators of ureteral obstruction: flank pain, nausea, vomiting, anuria.

2. Monitor I&O, and record the amount of urine output from the urinary diversion q2h for the first 24 hours postoperatively. Notify the MD of an output less than 60 mL during a 2-hour period because in the presence of adequate intake this can indicate a ureteral blockage, a leak in the urinary diversion, or impending renal failure.

3. To keep the urinary tract well irrigated, encourage an intake of at least 2–3 L/day in the nonrestricted patient.

4. For patients with ureterosigmoidostomies, anuria may result from obstruction by feces. If this occurs notify the MD. Usually, only the MD removes the tube during the first four postoperative days. At around the 7th day, the rectal tube is removed. Instruct the patient to empty the rectum q2–3h. The patient should be aware of rectal pressure, and will begin to note the difference between pressure caused by urine and that caused by feces. Teach the patient self-insertion of the rectal tube to prevent urinary incontinence at night. Because the anastomosis is only 15–20 cm (6–8 inches) from the anus, caution the patient about advancing the tube into the rectum farther than 10 cm (4 inches).

5. Be alert to oliguria in the presence of an adequate intake, paralytic ileus, abdominal distention, and patient complaints of abdominal discomfort, any of which can signal leakage of urine at the attachment of the ureters to the colon. If these occur, notify MD immediately.

See "Fecal Diversions" in Chapter 6 for the following: **Disturbance in self-concept** (related to alteration in body image), p. 317. See "Appendix One" for nursing diagnoses and interventions for the care of preoperative and postoperative patients, pp. 528–532, and for the care of patients with cancer and other life-disrupting illnesses, pp. 544–551.

C. Patient–Family Teaching and Discharge Planning

Provide patient and SOs with verbal and written information for the following:

1. Medications, including drug name, dosage, schedule, precautions, and potential side effects.

2. Indicators that necessitate medical intervention: fever, nausea, vomiting, cloudy urine, or abnormal changes in stoma shape or color.

3. Information regarding community resources, including local United Ostomy Association, the American Cancer Society, and an enterostomal therapy (ET) nurse in the area, if appropriate.

4. Maintenance of fluid intake of at least 2–3 L/day, including fruit juices made of cranberries, plums, and prunes, which acidify the urine and help prevent infection.

5. Care of stoma and application of urostomy appliances. The patient should be proficient in the application technique before discharge.

▶ Section Seven   **Urinary Disorders Secondary to Other Disease Processes**

I. Urinary Incontinence

Urinary incontinence is the physiologic or psychologic inability to control urine. Usually it results from an interruption in the signal from the musculature and sphincter of the bladder as it transmits through the spinal cord to the brain. General causes include diminished cerebral functioning, UTI, bladder weakness, medications (eg, anticholinergic drugs), and interference with the urethrobladder reflex. Diseases and trauma that can cause incontinence include cerebrovascular accident (CVA), traumatic brain injury, and meningitis. With stress incontinence, which occurs as the result of a weakness of the musculature and sphincter of the bladder, there is loss of urine with sneezing, laughing, coughing, or any other Valsalva-type activity. Urinary incontinence occurs most frequently in individuals over age 65.

A. Assessment

Signs and symptoms: Polyuria; dysuria; low back or flank pain; loss of urine with laughing, sneezing, coughing; inability to hold urine once the urge to void is felt; loss of urine without awareness of it.

History of: Recent CVA or cerebral injury, diminishing cerebral functioning, use of anticholinergic drugs.

B. Diagnostic Tests

1. <u>Urinalysis, urine culture, BUN, serum creatinine, and creatinine clearance:</u> To evaluate renal–urinary function and assess for infection.

2. <u>Urodynamic studies (urine flow studies, cystometry, pelvic floor sphincter electromyography, and urethral pressure measurement):</u> To evaluate cause and extent of the incontinence.

C. Medical Management and Surgical Interventions

1. **Bladder training program:** Focuses on emptying bladder at set times.

2. **Catheter drainage of urine:** Either intermittent or continuous.

3. **Kegel exercise program:** To increase strength of perineal muscles.

4. **Fluid intake:** At least 2–3 L/day in nonrestricted patients.

5. **External (condom) catheter:** For male patients, if appropriate.

6. **Marshall-Marchetti-Krantz procedure:** For stress incontinence. Via suprapubic transverse incision, the bladder is elevated in the abdominal cavity to lengthen the urethra, thereby creating resistence in the urethral lumen.

7. **Pereya procedure:** Same as that described above, but uses both vaginal and suprapubic approach.

8. **Artificial urinary sphincter:** See discussion in "Neurogenic Bladder," p. 140.

D. Nursing Diagnoses and Interventions

Potential impairment of skin integrity related to irritation of perineum secondary to incontinence of urine

Desired outcomes: Patient does not exhibit signs of impaired perineal skin integrity. Patient can verbalize knowledge of the rationale and importance for maintaining dryness and notifying staff as soon as wetness occurs.

1. Assess the patient for wetness of the perineal area at frequent intervals. Inform the patient that prolonged exposure to urine can cause excoriation and that staff should be alerted as soon as wetness occurs.

2. Keep bed linen dry. As necessary, use and change absorbent materials such as adult diapers or underpads.

3. Keep the perineum clean with mild soap and/or water; dry it well.

4. Expose the perineum to air whenever possible by using a sheet draped over a bed cradle; ensure the patient's privacy.

5. Make sure that plastic pads or sheet protectors do not contact the patient's skin directly because maceration can result from the increased perspiration they cause. Cover these pads with pillow cases or place them under the sheets.

6. Sprinkle cornstarch into patient's skin folds, but do not allow it to accumulate and cake into moisture-holding lumps.

Disturbance in self-concept related to odor and discomfort secondary to incontinence

Desired outcomes: Patient verbalizes feelings and frustrations without self-deprecating statements. Patient can verbalize knowledge of actions that will either control incontinence or control odor and discomfort.

1. Encourage patient to discuss feelings and frustrations. Allow sufficient time.

2. Offer reassurance and encouragement and provide information regarding treatment, especially about those activities that are within the patient's own control.

3. Be realistic with the patient; if incontinence cannot be controlled, reassure patient that odor and discomfort *can* be.

4. Explore with patient the methods for relief of discomfort and odor control: maintenance of good hygiene, frequent changes of undergarments, use and frequent changes of incontinence pads.

5. Although fluid intake of at least $2-3$ L/day is essential for minimizing the risk of UTI, suggest that the patient limit fluids when away from the home environment and increase them upon return. A decrease also should be incorporated into the evening hours to prevent nighttime incontinence.

Knowledge deficit: Procedure for bladder training and/or Kegel exercise programs

Desired outcome: Patient can verbalize and demonstrate knowledge of bladder training and/or Kegel exercise programs.

Bladder training program:

1. Assist patient with scheduling times for emptying the bladder, such as q1–2h when awake and q4h at night. If successful, attempt to lengthen the time intervals between voiding. Provide patient with a written copy of the schedule.

2. Teach patient to drink measured amounts of fluids about q2h and then attempt to void 30 minutes later. In nonrestricted patients, encourage a fluid intake of at least $2-3$ L/day.

3. For bedridden patients, keep call light within patient's reach and answer call quickly.

4. If patient is confused, attempt to reorient by keeping clock and calendar in room and reminding patient of the time and date.

Kegel exercise program to strengthen perineal muscles:

1. Instruct patient to tense perineal muscles by pressing the buttocks together, holding the position for at least 5 seconds, and relaxing. This exercise should be repeated $10-20$ times an hour. Remind patient that this exercise can be done anywhere.

2. Instruct patient to attempt to shut off urinary flow after beginning urination, hold for a few seconds, and then start the stream again.

Knowledge deficit: Use of external (condom) catheter

Desired outcome: Patient and/or SO can successfully return demonstration of condom catheter application and verbalize knowledge of the rationale for its use.

1. Instruct male patients and/or SO in the procedure for application of a condom catheter.

2. Teach the importance of keeping pubic hair trimmed or moved away from the penis to avoid contact with the adhesive used with the catheter.

3. Instruct patient to cleanse and dry the penis thoroughly before and after every condom application. With uncircumcised patients, the foreskin should be retracted to cleanse the area under the prepuce, and then returned to its original position.

4. For ambulatory patients, demonstrate connecting the condom catheter to a leg drainage bag; for patients on bed rest, demonstrate connecting the catheter to a bedside urinary collection container such as that used with an indwelling catheter.

5. Advise patient to remove and replace the catheter as directed. Most manufacturers recommend that external catheters be changed and replaced daily.

6. If appropriate for the patient, suggest that the condom catheter be used only during the night.

For surgical patients, see "Appendix One" for nursing diagnoses and interventions for the care of preoperative and postoperative patients, pp. $528-532$.

E. Patient–Family Teaching and Discharge Planning

Provide patient and SOs with verbal and written information for the following:

1. Medications, including drug name, dosage, purpose, schedule, precautions, and potential side effects.

2. Indicators that necessitate medical attention: fever, chills, cloudy or foul-smelling urine, hematuria, increasing or recurring incontinence.

3. Care of the incision, including cleansing and dressing, and indicators of infection: purulent drainage, persistent redness, swelling, warmth along incision line.

4. Care of catheters and/or drains if the patient is discharged with them.

5. Importance of maintaining fluid intake of at least 2–3 L/day.

6. Maintenance of schedule for bladder training program.

7. Use of perineal muscles to improve bladder tone.

8. Care of perineal skin.

9. Activity precautions for surgical patient: avoiding heavy lifting (>5 lb) and resting when fatigued. Explain that prolonged periods of sitting can cause relaxation of the musculature of the bladder and sphincter, leading to incontinence. Encourage mild activity such as walking to improve muscle tone.

II. Urinary Retention

When urine is produced and accumulates in the bladder but is not released, the condition is called urinary retention. The major cause is obstruction, for example, from benign obstructive hypertrophy, tumor, calculi, urethral stricture, fibrosis, or meatal stenosis. Other causes include decreased sensory stimulation to the bladder, anxiety, or muscular tension. Medications such as opiates, sedatives, antihistamines, antispasmodics, major tranquilizers and antidepressants, and antidyskinetics also can interfere with the normal micturition reflex.

A. Assessment

Signs and symptoms: Sudden inability to void, intense suprapubic pain, restlessness, diaphoresis, voiding small amounts (20–50 mL) at frequent intervals.

Physical exam: "Kettle drum" sound with bladder percussion, bladder distention, bladder displacement to one side of the abdomen.

B. Diagnostic Tests

1. Urinalysis, urine culture, serum electrolytes, BUN, serum creatinine, KUB, and IVP: All may be performed to evaluate renal–urinary function and structure and assess for infection and other problems.

2. Cystometrograms: To evaluate the neuromusculature of the bladder by measuring the efficiency of the detrusor muscle reflex, intravesical pressure and capacity, and the bladder's reaction to thermal stimulation. During this procedure the patient voids into a funnel attached to a machine that graphically measures the amount, time, and flow of voiding.

C. Medical Management

1. **Catheterization:** For drainage of urine.

2. **Pharmacotherapy**

   ☐ *Cholinergics:* To stimulate bladder contractions.

   ☐ *Analgesia:* For pain relief.

   ☐ *Antibiotics:* If infection is present.

3. **IV therapy:** For hydration of the acutely ill patient.

4. **Serial urine and serum electrolyte testing:** For ongoing evaluation of electrolyte and osmolality status.

5. **Surgery:** Performed if obstruction is the cause of the retention. (See "Urinary Tract Obstruction," p. 126.)

D. Nursing Diagnoses and Interventions

Alteration in pattern of urinary elimination related to acute retention

Desired outcomes: Patient can empty the bladder, optimally via noninvasive measures. If intermittent cathterization is performed, the patient remains free of infection and injury from rapid bladder decompression. If appropriate, the patient can successfully demonstrate self-catheterization.

1. Assess the bladder for distention by inspection, percussion, and/or palpation; measure and document I&O.

2. If appropriate, try noninvasive measures for release of urine: Have patient listen to the sound of running water or place hands in a basin of warm water. If these measures are ineffective, try pouring warm water over the perineum. Unless contraindicated, the *Crede* maneuver (pressure applied from the umbilicus to the pubis) may be used to stimulate a weak micturitional reflex.

3. Notify MD if patient is unable to void, has bladder distention, and/or has suprapubic or urethral pain.

4. If catheterization is prescribed, maintain aseptic technique and ensure that the bladder is slowly decompressed to prevent acute fluid and electrolyte imbalance, shock, and/or hemorrhage. Allow no more than 800-1000 mL of urine to drain during the first 5 minutes by clamping the catheter; unclamp after 15–30 minutes. For more information, see **Potential fluid volume deficit** related to excessive urinary loss and/or hemorrhage secondary to rapid bladder decompression, in "Urinary Tract Obstruction," p. 127.

5. Catheterization may be difficult beyond the prostate gland in men with benign prostatic hypertrophy. If this occurs, notify MD for intervention.

6. Teach patient the technique for intermittent self-catheterization, if appropriate. Catheterization should be accomplished on a set q4h schedule to prevent bladder distention, which can injure the bladder mucosa and increase the risk of infection. Teach the patient clean technique for use at home.

See "Urinary Tract Obstruction" for the following: **Alteration in comfort**, p. 127. See "Caring for Preoperative and Postoperative Patients" in "Appendix One" for **Potential for infection**, p. 532, for interventions for the care of patients with indwelling urethral catheters.

E. Patient–Family Teaching and Discharge Planning

Provide patient and SOs with verbal and written information for the following:

1. Medications, including drug name, purpose, dosage, schedule, precautions, and potential side effects.

2. Indicators that necessitate medical attention, including suprapubic or urethral pain, fever, recurring or increasing difficulty with voiding.

3. Self-catheterization technique, if appropriate.

III. Neurogenic Bladder

Neurogenic bladder is a bladder dysfunction caused by a congenital abnormality, injury, or neurologic disorder. Common disorders associated with this condition include multiple sclerosis, diabetic neuropathy, poliomyelitis, and spinal cord injury. When neurogenic bladder is caused by a lower motor neuron defect the bladder is flaccid, which can lead to bladder distention, infection caused by urinary stasis and bladder distention, and kidney infections. Upper motor neuron lesions can cause a spastic bladder, which results in urinary frequency.

A. Assessment

Signs and symptoms: Acute retention, lack of urinary control, dribbling of urine, presence of bladder calculi, recurrent UTIs.

History of: Spinal cord injury, spinal tumor, multiple sclerosis, diabetes mellitus.

B. Diagnostic Tests

Urinalysis, urine cultures, cystoscopy, IVP, cystography, BUN, serum creatinine, creatinine clearance: All may be used to evaluate renal–urinary structures and function.

C. Medical Management and Surgical Interventions

1. Pharmacotherapy

☐ *Anticholinergics such as propantheline bromide and oxybutynin chloride:* To treat hyperreflexive neurologic conditions.

☐ *Parasympathomimetics such as bethanechol chloride:* To treat hypotonic bladders.

☐ *Alpha-adrenergics such as phentolamine:* To treat spastic bladders.

☐ *Sympathomimetics such as ephedrine:* To improve bladder-neck and urethral tone.

☐ *Antibiotics:* For infection, if indicated.

2. Catheterization: Either intermittent or continuous.

3. Increase fluid intake: To prevent infection, minimize calcium concentration in urine, and prevent formation of urinary calculi.

4. Increase patient mobility: To augment renal blood flow and minimize urinary stasis.

5. Low-calcium diet: To prevent calculus formation.

6. Continent vesicostomy: Surgical closure of urethral neck of bladder to form an internal reservoir for urine and create an opening or valve in bladder wall so that patient can insert a catheter intermittently to remove urine.

7. Artificial urinary sphincter implantation: Surgical placement of a hydraulically activated sphincter mechanism around the bladder neck or urethra. To empty the bladder, patient activates the device by squeezing the bulbs, which are implanted under the labia or scrotum.

D. Nursing Diagnoses and Interventions

Alteration in pattern of urinary elimination related to retention (or frequency) secondary to bladder dysfunction

Desired outcomes: Patient is able to empty the bladder via an appropriate method. Patient and SO are able to verbalize rationale for the importance of urinary release and, if appropriate, can demonstrate procedure for same. Nonrestricted patients can verbalize knowledge of the rationale for a fluid intake of at least 2–3 L/day as well as the importance of increasing mobility as their condition warrants.

1. During admission history, assess the patient's ability to void. Ask about urinary history, such as past and present voiding patterns, difficulty with controlling or starting stream, awareness of the need to void, quantity of urine, and fluid intake in relation to voiding (time of intake and amount, time of voiding and amount).

2. Assess I&O, inspect the suprapubic area, and percuss and palpate the bladder for evidence of retention; document. Be alert to the presence of swelling above the level of the symphysis pubis, "kettle-drum" sound with percussion, and dribbling of urine.

3. As appropriate, teach the patient techniques that stimulate the voiding reflex, eg, tapping the suprapubic area with the fingers, pulling the pubic hair, or digitally stretching the anal sphincter. The latter is effective because the rectal nerves follow a path that is basically the same as that of the urethral nerves; however, it is contraindicated in patients with spinal cord injuries at or above T6 because it can cause autonomic dysreflexia. The Valsalva maneuver also can be used to stimulate voiding: The patient bears down as though having a bowel movement to increase intrathoracic and intra-abdominal pressure.

4. If an artificial inflatable sphincter is used, instruct the patient to deflate the valve q4h, which allows the bladder to empty. Remind the patient to wear a Medic-Alert tag or bracelet to alert emergency personnel to the presence and use of the device.

5. If a condom catheter is used, see **Knowledge deficit**: Use of external (condom) catheter, in "Urinary Incontinence," p. 137, for appropriate nursing interventions.

6. For males with extensive sphincter damage, a Cunningham (penile) clamp might be prescribed. Before and after use, instruct patient (or SO) to cleanse the penis with soap and water, dry it thoroughly, and sprinkle powder along the shaft. Explain that the clamp is placed horizontally behind the glans after voiding, and removed q4h. Stress the importance of inspecting the skin for redness along the area in which the clamp presses. If breakdown occurs (redness does not disappear after massage), use of the clamp must be discontinued. If swelling appears along the glans, advise patient to set the clamp at a looser setting. **Caution:** Minimize the potential for injury by alternating the clamp with a condom catheter.

7. If intermittent catheterization is prescribed, teach the procedure to the patient and/or SOs. Emphasize the necessity of following a routine, for example, q4h to minimize the potential for UTI caused by stasis and bladder distention.

8. If the *Crede* maneuver is prescribed, patients with arm and hand strength should be taught the procedure as an alternative to self-catheterization: Place the ulnar surface of the hand horizontally along the umbilicus; while bearing down with the abdominal muscles, press the hand downward and toward the bladder in a kneading motion until urination is initiated; continue q30 seconds until urination ceases.

9. Autonomic dysreflexia is a life-threatening condition that can occur in patients with neurogenic bladder, especially in those with spinal cord injuries at or above level T6. Be alert to the following indicators of this condition: headache, bradycardia, excessively high BP, blurred vision, flushing above the level of injury, and nausea. If signs of autonomic dysreflexia occur, assess for bladder distention and have the patient empty the bladder and/or rectum in the accustomed manner, or check for patency of the indwelling catheter. **Caution:** Do not irrigate the catheter because this increases bladder pressure and may exacerbate the condition. Give appropriate medications as prescribed, such as phenoxybenzamine hydrochloride, a long-acting vasodilator that increases blood flow to the skin, mucosae, and abdominal viscera and lowers both supine and erect BP. Notify MD if symptoms do not disappear after the bladder or rectum is emptied, if the bladder or rectum is full and cannot be emptied, or if the medication does not relieve symptoms. For further information see **Potential for injury** related to risk of autonomic dysreflexia, in "Spinal Cord Injury," p. 173.

10. Encourage a fluid intake of at least 2–3 L/day, which dilutes the urine and increases output, thereby minimizing the risk of developing an infection and calculi. Inform the patient that cranberry, plum, and prune juices leave an acid ash in the urine, inhibiting bacterial growth.

11. To help prevent urinary stasis, which can lead to UTI, and to increase cardiac output, which nourishes the kidneys, encourage as much mobility as the patient can tolerate.

Knowledge deficit: Care of long-term indwelling catheters after continent vesicostomy

Desired outcomes: Patient can verbalize knowledge of the rationale for the use of a suprapubic catheter and vesicostomy tube, including the approximate amount of time they will be indwelling. Patient and/or SO can demonstrate procedures such as tube irrigation and dressing changes.

1. Preoperatively, explain that the patient will return from surgery with a suprapubic catheter and vesicostomy tube in place.

2. Explain that the patient will be discharged with the catheter and readmitted for catheter removal in approximately 6 weeks. After removal of the indwelling catheter, intermittent catheterization will be performed hourly, progress to 2–4h, and ultimately to 4–6 hours. Continuous drainage will be used overnight.

3. Encourage patient's participation in care, including tube irrigation and dressing changes. Explain that backflow is normal and ensures patency of the tube. Demonstrate the procedure for irrigation once it has been prescribed. Typically, sterile normal saline (30–50 mL) is used for irrigation. Instruct the patient to wash hands before handling the catheters to help prevent contamination, and to cleanse around catheter site daily with an antimicrobial solution such as povidone-iodine.

As appropriate, see "Urinary Incontinence" for the following: **Potential impairment of skin integrity** related to irritation of perineum, p. 136, and **Disturbance in self-concept** related to odor and discomfort, p. 136.

E. Patient–Family Teaching and Discharge Planning

Provide patient and SOs with verbal and written information for the following:

1. For patients with artificial sphincters, the indicators of UTI and erosion: pain, swelling, urinary retention, or incontinence.

2. For other interventions, see discussion in "Urinary Incontinence," p. 138.

▶ Selected References

Balfe DM, McClellan BL: CT of the retroperitoneum in urosurgical disorders. *Surg Clin North Am* 1982; 62:919.

Binkley LS: Keeping up with peritoneal dialysis. *AJN* 1984; 84:729.

Broadwell DS, Jackson BS: *Principles of Ostomy Care.* Mosby, 1982.

Campbell JW, Frisse M (editors): *Manual of Medical Therapeutics*, 24th ed. Little, Brown, 1983.

Carpenito LJ: *Handbook of Nursing Diagnosis.* Lippincott, 1984.

Chambers JK: Bowel management in dialysis patients. *AJN* 1983; 83:1051.

Cianci J et al: Renal transplantation. *AJN* 1981; 81:354.

Fang LST: *Manual of Clinical Nephrology.* McGraw-Hill, 1983.

Flamenbaum W, Hamburger RJ: *Nephrology—An Approach to the Patient with Renal Disease.* Lippincott, 1982.

Hinker EA, Malasanos L (editors): *The Little Brown Manual of Medical-Surgical Nursing.* Little, Brown, 1983.

Houlihan, PJ: When your patient is a transplant recipient. *Canadian Nurse* 1982; 78:40.

Krupp MA, Chatton MJ (editors): *Current Medical Diagnosis and Treatment.* Lange, 1983.

Lerner J, Khan Z: *Mosby's Manual of Urologic Nursing.* Mosby, 1982.

Mars DR, Treloar D: Acute tubular necrosis—Pathophysiology and treatment. *Heart Lung* 1984; 13:194.

The Merck Manual of Diagnosis and Therapy, 14th ed. Merck, Sharp, and Dohme, 1982.

Methany N: Renal stones and urinary pH. *AJN* 1982; 82:1372.

Nissenson AR, Fine RN, Gentile DE (editors): *Clinical Dialysis.* Appleton-Century-Crofts, 1984.

Nurse's Clinical Library: *Renal and Urologic Disorders.* Springhouse, 1984.

Nurse's Reference Library Series. *Diagnostics.* Intermed, 1981.

Orr ML: Drugs and renal disease. *AJN* 1981; 81:969.

Pagana KD, Pagana TJ: *Diagnostic Testing and Nursing Implications: A Case Study Approach,* 2nd ed. Mosby, 1986.

Perinetti EP: Palliative urinary diversion. *Surg Clin North Am* 1982; 62:1025.

Reckling JB: Safeguarding the renal transplant patient. *Nursing 82* 1982; 12:47.

Roberts B, Ring EJ: Current status of percutaneous transluminal angioplasty. *Surg Clin North Am* 1982; 62:357.

Rose BD: *Pathophysiology of Renal Disease.* McGraw-Hill, 1981.

Saxton DF, et al: *The Addison-Wesley Manual of Nursing Practice.* Addison-Wesley, 1983.

Schrier RW (editor): *Manual of Nephrology.* Little, Brown, 1981.

Smith DR: *General Urology,* 10th ed. Lange, 1981.

Sorrels AJ: Peritoneal dialysis: A rediscovery. *Nurs Clin North Am* 1981; 16:515.

Surfin G: The challenge of renal adenocarcinoma. *Surg Clin North Am* 1982; 62:1101.

Swearingen PL: *The Addison-Wesley Photo-Atlas of Nursing Procedures.* Addison-Wesley, 1984.

Toner M: Urinary tract obstruction: The hidden threats in treatment. *RN* 1982; 45:58.

Whitehead DE, Leiter E: *Current Operative Urology,* 2nd ed. Harper and Row, 1984.

Wollam GL: Renovascular Hypertension. In: *Medicine for the Practicing Physician.* Hust JW (editor). Butterworth, 1983.

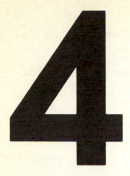
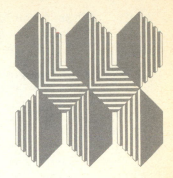

4

Neurologic Disorders

> ► Section One **Inflammatory Disorders of the Nervous System**

Inflammation of nervous system tissue results from a wide variety of causes, including bacterial or viral infections, autoimmune processes, and chemical toxins. The inflammatory response may cause increased vascular permeability with exudation of fluids from the vessels, resulting in swelling, which in turn can cause increased intracranial pressure (ICP).

I. Multiple Sclerosis

Multiple sclerosis (MS) is an inflammatory disorder of the central nervous system (CNS) myelin. In response to the inflammation, the myelin nerve sheaths peel off the axon cylinders. This demyelinization interrupts electric nerve transmission and causes the wide variety of symptoms associated with MS. If the myelin regenerates, electric nerve impulse transmission may be restored. Symptoms will decrease or disappear; that is, the patient may go into remission. If the inflammation is severe and causes irreversible destruction of myelin, the involved areas are replaced by dense glial scar tissue that forms areas of sclerotic plaque, which permanently damage the conductive pathways of the CNS.

Although the etiology of MS is unknown, slow-acting viral infections, allergic reactions to infectious agents such as viruses, and autoimmune processes are suspected causes. MS is 12–15 times more common among siblings of individuals who have the disease, suggesting a possible inheritance mechanism. Infection, trauma, and pregnancy are common precipitating factors, as are episodes of fatigue and physical or emotional stress. Heat and fever tend to aggravate symptoms.

A. Assessment

Onset of MS can be extremely rapid, causing disability within days, or it can be insidious, with exacerbations and prolonged remissions allowing an active life. Signs and symptoms vary widely, depending on the site and extent of demyelinization, and they can change from day to day. Usually, early symptoms are mild.

Signs and symptoms

□ *Damage to motor nerve tracts:* Weakness, paralysis, and/or spasticity. Fatigue is common. Diplopia may occur secondary to ocular muscle involvement.

□ *Damage to cerebellar or brain stem regions:* Intention tremor, nystagmus, or other tremors; uncoordination, ataxia; weakness of facial and throat muscles resulting in difficulty chewing, dysphagia, and dysarthria.

□ *Damage to sensory nerve tracts:* Decreased perception of pain, touch, and temperature; paresthesias such as numbness and tingling; decrease or loss of proprioception; and/or decrease or loss of vibratory sense. Optic neuritis may cause partial or total loss of vision.

□ *Damage to cerebral cortex (especially frontal lobes):* Mood swings, inappropriate affect, euphoria, apathy, irritability, depression, and/or hyperexcitability.

□ *Damage to motor and sensory control centers:* Urinary frequency, urgency, or retention; urinary and fecal incontinence; constipation.

□ *Sacral cord lesions:* Impotence; diminished sensations that result in inhibited sexual response.

Physical exam: Ophthalmoscopic inspection may reveal temporal pallor of optic disks. Reflex assessment may show increased deep tendon reflexes (DTRs) and diminished abdominal skin and cremasteric reflexes.

B. Diagnostic Tests

▶ **Note:** MS is sometimes called the "great masquerader." Diagnostic testing is often done to exclude disorders with similar symptoms.

---

1. Magnetic resonance imaging (MRI): To reveal presence of plaques.
2. EEG: Abnormal in a third of patients with MS. (See "Seizure Disorders," p. 202, for patient care.)
3. CT scan: To demonstrate presence of plaques and rule out mass lesions.
4. Lumber puncture and CSF analysis: To evaluate oligoclonal immunoglobulin G (IgG), protein, and gamma globulin levels, any of which may be elevated in the presence of MS. (See "Bacterial Meningitis," p. 153, for patient care.)

C. Medical Management and Surgical Interventions

1. **Bed rest:** During acute exacerbation.
2. **Pharmacotherapy**

   □ *Anti-inflammatory agents:* Prednisone, dexamethazone, adrenocorticotropic hormone (ACTH), etc. may be prescribed during an exacerbation in an attempt to decrease inflammation and associated edema of the myelin and hasten onset of a remission.

   □ *Antispasmodics and muscle relaxants such as baclofen or dantrolene sodium:* May be given to decrease spasticity.

   □ *Smooth muscle relaxants such as propantheline bromide:* To decrease urinary frequency and urgency.

   □ *Smooth muscle stimulants such as bethanechol chloride:* May be given to help prevent urinary retention.

   □ *Tranquilizers such as diazepam:* May be given for both their anxiety-reducing and muscle-relaxant effects.

3. **Physical medicine:** Physical therapy, occupational therapy, and assistive devices or braces may be prescribed so that patient can maintain mobility and independence with ADLs. Muscle-strengthening and conditioning exercises and gait training are also frequently indicated.
4. **ROM exercises:** To maintain or increase joint function and prevent contractures.
5. **Counseling and/or psychotherapy:** To help patient and SOs adapt to the disability and deal with emotions and feelings that are either a direct or indirect result of the disease process.
6. **Surgical interventions:** To treat complications such as contractures, spasticity, decreased mobility, and pain. Interventions may include tendotomy, myotomy, peripheral neurectomy, and rhizotomy.

D. Nursing Diagnoses and Interventions

Knowledge deficit: Factors that aggravate and/or exacerbate MS symptoms

Desired outcome: Patient can verbalize knowledge of factors that exacerbate, prevent, or ameliorate symptoms of MS.

1. Inform patient that heat, both external (hot weather, bath) and internal (fever), tends to aggravate weakness and other symptoms of MS.
2. Teach preventive measures such as avoiding hot baths and using acetaminophen or aspirin to reduce fever, if present.

3. Because infection often precedes exacerbations, caution patient to avoid exposure to persons known to have infections of any kind.

4. Teach the indicators of common infections and the importance of seeking prompt medical treatment should they occur.

Knowledge deficit: Precautions and potential side effects of prescribed medications

Desired outcome: Patient can verbalize accurate information regarding the prescribed medications.

1. Provide patient with verbal instructions and written handouts that describe the name, purpose, dosage, and schedule of the prescribed medications.

2. For patients taking prednisone or dexamethasone, provide additional instructions for the following:

□ *Common side effects:* fluid retention, hypertension, gastric ulcers, stomach upset, weakness, and mood changes.

□ Importance of monitoring weight and BP for evidence of fluid retention; taking the medication with food, milk, or buffering agents to help prevent gastric irritation; avoiding taking aspirin, indomethacin, caffeine, or other GI irritants while taking this medication as they will increase gastric irritation; and tapering rather than abruptly stopping the drug when it is discontinued.

3. If the patient is taking baclofen or dantrolene, provide instructions for the following:

□ *Common side effects:* drowsiness, dizziness, weakness, fatigue, and nausea. In addition, dantrolene can cause diarrhea, hepatitis, and photosensitivity.

□ Importance of taking the medication with food, milk, or a buffering agent to reduce gastric upset or nausea. Explain that although drowsiness is usually transient, patient should avoid activities that require alertness until their effect on the CNS is known. Patients on dantrolene should monitor for and report symptoms of fever and jaundice (which signal hepatitis) or severe diarrhea, avoid exposure to the sun, and use sunscreen lotions if exposure is unavoidable.

4. If bethanechol chloride has been prescribed, provide instructions for the following:

□ *Common side effects:* hypotension, diarrhea, abdominal cramps, urinary urgency, and bronchoconstriction.

□ Importance of taking the drug on an empty stomach to avoid nausea and vomiting, notifying MD if lightheadedness occurs as this can signal hypotension, and seeking medical attention if an asthmatic attack occurs.

5. If the patient is taking propantheline bromide, provide instructions for the following:

□ *Common side effects:* dryness of the mouth, blurred vision, constipation, palpitations, tachycardia, decreased sweating, and urinary retention or overflow incontinence.

□ Measures that relieve constipation; measures for remaining cool in hot or humid weather, as heat stroke is more likely to develop while on the medication; importance of notifying MD immediately if urinary retention or overflow incontinence occurs. In addition, if the patient can chew and swallow effectively, explain that sugarless gum, hard candy, and/or artificial saliva products may reduce mouth dryness.

Alteration in comfort: Pain and spasms related to motor nerve tract damage

Desired outcomes: Patient relates a reduction in discomfort and does not exhibit signs of uncontrolled pain. Patient and SOs can verbalize knowledge of preventive measures and demonstrate methods for controlling pain and spasms.

1. Because heat tends to aggravate MS symptoms, maintain a comfortable room temperature. Advise patient to keep environment cool in warm weather and avoid hot baths.

2. To reduce muscle tightness and spasms, provide passive, assisted, or active ROM q2h. Teach these exercises to patient and SOs.

3. For other interventions, see **Alteration In comfort**, p. 543, in "Caring for Patients with Neurologic Problems," "Appendix One."

See "Caring for Patients with Neurologic Disorders" in "Appendix One" for the following: **Potential for injury** related to unsteady gait, p. 537, **Potential for injury** related to impaired pain, touch, and temperature sensations, p. 538, **Potential for injury** related to corneal irritation/abrasions, p. 538, **Potential for injury** related to visual disturbances, p. 543, **Alteration in nutrition:** Less than body requirements, p. 538, **Potential fluid volume deficit** related to decreased intake, p. 539, **Ineffective airway clearance** related to coughing and swallowing deficits, p. 540, **Self-care deficit:** Inability to perform ADLs, p. 540, **Impaired verbal communication** related to dysarthria, p. 541, and **Alteration in bowel elimination:** Constipation related to inability to chew and swallow high-roughage foods, side effects of medications, and immobility, p. 541. See "Caring for Patients with Cancer and Other Life-Disrupting Illnesses" in "Appendix One" for the following, as appropriate: **Disturbance in self-concept**, p. 544, **Fear**, p. 544, **Alteration in family processes**, p. 546, and **Grieving**, p. 546. For patients who are immobile, see related nursing diagnoses in "Caring for Patients on Prolonged Bed Rest," pp. 533–537, "Appendix One." For patients who are experiencing renal–urinary dysfunction, see related discussions in Chapter 3, "Renal–Urinary Disorders."

E. Patient–Family Teaching and Discharge Planning

The patient with MS may have a wide variety of symptoms that cause disability, ranging from mild to severe. Provide patient and SOs with verbal and written information for the following, as appropriate:

1. Remission/exacerbation aspects of the disease process.

2. Referrals to community resources such as local and national MS society chapters, public health nurse, visiting nurse association, community support groups, social workers, psychological therapists, vocational rehabilitation agencies, home health agencies, and extended and skilled care facilities. The National Multiple Sclerosis Society is located at 205 East 42nd Street, New York, NY 10017.

3. Safety measures relative to decreased sensation, visual disturbances, and motor deficits.

4. Medications, including drug name, purpose, dosage, frequency, precautions, and potential side effects.

5. Exercises that promote muscle strength and mobility; measures for preventing contractures and skin breakdown; transfer techniques and proper body mechanics; use of assistive devices.

6. Measures for relieving pain, muscle spasms, or other discomfort.

7. Indications of constipation, urinary retention, or UTI; implementation of bowel and bladder training programs; self-catheterization technique or care of indwelling urinary catheters.

8. Indications of URI; implementation of measures that help prevent regurgitation, aspiration, and respiratory infection.

9. Importance of follow-up care, including visits to MD, PT, OT, as well as speech, sexual, or psychological counseling.

II. Guillain-Barré Syndrome

Guillain-Barré is a rapidly progressing polyneuritis of unknown etiology. An inflammatory process causes lymphocytes to enter the perivascular spaces and destroy the myelin sheath covering the peripheral and/or cranial nerves. Because posterior (sensory) and anterior (motor) nerve roots can be affected, the individual may experience both sensory and motor losses. In about 25% of cases, motor weakness progresses to total paralysis, a life-threatening situation. Remyelinization and return of complete function usually occur, but it may take months to years for a full recovery. Residual neurologic deficits tend to be mild motor or reflex alterations in the feet or legs.

Guillain-Barré syndrome may follow a febrile illness such as URI or gastroenteritis, a rabies or flu vaccination, lupus erythematosus, and Hodgkin's disease or other malignant process.

A. Assessment

Weakness is the most common indicator. Typically, numbness and weakness begin in the legs and ascend upward, progressing to the arms and facial nerves within 1–3 days. Peak severity usually occurs within 10–14 days of onset.

Anterior (motor) nerve root involvement: Weakness or flaccid paralysis. Weakness or paralysis of respiratory muscles can be life threatening. There is a loss of reflexes, muscle tension, and tone, but muscle atrophy usually does not occur.

Autonomic nervous system involvement: Sinus tachycardia, bradycardia, hypertension, hypotension, inability to perspire, loss of sphincter control, urinary retention, adynamic ileus, and increased pulmonary secretions. Autonomic nervous system involvement may occur unexpectedly and can be life threatening.

Cranial nerve involvement: Inability to chew, swallow, speak, or close the eyes.

Posterior (sensory) nerve root involvement: Paresthesia such as numbness and tingling, which are usually minor compared to the degree of motor loss. Ascending sensory loss often precedes motor loss. The patient generally does not experience pain.

Physical exam: Symmetrical motor weakness, impaired position and vibration sense, hypoactive or absent DTRs, hypotonia in affected muscles, and decreased ventilatory capacity.

B. Diagnostic Tests

Tests are performed to rule out other diseases such as acute poliomyelitis.

1. <u>CBC:</u> Will show presence of leukocytosis early in illness.
2. <u>Electromyography (EMG):</u> Reveals slowed nerve conduction velocities soon after paralysis appears. Denervation potentials appear later.
3. <u>Lumbar puncture and CSF analysis:</u> Usually show an elevated protein (especially immunoglobulin G) without pleocytosis. Although CSF pressure is usually normal, in severe disease it may be elevated. (See "Bacterial Meningitis," p. 153, for patient care.)

C. Medical Management

1. **Respiratory support:** Endotracheal tube, tracheostomy, or mechanical ventilation as necessary.
2. **Pharmacotherapy:** May include a 1-week trial with glucocorticosteroids such as prednisone to determine whether the symptoms decrease. In the absence of marked improvement, it is discontinued.
3. **Exercise and activity:** Activity other than passive ROM is restricted during the acute phase. After the patient stabilizes, active ROM or active assistive

ROM is implemented, and a physical therapy and rehabilitation program is initiated. Occupational therapy and assistive devices or braces are employed so that patient can maintain mobility and independence with ADLs. Muscle-strengthening exercises, conditioning exercises, and gait training are also frequently prescribed.

4. **Nutritional support:** If the patient cannot chew or swallow effectively due to cranial nerve involvement, NG or parenteral feedings may be prescribed.

5. **Management of acute autonomic dysfunction:** Short-acting antihypertensive agents for hypertension; intravascular volume expanders or vasopressors for hypotension; cardiac monitoring of dysrhythmias; NG suctioning and parenteral fluids for adynamic ileus; and catheterization and medications for urinary retention.

D. Nursing Diagnoses and Interventions

Alteration in nutrition: Less than body requirements related to decreased intake secondary to NPO status with adynamic ileus

Desired outcome: Patient does not exhibit signs of malnutrition or weight loss.

▶ **Note:** Patients with adynamic ileus generally require NG suctioning to decompress the stomach. Because these patients are unable to take foods orally, parenteral nutrition may be required. (See "Providing Nutritional Therapy," p. 521, in Chapter 11, "Metabolic Disorders," for a discussion of parenteral nutrition.)

For other interventions, see **Alteration in nutrition** in "Caring for Patients with Neurologic Problems," p. 538, "Appendix One."

Ineffective airway clearance related to coughing and swallowing deficits secondary to weakness or paralysis of the facial, throat, and respiratory muscles

Desired outcome: Patient does not exhibit signs of aspiration, URI, or impaired respiratory function.

1. Test for ascending loss of sensation by touching patient lightly with a pin or fingers at frequent intervals (qh or more frequently initially). Assess from the level of the iliac crest upward toward the shoulders. Measure the highest level at which decreased sensation occurs. Decreased sensation frequently precedes motor weakness, so if it ascends to the level of the T-8 dermatome, anticipate that intercostal muscles (used with respirations) will soon be impaired. Also monitor for upper arm and shoulder weakness, which precede respiratory failure. Alert MD to significant findings.

2. Monitor effectiveness of breathing by checking vital capacity results on pulmonary function tests. If the vital capacity is <1 L or if the patient exhibits signs of hypoxia such as tachycardia, increasing restlessness, mental dullness, or cyanosis, report findings immediately to MD. Monitor ABG levels to detect hypoxemia or hypercapnia.

3. The patient may require tracheostomy, endotracheal intubation, or mechanical ventilation to support respiratory function. Prepare patient emotionally for such procedures or for the eventual transfer to ICU or transition care unit for closer monitoring.

4. For other interventions, see **Ineffective airway clearance** in "Caring for Patients with Neurologic Problems," p. 540, "Appendix One."

Fear related to threat to biologic integrity

Desired outcome: Patient does not demonstrate use of ineffective coping mechanisms or exhibit signs of psychologic discomfort.

1. For the patient in whom the neurologic deficit is still progressing, arrange for a transfer to a room close to the nurses' station to help alleviate the fear of being suddenly incapacitated and helpless.

2. Be sure that patient's call light is within easy reach. Frequently assess patient's ability to use it.

3. For other interventions, see **Fear** in "Caring for Patients with Cancer and Other Life-Disrupting Illnesses," p. 544, "Appendix One."

See "Caring for Patients with Neurologic Disorders" in "Appendix One" for the following: **Potential for injury** related to unsteady gait, p. 537, **Potential for injury** related to impaired pain, touch, and temperature sensations, p. 538, **Potential for injury** related to visual disturbances, p. 543, **Potential for injury** related to corneal irritation/abrasions, p. 538, **Alteration in bowel elimination:** Constipation, p. 541, and **Impaired verbal communication** related to dysarthria, p. 541. For patients with urinary incontinence, retention, neurogenic bladder, or UTI, see related discussions in Chapter 3, "Renal–Urinary Disorders." For patients who are immobile, see related nursing diagnoses in "Caring for Patients on Prolonged Bed Rest," pp. 533–537, Appendix One. See "Caring for Patients with Cancer and Other Life-Disrupting Illnesses" in "Appendix One," for the following: **Disturbance in self-concept**, p. 544, **Ineffective individual coping**, p. 545, **Fear**, p. 544, **Alteration in family processes**, p. 546, and **Grieving**, p. 546.

E. Patient–Family Teaching and Discharge Planning

Most patients with Guillain-Barré syndrome eventually recover fully. Because the recovery period can be prolonged, the patient often goes home with some degree of neurologic deficit. Discharge planning and teaching will vary according to the degree of disability. Provide patient and SOs with verbal and written information for the following as appropriate:

1. The disease process, expected improvement, and importance of continuing in the rehabilitation or physical therapy program to promote as full a recovery as possible.

2. Referrals to community resources such as public health nurse, visiting nurse association, community support groups, social workers, psychologic therapy, home health agencies, and extended and skilled care facilities.

3. Safety measures relative to the decreased sensorimotor deficit.

4. Exercises that promote muscle strength and mobility; measures for preventing contractures and skin breakdown; transfer techniques and proper body mechanics; and use of assistive devices.

5. Indications of constipation, urinary retention, or UTI; and if appropriate, care of indwelling catheters or self-catheterization technique.

6. Indications of URI; measures for preventing regurgitation, aspiration, and respiratory infection.

7. Medications, including drug name, purpose, dosage, schedule, precautions, and potential side effects.

III. Bacterial Meningitis

Bacterial meningitis is an infection that results in inflammation of the meningeal membranes covering the brain and spinal cord. It can be transmitted in one of four ways: via airborn droplets from infected individuals; from direct contamination (eg, from a penetrating skull wound, lumbar puncture, ventricular shunt, or surgical procedure); via the bloodstream (eg, pneumonia, endocarditis); or from direct contact with an infectious process that invades the meningeal membranes such as that which can occur with osteomyelitis, sinusitis, otitis media, mastoiditis, or brain abscess. Common infecting agents include *Neisseria meningitidis, Diplococcus pneumoniae, Hemophilus influenzae, Staphylococcus aureus,* and *Escherichia coli.* The prognosis is good if the disorder is recognized early and antibiotic treatment is initiated promptly. However, if left untreated, the mortality rate is 70–100%. When *S aureus* is involved, the condition is often fatal.

A. Assessment

Infection: Fever, chills, malaise.

Increased ICP: Severe headache, irritability, drowsiness, stupor, coma, nausea and vomiting, decreased pupillary reaction to light, pupillary dilation or inequality.

Meningeal irritation: Back stiffness and pain, nuchal rigidity.

Other: Generalized seizures and photophobia; joint pain (in the presence of *H influenzae.*)

Physical exam: A positive Brudzinski's sign is elicited: When the neck is passively flexed forward, both legs flex involuntarily at the hip and knee. A positive Kernig's sign also may be found: When the thigh is flexed, the individual is unable to extend the leg completely without pain. In the presence of meningococcal meningitis, a pink macular rash, petechiae, ecchymoses, purpura, and increased DTRs also may occur.

B. Diagnostic Tests

1. Lumbar puncture, CSF analysis, and Gram stain and culture: To identify causative organism. Glucose is generally decreased and protein is usually increased. The CSF will be cloudy or milky if WBCs are increased, and increased CSF pressure may be noted if inflammation is causing an obstruction in outflow from the arachnoid villa.

    □ *Positioning:* Assist patient into a side-lying position, with chin tucked into the chest and knees drawn up to the abdomen. This position curves the spine and widens the intervertebral space for easier insertion of the spinal needle.

    □ *During the test:* Instruct patient to lie very still. Place your hands behind patient's knees and neck and pull gently to help maintain proper position. Assess for an elevated pulse, paleness, or clammy skin. Notify MD of significant findings.

    □ *After the test:* Minimize risk of headache by having patient lie flat for the amount of time prescribed by MD. Encourage turning from side to side. If prescribed, elevate HOB slightly. Encourage fluids and provide analgesics as prescribed. Monitor puncture site for redness, swelling, and drainage. Be alert to indicators of meningitis, including fever, nuchal rigidity, and irritability. If CSF pressure was elevated, check neurologic status and VS at frequent intervals for signs of brain herniation (decreased LOC; pupillary changes such as dilation, inequality, or decreased reaction; irregular respirations; and hemiparesis).

2. Culture and sensitivity testing of blood, urine, and other body secretions: To identify infective organism and determine appropriate antibiotic.

3. Counterimmunoelectrophoresis (CIE): For detection of antigens of pneumococci, meningococci, and *H influenzae* in the CSF, blood, and urine.

4. Sinus and chest x-rays: Taken after treatment is started to rule out sinusitis and pneumonia.

C. Medical Management

1. **Strict respiratory isolation:** For at least 24 hours after initiation of treatment for patients with *N meningitidis* or *H influenzae.* Patient is isolated when the causative organism is in doubt.

2. **Parenteral antibiotics:** Because treatment cannot be delayed until the results of the culture are returned, high doses are started immediately, based on Gram stain results. The antibiotic must penetrate the blood-brain barrier into the CSF. Adjustments in therapy can be made after CIE and culture and sensitivity test results are in. Antibiotics may include the following: penicillin G, ampicillin, nafcillin, oxacillin, chloramphenicol, gentamicin, kanamycin, or vancomycin.

3. **Prophylactic antibiotic treatment of SOs and close contacts:** Rifampin is administered.

4. **Other pharmacotherapy**

   □ *Osmotic diuretics (eg, mannitol):* To decrease cerebral edema.

   □ *Anticonvulsant agents (eg, diazepam and phenytoin):* To control seizures.

   □ *Analgesics and antipyretics (eg, aspirin and acetaminophen):* For headache and/or fever.

   □ *Sedatives and tranquilizers:* To promote rest.

5. **Bed rest:** During acute stage of the disease.

6. **Limitation of fluids to two-thirds maintenance (about 1500 mL):** To keep patient underhydrated and reduce cerebral edema and effects of inappropriate ADH secretion.

7. **Support respirations:** Via oxygen, suctioning, or intubation as necessary.

8. **Treatment of complications:** Examples include disseminated intravascular coagulation, respiratory or heart failure, and septic shock.

9. **Nutritional support:** Enteral or parenteral feedings as required for patients who are stuporous or comatose.

D. Nursing Diagnoses and Interventions

Knowledge deficit: Side effects and precautions for the prescribed antibiotics

Desired outcome: Patient and SOs can verbalize knowledge of the potential side effects and precautions for the prescribed antibiotics.

1. For SOs and contacts for whom rifampin is prescribed, explain the prescribed dosage and schedule. Rifampin should be taken 1 hour before meals for maximum absorption. Emphasize the importance of taking this drug as a preventive measure against meningitis, and describe potential side effects such as nausea, vomiting, diarrhea, orange urine, headache, and dizziness. Caution against wearing contact lenses, as the drug will permanently color them orange. In addition, rifampin reduces the effectiveness of oral contraceptives, and it is contraindicated in pregnancy.

2. For other interventions, see **Knowledge deficit:** Adverse side effects from prolonged use of potent antibiotics, p. 387, in "Osteomyelitis," Chapter 8.

Knowledge deficit: Rationale and procedure for respiratory isolation and/or secretion precautions

Desired outcome: Patient and SOs can verbalize knowledge of the rationale for isolation and/or secretion precautions and comply with the prescribed restrictions and precautionary measures.

▶ **Note:** Patients with *N meningitidis, H influenzae,* or unidentified organism will be placed in respiratory isolation for at least 24 hours from the initiation of appropriate antibiotic therapy. Patients with other organisms are usually placed on secretion precautions.

---

1. For patients on secretion precautions (as well as those in respiratory isolation), provide instructions for covering the mouth before coughing/sneezing and proper disposal of the tissue.

2. Instruct patients on respiratory precautions to stay in their room. However, if they must leave the room for a procedure or test, explain that a mask must be worn to protect others from contact with airborn droplets.

3. For individuals in contact with the patient in respiratory isolation, explain the importance of wearing a surgical mask and performing good handwashing. Usually, a gown and gloves are not necessary.

4. Reassure patient that respiratory isolation is temporary and will be discontinued once patient has been on the appropriate antibiotic for 24–48 hours.

See "Head injury" for the following: **Potential impairment of physical mobility** related to prolonged inactivity, p. 180. See "Seizure Disorders" for the following: **Potential for injury** related to oral, musculoskeletal, and airway vulnerability secondary to seizure activity, p. 203. See "Caring for Patients with Neurologic Disorders," "Appendix One," for the following: **Potential for injury** related to unsteady gait, p. 537, **Potential for injury** related to impaired pain, touch, and temperature sensations, p. 538, **Potential for injury** related to corneal abrasions/irritation, p. 538, **Self-care deficit:** Inability to perform ADLs, p. 540, **Alteration in nutrition:** Less than body requirements, p. 538, **Alteration in comfort**, p. 543, **Potential for injury** related to increased ICP, p. 542, **Potential fluid volume deficit**, p. 539, **Ineffective airway clearance**, p. 540, and **Alteration in bowel elimination:** Constipation, p. 541. For patients who are immobile, see related nursing diagnoses in "Caring for Patients on Prolonged Bed Rest," pp. 533–537, "Appendix One." See "Caring for the Patient with Cancer and Other Life-Disrupting Illnesses," in "Appendix One," for the following: **Ineffective individual coping**, p. 545, **Fear**, p. 544, **Alteration in family processes**, p. 546, and **Grieving**, p. 546.

E. Patient–Family Teaching and Discharge Planning

The extent of teaching and discharge planning will depend on whether or not patient has any residual damage. As appropriate, provide patient and SOs with verbal and written information for the following:

1. Referrals to community resources such as public health nurse, visiting nurse association, community support groups, social workers, psychologic therapy, vocational rehabilitation agency, home health agencies, and extended and skilled care facilities.

2. Medications, including purpose, dosage, schedule, precautions, and potential side effects.

In addition:

3. For patients with residual neurologic deficits, teach the following as appropriate: exercises that promote muscle strength and mobility; measures for preventing contractures and skin breakdown; transfer techniques and proper body mechanics; safety measures if the patient has decreased pain and sensation or visual disturbances; use of assistive devices; indications of constipation, urinary retention, or UTI; bowel and bladder training programs; and self-catheterization technique or care of indwelling catheters.

IV. Encephalitis

Encephalitis is an inflammation of the brain that can cause severe neuronal dysfunction. It is often the result of an arbovirus infection that is transmitted by an infected mosquito or tick. Post-infectious encephalitis occurs after a vaccination or as a complication of other infections such as measles, chickenpox, and herpesvirus. The prognosis varies according to the type of infection. Some cases of encephalitis leave few or no residual side effects, and the neurologic symptoms often subside in several weeks. Other types of encephalitis (eg, eastern equine encephalitis, an arbovirus infection) have a high mortality rate, and survivors frequently have severe residual damage. Herpes simplex encephalitis survivors are often left with seizures, aphasia, and/or severe mental deterioration such as dementia.

A. Assessment

Infection: Fever, chills, malaise.

Increased ICP: Headache; changes in LOC such as irritability, confusion, and drowsiness that can progress to stupor and coma; nausea and vomiting; pupillary changes such as inequality and decreased reaction to light.

Meningeal irritation: Neck stiffness/rigidity; pain.

Focal: Symptoms vary. Patient may have seizures or photophobia, ataxia, and sensorimotor deficits. Eastern equine encephalitis, for example, can destroy major portions of a lobe or hemisphere and leave the individual with hemiplegia, aphasia, blindness, deafness, and/or seizures. Herpes simplex encephalitis has a special affinity for the frontal and temporal lobes of the brain, resulting in alterations in the senses of smell and/or taste, seizures, aphasia, organic psychosis, and dementia.

B. Diagnostic Tests

1. <u>Lumbar puncture and CSF analysis:</u> May reveal increased CSF pressure, increased WBC and protein levels, and normal glucose. (See "Bacterial Meningitis," p. 153, for patient care.)

2. <u>CT scan:</u> To rule out other neurologic problems.

3. <u>EEG:</u> May show presence of abnormal electrical activity. (See "Seizure Disorders," p. 202, for patient care.)

C. Medical Management

Except for herpes encephalitis, the treatment is supportive only.

1. **Antiviral agent (eg, vidarabine):** For herpes encephalitis. Side effects may include tremor, dizziness, hallucinations, anorexia, nausea, vomiting, diarrhea, itching, rash, and anemia.

2. **Supportive pharmacotherapy**
   □ *Anticonvulsants such as phenytoin.*
   □ *Glucocorticosteroids such as dexamethasone:* To reduce cerebral edema and inflammation.
   □ *Sedatives:* For restlessness.
   □ *Analgesics and antipyretics such as aspirin and acetaminophen:* For headache and fever.

3. **Limitation of fluids to two-thirds maintenance (about 1500 ml):** To maintain a state of underhydration, which helps reduce cerebral edema.

4. **Support respirations:** Via oxygen, suctioning, or intubation.

5. **Nutritional support:** Enteral or parenteral feedings for stuporous or comatose patients, as needed.

D. Nursing Diagnoses and Interventions

See "Alzheimer's Disease" for the following: **Sensory-perceptual alterations** related to inability to evaluate reality, p. 163. See "Head Injury" for the following: **Potential impairment of physical mobility** related to prolonged inactivity, p. 180. See "Cerebrovascular Accident" for the following: **Impaired verbal communi-**

cation related to aphasia and/or dysarthria, p. 195. See "Seizure Disorders" for the following: **Potential for injury** related to oral, musculoskeletal, and airway vulnerability secondary to seizure activity, p. 203. For patients who have varying degrees of immobility, see related nursing diagnoses and interventions in "Caring for Patients on Prolonged Bed Rest," pp. 533–537, "Appendix One." See "Caring for Patients with Neurologic Problems," "Appendix One," for the following: **Self-care deficit**, p. 540, **Alteration in nutrition**, p. 538, **Alteration in comfort**, p. 543, **Potential for injury** related to unsteady gait, p. 537, **Potential for injury** related to risk of increased ICP, p. 542, **Ineffective airway clearance**, p. 540, **Alteration in bowel elimination:** Constipation, p. 541, **Potential fluid volume deficit**, p. 539, and **Potential for injury** related to impaired pain, touch, and temperature sensations, p. 538. See "Caring for Patients with Cancer and Other Life-Disrupting Illnesses" in "Appendix One" for the following: **Disturbance in self-concept**, p. 544, **Ineffective individual coping**, p. 545, **Fear**, p. 544, **Alteration in family processes**, p. 546, and **Grieving**, p. 546.

E. Patient–Family Teaching and Discharge Planning

The amount of teaching and discharge planning will depend on the degree of neurologic deficit. See teaching/discharge planning interventions 2–9 in "Multiple Sclerosis," p. 149, as appropriate.

▶ Section Two   **Degenerative Disorders of the Nervous System**

The central nervous system (CNS), peripheral nervous system, and autonomic nervous system are responsible for controlling and coordinating functions of all body systems. With degenerative nerve disorders, the function of the nerve cells, dendrites, and/or axons is progressively altered or decreased. A variety of mechanisms, including outright destruction of the neurons or decreases in neurotransmitter synthesis uptake or release, account for this change in neuronal function.

I. Parkinsonism

Parkinson's disease is a slowly progressive, degenerative disorder of the CNS affecting the brain centers that regulate movement. For unknown reasons, cell death occurs in the substantia nigra of the midbrain. This leads to an abnormally low concentration of dopamine in the corpus striatum, which causes symptoms of Parkinson's disease. Possible causes include viral encephalitis, neurotoxins, cerebrovascular disease, head injury, phenothiazide use, and exposure to carbon monoxide. Approximately 1% of all individuals over age 50 have this disease. Parkinsonism is usually progressive, and death can result from aspiration pneumonia or choking. *Parkinsonian crisis*, a medical emergency, is usually precipitated by emotional trauma or failure to take the prescribed medications.

A. Assessment

Initially, symptoms are mild and include stiffness or slight hand tremors. They gradually increase and can become disabling.

Bradykinesia: Slowness, stiffness, and difficulty with initiating movement. The patient may have a mask-like facial expression, unblinking stare, difficulty chewing and swallowing, drooling, and a high-pitched, monotone, weak voice. The patient also has loss of automatic associated movements, such as swinging the arms when walking. In addition, *oculogynic crisis* can occur, causing the eyes to become fixed in one position, generally upward, sometimes for several hours.

Loss of postural reflexes: Causes the typical shuffling, propulsive gait with short steps; stumbling; falling.

Increased muscle rigidity: Limb muscles become rigid on passive motion. Typically, this rigidity results in jerky ("cogwheel") motions.

Tremors: Increase when the limb is at rest and stop with voluntary movement and during sleep (non-intention tremor). "Pill-rolling" tremor of the hands and "to and fro" tremor of the head are typical.

Autonomic: Excessive diaphoresis, seborrhea, postural hypotension, and decreased libido.

Physical exam: Usually a positive blink reflex is elicited by tapping a finger between the patient's eyebrows. A positive palmomental reflex (contraction of muscles of the chin and corner of mouth) can be elicited by stroking patient's palm. Diminished postural reflexes are present on neurologic exam; however, there is risk of injury with this test because the patient may quickly lose balance and fall.

Parkinsonian crisis: This sudden and severe increase in bradykinesia, rigidity, and tremors can lead to tachycardia, hyperpnea, and inability to swallow or maintain a patent airway.

B. Diagnostic Tests

Diagnosis is usually made on the basis of physical exam and characteristic symptoms, and after other neurologic problems have been ruled out.

1. <u>Urinalysis:</u> May reveal decreased dopamine level, which supports the diagnosis.

2. <u>Medication withdrawal:</u> Long-term therapy with large doses of medications such as haloperidol or phenothiazines can produce Parkinson-like symptoms. If caused by these medications, symptoms will disappear when the drug is discontinued.

3. <u>EEG:</u> Often shows abnormalities. (See "Seizure Disorders," p. 202, for patient care.)

C. Medical Management and Surgical Interventions

1. **Pharmacotherapy**

   □ *Dopamine replacement, eg, levodopa or levodopa-carbidopa combination:* Given in increasing amounts until symptoms are reduced or patient's tolerance is reached. Side effects include anorexia, nausea, postural hypotension, urinary retention, GI bleeding, cardiac dysrhythmias, insomnia, hallucinations, and depression. Vitamin B_6 (pyridoxine) can reverse the effects of levodopa.

   □ *Antiviral agents, eg, amantadine hydrochloride:* Less effective than levodopa, but has less severe side effects. Side effects include dizziness, insomnia, orthostatic hypotension, and ataxia.

   □ *Anticholinergics, eg, trihexyphenidyl hydrochloride, cycrimine hydrochloride, and procyclidine hydrochloride:* To help relieve tremors and rigidity. Side effects include dryness of the mouth, blurred vision, constipation, mental dullness, confusion, and urinary retention or overflow incontinence.

2. **Physical therapy:** Massage; muscle stretching; active/passive ROM, especially on hands and feet; and walking and gait–training exercises.

3. **Treatment for Parkinsonian crisis:** This crisis necessitates respiratory and cardiac support. The patient is placed in a quiet, calm environment with subdued lighting. Sodium phenobarbital or sodium amobarbital is given IM or IV.

4. **Stereotaxic surgery:** Performed in selected patients. Electrical coagulation, freezing, radioactivity, or ultrasound is used to destroy portions of the globus

pallidus of the ventrolateral nucleus of the thalamus to prevent involuntary movement and help relieve tremors and rigidity of the extremities.

D. Nursing Diagnoses and Interventions

Potential for injury related to unsteady gait secondary to bradykinesis, tremors, and rigidity

Desired outcome: Patient demonstrates compliance with the therapeutic regimen and preventive measures, and does not exhibit signs of injury.

1. During ambulation, encourage patient to deliberately swing the arms to assist with the gait and raise the feet to help prevent falls.
2. Have patient practice movements that are especially difficult, eg; turning.
3. Teach head and neck exercises to help improve patient's posture.
4. For other interventions, see **Potential for injury** related to unsteady gait in "Caring for Patients with Neurologic Problems," p. 537, "Appendix One."

Knowledge deficit: Precautions for taking levodopa

Desired outcome: Patient can verbalize knowledge of the precautionary measures for taking levodopa.

1. Instruct patient to take levodopa with meals to decrease the potential for nausea and stomach upset. Provide instructions for avoiding alcohol and vitamin preparations that contain vitamin B_6, as they reduce the effectiveness of levodopa.
2. To help prevent postural hypotension, advise patient to wear elastic stockings and change positions slowly.
3. Encourage sugarless chewing gum and hard candy or the liberal use of artificial saliva products so that dryness of the mouth will be lessened and integrity of the oral mucous membranes will be maintained. **Note:** This measure also applies if the patient is taking anticholinergic drugs.

Knowledge deficit: Facial and tongue exercises that enhance verbal communication and help prevent choking

Desired outcome: Patient can demonstrate knowledge of facial and tongue exercises and state the rationale for their use.

1. Explain to patient that special exercises can help strengthen and control facial and tongue muscles, which in turn will improve verbal communication and help prevent choking. Emphasize that routine exercises of the facial and tongue muscles, along with the prescribed medications, may prevent or delay disability.
2. Teach the following exercises and have patient return the demonstration: Hold a sound for 5 seconds, sing the scale, read aloud, and extend the tongue and try to touch the chin, nose, and cheek.
3. Provide a written handout that lists and describes the above exercises. Encourage patient to perform them hourly while awake.
4. Teach patient the importance of stating feelings verbally, as monotone speech and lack of facial expression impede verbal and nonverbal communication.

See "Caring for Patients with Neurologic Disorders" in "Appendix One" for the following: **Potential fluid volume deficit**, p. 539, **Self-care deficit**, p. 540, **Ineffective airway clearance**, p. 540, **Potential for injury** related to risk of corneal irritation/abrasion, p. 538, **Impaired verbal communication** related to dysarthria, p. 541, and **Alteration in nutrition**, p. 538. For patients with varying degrees of immobility, refer to related nursing diagnoses in "Caring for Patients on Prolonged Bed Rest," pp. 533–537, "Appendix One." See

"Caring for Patients with Cancer and Other Life-disrupting Illnesses" in "Appendix One" for the following: **Ineffective individual coping**, p. 545, **Fear**, p. 544, **Disturbance in self-concept**, p. 544, **Alteration in family processes**, p. 546, and **Grieving**, p. 546.

E. Patient–Family Teaching and Discharge Planning

Provide patient and SOs with verbal and written information for the following:

1. Referrals to community resources such as local and national Parkinson's Society chapters, public health nurse, visiting nurses association, community support groups, social workers, psychologic therapy, vocational rehabilitation agency, home health agencies, and extended and skilled care facilities. Provide the address of United Parkinsonism Foundation: 220 South State Street, Chicago, IL 60604, and Parkinson's Disease Foundation, Inc: 640 West 168th Street, New York, NY, 10032.

2. Related safety measures for patients with bradykinesia, muscle rigidity, and tremors.

3. Emphasis that disability may be prevented or delayed through exercises and medications.

4. For other interventions, see the same section in "Multiple Sclerosis," p. 149.

II. Alzheimer's Disease

Alzheimer's disease is a progressive, degenerative disorder of the brain characterized by changes and degeneration of the cerebral cortical nerve cells and nerve endings, resulting in abnormal neurofibrillary tangles and neuritic plaques. This process causes irreversible impairment of memory and degeneration of intellectual functions. Although etiology is unknown, aluminum poisoning, viruses, genetics, autoimmune disease, and neurotransmitter deficiency of choline acetyltransferase are possible causes, of which the last is considered the most probable. The onset of Alzheimer's disease is insidious, and it can strike individuals as young as 40 years of age. The disease progresses to total disability and eventually results in death from problems such as infection or aspiration, usually within 3–15 years.

A. Assessment

The appearance and severity of signs and symptoms vary from individual to individual. Initial indicators are mild, and it may take several years before a definite diagnosis can be made.

Memory: Early short-term memory loss, with longer retention of long-term memory; the past can become "the present." Eventually, long-term memory is lost as well.

Cognitive process: Inability to think through problems, poor decision-making ability, shortened attention span, lack of insight, inability to perform arithmetic calculations, inability to recognize or name common objects, disorientation to time and place, inability to recognize relatives or recall names, getting lost in own home or familiar places, not recognizing own reflection in the mirror. Hallucinations also may occur.

Mood: Apathy, lack of initiative, irritability, emotional lability, panic, fear, bewilderment, perplexity, exaggeration of any previous psychotic traits, depression, and anxiety. As the ability to communicate lessens and the world becomes more frightening, the potential for violence and agitation increases. The patient may have catastrophic reactions and emotional outbursts when faced with a complex task.

Social behavior: Decreased ability to handle social interaction, loss of social graces, loss of inhibitions, helplessness, dependency.

Speech patterns: Difficulty finding words, loss of spontaneity in speech, inability to express thoughts, incoherent speech.

Sleep pattern: Restlessness, pacing, decreased need for sleep, nocturnal awakening, reversal of normal sleep pattern.

Self-care: Neglect of routine tasks and personal hygiene; weight loss; increasing inability to dress, bathe, toilet, and feed self or recognize where to urinate or defecate.

Mobility/posture: Stooped and shuffling gait, balance and coordination problems, falling, inability to walk.

B. Diagnostic Tests

Many disorders that can cause a progressive dementia syndrome (eg, head injuries, brain tumors, depression, arteriosclerosis, drug toxicity, and alcoholism) need to be ruled out. This is especially important because some dementias are reversible.

1. Mental status exam: To test orientation, memory, calculation, abstraction, judgment, and mood.

2. Magnetic resonance imaging (MRI): Because of its ability to detect both biochemical and anatomic changes, this test may identify Alzheimer's disease at a very early stage.

3. EEG: May reveal slowed brainwave activity. (See "Seizure Disorders," p. 202, for patient care.)

4. CT scan: May reveal brain atrophy and ventricular enlargement. It also helps rule out other neurologic problems, particularly mass lesions.

5. In addition: The following tests may be performed to rule out other causes of dementia: skull and chest x-rays, lumbar puncture, serum tests, urinalysis, arteriograms, drug screen, and brain scan.

C. Medical Management

Generally, the treatment is supportive only.

Pharmacotherapy: Medications, if prescribed, are used to treat behavioral manifestations. These include:

☐ *Tricyclic or other antidepressants such as doxepin hydrochloride and trazodone hydrochloride.*

☐ *Antipsychotic agents such as haloperidol:* Used for combative patients.

☐ *Tranquilizers or sedatives such as chloral hydrate, triazolam, and oxazepam.*

D. Nursing Diagnoses and Interventions

Potential for injury related to lack of awareness of environmental hazards secondary to cognitive deficit

Desired outcomes: Patient does not exhibit signs of injury caused by cognitive deficit. SOs identify and eliminate or control potentially dangerous factors in the patient's home environment.

1. Orient patient to new surroundings. Reorient as needed. Keep necessary items, including water, telephone, and call light within easy reach. Assess patient's ability to use these items. Keep siderails up and the bed in its lowest position.

2. Maintain an uncluttered environment to minimize the risk of tripping. Ensure adequate lighting to help prevent falls in the dark.

3. Prevent exposure to hot food or equipment such as hot pads, which can burn the skin. Discourage use of heating pads. Check temperature of heating device and bath water before patient is exposed to them.

4. Encourage patient to use low-heeled, nonskid shoes for walking. Teach the use of wide-based gait to give unsteady patients a broader base of support. Assess patient for the presence of ataxia, and assist with walking as necessary.

Canes and walkers may be too complicated for patients with Alzheimer's disease.

5. Request that SOs assist with watching restless patients. Provide attendant care if necessary. Avoid restraining patient, because this usually increases agitation. If retraints are unavoidable, reassure patient that he or she is not being punished, that you are trying to help him or her regain control, and the restraints will be removed when the staff is certain he or she will not cause self-injury.

6. Check patient at frequent intervals. If necessary, move patient closer to the nursing station or seat patient in a chair at the nursing station.

Suggestions for home safety:

7. Encourage SOs to evaluate the home environment carefully for potential safety hazards. Caution them to remove harmful objects (eg, matches and scissors) from the bedside and store medications and chemicals in locked cabinets to prevent accidental ingestion. Remind SOs to check the house carefully before leaving, because the patient may leave the stove on or water running.

8. If patient tends to wander, encourage SOs to have an identification bracelet made.

9. Caution SOs that patients who are disoriented should be allowed to smoke only while being observed. Advise them to get a smoke detector and take control of matches.

10. Advise SOs that when the patient is no longer able to drive safely, the state automobile licensing bureau should be informed of the need for retesting. This will take the burden of restriction off the family. Suggest that SOs hide car keys if necessary to prevent patient from driving.

Alteration in nutrition: Less than body requirements related to decreased intake secondary to cognitive and motor deficit; and increased nutritional need secondary to constant pacing and restlessness

Desired outcome: Patient does not exhibit signs of weight loss or malnutrition.

1. Because patient may not eat food that does not look familiar or is on hospital plates, request that SOs assist with menu planning or bring in meals and dishes the patient will recognize.

2. When patient is no longer able to handle a fork, knife, and spoon, supply finger foods.

3. For the patient who is in constant motion, provide a diet that is high in calories unless contraindicated.

4. Try to limit the number of foods on the plate, as too many foods can be overwhelming for patient.

5. For other interventions, see **Alteration in nutrition** in "Caring for Patients with Neurologic Problems," p. 538, "Appendix One."

Alteration in pattern of urinary elimination related to incontinence or retention secondary to cognitive deficit

Desired outcome: Patient does not exhibit signs of incontinence or urinary retention.

1. Take patient to the bathroom q1–2h; restrict fluids in the evenings to minimize the risk of enuresis.

2. Identify bathroom door with a picture of a toilet stool to help patient locate the bathroom.

3. Assess for restlessness, which can signal the need to void.

4. As appropriate, provide male patients with condom catheters to help manage incontinence.

Self-care deficit: Inability to perform ADLs related to memory loss and coordination problems secondary to cognitive and motor deficits

Desired outcome: Patient demonstrates independence with performing ADLs.

1. Provide care for the totally dependent patient, and assist those who are not totally dependent. Do not hurry patient. Involve SOs with care activities if they are comfortable with doing so.
2. Place a stool in the shower if sitting will enhance self-care.
3. To facilitate dressing and undressing, encourage SOs or patient to buy shoes without laces and clothing that is loose fitting or has snaps or Velcro closures.
4. Provide a commode chair or elevated toilet seat as needed.

Sensory-perceptual alterations related to inability to evaluate reality secondary to degeneration of intellectual functioning

Desired outcome: Patient can verbalize orientation to person, place, and time.

1. Monitor for and record short-term memory deficit. At frequent intervals, orient patient to reality, time, and place in the following ways: Keep clocks and calendars in the room; inform patient of the day and time; correct patient gently; minimize disturbing noises; ensure adequate lighting to prevent shadow formation; request that SOs bring in familiar objects; speak with patient about his or her interests, both present and past; ensure that staff members show name tags and identify themselves; explain upcoming events; and set up regular schedules for hygiene, eating, and elimination.
2. Approach patient in a calm, relaxed, nonthreatening, and friendly manner. Treat patient with dignity and respect. Remain calm and patient when having to repeat questions. Be nonjudgmental and objective, even when confronted with unacceptable or inappropriate behaviors.
3. Keep patient's personal belongings where they can be used and seen.
4. Evaluate patient's cognitive impairment for any relation to medication usage such as sedatives or tranquilizers. If found, inform MD.
5. Explain activities in short, easily understood sentences. Point to objects or use demonstration if possible. When giving directions, be sure tasks have been broken into small, understandable units. Give patient time to accomplish one task before progressing to the next.
6. Be sure that you have the patient's attention. Repeat patient's name or gently touch patient to get his or her attention. Use a clear, low-pitched voice and simple words and sentences, but speak as though patient understands you. Ask only one question at a time, and formulate questions that can be answered by "yes" or "no." Wait for a response. If patient does not respond, repeat the question again, exactly as before, to help patient mentally process the question.

Sensory-perceptual alterations related to sensory overload secondary to degeneration of intellectual functioning

Desired outcome: Patient does not exhibit signs of sensory overload.

1. Provide a quiet, calm environment.
2. Provide stimulation the patient can handle. Soft music may be fine, while television might be too overwhelming.
3. If patient becomes agitated, reduce environmental stimuli. Use a soft, reassuring voice and gentle touch. Avoid quick, unexpected movements.

Anxiety related to actual or perceived threats or changes (eg, from bewildering hospital environment and multiple tests and procedures) secondary to degeneration of intellectual functioning

Desired outcome: Patient does not exhibit signs of uncontrolled or harmful anxiety.

1. Remain calm with patient. Use slow, deliberate gestures. Patients with Alzheimer's disease frequently mirror the emotions of others.

2. Provide time for patient to verbalize feelings of fear, concern, and anxiety. Patients with Alzheimer's disease often have trouble finding the correct words and may not be capable of stringing more than a few words together. Provide calm, realistic assurance, and stay with patient during periods of acute anxiety.

3. To help reduce anxiety and establish ongoing rapport, provide patient with a consistent caregiver.

Potential for violence related to irritability, frustration, and disorientation secondary to degeneration of cognitive thinking

Desired outcome: Patient does not become violent or demonstrate lack of control over his or her behavior.

1. Monitor patient for signs of increasing anxiety, eg, inability to verbalize feelings, suspiciousness of others, fear of others or self, irritability, and agitation, any of which can precede a violent act.

2. Encourage verbalization of feelings rather than suppression, as frustration can lead to violence.

3. Try to identify what is immediately distressing to patient and attempt to remedy it. Respond to the emotion. Do not confront patient and become authoritarian. If the situation cannot be remedied by calming the patient, use distraction and try to defuse the situation.

4. Remain calm and keep gestures slow and deliberate. Keep your hands where they can be seen. Approach patient slowly in a relaxed and open manner. Some patients may respond positively to gentle touch.

5. Reduce environmental stimuli.

6. Do not give routine care when patient is upset or agitated.

7. If patient is upset or agitated, avoid turning your back on patient. Think of escape routes for yourself, and be alert to potential weapons patient may use. Get help; protect yourself.

Alteration in family processes related to illness of family member

Desired outcome: SOs can verbalize knowledge of measures that will assist with coping for the care of the patient after hospital discharge.

1. Encourage patient's major caregiver to have other SOs or hired help take care of patient regularly so that he or she can have scheduled respites. Local day care programs also may be useful.

2. If SO is unaccustomed to handling finances, refer him or her to a place in which assistance with financial management is given. Often, patients with Alzheimer's disease lose the ability to manage finances and balance checkbooks and may give away money inappropriately.

3. Encourage early family legal planning and consultation. This is especially important because an individual must have mental capacity and competence to sign documents. Legal planning may involve wills, trusts, subpayee assignment for social security, power of attorney, and conservatorship, among others.

4. Encourage participation in local or national support groups such as Alzheimer's Disease and Related Disorders Association (ADRDA): 360 North Michigan Avenue, Chicago, IL 60601.

5. For other interventions, see **Alteration in family processes** in "Caring for Pa-

tients with Cancer and Other Life-Disrupting Illnesses," p. 546, "Appendix One."

See "Caring for Patients with Cancer and Other Life-Disrupting Illnesses" in "Appendix One," for the following: **Grieving**, p. 546. See "Caring for Patients with Neurologic Problems," in "Appendix One," for the following: **Potential fluid volume deficit**, p. 539, and **Ineffective airway clearance**, p. 540. For patients experiencing varying degrees of immobility, see related nursing diagnoses in "Caring for Patients on Prolonged Bed Rest," pp. 533–537, Appendix One.

E. Patient–Family Teaching and Discharge Planning

The degree and scope of discharge teaching and planning will depend on the severity of the patient's condition. Provide patient and SOs with verbal and written information for the following, as appropriate:

1. Referrals to community resources, local and national Alzheimer's disease chapters, public health nurse, visiting nurses association, community support groups, social workers, psychologic therapy, home health agencies, and extended and skilled care facilities.

2. Safety measures for preventing injury relative to cognitive deficits.

3. Measures that assist in reorienting and communicating with patient, in view of cognitive deficits.

4. Importance of scheduled respites and involvement in support groups for SOs.

5. Medications, including drug name, purpose, dosage, frequency, precautions, and potential side effects.

6. Exercises that promote muscle strength and mobility; measures for preventing contractures and skin breakdown; transfer techniques and proper body mechanics; and use of assistive devices, if appropriate.

7. Indications of constipation or infection; implementation of bowel and bladder training programs; and indwelling catheter care, if appropriate.

8. Indications of URI and measures that prevent regurgitation, aspiration, and infection.

▶ Section Three   **Traumatic Disorders of the Nervous System**

I. Herniated Nucleus Pulposus

Herniated nucleus pulposus is a rupture or bulging of an intervertebral disk that presses on and irritates the spinal nerve roots and/or spinal cord itself. This disorder is usually the result of injury or a series of insults to the vertebral column from lifting or twisting. Deterioration can occur suddenly, or it may happen gradually, with symptoms occurring months or years after the initial injury. Almost all herniated disks occur in the lumbar spine, with 90% of the problems occurring at L4–5. Cervical disk problems most frequently occur at C5–6 and C6–7.

A. Assessment

General indicators: Onset can be sudden, with intense unilateral pain, or pain that is dull, diffuse, deep, and aching. Symptoms vary according to the level of injury and nerves involved. Usually, pain is increased with sneezing, coughing, straining, and other activities that increase intra-abdominal or intrathoracic pressure. Immediate medical attention is essential if there is paralysis, extreme sensory loss, or altered bowel or bladder function.

□ *Cervical disk disease:* Pain and/or numbness in the upper extremities and/or back of the neck. Pain can radiate down the forearms and into the hands and fingers. Usually, the neck has restricted mobility, and there can be cervical muscle spasm as well. The patient may have upper extremity muscle weakness with decreased biceps or triceps reflex.

□ *Lumbar disk disease:* Pain in the lumbosacral area, with possible radiculopathy to the buttock, down the posterior surface of the thigh and calf, to the lateral border of the foot. Frequently, there is altered mobility, as evidenced by decreased ability to stand upright, listing to one side, asymmetrical gait, limited ability to flex forward, and restricted side movement caused by pain and muscle spasms. Reflex muscle spasms can cause bulging of the back, with concomitant flattening of the lumbar curve and possible scoliosis at the level of the affected disk. Usually, there is depression of the patellar and Achilles tendon reflexes.

Physical exam: Possible findings include depressed reflexes, muscle atrophy, paresthesia (described as "pins and needles"), or anesthesia in the dermatome of the involved nerves. The following tests are two of several that are performed to confirm the presence of lumbar disk disease:

□ *Straight leg raise test:* Examiner extends and raises patient's leg. The test is positive if patient has pain on the posterior aspect of the leg.

□ *Sciatic nerve test:* Examiner extends and raises patient's leg until pain is elicited and then lowers the leg to a comfortable level. The examiner then dorsiflexes the foot to stretch the sciatic nerve. If this causes pain, the test is positive for sciatic nerve involvement.

B. Diagnostic Tests

1. <u>X-ray of the spine:</u> May show narrowing of the vertebral interspaces in affected areas and loss of curvature of the spine.

2. <u>Magnetic resonance imaging (MRI):</u> May reveal that the disk is impinging on the spinal cord or nerve root.

3. <u>CT of the spine:</u> May reveal disk protrusion/prolapse.

4. <u>Myelogram:</u> May show characteristic deformity or filling defect. (See "Spinal Cord Injury," p. 172, for patient care.)

5. <u>Electromyelogram:</u> May show denervation patterns of specific nerve roots to indicate the level and site of injury.

C. Medical Management and Surgical Interventions

1. **Bed rest:** To limit motion of vertebral column, relieve nerve root compression, and enhance shrinkage of the disk.

2. **Bedboards under the mattress:** To support normal spine curvature and minimize spinal flexion.

3. **Orthotics such as splints, braces, girdles, and cervical collars:** To limit motion of the vertebral column. Braces are generally discouraged because they prohibit development of necessary musculature. If used, patient is weaned from them quickly so that adequate musculature can be developed to support the back.

4. **Pelvic/cervical skin traction:** To reduce muscle spasm and distract vertebral bodies to reduce bulging or rupture of the disk.

5. **Pelvic traction girdle:** Device used in an attempt to widen the interverterbral space. The patient pulls the side handles in an axial direction to flex the pelvis. Alternatively, the handles can be attached to weights.

6. **Other therapeutic modalities:** Include thermotherapy, massage, and dia-thermy/ultrasound electrotherapy.

7. **Physical therapy and a graded exercise program:** To strengthen the legs, back, and abdominal muscles. It is initiated once acute symptoms subside.

8. **Local injection of anesthetic or cortisone into paraspinal or paravertebral regions and epidural or subarachnoid spaces:** To reduce pain and muscle spasms and increase function.

9. **Pharmacotherapy**

   □ *Analgesics such as aspirin and acetaminophen.*

   □ *Muscle relaxants such as carisoprodol, methocarbamol, and diazepam.*

   □ *Corticosteroids such as dexamethasone:* May be given for a short period of time to reduce cord edema, if present.

   □ *Nonsteroidal anti-inflammatory agents.* See Table 8-1 in "Musculoskeletal Dis-orders," p. 370, for names and usual dosage.

10. **Chemonucleolysis:** Injection of the enzyme chymopapain directly into the disk to dissolve the nucleus pulposus in an attempt to relieve pressure on the spinal cord and/or nerve roots. Fluoroscopy is used to confirm proper posi-tion of the needle. Because of the 1% incidence of allergic reaction and po-tential for severe anaphylaxis, chymopapain is injected in the operating room with an anesthesiologist or nurse anesthetist in attendance.

    □ *Before the procedure:* Evaluate for patient allergies to papaya and meat ten-derizer.

    □ *After the procedure:* Be alert to signs of a delayed reaction: urticaria; itching; edema; nausea; vomiting; diarrhea; numbness; respiratory distress with rhi-nitis, wheezing, laryngospasm, and bronchospasm; hypotension; dysrhyth-mias; and loss of consciousness. Cardiac arrest can ensue if patient is not treated immediately. In addition, monitor for bowel and bladder dysfunc-tions, which are other potential complications of this procedure. Alert MD if patient does not have bowel sounds, has abdominal distention, and/or does not void within 8 hours of the procedure.

11. **Discectomy/laminectomy:** An incision is made, allowing removal of part of the vertebra (laminectomy) so that the herniated portion of the disk can be removed (discectomy). If multiple intervertebral disk spaces are explored, a drain may be present when the patient returns to the room.

    □ Monitor VS and perform neurovascular checks, including color, capillary refill, pulse, warmth, muscle power, movement, and sensation. Inspect dress-ing for excess drainage.

    □ Monitor for bowel and bladder dysfunction, which are potential complica-tions of this procedure. If patient does not have bowel sounds, has abdominal distention, and/or has not voided within 8 hours of the surgery, notify MD.

12. **Spinal fusion:** May be indicated for patients with recurrent low back pain, spondylolisthesis, or subluxation of the vertebra. Bone chips are taken from the iliac crest or tibia and placed in the prepared area of the unstable spine to fuse and stabilize the area. Internal fixation may be necessary to provide added stability until the fusion has healed fully.

    □ Monitor patients undergoing anterior cervical laminectomy and/or fusion for difficulty with swallowing, which can occur because of postoperative edema and hematoma formation secondary to retraction of the trachea and esophagus during surgery. Hoarseness also can occur secondary to nerve irritation.

D. Nursing Diagnoses and Interventions

Knowledge deficit: Proper body mechanics and other measures that prevent back injury

Desired outcome: Patient can verbalize knowledge of measures that prevent back injury and demonstrate proper body mechanics.

1. Teach patient proper body mechanics: Stand and sit straight with the chin and head up and the pelvis and back straight; bend at the knees and hips rather than at the waist, keeping the back straight; when carrying objects, hold them close to the body, avoiding twisting when lifting. Have patient demonstrate proper body mechanics, if possible, before hospital discharge.

2. Teach patient about the following measures for keeping the body in alignment: Sit close to the pedals when driving a car, and use a seat belt and firm back rest to support the back; support the feet on a footstool when sitting so that the knees are at hip level or higher; obtain a firm mattress or bedboard; use a flat pillow when sleeping to avoid strain on the neck, arms, and shoulders; sleep in a side-lying position with the knees bent or in a supine position with the knees and legs supported on pillows; avoid sleeping in a prone position.

3. Encourage patient to perform the following measures for relieving pressure on the back: Reduce to a proper weight for age, height, and sex; continue the exercise program prescribed by MD for strengthening abdominal, thoracic, and back muscles; use the thoracic and abdominal muscles when lifting to keep a significant portion of the weight off the vertebral disks.

4. Teach patient the rationale and procedure for Williams flexion exercises, which are performed while lying down on the floor with the knees flexed.

   □ *Pelvic tilt:* To strengthen the abdominal muscles. Stomach and buttock muscles are tightened and the pelvis is tilted with the lower spine kept flat against the floor.

   □ *Knee-to-chest raise:* To help make a stiff back limber. Each knee is individually raised to the chest, returned to the starting position, and then both knees are raised simultaneously to the chest.

   □ *Nose-to-knee touch:* To stretch hip muscles and strengthen abdominal muscles. Raise the knee to the chest and then pull the knee to the chest with the hands. Raise the head and try to touch the nose to the knee. Keep the lower back flat on the floor.

   □ *Half situps:* To strengthen abdomen and back. Slowly raise the head and neck to the top of the chest. Reach both hands forward to knees and hold for a count of 5. Repeat, keeping lower back flat on the floor.

5. Instruct patient to wear supportive shoes with a moderate heel height for walking.

6. Teach patient the following technique for sitting up at the bedside from a supine position: Logroll to the side, and then raise to a sitting position by pushing against the mattress with the hands while swinging the legs over the side of the bed. Instruct patient to maintain alignment of the back during the procedure.

7. Caution patient that pain is the signal to stop or change an activity or position.

8. Teach patient the following indicators that necessitate medical attention: increased sensory loss, increased motor loss/weakness, and loss of bowel and bladder function.

Knowledge deficit: Pain control measures

Desired outcome: Patient verbalizes knowledge of pain control measures.

1. Teach patient about the physiologic mechanisms of pain.

2. Instruct patient about methods of controlling pain and their individual applications. Methods include distraction, use of counterirritants, massage, use of

a transcutaneous electrical nerve stimulator (TENS), behavior modification, relaxation techniques, hypnosis, imagery, biofeedback, and diathermy. In addition, suggest the application of local heat or cold massage to painful areas. The latter can be achieved by freezing water in a paper cup, tearing off the top of the cup to expose the ice, and massaging in a circular motion, using the remaining portion of the cup as a handle.

3. Suggest that patient use a stool to rest the affected leg when standing.

4. Advise patient to sit in a straight-back chair that is high enough to get out of easily. Elevated toilet seats also may be useful, and straddling a straight-back chair and resting the arms on the chair back is comfortable for many individuals.

5. Encourage use of a firm mattress to support normal spinal curvature and extra pillows as needed for positioning. Some patients find normal bed height too low and use blocks to raise the bed to a more comfortable height.

6. Instruct patient on bed rest to roll rather than lift off the bedpan. The patient may find a fracture bedpan more comfortable than a regular bedpan.

7. Caution patient to avoid sudden twisting or turning movements. Explain the importance of logrolling when moving from side to side.

8. Advise patient to avoid factors that enhance spasms such as staying in one position too long, fatigue, chilling, and anxiety.

9. Suggest positions of comfort, such as lying on the side with the knees bent or lying supine with the knees supported on pillows.

10. Inform patient that applying a heating pad to the back 15–30 minutes before getting out of bed in the morning will help allay stiffness and discomfort. Heating pads should be used only for short intervals and only if patient's temperature sensations are intact. Remind patient to place a towel or cloth between heating pad and skin to prevent burns.

Knowledge deficit: Surgical procedure, preoperative routine, and postoperative regimen

Desired outcome: Patient can verbalize knowledge of the surgical procedure, preoperative routine, and postoperative regimen.

1. Assess patient's knowledge of the surgical procedure, preoperative routine, and postoperative regimen. Provide ample time for instruction and clarification.

2. Teach patient the technique for deep breathing (coughing may be contraindicated in the immediate postoperative period to prevent disruption of the fusion or surgical repair).

3. Explain that VS and neurologic status will be evaluated at frequent intervals after the surgery.

4. Teach patient the following logrolling technique for turning: Position a pillow between the legs, cross the arms across the chest while turning, and contract the long back muscles to maintain the shoulders and pelvis in straight alignment. Explain that initially, patient will be assisted in this procedure.

5. Teach patient the following technique for getting out of bed: Logroll to the side, splint the back, and raise to a sitting position by pushing against the mattress while swinging the legs over the side of the bed.

6. Explain that antiembolism hose will be applied after surgery to prevent thrombus formation. Teach techniques for ankle circling and calf pumping to promote venous circulation in the legs.

7. Advise patient that in the postoperative period, sitting for limited, prescribed periods of time will be permitted in a straight-back chair.

8. If patient is scheduled for a cervical laminectomy, explain that a cervical collar will be worn postoperatively.

9. Instruct patient in use of braces or corsets, if prescribed.

Potential Impairment of skin integrity related to irritation or pressure secondary to cervical or pelvic traction

Desired outcome: Patient does not exhibit signs of skin irritation or breakdown.

1. *Pelvic traction:* Ensure that patient is positioned correctly, with the HOB elevated 30° and the knees flexed. Be especially alert to the condition of the skin at the iliac crests, coccyx, and intergluteal fold. Inspect and massage these areas at least q4h.

2. *Cervical traction:* Maintain bed in low Fowler's position, and keep a small rolled towel under patient's shoulders to enhance hyperextension. Apply cornstarch to skin that is in contact with the halter. Check the chin, ears, and occipital areas for the presence of redness or irritation. Inspect and massage these areas at least q4h.

For surgical patients, see "Caring for Preoperative and Postoperative Patients," pp. 528–532, "Appendix One," for related nursing diagnoses and interventions. For patients experiencing varying degrees of immobility, see "Caring for Patients on Prolonged Bed Rest," pp. 533–537, "Appendix One," for related nursing diagnoses and interventions.

E. Patient–Family Teaching and Discharge Plannning

Provide patient and SOs with verbal and written information for the following:

1. Prescribed exercise regimen, including rationale for each exercise, technique for performing the exercise, number of repetitions of each, and frequency of the exercise periods. If possible, ensure that patient demonstrates understanding of the exercise regimen and proper body mechanics before hospital discharge.

2. Indicators of postoperative wound infection that necessitate medical attention including swelling, discharge, persistent redness, local warmth, fever, and pain.

3. Use and care of a brace or immobilizer, if appropriate.

4. Medications, including name, rationale, dosage, schedule, precautions, and potential side effects.

5. Anticonstipation routine, which should be initiated during hospitalization.

6. Pain control measures.

7. Telephone number of a resource person, should questions arise after hospital discharge.

8. Postsurgical activity restrictions as directed by MD. These may include the following: driving and riding in a car, sexual activity, lifting and carrying, tub bathing, going up and down steps, and the amount of time spent in or out of bed.

II. Spinal Cord Injury

The spinal cord injuries (SCIs) discussed in this section are caused by vertebral fractures and/or dislocations that sever, lacerate, or compress the spinal cord and interrupt neuronal function and transmission of nerve impulses. The spinal cord swells in response to injury, and this, along with hemorrhage, can cause additional compression and compromised function. Neurologic deficits resulting from compression may be reversible if the resulting edema and ischemia do not lead to spinal cord degeneration. Common causes of injury include motor vehicle accidents, diving or other sporting accidents, falls, and gunshot wounds.

Prognosis: Any evidence of voluntary motor function, sensory function, or sacral sensation below the level of injury is indicative of an incomplete SCI, with the potential for partial or complete recovery. After an acute injury, the spinal cord may go into a condition called *spinal shock*, in which there can be total loss of spinal cord function below the level of injury. During spinal shock there is no reflex activity, but it generally returns within 6 weeks. If there is no evidence of returning motor function after local reflexes have returned, the spinal cord is considered irreversibly damaged. Generally, an SCI does not cause immediate death unless it is at C-1 through C-3, which results in respiratory muscle paralysis. Individuals who survive these injuries require a ventilator for the rest of their lives. If the injury occurs at C-4, respiratory difficulties may result in death, although some patients who have survived the initial injury have been successfully weaned from the ventilator. Injuries below C-4 also can be life-threatening because of ascending cord edema, which can cause respiratory muscle paralysis. Other potential complications of SCIs include autonomic dysreflexia, decubitus ulcers, and UTI, any of which can be life-threatening.

A. Assessment

Acute indicators: Loss of sensation, weakness, and/or paralysis below the level of the injury; localized pain or tenderness over the site of injury; headache; hypothermia or hyperthermia; and alterations in bowel and bladder function.

☐ *Cervical injury:* Possible alterations in LOC, weakness or paralysis in all four extremities (quadriparesis or quadriplegia), paralysis of respiratory muscles or signs of respiratory problems such as flaring nostrils and use of accessory muscles for respirations. Any cervical injury can result in a low body temperature (to 96F), slowed pulse rate caused by vagal stimulation of the heart, hypotension caused by vasodilation, and decreased peristalsis.

☐ *Thoracic and lumbar injuries:* Paraparesis/paraplegia or altered sensation in the legs; hand and arm involvement in upper thoracic injuries.

☐ *Acute spinal shock:* Can last from 2 days to 6 months. Indicators depend on the severity of the injury, and include total loss of spinal cord function, flaccidity and/or absence of reflexes below the level of injury, paralytic ileus secondary to atonic bowel, bladder distention secondary to atonic bladder, low/falling BP secondary to loss of vasomotor tone, and anidrosis (absence of sweating) below level of injury.

Chronic indicators: As spinal shock resolves, muscle tone, reflexes, and some function may return, depending on severity and level of injury. The return of reflexes usually results in muscle spasticity. Chronic autonomic dysfunction may be manifested as fever; mild hypotension; anidrosis; and alterations in bowel, bladder, and sexual function. Injuries below L-1 or L-2 may result in permanent flaccid paralysis.

☐ *Bowel and bladder dysfunction:* With a spastic (upper motor neuron) bladder, there is loss of conscious sensation. But contraction does occur, which permits reflex emptying. Similarly, return of reflexes to the bowel permits reflex evacuation. The bowel and bladder with intact reflexes, even though the patient is incontinent, are generally considered trainable with reflex stimulation techniques and increased intra-abdominal pressure. A flaccid (lower motor neuron) bladder will distend and periodically overflow. Spinal cord lesions at or below the reflex arc of micturition (S-2 to S-4) usually result in this type of bladder. This bladder cannot be trained. Intermittent catheterization is usually indicated and the patient may be a candidate for urinary diversion.

Autonomic dysreflexia: For patients with injuries at or above T-6, the uninhibited autonomic reflex response to stimuli can be life-threatening as reflex activity returns. Signs and symptoms include hypertension, headache, blurred vision, sweating, flushing, nausea, low pulse rate, and nasal congestion.

Physical exam

□ *Acute (spinal shock):* Absence of DTRs below level of injury, absence of cremasteric reflex (scratching or light stroking of the inner thigh for male patients causes the testicle on that side to elevate) for T-12 and L-1 injuries; absence of penile reflex.

□ *Chronic:* Generally, increased DTRs occur if the spinal cord lesion is of the upper motor neuron type.

B. Diagnostic Tests

1. <u>X-ray of spine:</u> To delineate fracture, deformity, or displacement of vertebrae, as well as soft tissue masses such as hematomas.

2. <u>Magnetic resonance imaging (MRI):</u> Reveals changes in the spinal cord and surrounding soft tissue.

3. <u>Myelography:</u> Shows blockage or disruption of the spinal canal and is used if other diagnostic exams are inconclusive.

   □ *General pretest guidelines:* Assess for sensitivity to iodine, shellfish, and contrast medium; keep patient NPO for 8 hours.

   □ *Posttest guidelines:* Keep patient flat if isophendylate contrast medium was used; if metrizoate sodium was used, keep HOB elevated to 60° and do not allow patient to lie flat for 8 hours to minimize irritation to cranial nerves and cranial structures.

4. <u>ABG/pulmonary function tests:</u> To assess effectiveness of respirations.

5. <u>Cystometry:</u> To assess capacity and function of the bladder.

6. <u>CT scan:</u> To reveal changes in the spinal cord, vertebrae, and soft tissue surrounding the spine.

C. Medical Management and Surgical Interventions

Acute care:

1. **Immobilization of injury site:** See No. 7 below.

2. **Bed rest on a firm surface:** For example, Strykor wedge turning frame or Roto Rest Kinetic Treatment Table.

3. **Pharmacotherapy**

   □ *Anti-inflammatory agents and corticosteroids such as dexamethasone:* To reduce cord edema after the initial injury and minimize ascending cord edema.

   □ *Osmotic diuretics such as 20% mannitol:* Sometimes used for 10 days to reduce cord edema after the initial injury and minimize ascending cord edema.

   □ *Analgesics and sedatives:* To decrease pain and anxiety.

4. **Aggressive respiratory therapy:** For all patients with SCIs. Patient with injuries above C-5 are intubated and put on a ventilator.

5. **Nasogastric decompression during spinal shock phase**: Necessitated by the presence of paralytic ileus.

6. **Bladder decompression during spinal shock phase:** Either intermittent catheterization or continuous drainage.

7. **Surgery/immobilization:** May include traction, fusion, laminectomy, and closed or open reduction of fractures. The surgical goal is to immobilize the spine and, if indicated, decompress the spinal cord to help prevent additional neurologic deficit. If indicated, bone fragments are removed and the spine is surgically fused within 5–10 days of the injury.

   □ *Cervical spine:* Immobilized with Crutchfield tongs, Vinke Gardner-Wells tongs, or halo traction.

    □ *Thoracic spine:* May be immobilized with a surgical corset, plaster Minerva jacket, plastic body jacket, or spinal fusion.

    □ *Lumbar spine injuries:* Usually treated with closed reduction and hyperextension or extension with traction techniques, followed by immobilization in a plastic jacket or spica cast. If these interventions are unsuccessful or if neurologic symptoms occur, a laminectomy is usually performed.

    □ *Sacral (cauda equina) fracture:* Usually treated with a laminectomy and spinal fusion.

8. **Physical and occupational therapy:** Passive ROM is started on all joints. After the injury is stabilized, an aggressive rehabilitation program is initiated, including muscle-strengthening exercises; conditioning exercises; massage; and instruction in adaptive devices, equipment, and transfer techniques as appropriate. Patients with sacral injuries have the potential to walk and should be instructed in the use of braces, crutches, or a cane as appropriate.

9. **Counseling and psychotherapy:** To help patient and SOs adjust to the disability.

Chronic care:

1. **Pharmacotherapy**

    □ *Muscle relaxants such as diazepam.*

    □ *Antispasmodics such as baclofen and dantrolene:* To decrease spasms. Common side effects include drowsiness, dizziness, weakness, fatigue, and nausea. In addition, dantrolene may cause diarrhea, hepatitis (monitor patient for fever and jaundice), and photosensitivity.

    □ *Antibiotics:* To prevent bladder infection.

2. **Dietary management:** Limiting milk and other dairy products to minimize the risk of renal calculi, and promoting juices (eg, cranberry, plum, and prune) that leave an acid ash in the urine and decrease urinary pH, which reduces the potential for infection.

3. **Management of autonomic dysreflexia:** A medical emergency that can occur for patients with SCIs at or above level T-6. The noxious stimulus must be found and alleviated as quickly as possible. The following may be administered during crisis to control hypertension: adrenergic blockers such as IV phentolamine, vasodilators such as hydralazine, and ganglionic blocking agents such as reserpine or guanethidine. Tetracaine or lidocaine may be instilled into the bladder to reduce bladder excitability.

For nursing interventions, see **Potential for injury** related to autonomic dysreflexia secondary to noxious stimulus, directly following.

D. Nursing Diagnoses and Interventions

Potential for injury related to risk of autonomic dysreflexia secondary to noxious stimulus

Desired outcome: If autonomic dysreflexia occurs, it is detected and treated promptly, resulting in absence of injury to the patient.

1. Monitor for indicators of autonomic dysreflexia, including hypertension, headache, blurred vision, diaphoresis, flushing, nausea, bradycardia, and nasal congestion.

2. If autonomic dysreflexia is suspected, raise HOB immediately or assist patient into a sitting position to lower the BP.

3. Call for someone to notify MD; stay with patient and try to find and ameliorate the noxious stimulus. Speed is essential. Monitor BP q5 min during the hypertensive episode.

4. Assess the following sites for causes and implement measures for removing the noxious stimulus:

Bladder: Potential causes include distention, UTI, and calculus and other obstructions.

☐ Do not perform the Credé maneuver for a distended bladder.

☐ If the bladder is distended, catheterize patient using anesthetic jelly and notify MD *stat*.

☐ If a catheter is already in place, check the tubing for kinks and lower the drainage bag. If catheter patency is uncertain, recatheterize patient using anesthetic jelly.

☐ If the bladder is not distended, check for signs of UTI and/or urinary calculi, including cloudy urine, hematuria, and positive lab or x-ray results.

Bowel: Potential causes include constipation, impaction, insertion of suppository or enema, and rectal exam.

☐ Do not attempt rectal examination without first anesthetizing the rectal sphincter with anesthetic jelly.

☐ Use large amounts of anesthetic jelly in the anus and rectum before disimpacting patient to remove the potential stimulus.

Skin: Possible causes include pressure, heat, and cold.

☐ For male patients, check for a pressure source on the penis, and remove the pressure if present.

☐ Check the skin surface below level of injury. Monitor for the presence of a pressure area or sore, rash, ingrown toenail, or infected area. If indicated, apply a topical anesthetic.

☐ Observe for and remove the source of heat or cold (eg, ice pack or heating pad).

5. Administer antihypertensive agents as prescribed.

▶ **Note:** Prevention is the best way of dealing with autonomic dysreflexia. A good bowel regimen and skin integrity program are key factors in preventing the noxious stimuli that constipation or pressure areas may cause. Measures should be instituted to reduce the potential for UTI and urinary calculi, and the patient should be taught self-inspection of skin and urinary catheter and the importance of using anesthetic jelly for catheterization and disimpaction.

Alteration in bowel elimination: Constipation related to immobility and decreased peristalsis, atonic bowel, and loss of voluntary function secondary to sensorimotor deficit

Desired outcome: Patient has bowel movements that are soft and easily evacuated.

1. During acute phase of spinal shock, assess patient's bowel function by auscultating for bowel sounds, inspecting for the presence of abdominal distention, and monitoring for nausea and vomiting. Notify MD of significant findings. In the presence of fecal impaction, a small cleansing enema may be prescribed. Because the atonic intestine distends easily, administer small-volume enemas only. Avoid long-term use of enemas.

2. Once bowel activity returns, teach patient to attempt bowel movement 30 minutes after a meal or warm drink. This will allow patient's gastrocolic and duodenalcolic mass peristalsis reflexes to assist with evacuation. Increasing intra-abdominal pressure will also help promote bowel evacuation.

3. For patients with injuries at T-6 or above, promote use of stool softeners and high-fiber diet. Use suppositories and enemas only when essential and with extreme caution because they can precipitate autonomic dysreflexia.

4. For patients with hand mobility (who are not at risk for autonomic dysreflexia), teach the technique for digital stimulation of the anus to promote reflex bowel evacuation.

5. For other interventions, see the same nursing diagnosis in "Caring for Patients on Prolonged Bed Rest," p. 536, "Appendix One."

Potential alteration in respiratory function related to immobility, embolus, and/or increased secretions secondary to paresis or plegia of the respiratory muscles and/or restriction of chest expansion secondary to halo vest traction

Desired outcome: Patient does not exhibit signs of respiratory dysfunction.

1. Monitor ventilation capability by checking vital capacity, tidal volume, and pulmonary function tests. If vital capacity is less than 1 liter or if patient exhibits signs of hypoxia (tachycardia, increased restlessness, mental dullness, cyanosis), notify MD immediately.

2. Monitor for indicators of pulmonary embolus, including tachycardia, SOB, hemoptysis, and decreased or adventitious breath sounds. Pain may or may not be present, depending on the level of injury. Report significant findings to MD.

3. If indicated, prepare patient for a tracheostomy, endotracheal intubation, and/or mechanical ventilation to support respiratory function. If appropriate, arrange for a transfer to ICU for continuous monitoring.

4. If patient is wearing halo vest traction, assess respiratory status at least q4h. Ensure that the vest is not restricting chest expansion. Teach the use of incentive spirometry. Be alert to the indicators of pulmonary emboli.

5. For additional interventions, see **Potential alteration in respiratory function** related to prolonged inactivity in "Atelectasis," p. 12, in Chapter 1, "Respiratory Disorders."

Potential impairment of physical mobility related to inactivity and/or spasticity secondary to sensorimotor deficits

Desired outcomes: Patient does not exhibit signs of joint contractures and/or muscle atrophy. If possible, patient can demonstrate measures that enhance mobility and prevent complications and verbalize knowledge of their rationale and importance.

1. Once the injury is stabilized, assist patient with position changes. For example, a prone position, if not contraindicated, will help prevent sacral decubiti and hip contractures. Assist patient into this position on a regularly scheduled basis.

2. For patients with spasticity, use hand splints or cones to assist with maintaining a functional grasp.

3. To help prevent foot contractures for patients with spasticity, it may be helpful to fit patient with splints or high-top tennis shoes that are cut off at the toes so that each shoe ends just proximal to the metatarsal head. These shoes will help keep the feet dorsiflexed yet prevent the contact of the balls of the feet with a hard surface, which can cause spasticity. Avoid footboards for these patients because the hard surface may trigger spasticity and promote plantarflexion.

4. Elevate the extremities to reduce or prevent peripheral dependent edema.

5. For additional interventions, see **Potential impairment of physical mobility** in "Caring for Patients on Prolonged Bed Rest," p. 535, "Appendix One."

Potential for injury related to lack of access for external cardiac compression, incorrect neck position, irritation of cranial nerves, and impaired lateral vision secondary to use of halo vest traction

Desired outcomes: Patient does not exhibit signs of injury from wearing halo vest traction. If complications do occur, they are detected and reported promptly, resulting in immediate treatment and absence of injury to the patient.

1. Ensure that an open-end wrench is taped to the halo vest so that if external cardiac compression is needed the bolts can be released and the vest removed promptly

2. Assess position of the patient's neck relative to the body. Alert MD to the presence of flexion or hyperextension. Keep a torque screwdriver in a secure place so that MD can readily adjust tension on bars to return the patient's neck position to neutral.

3. Evaluate degree of sensation and movement of the upper extremities, and assess cranial nerve function. Changes in cranial nerve function can occur if the cranial pins compress or irritate a nerve. Notify MD of significant findings.

4. If patient is ambulatory, teach him or her how to survey the environment while walking, either by using a mirror or turning the eyes to their extreme lateral positions.

Potential impairment of skin integrity related to irritation and pressure secondary to presence of halo vest traction

Desired outcome: Patient does not exhibit signs of skin irritation or breakdown.

1. Inspect the skin around the vest edges for redness and other signs of irritation. Massage these areas routinely to promote circulation and help prevent breakdown.

2. Investigate complaints of discomfort or uncomfortable fit. Pad the vest as needed until it can be properly adjusted by MD. Protect the vest from moisture and soiling. Be alert to foul odor from the cast openings, which can signal pressure necrosis beneath the vest.

3. Instruct/assist patient with changing body positions q2h.

Note: For a discussion of pin care, see "Fractures" in Chapter 8, "Musculoskeletal Disorders," for the following: **Knowledge deficit:** Function of external fixation, pin care, and signs and symptoms of pin site infection, p. 395.

See "Multiple Sclerosis" for the following: **Knowledge deficit:** Precautions and potential side effects of prescribed medications, p. 148. If the patient has bladder dysfunction, see related nursing diagnoses in Chapter 3, "Renal–Urinary Disorders," in the following: "Urinary Incontinence," pp. 136–137, "Urinary Retention," p. 139, and "Neurogenic Bladder," pp. 140–142. See "Caring for Patients with Neurologic Problems" in "Appendix One," for the following: **Potential fluid volume deficit**, p. 539, **Self-care deficit**, p. 540, **Potential for injury** related to unsteady gait, p. 537, **Potential for injury** related to impaired pain, touch, and temperature sensations, p. 540, **Alteration in comfort:** Pain and/or spasms, p. 543, and **Alteration in nutrition:** Less than body requirements, p. 538. See "Caring for Patients with Cancer and Other Life-Disrupting Illnesses" in "Appendix One" for the following: **Disturbance in self-concept**, p. 544, **Fear**, p. 544, **Alteration in family processes**, p. 546, and **Grieving**, p. 546. For patients with varying degrees of immobility, see related nursing diagnoses and interventions in "Caring for Patients on Prolonged Bed Rest," pp. 533–537, "Appendix One."

E. Patient–Family Teaching and Discharge Planning

Provide patient and SOs with verbal and written information for the following:

1. Referrals to community resources such as public health nurse, visiting nurses association, community support groups, social workers, psychologic therapy, vocational rehabilitation agency, home health agencies, and extended and skilled care facilities. As appropriate, provide the following addresses: Infor-

mation Center for Individuals with Disabilities: 20 Park Plaza, Suite 330, Boston, MA 02116; National Spinal Cord Injury Association: 369 Elliot Street, Newton Upper Falls, MA 02164; and American Spinal Injury Association: 250 East Superior, Room 619, Chicago, IL 60611.

2. Safety measures relative to decreased sensation and motor deficits and the symptoms, preventive measures, and interventions for autonomic dysreflexia.

3. For additional information, see teaching/discharge planning interventions 4–9 in "Multiple Sclerosis," p. 149.

III. Head Injury

Head injuries can cause varying degrees of damage to the skull and/or brain tissue. Primary injuries that result from head injury include skull fracture, concussion, contusion, scalp laceration, brain tissue laceration, and tear or rupture of cerebral vessels. Problems that arise soon after the primary injury and are the result of that injury include hemorrhage and hematoma formation from the tear or rupture of vessels, ischemia from interrupted blood flow, cerebral swelling and edema, and infection, any of which can interrupt neuronal function.

A. Assessment

Concussion: Mild head injury in which there is temporary neurologic impairment involving loss of consciousness and possible amnesia of the event. After the concussion, the patient may have headache, dizziness, nausea, lethargy, and irritability. Although full recovery usually occurs in a few days, a postconcussion syndrome with headaches, dizziness, and lethargy may continue for several weeks.

Contusion: Bruising of the brain tissue producing a longer-lasting neurologic deficit than concussion. Traumatic amnesia often occurs, causing loss of memory not only of the trauma, but also of events occurring prior to the incident. Loss of consciousness is common, and it is generally more prolonged than that with concussion. Changes in behavior such as agitation or confusion can last for several hours to days. Headache, nausea, lethargy, motor paralysis, paresis, and possibly seizures can occur as well. Depending on the extent of damage, there is the potential for either full recovery or permanent neurologic deficit such as seizures, paralysis, paresis, or even coma and death.

Skull fracture: Can be *closed* (simple) or *open* (compound). Skull fractures are further classified as *linear* (hairline), *comminuted* (fragmented, splintered), or *depressed* (pushed inward toward the brain tissue). A blow forceful enough to fracture the skull is capable of causing significant brain tissue damage, and therefore, close observation is essential. With a penetrating wound or basilar fracture (see below), there is the potential for meningitis, encephalitis, brain abscess, cellulitis, or osteomyelitis.

□ *Basilar fractures:* Do not show up easily on skull/cervical x-rays. Indicators include blood from the nose, throat, ears; serous or serosanguinous drainage from the nose, throat, ears, eyes; Battle's sign (bruising noted behind the ear); "raccoon's eyes" (bruising around the eyes in the absence of eye injury); and bleeding behind the tympanum noted on otoscopic exam. Glucose in serous drainage signals the presence of CSF.

□ *Temporal fractures:* May result in deafness or facial paralysis.

□ *Occipital fractures:* May cause visual field and gait disturbances.

□ *Sphenoidal fractures:* May disrupt the optic nerve, possibly causing blindness.

Rupture of cerebral blood vessels

□ *Epidural (extradural) hematoma or hemorrhage:* Bleeding, usually arterial, between dura mater (outer meninges) and skull. Indicators are primarily those of increased ICP: headache, unilateral pupil dilation (on same side as the lesion), and possibly hemiparesis. Typically, the patient loses consciousness for a short period of time immediately after injury, regains consciousness, and has a lucid period; however, because arterial bleeding causes a rapid rise in ICP, a rapid decrease in LOC often ensues. These patients are at high risk for brain stem herniation.

□ *Subdural hematoma or hemorrhage:* Accumulation of venous blood between dura mater (outer meninges) and arachnoid membrane (middle meninges) that is not reabsorbed. This type of hematoma is classified as acute, subacute, or chronic depending on how quickly indicators arise. In acute subdural hematomas, indicators appear within 24 hours, resulting from focal neurologic deficit (hemiparesis, pupillary dilation) and increased ICP (headache, decreased LOC). When indicators occur 2–10 days later, the hematoma is considered subacute. When indicators occur several weeks or more later, it is considered chronic. Early indicators can include headache, progressive personality changes, decreased intellectual functioning, and drowsiness. Later indicators may include unilateral weakness or paralysis and loss of consciousness.

□ *Intracerebral hemorrhage:* Arterial or venous bleeding into the white matter of the brain. Signs of increased ICP may develop early if the bleeding causes a rapidly expanding space-occupying lesion. If the bleeding is slower, signs of increased ICP can take 36–72 hours to develop. Indicators depend on location of the hematoma and can include aphasia, hemiparesis, hemiplegia, hemisensory deficits, and loss of consciousness.

□ *Subarachnoid hemorrhage:* Bleeding into the subarachnoid space below the arachnoid membrane (middle meninges) and above the pia mater (inner meninges next to brain). The patient often has a severe headache. Other general indicators include vomiting, restlessness, seizures, and loss of consciousness. Signs of meningeal irritation include nuchal rigidity and a positive Kernig's sign. This patient may be a candidate for a shunt because of hemorrhagic interference with CSF circulation.

Indicators of increased intracranial pressure: Sudden onset or worsening of headache, renewed or worsening nuchal rigidity, renewed or persistant nausea and vomiting, increasing BP, widening pulse pressure, decreased pulse rate (initially may increase), transient loss of vision, alteration in LOC ranging from irritability and restlessness to confusion to coma, seizures, and onset or increase in sensorimotor changes or deficits.

Indicators of impending/occurring brain stem herniation: Change in mental status or decreased LOC such as lethargy, stupor, coma; irregular respirations (eg, Cheyne-Stokes); hemiparesis; and pupillary changes such as inequality, nonreactivity to light, or dilation and fixation. Signs are generally related to brain stem compression and disruption of cranial nerves and vital centers.

B. Diagnostic Tests

1. Skull and cervical spine x-rays: To locate skull and neck fractures. If the fracture crosses the groove of the meningeal artery, epidural hematoma is likely to be found.

2. Magnetic resonance imaging (MRI): To identify the presence of blood in the intracranial area.

3. CT scan: To identify any accumulation of blood and/or a shift of midline structure caused by increased ICP.

4. Brain scan: To identify hematoma with chronic subdural hematoma. Generally, it is not done for more acute disorders because of the lengthy uptake time of the radioactive isotope.

5. EEG: May reveal electrical activity, indicating the presence of a hematoma. (See "Seizure Disorders," p. 202, for patient care.)

6. Cerebral angiography: To reveal presence of a hematoma and status of blood vessels secondary to rupture or compression. (See "Cerebral Aneurysm," p. 188, for patient care.)

C. Medical Management and Surgical Interventions

1. **Support respirations and other vital functions:** Oxygen delivery, suction, intubation, and ventilation. Initially, patient may have an NG tube for gastric decompression to prevent vomiting and aspiration.

2. **Monitor vital signs/neurologic status:** Baseline assessment is established and patient is monitored frequently for changes.

3. **Bed rest with HOB elevated** (or as prescribed): To promote venous drainage and help reduce cerebral congestion and edema.

4. **Fluid restrictions:** NPO status for 8–24 hours (or longer if patient is unresponsive). Then, fluids are limited to decrease cerebral edema. Hypotonic IV solutions such as 5% dextrose in water are contraindicated because they increase cerebral edema.

5. **Diet:** Hyperalimentation/intralipids or progressive diet, depending on patient's LOC and ability to swallow.

6. **Treat secondary complications:** For example, cerebral edema, increased ICP, inappropriate ADH secretion, disseminated intravascular coagulation (DIC), adult respiratory distress syndrome (ARDS), and diabetes insipidus.

7. **Pharmacotherapy: Note:** Narcotics and other medications that alter mentation are contraindicated.

   □ *Anticonvulsants:* Prophylaxis for seizures with or following penetrating wounds. These drugs may include phenytoin, phenobarbital, and IV diazepam.

   □ *Glucocorticosteroids such as dexamethasone and osmotic diuretics such as mannitol:* To decrease cerebral edema.

   □ *Antibiotics and tetanus prophylaxis:* In the presence of penetrating wounds and basilar fractures.

   □ *Antipyretics:* For fever.

   □ *Analgesics such as acetaminophen:* For pain.

   □ *Mild sedatives such as chloral hydrate or diphenhydramine:* For restlessness.

8. **Hypothermia:** If indicated, a hypothermia blanket is used to reduce body temperature to 87–90F and thereby minimize metabolic needs.

9. **Surgical procedures**

   □ *Suturing:* To repair superficial laceration or dural tears.

   □ *Craniotomy:* To remove bone fragment or elevate depressed fractures. (See "Brain Tumors," p. 183, for patient care.)

   □ *Craniotomy or trephination ("burr" holes):* To evacuate hematomas, control hemorrhage, remove foreign objects, or debride necrotic tissue.

   □ *Cranioplasty:* To repair traumatic or surgical defects in the skull.

   □ *Ventricular puncture:* To remove excess CSF.

   □ *Ventricular shunt:* To provide drainage of CSF and reduce ICP.

D. Nursing Diagnoses and Interventions

Knowledge deficit: Caretaker's responsibilities for observing the patient who is sent home with a concussion

Desired outcome: Caretaker can verbalize knowledge of the observation regimen and returns the patient to the hospital if neurologic deficits are noted.

If patient goes home for observation, provide caretaker with verbal and written instructions for the following:

1. Avoid giving patient anything stronger than acetaminophen to relieve headache. Aspirin is usually contraindicated because it can prolong bleeding, if it occurs.

2. Assess patient at least qh for the next 24 hours as follows: Awaken patient; ask patient's name, where he or she is, and caretaker's name; monitor for twitching or seizure activity. Return patient to the hospital immediately if he or she becomes increasingly difficult to awaken; cannot answer questions appropriately; cannot answer at all; develops seizures; develops or reports worsening headache or nausea/vomiting; or has visual disturbances, twitching, seizures, or walking difficulties.

3. Ensure that patient rests and eats lightly for the first day or so after the concussion or until he or she feels well.

Potential for infection related to increased susceptibility secondary to penetrating or open head injuries and/or surgical wounds

Desired outcomes: Patient does not develop a CNS infection, or, if it occurs, it is detected and treated promptly. Patient can verbalize knowledge of the signs and symptoms of infection and the importance of reporting them promptly.

1. Monitor injury site or surgical wounds for indicators of infection, such as persistent redness, warmth, pain, hardness, and purulent drainage. Notify MD of significant findings.

2. Be alert to indicators of meningitis (p. 153) or encephalitis (p. 156), which can occur after a penetrating, open head injury, or cerebral surgical wound.

3. When examining scalp lacerations and assessing for foreign bodies or palpable fractures, wear sterile gloves and follow aseptic technique. Cleanse the area gently, and cover scalp wounds with sterile dressings.

4. If CSF leakage occurs, do not clean the ears unless prescribed by MD. Place a sterile pad over the affected ear, but do not pack it. Position patient so that fluids can drain. Change dressings when they become damp, using aseptic technique.

5. To prevent introduction of bacteria into the nervous system in the presence of CSF leakage or possible basilar fracture, avoid nasal suction and instruct patient to avoid nose blowing.

6. Teach patient to report promptly any indicators of infection.

Potential impairment of physical mobility related to prolonged inactivity secondary to sensorimotor deficits and decreased LOC

Desired outcome: Patient does not exhibit signs of joint contractures or muscle atrophy.

1. For patients at risk of increased ICP, perform passive ROM exercises rather than allow active or assisted ROM exercises, which can increase intra-abdominal or intrathoracic pressure, and hence, ICP. For the same reason, avoid using the prone position.

2. Once the risk of increased ICP is no longer significant, additional measures to enhance mobility and strength may be implemented. For discussion, see **Potential impairment of physical mobility** in "Caring for Patients on Prolonged Bed Rest," pp. 535–536, "Appendix One."

Alteration in comfort: Headache related to head injury

Desired outcome: Patient relates a reduction in discomfort and does not exhibit signs of uncontrolled pain.

1. Administer analgesics as prescribed. Patients with head injuries generally do not have much pain, and the pain is usually relieved by analgesics such as acetaminophen. Narcotics are contraindicated because they can mask neurologic indicators of increased ICP and cause respiratory depression.

2. For other interventions, see **Alteration in comfort** in "Caring for Patients with Neurologic Problems," p. 543, "Appendix One."

If the patient has bladder dysfunction, see "Renal–Urinary Disorders," pp. 135–142, for related discussions. **Caution:** The Credé maneuver and other measures that can increase intra-abdominal and intrathoracic pressure are contraindicated for patients who are at risk of increased ICP.

See "Alzheimer's Disease" for the following: **Sensory-perceptual alterations** related to inability to evaluate reality, p. 163. See "Cerebrovascular Accident" for the following: **Impaired verbal communication** related to aphasia and/or dysarthria, p. 195. See "Seizure Disorders" for the following: **Potential for injury** related to oral, musculoskeletal, and airway vulnerability secondary to seizure activity, p. 203. For patients with varying degrees of immobility, see related nursing diagnoses in "Caring for Patients on Prolonged Bed Rest," pp. 533–537, "Appendix One." See "Caring for Patients with Neurologic Problems" in "Appendix One" for the following: **Potential for injury** related to risk of increased ICP, p. 542, **Alteration in nutrition**, p. 538, **Self-care deficit**, p. 540, **Potential fluid volume deficit**, p. 539, **Potential for injury** related to unsteady gait, p. 537, **Potential for injury** related to visual disturbances, p. 543, **Potential for injury** related to corneal irritation/abrasion, p. 538, **Ineffective airway clearance**, p. 540, and **Alteration in bowel elimination:** Constipation, p. 541. See "Caring for Patients with Cancer and Other Life-Disrupting Illnesses" in "Appendix One" for the following: **Disturbance in self-concept**, p. 544, **Fear**, p. 544, **Alteration in family processes**, p. 546, and **Grieving**, p. 546.

E. Patient–Family Teaching and Discharge Planning

The head-injured patient can have varying degrees of neurologic deficit, ranging from mild to severe. As indicated by the patient's condition and prognosis, provide patient and SOs with verbal and written information for the following:

1. Referrals to community resources such as visiting nurses association, community support groups, social workers, psychologic therapy, vocational rehabilitation agency, home health agencies, and extended and skilled care facilities. In addition, provide the following address: National Head Injury Foundation: 18 A Vernon Street, Framingham, MA 01701.

2. Safety measures related to decreased sensation, visual disturbances, motor deficits, and seizure activity.

3. For other information, see teaching/discharge planning interventions 4–9 in "Multiple Sclerosis," p. 149.

▶ Section Four   **Nervous System Tumors**

I. Brain Tumors

The abnormal and uncontrolled cell growth of neoplastic or benign tumors can have a wide variety of effects on the brain. Most significant is the disruption of neuronal function caused by infiltration of the tissue, compression of brain tissue and blood vessels, and/or obstruction of normal flow of CSF. *Primary brain tumors*, composed of nervous system tissue, rarely metastasize outside the CNS. *Secondary brain tumors* arise from cells that have metastasized from other parts of the body such as the lung, breast, and skin. Although benign tumors tend to be more treatable than neoplastic tumors, they are considered as serious because they are equally capable of increasing ICP, which in turn compromises vital centers.

Tumor classification

□ *Gliomas:* Constitute 45% of all brain tumors, are neoplastic, arise from brain connective tissue, and are generally infiltrative and cannot be removed totally by surgery. The most common and most malignant glioma is glioblastoma multiforme. It comprises 20% of all brain tumors.

□ *Secondary (metastatic):* Most often occurs in the cerebrum, may be multiple because of the "seeding" effect, and resembles the primary neoplasm histologically.

□ *Meningiomas:* Originate from pia or arachnoid membranes, comprise around 15% of all brain tumors, and, while technically benign, can invade the skull and cause brain tissue compression.

□ *Schwannomas (eg, acoustic neuroma):* Account for about 10% of brain tumors, affect the craniospinal nerve sheath, and are slow growing and technically benign.

A. Assessment

Onset of signs and symptoms is usually insidious.

General indicators: Headache, nausea, projectile vomiting, lethargy, forgetfulness, disorientation, and seizure activity.

Focal symptoms

□ *Frontal lobe:* Personality/mood changes, impaired judgment, weakness or paralysis (usually unilateral), apraxia, aphasia.

□ *Parietal lobe:* Visual field deficit, sensory disturbance, impaired position sense, perceptual problems such as altered stereognosis and dyslexia.

□ *Temporal lobe:* Auditory changes, tinnitus, visual field deficit, sensory aphasia, impaired memory, personality changes, psychomotor seizures.

□ *Occipital lobe:* Seizures, visual agnosia, visual field deficit.

□ *Cerebellar:* Tremors, nystagmus, uncoordination, loss of balance, gait disturbances, nuchal headache.

□ *Ventricular or hypothalamic:* Diabetes insipidus, weight gain, somnolence, headache, disturbance of temperature regulation.

□ *Cranial nerve:* Sense of smell alterations, ptosis, diplopia, alterations in ocular movement, drooping of facial muscles on the same side as the tumor, difficulty swallowing, loss of cough/gag reflex, loss of corneal reflex, protrusion of the tongue toward the side of the tumor.

□ *Schwannoma:* Unilateral hearing loss with or without tinnitus, stiff neck. Other symptoms may include decreased facial sensation, facial muscle weakness or paralysis on same side as the hearing loss, and diplopia. Late symptoms include ataxia and arm coordination problems secondary to brain stem and cerebellar compression.

Indicators of increased ICP: See discussion in "Head Injury," p. 178.

Indicators of impending/occurring brain stem herniation: See discussion in "Head Injury," p. 178.

Physical exam: Ophthalmoscopic examination may reveal papilledema if ICP is increased; visual field exam may reveal impairment such as hemianopia (blindness in part of the field of vision); and audiometry or vestibular function studies may show abnormalities as well.

B. Diagnostic Tests

Tests are performed to rule out vascular etiology, such as hemorrhage, abscess, and trauma, as well as diagnose brain tumor. Any one or a combination of the following tests may be performed.

1. Magnetic resonance imaging (MRI): May reveal presence of tumor, tissue shift, and hydrocephalus. This diagnostic tool, because of its ability to detect biochemical changes, can help diagnose tumors at an early stage.

2. CT scan: May detect mass, tissue shift, and hydrocephalus.

3. <u>X-rays of the skull and spinal cord:</u> May reveal shift of brain structure, mass, and calcification.

4. <u>EEG:</u> May localize abnormal brain wave activity. (See "Seizure Disorders," p. 202, for patient care.)

5. <u>Brain scan:</u> May demonstrate presence of a space-occupying lesion via uptake of radioisotope.

6. <u>Echoencephalography of the cranium:</u> May show shift of brain structure.

7. <u>Cerebral angiography:</u> To outline the tumor and reveal alterations in position of the vessels. (See "Cerebral Aneurysm," p. 188, for patient care.)

8. <u>Lumbar puncture and CSF analysis:</u> May be performed in the absence of any indicators of increased ICP. CSF may be clear to bloody; protein values and WBC count may be increased; glucose values may be decreased; and cytology may reveal the presence of cancer cells. (See "Bacterial Meningitis," p. 153, for patient care.)

9. <u>Lesion biopsy:</u> Identifies pathologic cells and confirms diagnosis.

C. Medical Management and Surgical Interventions

The mode of treatment depends on the tumor's histologic type, anatomic location, and sensitivity to radiation. Treatment usually includes surgery, often in combination with radiation and/or chemotherapy. The location and accessibility of the tumor determines whether or not surgery can be performed.

1. **Craniotomy:** Surgical opening into the skull. The dura and boneflap may be left open postoperatively to accommodate cerebral edema and prevent compression. Typically, the patient is in ICU immediately after surgery, where the following interventions are performed:

   ☐ Frequent VS and neurologic assessment to monitor for changes and trends.

   ☐ Assessment of the dressing for the presence of abnormal bleeding or CSF leakage. Nonsanguineous drainage is tested with a glucose reagent stick, which is positive in the presence of CSF. Sterile technique is maintained to prevent wound infection and meningitis.

   ☐ If surgery was performed with the patient in Fowler's position, the same position (usually a 30–35° angle) is maintained as prescribed.

   ☐ Patients with supratentorial craniotomies are maintained with HOB elevated and are kept off the operative site.

   ☐ Patients with infratentorial craniotomies for cerebellar or brain stem tumors are usually kept flat for 48 hours. To prevent pressure areas with subsequent skin breakdown, the patient is logrolled q2h to the side, with the head kept in alignment. Pressure is kept off the operative site.

   ☐ Oral temperatures are avoided because of the patient's decreased cognitive function. Rectal temperature is taken q2–4h, and the staff is alert to the presence of hyperthermia. 102F is considered a dangerous level, and the patient is sponged with tepid water and/or placed on a hypothermia blanket if this occurs.

   ☐ Usually the patient is kept NPO for the first 36–48 hours because of the risk of vomiting and choking. Fluids are generally restricted to reduce cerebral edema. Usually, an indwelling catheter is inserted to allow more accurate monitoring of urine output.

   ☐ In the presence of periorbital edema, petroleum jelly and cold compresses are lightly applied around patient's eyes. Maximum swelling usually occurs within 24–48 hours of surgery.

   ☐ Measures are taken to reduce increased ICP (see **Potential for injury** related to risk of increased ICP in "Caring for Patients with Neurologic Problems," p. 542, "Appendix One.") Precautions are taken for seizures (see **Potential for**

injury related to oral, musculoskeletal, and airway vulnerability secondary to seizure activity, p. 203, in "Seizure Disorders").

2. **Ventricular shunt for ventricular drainage:** May be done to allow drainage of CSF. Shunt types vary but can extend from the lateral ventricle of the brain to one of the following: subarachnoid space of the spinal canal, right atrium of the heart, a large vein, or the peritoneal cavity. This procedure is usually performed if the brain tumor is inoperable and obstructs the flow of CSF.

3. **Supportive pharmacotherapy**

   □ *Anticonvulsants:* If indicated.

   □ *Diuretics:* To decrease cerebral edema and ICP.

   □ *Corticosteroids such as dexamethasone:* To reduce cerebral edema.

   □ *Antacids and H_2 receptor antagonists:* To prevent/treat stress ulcers.

   □ *Analgesics:* For headaches.

4. **Radiation therapy:** Frequently begun as soon as the surgical incision has healed. It can be localized or include the entire brain and part of the spinal cord, depending on the type, location, and extent of the tumor. Radiation can cause inflammation of the brain, which in turn increases ICP and neurologic symptoms.

5. **Chemotherapy:** Carmustine, lomustine, and methyl-CCNU cross the blood–brain barrier, and because of this are particularly useful for patients with brain tumors.

Depending on the presence and severity of neurologic deficits, the patient also may need the following:

6. **Respiratory support and intubation**: To maintain the airway and supply oxygen as needed.

7. **Fluid and nutritional support**: The patient may require high-calorie, high-protein supplements, enteral feedings or parenteral nutrition because of swallowing/chewing deficits or side effects of radiation and chemotherapy, and IV fluids to prevent dehydration.

8. **Physical medicine:** For example, PT, OT, and assistive devices or braces, so that the patient can maintain mobility and independence with ADLs. Muscle-strengthening exercises, conditioning exercises, and gait training are also frequently prescribed.

9. **ROM exercises:** To maintain or increase joint function and prevent contractures. While the patient is at risk of increased ICP, the exercises are passive only. Once the risk of increased ICP is minimized, active or active-assistive ROM is employed.

D. Nursing Diagnoses and Interventions

See "Alzheimer's Disease" for the following: **Sensory-perceptual alterations** related to inability to evaluate reality, p. 163. See "Head Injury" for the following: **Potential impairment of physical mobility**, p. 180. See "Cerebrovascular Accident" for the following: **Impaired verbal communication** related to aphasia and/or dysarthria, p. 195. See "Seizure Disorders" for the following: **Potential for injury** related to oral, musculoskeletal, and airway vulnerability secondary to seizure activity, p. 203. For patients with varying degrees of immobility, see related nursing diagnoses in "Caring for Patients on Prolonged Bed Rest," pp. 533–537, "Appendix One." See "Caring for Patients with Neurologic Problems" in "Appendix One" for the following: **Potential for injury** related to risk of increased ICP, p. 542, **Potential for injury** related to unsteady gait, p. 537, **Potential for injury** related to visual disturbances, p. 543, **Potential for injury** related to risk of corneal irritation/abrasion, p. 538, **Alteration in bowel elimination:** Constipation, p. 541, **Ineffective airway clearance**, p. 540, **Potential fluid volume deficit**, p. 539, **Alteration in comfort**, p. 543, **Self-care deficit**, p. 540, and **Alteration in nutrition**, p. 538. See "Caring for Patients with Cancer and Other Life-Disrupting Illnesses," pp. 544–551, and "Caring for Preoperative and Postoperative Patients," pp. 528–532, "Appendix One," as appropriate.

E. Patient—Family Teaching and Discharge Planning

Provide patient and SOs with verbal and written information for the following as appropriate:

1. Safety measures specific to sensory deficits, motor deficits, uncoordination, cognitive deficits, and seizures.

2. Measures to promote communication in the presence of aphasia.

3. Appropriate referrals to community resources such as public health nurse, visiting nurses association, community support groups, social workers, psychologic therapy, vocational rehabilitation agency, home health agencies, and extended and skilled care facilities. In addition, provide the address for the American Cancer Society: 777 Third Avenue, New York, NY 10017.

4. Care of postoperative or postprocedure wounds.

5. Potential side effects and precautions for patients undergoing radiation therapy.

6. Medications, including drug name, purpose, dosage, frequency, precautions, and potential side effects, especially for chemotherapeutic agents.

7. Exercises that promote muscle strength and mobility, measures for preventing contractures and skin breakdown, transfer techniques and proper body mechanics, use of assistive devices.

8. Measures for relieving pain, nausea, or other discomfort.

9. Indications of constipation, urinary retention, or UTI; implementation of bowel and bladder training programs; and if appropriate, care of indwelling catheters.

10. Indications of URI and measures to prevent regurgitation, aspiration, and respiratory infection.

11. Importance of follow-up care, including MD visits, PT, OT, speech therapy, pyschologic counseling, and laboratory monitoring for side effects of radiation/chemotherapy.

II. Spinal Cord Tumors

The majority of spinal cord tumors interrupt neuronal function and nerve impulse transmission by compressing the spinal cord and its roots and eventually causing degeneration of the cord. Spinal cord tumors can occur anywhere along the length of the spinal cord, and, if untreated, lead to paralysis and sensory deficits. *Intramedullary tumors* occur within the cord itself and are fairly rare. *Extramedullary tumors* occur outside the spinal cord and are further classified as intradural or extradural. *Intradural tumors*, such a meningiomas and schwannomas, account for the majority of all primary spinal cord tumors. *Extradural tumors* are usually secondary (metastatic) tumors that have been "seeded" from other sites in the body such as the prostate, bone marrow, lymph tissue, breast, or lungs. They occur in the epidural space or in the vertebrae that surround the spinal cord and related tissue.

A. Assessment

Indicators vary according to tumor site.

Motor involvement: Weakness or paralysis of one or more body parts, with the potential for spasticity below the level of the tumor. If the tumor interrupts the spinal cord reflex arc (eg, a tumor at the level of the cauda equina), decreased or loss of reflexes, flaccidity, muscle atrophy, and fasciculations can occur.

Sensory involvement: Decreased sensation to pain, touch, and temperature, with potential loss of position and vibration sense.

Pain: Neck or back pain that persists despite bed rest, is most severe over the tumor site, and potentially radiates around the trunk or down the affected side because of nerve root irritation.

Bladder and bowel dysfunction: The patient may have a spastic bladder, causing urinary retention; a flaccid bladder, causing incontinence; and/or bowel incontinence from loss of control.

Physical exam: Depending on location of the tumor, patient may exhibit increased or decreased/absent DTRs.

B. Diagnostic Tests

1. <u>X-ray:</u> May show changes in vertebrae such as destruction and collapse of bony matrix.

2. <u>Magnetic resonance imaging (MRI):</u> To show tumor location and the presence of cord compression. Because it can detect biochemical abnormalities, it may detect the tumor at a very early stage.

3. <u>CT scan:</u> To reveal tumor location and presence of cord compression.

4. <u>Bone scan:</u> Shows increased radioactive tracer uptake where there is metastatic invasion of the vertebrae causing increased osteoblastic activity. **Note:** Check for pregnancy in appropriate patients, and notify MD accordingly. After procedure, patient should drink several glasses of water to facilitate clearance of free-circulating isotope.

5. <u>Lumbar puncture and CSF analysis:</u> May show malignant cells in CSF. With partial blockage, there may be slightly increased levels of protein and a yellow tinge to the fluid; with complete blockage, there are definite increases in protein and the fluid is yellow. (See "Bacterial Meningitis," p. 153, for patient care.)

   □ *Queckenstedt's test:* Performed by compressing the jugular vein for 10 seconds during the LP. Normally, a rise in CSF pressure occurs. For patients in whom a tumor is partially blocking the spinal cord above the level of the LP, the test may cause a sluggish rise in CSF. With complete blockage, there will be no rise in CSF pressure.

6. <u>Myelography:</u> Shows level at which the tumor is located if the spinal canal is not totally obstructed. This procedure can be dangerous because withdrawal of CSF may cause increased compression of the cord by the tumor. (See "Spinal Cord Injury," p. 172, for pre- and postprocedure care.)

7. <u>Tissue biopsy:</u> Confirms presence of a tumor.

C. Medical Management and Surgical Interventions

1. **Bed rest:** For patients with cancer that has invaded the bony vertebral body.

2. **Pharmacotherapy**

   □ *Steroids:* To decrease compression caused by cord edema.

   □ *Hormone therapy:* For hormone-mediated metastatic tumor.

   □ *Analgesics:* For pain.

3. **Transcutaneous electrical nerve stimulation (TENS):** Battery-operated device that delivers electrical impulses to the body to relieve pain.

4. **Surgery:** May include a laminectomy or decompression and/or excision of primary tumors. Generally, surgery is not indicated for metastatic tumors. Emergency surgical decompression of the spinal cord may save function in instances of sudden onset of partial paralysis. (See "Herniated Nucleus Pulposus," p. 167, for care of patient with a laminectomy.)

5. **Radiation therapy:** May be performed pre- and postoperatively to reduce tumor mass and symptoms and help prevent recurrence. Cord inflammation and edema caused by radiation therapy can result in an increase in the neurologic deficit .

6. **Physical medicine:** May include PT, OT, and assistive devices or braces so that patient can maintain mobility and independence with ADLs. Muscle-strengthening exercises, conditioning exercises, and gait training are also frequently prescribed.

7. **ROM exercises**: To maintain or increase joint function and prevent contractures.

D. Nursing Diagnoses and Interventions

Alteration in comfort: Pain related to tumor growth

Desired outcome: Patient relates a decrease in discomfort and does not exhibit signs of uncontrolled pain.

1. Advise patient that moving slowly with good body alignment may help minimize pain.

2. Suggest that keeping knees and hips slightly flexed when in bed will help reduce pain by preventing full extension of the spinal cord.

3. Inform patient that sneezing and straining can cause pain.

4. For other interventions, see **Alteration in comfort** in "Caring for Patients with Neurologic Problems," p. 543, Appendix One.

See "Spinal Cord Injury," pp. 173–176, for nursing diagnoses and interventions related to the care of patients with disorders of the spinal cord. If patient has bladder dysfunction, see related discussions in Chapter 3, "Renal–Urinary Disorders," pp. 135–142. See "Caring for Patients on Prolonged Bed Rest," pp. 533–537, "Appendix One," for nursing diagnoses and interventions for patients who are immobile. See "Caring for Patients with Cancer and other Life-Disrupting Illnesses," pp. 544–551, "Appendix One," for additional nursing diagnoses and interventions.

E. Patient–Family Teaching and Discharge Planning

Provide patient and SOs with verbal and written information for the following, as appropriate:

1. Safety measures relative to sensorimotor deficits.

2. For more informaton, see teaching/discharge planning interventions 3–11 in "Brain Tumors," p. 185.

► Section Five   **Vascular Disorders of the Nervous System**

I. Cerebral Aneurysm

An aneurysm is a localized weakness and dilation of an artery. With cerebral aneurysms, this dilation generally takes one of two forms: *fusiform*, in which the entire circumference of a vessel section is dilated, or *saccular*, in which there is dilation of the side of a vessel. Saccular aneurysms, also called "berry" aneurysms, are the most common. Depending on their size and location, unruptured aneurysms can produce neurologic symptoms by compressing brain tissue or cranial nerves. Usually, however, the aneurysm causes no symptoms until it ruptures. When this occurs, hemorrhage into the subarachnoid space prevents adequate circulation of CSF, which increases ICP. In addition, interruption of blood flow to the areas supplied by the ruptured artery can cause brain ischemia and, possibly, infarction.

Aneurysm can be caused by congenital defect in the arterial wall, degenerative processes such as hypertension or atherosclerosis, or vessel trauma. Prognosis depends on the site and size of the ruptured aneurysm, but 45–50% of affected individuals die immediately. In survivors, rebleeding tends to occur 3–11 days following the initial rupture because of the body's normal process of lysis of the clot at the rupture site. Common causes of death for individuals who survive the initial rupture include increased ICP, rebleeding, and vasospasm of the blood vessels.

A. Assessment

Indicators vary, depending on the site and amount of bleeding.

Signs and symptoms

□ *Prodromal (as the aneurysm enlarges but before it ruptures):* Periodic headaches, transitory weakness, numbness, tingling on one side, and transitory speech disturbances.

□ *Acute (with leakage and rupture):* Sudden and severe headache, nausea and/or vomiting, and neck stiffness are among the most common symptoms.

Increased ICP: Sudden, severe headache; nausea and/or vomiting; changes or alteration in LOC ranging from confusion, irritability, and restlessness to coma; pupillary dilation and changes in their size and reaction to light; VS changes such as increasing BP with widening pulse pressure and decreased pulse rate; irregular respiratory pattern.

Meningeal irritation (caused by blood in the subarachnoid space): Neck stiffness; neck, back, and leg pain; fever; seizures.

Cranial nerve irritation/compression: Blurred vision and other visual disturbances, ptosis, inability to rotate the eyes, difficulty with swallowing or speaking, tinnitus.

Focal symptoms: Sensory loss, motor weakness, or paralysis on one side of the body.

Physical exam: Positive Kernig's and Brudzinski's signs confirm presence of meningeal irritation. (See description with "Bacterial Meningitis," p. 153.)

Grading: Individuals with ruptured aneurysms are often graded according to the severity of the bleeding or injury:

□ *Grade I (minimal bleeding):* Patient alert, with no neurologic deficit; may have slight headache and stiff neck.

□ *Grade II (mild bleeding):* Patient alert, with mild to severe headache; presence of stiff neck; may have minimal neurologic deficit such as third nerve palsy.

□ *Grade III (moderate bleeding):* Patient drowsy or confused; presence of stiff neck; may have mild focal neurologic deficit.

□ *Grade IV (moderate to severe bleeding):* Patient stuporous or semi-comatose; presence of stiff neck; may have neurologic deficit such as hemiparesis.

□ *Grade V (severe bleeding):* Patient in deep coma; may have decerebrate movements; often fatal.

B. Diagnostic Tests

1. Cerebral angiography: To pinpoint site, structure, and size of aneurysm and presence of vasospasm. This test provides the definitive diagnosis of aneurysm. Before the test, keep patient NPO for 8–10 hours, or as prescribed; and assess for and notify MD of allergies to iodine, shellfish, or radiopaque dyes. After the test follow these guidelines:

□ Maintain patient on strict bed rest for 6–24 hours, followed by a specified period of "bathroom privileges only."

□ If bleeding occurs, apply manual pressure until it has ceased, and then apply a pressure dressing to prevent further bleeding. Notify MD, and reinstate frequent monitoring of VS and puncture site.

☐ If the femoral approach was used, keep leg straight for the prescribed amount of time (usually 6–12 hours) to minimize risk of bleeding. Patient will need to use bedpan and eat on the side during this time period. At frequent intervals, assess pedal pulses and temperature, color, and tactile sensation of the leg. Notify MD of loss or weakening of pulses; numbness; tingling; and cool, pale, or cyanotic feet, which can occur with thrombus formation or obstruction of the artery.

☐ If the brachial approach was used, immobilize arm 6–12 hours or as prescribed. Check radial pulses frequently and be alert to loss or weakening of pulses, numbness, tingling; or coolness, pallor, cyanosis in the hand. If these occur, notify MD because they are indicative of thrombus formation and obstruction of the artery. Do not measure BP in affected arm; post a sign over patient's bed to alert other staff members.

☐ If the carotid artery was the puncture site, check for tracheal displacement, difficulty with swallowing or breathing, weakness, numbness, confusion, or neurologic deficits, any of which can occur with bleeding, hematoma formation, or thrombus obstruction in the artery. Notify MD of significant findings.

2. <u>Magnetic resonance imaging (MRI):</u> Can reveal presence of even small amounts of blood.

3. <u>CT scan:</u> To reveal presence of aneurysm and location and extent of blood.

4. <u>Lumbar puncture and CSF analysis:</u> May reveal presence of bloody CSF, increased CSF pressure, and increased protein. This procedure is contraindicated for patients with increased ICP. (See "Bacterial Meningitis," p. 153, for patient care.)

5. <u>Skull x-ray:</u> May reveal calcification in the wall of a large aneurysm.

C. Medical Management and Surgical Interventions

1. **Respiratory support:** Airway maintenance, intubation, and ventilation as necessary. ABG values are often monitored for evidence of hypoxemia. If indicated, oxygen is administered to prevent hypoxia and carbon dioxide retention, which can cause vasodilation of the cerebral arteries and cerebral edema.

2. **Activity restrictions:** Strict bed rest in a quiet, dark room; limitation of visitors; restriction of ADLs. Although active ROM is occasionally permitted, even the alert patient is usually limited to passive ROM. Restraints are avoided because they can result in increased ICP if the patient struggles against them.

3. **Elevation of HOB:** To 30° or less to reduce cerebral congestion.

4. **Pharmacotherapy**

   ☐ *Antifibrinolytic agent, eg, aminocaproic acid:* To decrease the risk of rebleeding at the site of aneurysm by delaying the body's lysis of the blood clot. Generally, a loading dose of 5 g in 50 mL D_5W is given over an hour; 24–30 g in 500 mL D_5W is given by constant IV infusion for 10 days. This is followed by 3 grams orally q2h for 21 days or until surgical repair is performed. Rapid IV infusion may cause hypotension, bradycardia, or dysrhythmias. Side effects include phlebitis at the insertion site (IV route) and nausea and diarrhea (oral route). Other side effects include headache, tinnitus, dizziness, fatigue, and generalized thrombosis.

   ☐ *Corticosteroids such as dexamethasone:* To help decrease cerebral edema and ICP.

   ☐ *Antihypertensives such as hydralazine:* If indicated, to treat underlying hypertension.

   ☐ *Laxatives and stool softeners:* To prevent straining with bowel movements.

   ☐ *Sedatives/tranquilizers such as phenobarbital:* To reduce stress and promote rest.

    □ *Osmotic diuretics such as mannitol:* To reduce cerebral edema.

    □ *Analgesics such as codeine:* To manage pain. Aspirin is contraindicated because it prevents platelet adhesion.

5. **Fluid limitation:** Generally, fluids are limited to keep patient slightly underhydrated and reduce cerebral congestion and ICP.

6. **Nutrition:** Coffee and other stimulants are restricted. For patients with dysphagia, enteral or parenteral feedings may be necessary. A low-sodium, low-cholesterol diet is often prescribed to control hypertension.

7. **Antiembolism hose:** To help prevent deep-vein thrombosis.

8. **ICU monitoring:** May be necessary. If indicated, a cannula is inserted into the ventricle to monitor ICP and provide ventricular drainage.

9. **Surgical management:** For patients graded I–III, repair of the aneurysm by clipping, ligating, or wrapping the aneurysm neck with muscle may be indicated. The patient's surgical candidacy depends on LOC, extent of neurologic deficit, nature and location of the aneurysm, and presence of vasospasm. (For information on postoperative care, see craniotomy discussion, p. 183, in "Brain Tumors.")

D. Nursing Diagnoses and Interventions

The following relate primarily to the patient whose aneurysm is graded I–III. If the patient's aneurysm is graded IV or V, see nursing diagnoses in "Cerebrovascular Accident," p. 194, for patient care.

Knowledge deficit: Potential for rebleeding, rupture, vasospasm, and negative side effects of drug therapy (aminocaproic acid)

Desired outcomes: Patient can verbalize knowledge of the potential for rebleeding, vasospasm, and negative side effects of aminocaproic therapy and can relate preventive measures, as appropriate.

1. Assess patient for sensorimotor deficits such as decreased or absent vision, impaired temperature and pain sensation, unsteady gait, weakness, and/or paralysis. Document baseline neurologic and physical assessments so that changes in patient status are detected promptly. Teach patient and SOs these indicators and explain the importance of reporting them to the staff promptly should they occur.

2. Teach patient the importance of maintaining strict bed rest and reducing activity level to avoid rebleeding or rupture. Explain that the number and frequency of visitors, as well as other stimuli such as television and radio, will be limited.

3. Teach patient and SOs the indicators of cerebral vasospasm, which can lead to ischemia and infarction. These include visual disturbances, hemiparesis, seizures, and deteriorating LOC. Instruct patient and SOs to alert the staff immediately should they occur. At this time there is no effective treatment for vasospasm.

4. Teach patients on aminocaproic acid therapy the indicators of pulmonary embolus, including SOB, chest pain (especially that which increases with inspiration), and blood-tinged sputum, as well as indicators of deep-vein thrombosis such as calf pain or tenderness and increased heat, swelling, or redness of the leg. Stress the importance of notifying staff immediately should they occur.

5. Alert patient to the potential for loose stools, frequent stools (more than 3/day), cramps, and weakness with aminocaproic therapy. Instruct patient to report these problems promptly, because if the diarrhea is a side effect of oral aminocaproic therapy, MD may switch patient to IV medication.

Potential alteration in respiratory function related to imposed inactivity secondary to the risk of aneurysm rupture or rebleeding

Desired outcome: Patient does not exhibit signs of respiratory dysfunction.

1. Assess patient for increased work of breathing or a change in the rate or depth of respirations. Auscultate lung fields for breath sounds, noting presence of crackles (rales), rhonchi, and diminished or adventitious sounds. Assess for cyanosis, and monitor patient's ABG values for evidence of hypoxemia or hypercapnia. Notify MD of significant findings.

2. Encourage patient to breathe deeply and change positions q2h to help expand the lungs. Instruct patient to avoid coughing or sneezing, as these activities increase intra-abdominal and intrathoracic pressure, which in turn increases ICP and the risk of aneurysm rupture. Explain that if sneezing is unavoidable, it should be done with an open mouth.

3. Maintain patient on oxygen as prescribed.

Potential impairment of physical mobility related to imposed activity restrictions secondary to risk of aneurysm rupture or rebleeding

Desired outcome: Patient does not exhibit signs of joint contracture or muscle atrophy.

1. To maintain joint mobility, perform passive ROM exercises during the period of activity restriction. Even if the patient feels well enough to perform assisted or active ROM, these activities are contraindicated because they increase ICP and the risk of rupture or rebleeding.

2. Maintain joint alignment, and provide support to the joints and extremities with pillows, trochanter rolls, sand bags, and other positioning devices.

3. When the patient is no longer on bed rest and activity restrictions, additional strengthening and conditioning exercises may be necessary to counteract the effects of prolonged bed rest. In addition, the patient may have residual neurologic deficits that necessitate gait training or the use of assistive devices to promote mobility. Obtain a PT/OT referral as appropriate. For additional interventions, see **Potential impairment of physical mobility** in "Caring for Patients on Prolonged Bed Rest," p. 535, "Appendix One."

Self-care deficit: Inability to perform ADLs related to imposed activity restrictions secondary to risk of aneurysm rupture or rebleeding

Desired outcome: Patient expresses satisfaction with care activities that are completed for him or her.

1. During the period of strict bed rest and activity restrictions, perform care activities, even for patients who do not exhibit signs of neurologic deficit.

2. If patient has bathroom privileges, provide a commode as appropriate, and assist patient with transferring as necessary.

See "Seizure Disorders" for the following: **Potential for injury** related to oral, musculoskeletal, and airway vulnerability secondary to seizure activity, p. 203. See "Caring for Preoperative and Postoperative Patients," pp. 528–532, and "Caring for Patients on Prolonged Bed Rest," pp. 533–537, "Appendix One," as appropriate. See "Caring for Patients with Neurologic Problems" in "Appendix One" for the following: **Potential for injury** related to risk of increased ICP, p. 542, **Alteration in comfort**, p. 543, **Potential fluid volume deficit**, p. 539, and **Alteration in bowel elimination:** Constipation, p. 541. See "Caring for Patients with Cancer and Other Life-Disrupting Illnesses" in "Appendix One" for the following, as appropriate: **Disturbance in self-concept**, p. 544, **Ineffective individual coping**, p. 545, **Fear**, p. 544, **Alteration in family processes**, p. 546, and **Grieving**, p. 546.

E. Patient–Family Teaching and Discharge Planning

Provide patient and SOs with verbal and written information for the following:

1. Wound care and indicators of wound infection for patients who have undergone surgery.
2. Importance of avoiding strenous physical activity. Check with MD regarding activity restrictions/limitations; instruct patient accordingly.
3. Low-sodium, low-cholesterol diet if prescribed to control hypertension and atherosclerosis.
4. Medications, including drug name, rationale, schedule, dosage, precautions, and potential side effects.

In addition:

5. See the teaching/discharge planning section in "Cerebrovascular Accident," p. 200, for additional interventions for patients who have residual neurologic deficits.

II. Cerebrovascular Accident

A cerebrovascular accident (CVA) is the sudden disruption of oxygen supply to the nerve cells caused by obstruction or rupture in one or more of the blood vessels that supply the brain. *Occlusive CVA*, which can be caused by thrombosis or embolism, results in blockage of blood supply to the brain tissue. The resulting ischemia, if prolonged, causes brain tissue necrosis (infarction) as well as cerebral edema and increased ICP. A transient ischemic attack (TIA), which is a temporary neurologic deficit that resolves completely, may precede a thrombotic CVA. *Hemorrhagic CVA* causes neural tissue destruction because of the infiltration and accumulation of blood. Although a cerebral hemorrhage usually results from hypertension or an aneurysm, trauma also can cause hemorrhagic CVA. CVA is the third most common cause of death and the most common cause of neurologic disability. Half the survivors are left permanently disabled or experience another CVA.

A. Assessssment

General findings: Classically, symptoms appear on the side of the body opposite that of the damaged site. For example, a CVA in the left hemisphere of the brain will produce symptoms in the right arm and leg. However, when the CVA affects the cranial nerves, the symptoms of cranial nerve deficit will appear on the same side as the site of injury. An obstruction of an anterior cerebral artery may produce bilateral symptoms, as will severe bleeding or multiple emboli. Hemiplegia is fairly common. Initially, the patient usually has flaccid paralysis. As spinal cord depression resolves, more normal tone is seen and hyperactive reflexes occur.

Signs and symptoms: Vary with the size and site of injury and may improve in 2–3 days as the cerebral edema decreases. Headache; neck stiffness and rigidity; vomiting; seizures; dizziness and/or syncope; fever; changes in mentation, including apathy, emotional lability, irritability, disorientation, memory loss, withdrawal, drowsiness, stupor, or coma; bowel and bladder incontinence; numbness or loss of sensation; weakness or paralysis on part or one side of the body; and aphasia can occur.

☐ *Cranial nerve involvement:* Visual disturbances, including diplopia, blindness, hemianopia; inequality or fixation of the pupils; nystagmus; tinnitus; difficulty chewing and swallowing.

Physical exam: Papilledema, arteriosclerotic retinal changes, and/or hemorrhagic retinal areas on ophthalmic exam. Hyperactive DTRs, decreased superficial reflexes, and positive Babinski's sign also may be present. To check for Babinski's response, stroke the lateral aspect of the sole of the foot (from the heel to the ball of the foot) with a hard object. Dorsiflexion of the great toe with fanning of the other toes is a positive sign. A positive Kernig's sign (see "Bacterial Meningitis," p. 153) is indicative of meningeal irritation.

History of: Rheumatic heart disease, TIAs, hypertension, atherosclerosis, high serum cholesterol and/or triglycerides, diabetes mellitus, gout, smoking, heart disease, oral contraceptive use, family predisposition for arteriovenous malformation (AVM), aneurysm, or previous CVA.

B. Diagnostic Tests

1. <u>Magnetic resonance imaging (MRI):</u> To reveal site of infarction, hematoma, shift of brain structure, and cerebral edema.

2. <u>CT scan:</u> To reveal site of infarction, hematoma, and shift of brain structures.

3. <u>Phonoangiography/Doppler ultrasonography:</u> May identify presence of bruits if there is a partial occlusion of the blood vessels.

4. <u>Oculoplethysmography:</u> To obtain indirect measurement of carotid blood flow.

5. <u>Skull x-ray:</u> May show calcification of the pineal gland.

6. <u>EEG:</u> To show abnormal nerve impulse transmission, which will help locate the lesion and/or indicate the amount of brain wave activity present. (See "Seizure Disorders," p. 202, for patient care.)

7. <u>SGOT:</u> Often increased 1 week after the CVA.

8. <u>Brain scan:</u> Reveals ischemic areas; however, results may not be positive until two weeks after the CVA.

9. <u>Lumbar puncture and CSF analysis:</u> May reveal increase in CSF pressure; clear to bloody CSF, depending on the type of stroke; and presence of infection or other nonvascular cause for bleeding. CSF glutamic oxalacetic transaminase (GOT) will be increased for 10 days postinjury. (See patient care in "Bacterial Meningitis," p. 153.)

10. <u>Cerebral angiography:</u> To pinpoint site of rupture or occlusion and identify collateral blood circulation, aneurysms, or AVM. (See "Cerebral Aneurysm," p. 188, for patient care.)

C. Medical Management and Surgical Interventions

1. **Respiratory support:** Maintenance of airway and delivery of oxygen, as needed.

2. **IV fluids:** To maintain fluid and electrolyte balance.

3. **Bed rest during acute stage:** Activity level is increased as patient's condition improves.

4. **Diet:** NPO status if swallow and gag reflexes are diminished or if patient has decreased LOC. A low-sodium and/or low-fat, low-cholesterol diet may be prescribed to minimize other risk factors. Diet may consist of fluids and pureed, soft, or chopped foods, or tube feedings, depending on patient's LOC and ability to chew and swallow.

5. **Pharmacotherapy**

   □ *Anticoagulants:* May be used for patients with thrombotic CVAs. Medications include aspirin, heparin sodium, and warfarin sodium to help prevent further thrombosis. If the stroke or neurologic deficit is in evolution (still progressing), anticoagulants may be useful for 24–72 hours. Once the stroke is completed and neurologic status is stable, anticoagulants are no longer useful. Anticoagulants are contraindicated with hemorrhagic CVA.

   □ *Antihypertensive agents:* To control high BP.

   □ *Vasopressors:* To treat low BP.

   □ *Corticosteroids (eg, dexamethasone) and osmotic diuretics (eg, mannitol):* To prevent or reduce cerebral edema.

   □ *Cimetidine or antacids:* To reduce the risk of GI hemorrhage from gastric ulcer caused by stress or corticosteroid therapy.

   □ *Anticonvulsants such as phenytoin or phenobarbital:* To control and prevent seizures.

   □ *Sedatives/tranquilizers:* To promote rest. These are used cautiously to avoid further impairment of neurologic function.

□ *Analgesics such as acetaminophen:* To control headache. If CVA is hemorrhagic, aspirin is avoided because it can cause an increase in bleeding.

□ *Stool softeners:* To prevent straining, which can result in increased ICP.

6. **Physical medicine:** May include PT, OT, and assistive devices or braces so that patient can maintain mobility and independence with ADLs. Muscle-strengthening exercises, conditioning exercises, and gait training are also frequently prescribed.

7. **ROM:** To maintain or increase joint function and prevent contractures. Exercises may include passive ROM, active ROM, or active-assistive ROM. Passive ROM is started immediately for all joints.

8. **Speech therapy:** For aphasic patients.

9. **Carotid endarterectomy:** Surgical removal of plaque in the obstructed artery to increase blood supply to the brain.

Postoperative assessments should include the following:

□ At least every hour, assess VS and neurologic status, especially of cranial nerves. Note and document patient's ability to swallow, move the tongue, smile, and speak. Monitor for facial drooping, tongue deviation, hoarseness, or loss of facial sensation. Stretching of cranial nerves during surgery is not uncommon and may cause temporary deficit. Monitor for the presence of hypertension, which if not controlled, can lead to cerebral infarction.

□ Palpate superficial temporal and facial pulses to evaluate patency of the external carotid artery.

10. **Cerebral artery bypass surgery:** Anastomosis of the superficial temporal artery to the middle cerebral artery to increase blood flow to the brain.

Postoperative assessments/interventions should include the following:

□ Assess VS and neurologic status at least hourly. Be alert to any neurologic deficit, especially differences on either side of the body or face.

□ To prevent impaired circulation to the temporal area, position patient away from operative side. Elevate HOB 30°.

□ Ensure that patient maintains bed rest for 24–48 hours.

□ Monitor for indicators of increased ICP. Check head dressing for drainage. Be aware that the scalp may swell. Be alert to patient complaints of "burning" scalp, which can occur with ischemia. (For additional interventions, see **Potential for injury** related to risk of increased ICP, in "Caring for Patients with Neurologic Problems," p. 542, "Appendix One.")

11. **Craniotomy:** May be performed for evacuation of a hematoma, repair of a ruptured aneurysm, or application of arterial clips or plastic spray to the involved vessel to prevent further rupture. (See "Brain Tumors," p. 183, for patient care.)

D. Nursing Diagnoses and Interventions

Sensory-perceptual alterations related to neglect of the affected side secondary to neurologic deficit

Desired outcome: Patient does not neglect the affected side.

1. Assess patient's ability to recognize objects to the right or left of his or her visual midline; perceive body parts as his or her own; perceive pain, touch, and temperature sensations; judge distances; orient self to changes in the environment; differentiate left from right; maintain posture sense; and identify objects by sight, hearing, or touch. Document deficits.

2. Neglect of the affected side occurs more often with right hemisphere injury. Neglect cannot be totally accounted for on the basis of loss of physical senses. For example, both ears are used in hearing, but with auditory neglect, patient

may ignore conversation or noises that occur on the affected side. Assess patient for neglect of the affected side as follows:

□ *Visual neglect:* Patient does not turn his or her head to see all parts of an object, eg, he or she may read only half of a page or eat from only one side of the plate. When the patient exhibits signs of visual neglect, continue to place objects necessary for ADLs on the unaffected side and approach patient from that side, but gradually increase stimuli on the affected side. For example, while communicating with patient, physically move across her or his visual boundary.

□ *Self-neglect:* Patient does not perceive his or her arm or leg as being a part of the body. For example, when combing or brushing the hair, patient attends to only one (the unaffected) side of the head. Encourage patient to make a conscious effort to care for neglected body parts and/or check them for proper position to ensure against contractures and skin breakdown. When patient is in bed or up in a chair, provide safety measures such as bedrails and restraints to prevent patient from attempting to get up, which can occur because of unawareness of the affected side. Teach patient to use unaffected arm to perform ROM exercises on the affected side.

□ *Auditory neglect:* Patient ignores individuals who approach and speak from his or her affected side, but communicates with those who approach or speak from the unaffected side. To stimulate patient's attention to the affected side, move across the auditory boundary while speaking.

3. Arrange the environment to maximize performance of ADLs by keeping necessary objects on patient's unaffected side. Perform activities on the unaffected side unless you are specifically attempting to stimulate the neglected side. After attempting to stimulate the neglected side, return to patient's unaffected side for activities and communication.

Impaired physical mobility related to alterations in the upper or lower limbs secondary to hemiparesis or hemiplegia

Desired outcome: Patient can demonstrate techniques that enhance ambulating and transferring.

1. Teach patient methods for turning and moving, using the stronger extremity to move the weaker extremity.

2. Instruct patient always to lead with the stronger side when transferring by maintaining weight on the stronger side and pivoting, using the stronger arm for support.

3. Encourage patient to make a conscious attempt to look at the extremities and check their position before moving. Remind patient to make a conscious effort to lift and then extend the foot when ambulating.

4. Instruct patient with impaired sense of balance to compensate by leaning toward the stronger side. (The tendency is to lean toward the weaker or paralyzed side.) If necessary, remind patient to keep body weight forward over the feet when standing.

Impaired verbal communication related to aphasia and/or dysarthria secondary to cerebrovascular insult

Desired outcome: Patient demonstrates ability for self-expression and two-way communication.

1. Evaluate the nature and severity of the patient's aphasia. When doing so, avoid giving nonverbal cues. Assess patient's ability to point or look toward a specific object, follow simple directions, understand yes/no questions, understand complex questions, repeat both simple and complex words, repeat sentences, name objects that are shown, demonstrate or relate the purpose or action of the object, fulfill written requests, and write requests. Use this assessment as the basis for a communication plan.

2. One example of an intervention in a communication plan for a patient who has difficulty expressing words is to provide practice by having patient repeat words after you. See Table 4-1 for additional information.

3. Obtain a referral to a speech therapist/pathologist as needed. Provide therapist with a list of words that would enhance patient's independence and/or care. In addition, ask for tips that will help improve communication with patient.

Table 4-1 Selected Hemispheric-Related Problems Associated with CVA*

Deficit	Comments	Suggestions
I. Dominant (left) hemisphere damage		
A. *Impaired verbal communication*		
1. Aphasia: Partial or complete inability to use or comprehend language and symbols	Aphasia is not the result of impaired hearing or intelligence	Treat patient as an adult. It is not necessary to raise your voice unless patient is indeed deaf
	There are many different types of aphasia. The patient generally has a combination of types which vary in severity.	Describe aphasia symptoms to patient, using simple terms. Communicate simply; ask questions that have yes or no answers. Progress to more complex statements as indicated
☐ Word deafness: May not recognize or comprehend spoken word (as if a foreign language were being spoken)	Patient is frequently good at responding to nonverbal cues such as gestures and facial expressions	When evaluating patient for aphasia, be aware that patient may be responding to nonverbal cues and may understand less than you think. Use gestures, nonverbal cues, and pantomime to enhance day-to-day communication. Give short, simple directions, and repeat as needed to ensure understanding
☐ Difficulty expressing words, naming objects	Patient may use gestures, groans, swearing, nonsense words. Patient has difficulty with symbols and their meaning, not with the muscles used in speaking. Patient knows what she or he wants to say but cannot say it. May mix appropriate/inappropriate words or have problems finding words	Give patient practice in verbal expression by encouraging him/her to repeat words after you. Listen and respond to patient's communication efforts; otherwise patient may give up. Give practice in receiving word images by pointing to an object and clearly stating its name. Watch signals patient gives you

Table 4-1 (continued)

Deficit	Comments	Suggestions
☐ Loss of ability to monitor verbal output	Patient may not produce sensible language, but may think she or he is making sense. Patient will not understand why no one understands or responds appropriately	Avoid labeling patient "belligerent" or "confused" when the problem is aphasia and frustration
☐ Nonrecognition of number symbols or relationships	Impaired ability to do math, calculations. Difficulty understanding time concept, telling time	Avoid instructing patient to "wait 5 minutes," as this may not be meaningful
B. *Sensory-perceptual alterations*	Patient has a better grasp of the "general" scope than of specifics (can see the forest but not the trees)	
1. Perceptions/reactions	Can be slow, cautious, and/or disorganized when approaching an unfamiliar problem	Provide frequent, accurate, and immediate feedback on performance
☐ Impaired ability to think logically, reason (deduction/induction), and make decisions		Give step-by-step instructions Keep questions simple initially
☐ Poor abstract thinking		Keep conversation on concrete level (use "water" instead of the term "fluid," "leg" instead of the term "limb")
☐ Short attention span		Keep messages short
2. Impaired contralateral sensory interpretation/ association	Inability to recognize items by touch	Give patient item to feel and name it as you do (eg, give patient a washcloth and name it as such)
3. Visual field deficit	Sees only a portion of normal visual field	Instruct patient to make a conscious effort to scan the rest of the environment by turning head from side to side
	May also have visual "neglect," but this does not happen as often as with right hemisphere damage	Approach patient on unaffected side. Place commonly used items on unaffected side. Check toward end of meal to be sure patient has eaten from both sides of the plate

Table 4-1 (continued)

Deficit	Comments	Suggestions
II. Nondominant (right) hemi-sphere damage		
A. *Impaired verbal communication*		
1. Copious speech	When speaking, patient may use excessive detail, with irrelevant information. Gets off on a tangent	Bring patient back to the subject by saying, "Let's come back to what we were talking about"
B. *Sensory-perceptual alterations*		
1. Perceptions/reactions	Denial of disability or loss of abilities; over-estimation of abilities; tends to be impulsive and too quick with movements. May lack motivation	Encourage patient to slow down. Encourage patient to check each step or task as completed
	Unawareness of deficits; impaired judgment	Patient may need to be restrained from attempting unsafe activities
	Patient may be able to describe a task in detail but cannot necessarily perform it	Have patient return demonstrate skills. Patient may be able to be "talked through" a task step-by-step. Patient may be able to talk self through a task with verbal cues; encourage this
	Generally retains ability to think logically; sees specifics rather than global picture (sees the trees, but not the forest)	
☐ Literal association	If, for example you say you ate the "lion's share," patient may take it literally and think there was a lion at the meal	Be careful what you say, as it may be taken literally
☐ Impaired ability to make subtle distinctions	The distinction between a fork and a spoon may be too subtle	
2. Impaired ability to recognize, associate, or interpret sounds	May not recognize voice qualities, animal noises, musical pieces, types of instruments	If, for example, the sound of a cat appears on television, verbally state that it is the sound a cat makes, and point to the cat on the screen

Table 4-1 (continued)

Deficit	Comments	Suggestions
3. Visual-spatial misperception; difficulty comprehending spatial relationships	May underestimate distances and bump into doors. May confuse the inside and outside of an object such as an article of clothing. May lose place when reading or adding up numbers, and thus never complete the task	
4. Difficulty recognizing and associating familiar objects, environments, or faces. Inability to orient self in space	May not recognize dangerous or hazardous objects. Purpose of object is unknown to the patient. May not know if she or he is sitting, standing, or leaning.	May need assistance eating, as will not know purpose of silverware; monitor the environment for safety hazards and remove objects such as scissors from the bedside
5. Misperception of own body and body parts	Potential for self-care deficits. May not perceive foot as being a part of the body	Needs to be taught to make a conscious effort to keep track of body parts, for example, by watching feet very carefully while walking
6. Impaired contralateral sensory interpretation/ association: Impaired ability to recognize objects by means of hearing, vision, touch	Patient has difficulty with visual cues	Keep environment simple to reduce sensory overload and enable patient to concentrate on visual cues. Remove distracting stimuli
7. Visual field deficit	May only see a portion of normal visual field	See "Visual field deficit" in "Dominant (left) hemisphere damage," p. 197
8. Often has problems with "neglect": auditory/visual field and involved body part		See nursing diagnosis "**Sensory-perceptual alterations** related to neglect of affected side," p. 194
9. Impaired conceptualization of motor movement pattern	*Apraxia:* inability to perform purposeful movement in the absence of paresis, paralsysis, ataxia, and sensory dysfunction, resulting in difficulty making voluntary muscle movements needed for speech, eating, or dressing	

*Problems will vary, depending on the portion of the brain that has been damaged as well as the severity and type of injury.

4. Communicate with patient as much as possible. General principles include the following: Speak slowly and clearly; give patient time to process your communication and answer; keep messages short and simple; stay with one clearly defined subject; avoid questions with multiple choices; phrase questions so that they can be answered "yes" or "no"; and use the same words each time you repeat a statement or question. If patient does not understand after repetition, try different words. Use gestures and facial expressions liberally to supplement and reinforce your message.

5. When helping patients regain use of symbolic language, start with nouns first, and then progress to verbs, pronouns, adjectives.

6. Dysarthria can complicate aphasia. Encourage patient to perform exercises that will increase the ability to control facial muscles and tongue. This includes holding a sound for 5 seconds, singing the scale, reading aloud, and extending tongue and trying to touch the chin, nose, or cheek.

7. Provide a supportive and relaxed environment for those patients who are unable to form words or sentences, or who are unable to speak clearly or appropriately. Address and acknowledge patient's frustration over the inability to communicate. Maintain a calm and positive attitude. Ask patient to repeat unclear words. Observe for nonverbal cues, and anticipate patient's needs.

8. For additional interventions for patients with dysarthria, see **Impaired verbal communication** related to dysarthria in "Caring for Patients with Neurologic Problems," p. 541, "Appendix One."

See "Alzheimer's Disease" for the following: **Sensory-perceptual alterations** related to inability to evaluate reality, p. 163. See "Head Injury" for the following: **Potential impairment of physical mobility** related to prolonged inactivity, p. 180. See "Seizure Disorders" for the following: **Potential for injury** related to oral, musculoskeletal, and airway vulnerability secondary to seizure activity, p. 203. See "Pulmonary Embolism" in Chapter 1, "Respiratory Disorders," for the following: **Potential for injury** related to increased risk of bleeding secondary to anticoagulant therapy, p. 9.

See Chapter 3, "Renal–Urinary Disorders," for a discussion of disorders specific to patient's bladder condition. **Caution:** The Credé maneuver and other interventions that increase intrathoracic or intra-abdominal pressure are contraindicated until the risk of increased ICP is no longer a factor.

See "Caring for Patients on Prolonged Bed Rest" in "Appendix One," pp. 533–537, for nursing diagnoses and interventions related to immobility. Adjust interventions accordingly if patient has increased ICP or is at risk for this problem. See "Caring for Patients with Neurologic Problems" in "Appendix One" for the following: **Ineffective airway clearance**, p. 540, **Alteration in bowel elimination:** Constipation, p. 541, **Potential for injury** related to unsteady gait, p. 537, **Potential for injury** related to visual disturbances, p. 543, **Potential for injury** related to risk of corneal irritation/abrasion, p. 538, **Potential for injury** related to risk of increased ICP, p. 542, **Self-care deficit**, p. 540, **Potential fluid volume deficit**, p. 539, and **Alteration in nutrition:** Less than body requirements, p. 538. See "Caring for Patients with Cancer and Other Life-Disrupting Illnesses" in "Appendix One" for the following: **Disturbance in self-concept**, p. 544, **Ineffective individual coping**, p. 545, **Alteration in family processes**, p. 546, and **Grieving**, p. 546.

E. Patient–Family Teaching and Discharge Planning

Provide patient and SOs with verbal and written information for the following:

1. Importance of minimizing or treating the following risk factors: diabetes mellitus, hypertension, high cholesterol, high sodium intake, obesity, inactivity, smoking, prolonged bed rest, and stressful lifestyle.

2. Interventions that increase effective communication in the presence of aphasia or dysarthria.

3. Referrals to the following as appropriate: public health nurse, visiting nurses association, psychologic therapy, vocational rehabilitation agency, home health agencies, and extended and skilled care facilities.

4. For other information, see teaching/discharge interventions 3–9 in "Multiple Sclerosis," p. 149.

▶ Section Six **Seizure Disorders**

Seizures result from an abnormal, uncontrolled, electrical discharge from the neurons of the cerebral cortex in response to a stimulus. If the activity is localized in one portion of the brain the individual will have a partial seizure, but when it is widespread and diffuse a generalized seizure occurs. Symptoms vary widely, depending on the involved area of the cerebral cortex.

Seizure threshold refers to the amount of stimulation needed to cause the neural activity. Although anyone can have a seizure if the stimulus is sufficient, the seizure threshold is lowered in some individuals and this may result in spontaneous seizures. Potential causes for lowered seizure threshold include congenital defects; head injury; intracranial tumors; infections such as meningitis and encephalitis; exposure to toxins such as lead; hypoxia; and metabolic and endocrine disorders such as hypoglycemia, hypocalcemia, uremia, hypoparathyroidism, and excessive hydration. For susceptible individuals, "triggers" may include physical stimulation such as loud music or bright, flashing lights; lack of sleep or food; fatigue; emotional tension or stress; and excessive drug/alcohol use. Although a seizure itself is generally not fatal, instances of prolonged and repeated generalized seizures, *status epilepticus*, can be life–threatening because exhaustion, respiratory arrest, and cardiovascular collapse can occur.

A. Assessment for Generalized Seizures

There are a great variety of seizures, but the following are the most serious and/or common:

Tonic-clonic (grand mal): Possible presence of an aura (visceral sensation, visual disturbances, sounds, or odors preceding the seizure); seizure can last 2–5 minutes and includes the following phases:

□ *Tonic (rigid/contracted):* Can last 1–2 minutes. Symptoms include loss of consciousness, eyes rolling upward, clenched jaws (potential for tongue to be bitten), apnea (may hear cry as air is forced out of the lungs), cyanosis, and excessive salivation resulting in foaming at the mouth.

□ *Clonic (rhythmic contraction and relaxation of the extremities and muscles):* Can last 1–2 minutes. Patient may be incontinent. During this phase, the potential is greatest for biting the tongue.

□ *Post-ictal:* Patient may be sleepy, semiconscious, confused, unable to speak clearly, uncoordinated, have a headache, and/or have little recollection of the seizure event.

Absence (petit mal): Patient has momentary loss of awareness, may appear to be daydreaming, and ceases voluntary muscle activity. Patient may experience facial, eyelid, or hand twitching. There is usually no memory of the seizure, and the patient may have difficulty reorienting after the seizure event. This type of seizure can last 1–10 seconds and may occur up to 100 times a day.

Myoclonic: Sudden, very brief contraction of muscles or muscle groups with no loss of consciousness or post-ictal state.

Status epilepticus: State of continous or rapidly recurring seizures. This is a medical emergency, resulting in potential complications such as cerebral edema, aspiration, hyperthermia, exhaustion, and respiratory and cardiovascular collapse. Patient may not regain consciousness between seizures. Death may result.

B. Diagnostic Tests

Because a variety of problems can precipitate seizures, testing may be extensive. Common tests include the following:

1. Serum electrolytes: To rule out metabolic causes such as hypoglycemia or hypocalcemia.

2. EEG, both sleeping and awake: May reveal abnormal patterns of electrical activity, particularly with stimuli such as flashing lights.

   □ *Before the test:* As directed, withhold anticonvulsants, sedatives, and tranquilizers for 24–48 hours. Alert EEG staff to drugs the patient is taking, and provide a normal diet to prevent hypoglycemia. If a sleep EEG is prescribed, keep patient awake the night before the test.

   □ *After the test:* Check with MD regarding reinstatement of medications. If needed, provide hairwashing or acetone swabs to remove the paste used for attaching the electrodes.

3. Skull x-rays: To reveal fractures, tumors, calcifications, or congenital anomalies (pineal shift, ventricular deformity).

4. CT scan: May reveal presence of a space-occupying lesion such as a tumor or hematoma.

5. Brain scan: To rule out lesions such as a tumor.

6. Lumbar puncture and CSF analysis: To rule out increased ICP or infection. (See "Bacterial Meningitis," p. 153, for patient care.)

C. Medical Management and Surgical Interventions

1. **Anticonvulsants and sedatives:** To help prevent seizure activity.

   □ *Hydantoin derivatives such as phenytoin, mephenytoin, or ethotoin:* For grand mal seizures.

   □ *Carbamazepine:* For grand mal seizures.

   □ *Valproic acid:* For petit mal seizures.

   □ *Succinimide derivatives such as ethosuximide:* For petit mal seizures.

   □ *Barbiturate derivatives such a phenobarbital or primidone:* May be used in conjunction with one of the anticonvulsants above.

2. **Treatment of underlying causes:** Such as metabolic disorder or infectious process.

3. **Counseling or psychotherapy:** For patients with poor self-concept or coping difficulties related to the diagnosis.

4. **Surgery:** May include a craniotomy (see "Brain Tumors," p. 183) to remove a hematoma or focal lesion such as a tumor.

5. **Management of status epilepticus**

   □ *Maintenance of patent airway.*

   □ *Assessment of serum glucose and administration of IV glucose:* If indicated.

   □ *Slow administration of IV diazepam, 1 mg/min.* **Note:** Monitor for signs of respiratory depression and hypotension.

   □ *Administration of IV phenytoin:* If diazepam is unsuccessful. **Note:** Do not mix this medication; give it slowly, at no more than 50 mg/min; monitor for hypotension, apnea, and cardiac dysrhythmias.

   □ *Administration of IV phenobarbital:* If diazepam and phenytoin are unsuccessful. **Note:** Monitor for signs of respiratory depression.

   □ *Administration of thiamine:* If alcohol withdrawal occurs.

□ *Administration of paraldehyde:* May be given if other medications are unsuccessful. **Note:** Because the solution reacts negatively with plastic, use a glass syringe for IM and IV routes or a rubber catheter if it is given via retention enema.

□ *Intubation and general anesthesia with large doses of short-acting barbiturate or neuromuscular blocking agent:* For severe cases.

D. Nursing Diagnoses and Interventions

Potential for injury related to oral, musculoskeletal, and airway vulnerability secondary to seizure activity

Desired outcomes: Patient does not exhibit signs of oral and/or musculoskeletal injury or airway compromise. SOs can verbalize knowledge of actions that are necessary during seizure activity.

Seizure precautions:

1. Pad siderails with blankets or pillows.
2. Tape an airway or padded tongue blade to the bedside.
3. Avoid using glass or other breakable oral thermometers when taking patient's temperature.

During the seizure:

4. Remain with patient. Observe for, record, and report type, duration, and characteristics of seizure activity and any postseizure response.
5. Prevent or break the fall, and ease patient to the floor if the seizure occurs while patient is out of bed. Keep patient in bed if the seizure occurs while he or she is there.
6. If the patient's jaws are clenched, do not force an object between the teeth as this can break teeth or lacerate oral mucous membranes. If able to do so safely and without damage to oral tissue, insert an airway or tongue blade.
7. Protect patient's head from injury during seizure activity. A towel folded flat may be used to cushion the head from striking the ground. Be sure the head's position does not occlude the airway.
8. Do not restrain patient.
9. Roll patient into a side-lying position to promote drainage of secretions and maintain a patent airway.
10. Loosen tight clothing.
11. Reassure and reorient patient after the seizure. Ask patient if an aura preceded the seizure activity; record this information.
12. Provide SOs with verbal and written information for the above interventions.

Knowledge deficit: Life-threatening environmental factors and preventive measures for seizures

Desired outcomes: Patient can verbalize accurate information regarding measures that may prevent seizures and environmental factors that can be life-threatening in the presence of seizures.

1. Assess patient's knowledge of measures that can prevent seizures and/or environmental hazards that can be life-threatening in the presence of seizure activity. Provide or clarify information as indicated.
2. Advise patient to check into state regulations regarding automobile operation. Most states require 3–6 months of being seizure-free before an individual can obtain driver's license.
3. Caution patient to refrain from operating heavy or dangerous equipment, swimming, and possibly even tub bathing until he or she is seizure-free for

the amount of time specified by MD. Teach patient never to swim alone, regardless of the amount of time he or she has been seizure-free.

4. Teach patient that withdrawal from stimulants (eg, caffeine) and depressants (eg, alcohol) can increase the likelihood of seizures and therefore these drugs should be avoided. In addition, depressants can potentiate the effects of the anticonvulsant medication.

5. Teach patient that getting adequate amounts of rest, avoiding physical and emotional stress, and maintaining a nutritious diet may help prevent seizure activity. If stimuli such as flashing lights appear to trigger seizures, advise patient to avoid environments that are likely to have these stimuli.

6. Encourage patient to wear a Medic-Alert bracelet or similar identification.

Knowledge deficit: Purpose, precautions, and side effects of anticonvulsant medications

Desired outcome: Patient can verbalize accurate information regarding the prescribed anticonvulsant medication.

1. Stress the importance of taking the prescribed medication regularly and on schedule and not discontinuing the medication without MD guidance. Explain that missing a scheduled dose can precipitate a seizure several days later. Stress that abrupt withdrawal of any anticonvulsant medication can precipitate seizures and that discontinuing these medications is the most common cause of status epilepticus. Assist patients with finding methods that will help them remember to take the medication and monitor their drug supply to avoid running out.

2. Reinforce prescribed drug dosage instructions.

3. Stress the importance of informing MD of side effects and keeping appointments for periodic lab work, which determines whether blood levels are therapeutic and assesses for side effects. See Table 4-2 for common side effects and precautions.

4. Explain that anticonvulsants may make people drowsy. Advise patient to avoid activities that require alertness until his or her CNS response to the medication has been determined.

5. Caution patients who are taking phenytoin that there are two types of this drug. Dilantin Kapseal is absorbed more slowly and is longer acting. It is important not to confuse this extended-release phenytoin with prompt-release phenytoin. Doing so may cause dangerous underdosage or overdosage. Generic phenytoin should not be substituted for Dilantin Kapseal.

6. Instruct patient to notify MD if a significant weight gain or weight loss occurs, because it may necessitate a change in dosage or scheduling.

Noncompliance with the therapy related to frustration secondary to negative side effects of anticonvulsant medications and difficulty with making necessary lifestyle changes, and/or denial of the illness

Desired outcome: Patient can verbalize knowledge and feelings about the disease process and treatment plan and complies with the therapeutic regimen.

1. Assess patient's understanding of the disease process, medical management, and treatment plan. Explain or clarify information as indicated.

2. Assess for causes of noncompliance, such as medication side effects and/or difficulty with making significant lifestyle changes or with following the medication schedule.

3. Evaluate patient's perception of his or her vulnerability to the disease process, and be alert to signs of denial of the illness. In addition, evaluate patient's perception of the effectiveness or noneffectiveness of treatment.

4. Determine if a value, cultural, or spiritual conflict is causing noncompliance.

Table 4-2 Common Anticonvulsants

Name	Seizure Type	Side Effects	Precautions
phenytoin (Dilantin)	Grand mal	Mental dullness, ataxia diplopia, gingival hypertrophy, nystagmus, nausea, vomiting, increased body hair	Ensure frequent oral hygiene, gum massage, and gentle flossing. Take drug with food or large amounts of liquid
carbamazepine (Tegretol)	Grand mal	Blood dyscrasias, ataxia, rash, nystagmus, diplopia, nausea, vomiting, liver damage	Check CBC frequently. Patient should report fever, mouth ulcers, sore throat, bruising, or bleeding immediately. Take drug with food
mephenytoin (Mesantoin)	Grand mal	Blood dyscrasias, rash, drowsiness, ataxia, diplopia, gastric distress, gingival hyperplasia	Check CBC frequently. Patient should report fever, mouth ulcers, sore throat, bruising, or bleeding immediately. Take drug with food. Good oral hygiene, gum massage, and gentle flossing are important
phenobarbital (Luminal)	All types, generally in combination with other medications	Drowsiness, lethargy	Do not stop abruptly as this may cause withdrawal seizures
primidone (Mysoline)	Grand mal, generally in combination with other drugs	Drowsiness, emotional changes including depression, irritability, ataxia, decreased muscle coordination, nausea, vomiting, impotence	Do not stop abruptly as it may cause withdrawal seizures. Take with food or large amounts of fluid
ethosuximide (Zarontin)	Petit mal	Gastric distress, nausea, vomiting, dizziness, drowsiness	Take with food or large amounts of fluid
valproic acid (Depakene)	Petit mal	Sedation, dizziness, nausea/vomiting, anorexia, liver damage	Do not chew as it may irritate mucous membranes. Take with food. Monitor liver function through periodic lab tests. May produce false-positive test for ketones in the urine

5. Assess patient's support systems. Determine whether the presence of a family disruption pattern (whether or not it is caused by the patient's illness), is making compliance difficult and "not worth it."

6. Once the reason for noncompliance is found, intervene accordingly to ensure compliance. If it appears that a change in the medical treatment plan (eg, in

scheduling medications) may promote compliance, discuss this with MD. Provide patient with information regarding interventions that can minimize the drug side effects. (See Table 4-2.) Encourage involvement with support systems such as local epilepsy centers and/or national organizations.

See "Caring for Patients with Cancer and Other Life-Disrupting Illnesses" in "Appendix One" for the following: **Disturbance in self-concept**, p. 544, **Ineffective individual coping**, p. 545, and **Alteration in family processes**, p. 546.

E. Patient-Family Teaching and Discharge Planning

Provide patient and SOs with verbal and written information for the following:

1. Reinforcement of knowledge of the disease process, pathophysiology, symptoms, and the precipitating or aggravating factors.
2. Medications, including purpose, dosage, schedule, and potential side effects. See Table 4-2, "Common Anticonvulsants."
3. Importance of follow-up care and keeping medical appointments. Stress that use of anticonvulsant agents necessitates periodic monitoring of blood levels to ensure therapeutic medication levels and assessment for side effects.
4. Environmental factors that can be life-threatening in the presence of seizures and measures that may help prevent seizures.

In addition,

5. Provide the following address, as appropriate: Epilepsy Foundation of America, 4351 Garden City Drive, Suite 406, Landover, MD 20785.

▶ Section Seven **Chemical Dependency**

Addiction to alcohol or drugs can be defined as follows: compulsive use, loss of control of the amount used, and continued use despite adverse consequences. The abuse of alcohol and drugs has physiologic, psychologic, and socioeconomic effects. Knowledge of what to expect and how to care for affected patients to prevent or minimize complications is important.

I. Alcohol Abuse (CNS Depressant)

Alcoholism ranks as the country's third greatest health care problem, and it is estimated that 10 million Americans are affected by the toxic effects of alcohol. It is a progressive disease that may take 5–20 years to develop. There is proof of genetic predisposition to alcoholism, and it is important to consider the sociocultural factors that are likely to influence its development.

There are numerous medical problems associated with alcohol use and abuse, including neurologic disorders such as polyneuropathy and Wernicke-Korsakoff syndrome, gastrointestinal disorders such as megaloblastic anemia and platelet abnormalities, and cardiovascular disorders such as hypertension and cardiomyopathy. Excessive use of alcohol can cause chronic debilitation and concomitant illnesses such as pneumonia. Alcohol use during pregnancy is linked with increased perinatal morbidity and mortality to both the mother and infant.

A. Assessment

Nursing history should include the following: Time of last drink, amount and type of beverage consumed, length of time individual has consumed alcohol, other drug use, seizure history, and presence of other disease states. The length of time drinking has occurred and the amount of alcohol consumed on a consistent basis are important factors in determining the type of withdrawal to expect. There is a positive correlation between past withdrawal symptoms and their recurrence. Alcohol withdrawal is usually complete within 5−7 days.

Indicators of minor withdrawal: Onset within 6−12 hours after cessation of drinking, with duration of 24 hours or less. Signs and symptoms may include anxiety, agitation, irritability, tremors, diaphoresis, tachycardia, systolic hypertension, increased respirations, nausea, vomiting, diarrhea, anorexia, insomnia, and vivid dreams. **Note:** Seizures can occur during this period but they are not considered minor withdrawal symptoms. They are related to a decreased seizure threshold, are a part of the withdrawal progression, and precede delirium tremens.

Indicators of major withdrawal: Develop 2−4 days after the last drink and continue for more than 24 hours. Signs and symptoms may include progressive tremors, diaphoresis, anxiety, and tachycardia. Disorientation, clouding of sensorium, hallucinations (most commonly visual and tactile), and delusions also can occur.

□ *Delirium tremens (DTs):* The most severe progression of withdrawal and they can result in death. Signs and symptoms can develop 72−96 hours after cessation of drinking and can include disorientation, delirium, agitation, severe diaphoresis, tachycardia, cardiovascular collapse, and fever. Generally, DTs resolve within 3−5 days.

Criteria for diagnosis of alcoholism

1. Possible physiologic dependence (withdrawal symptoms seen with cessation of drinking).
2. Tolerance to the effects of alcohol.
3. Evidence of alcohol-associated illnesses.
4. Continued drinking in spite of consequences.
5. Impaired functioning (social and occupational).
6. Depression.
7. Inability to control the amount used.

B. Diagnostic Tests

1. Serum tests: A concentration of blood alcohol 0.10% or more indicates intoxication. If the concentration is greater and the patient does not appear intoxicated, this is evidence of tolerance. Mean corpuscular volume (MCV) and high-density lipoprotein cholesterol (HDL) will be increased; and SGOT (AST) and SGPT (ALT) will be elevated with liver disease. Increased amylase can signal the presence of pancreatitis. CBC is done to rule out anemia, and glucose levels are obtained to rule out hypoglycemia. Electrolytes are measured to rule out abnormalities (hypokalemia and hypomagnesemia may be seen), and PT is obtained to rule out clotting disorders.
2. Stool hemoccult: To rule out GI bleeding.
3. Chest x-ray: To rule out pneumonia.
4. EKG: To determine presence of cardiac abnormalities.

C. Medical Management

1. **Complete physical examination:** Special emphasis on liver and nervous system.
2. **Pharmacotherapy**

   □ *Sedation:* Substitution of long-acting CNS depressant (benzodiazepine) for short-acting CNS depressant (alcohol) to produce a state of calm wakefulness. **Note:** Withholding sedation until severe symptoms develop is not effective with alcohol withdrawal. Increase in VS, especially pulse rate, is the most sensitive indicator of the need for medication. Dosage is tapered daily until it reaches zero, with each daily dosage at least half as much as that of the previous day.

□ *IM thiamine on admission; supplemental po thiamine and multivitamins and multi-minerals high in C, B-complex, zinc, and magnesium:* Thiamine is given to prevent Wernicke-Korsakoff syndrome; multivitamins and multiminerals are given because of the potential for malnutrition related to inadequate food intake and malabsorption caused by alcohol's irritating effect on the GI tract.

□ *Disulfiram (Antabuse):* Often given as a deterrent for alcohol consumption in long-term treatment. It blocks the metabolism of alcohol, causing acetaldehyde to accumulate and produce unpleasant reactions such as flushing, sweating, palpitations, dyspnea, tachycardia, hyperventilation, hypotension, nausea, and vomiting with alcohol consumption.

3. **Dietary management:** Foods high in protein and vitamins. Parenteral therapy with electrolytes may be indicated if the patient has had severe diarrhea, vomiting, and malnutrition. Electrolytes are not administered in all cases, however, because although alcohol is a diuretic as its concentration in the blood increases, the body retains fluids after levels decrease.

4. **Promote rest and relaxation:** Provide a calm, dimly lit environment.

5. **Treatment of complications**

□ *Seizures:* Because alcohol-withdrawal seizures occur during the first 2 days, benzodiazepine is given to lower the seizure threshold during the withdrawal period. In the event of a seizure, IV diazepam or other anticonvulsant agent may be given.

□ *Alcoholic hallicinosis (auditory hallucinations that are usually persecutory in nature in a person who is otherwise well-oriented):* Reassurance, sleep, and continued treatment with benzodiazepines are usually therapeutic.

□ *Delirium tremens (DTs):* Continued sedation with benzodiazepines; rest and sleep; and frequent orientation to reality, using familiar terms.

□ *Wernicke-Korsakoff syndrome:* Caused by thiamine deficiency and manifested by diplopia (the first real diagnostic clue), confusion, excitation, peripheral neuropathy, severe recent memory loss, impaired thought processes, and confabulation. The prophylactic administration of thiamine is recommended. **Caution:** Ingestion of carbohydrates, either oral or parenteral, increases the body's demand for thiamine. In patients with minimal thiamine levels, use of IV glucose can precipitate the syndrome. If the syndrome progresses, lifetime custodial care might be the only treatment.

6. **Detoxification:** Although not a treatment in itself, it provides the opportunity to begin treatment. It entails withdrawing the patient from alcohol in a controlled environment, using a protocol specified by the institution. Generally, sedation is used (see discussion with pharmacotherapy).

D. Nursing Diagnoses and Interventions

Potential for injury related to tremors, disorientation, and hallucinations secondary to alcohol withdrawal

Desired outcome: Patient does not exhibit signs of injury related to alcohol withdrawal.

1. Assess and document patient's orientation to reality to determine safety needs.

2. Admit patient into a room near the nurses' station.

3. Monitor VS at frequent intervals. Be alert to indicators of increasingly severe withdrawal, including increasing pulse rate, respirations, and BP; and tremors, diaphoresis, and anxiety. Describe potential withdrawal symptoms to patient and SOs, and request that they alert you when they occur.

4. Administer benzodiazepines as prescribed, usually as VS increase.

5. Provide an electric rather than manual razor for shaving.

6. Keep frequently used objects within patient's reach to minimize need for getting out of bed.

7. As necessary, assist patient with activities such as ambulation.

8. Obtain a prescription for restraints if indicated.

Sleep pattern disturbance related to agitation secondary to withdrawal from short-acting CNS depressant

Desired outcome: Patient relates the attainment of adequate amount of sleep and rest.

1. Decrease environmental stimuli and minimize care activities, as appropriate, when patient is trying to sleep.

2. Consider use of low-volume, relaxing music during patient's awake time.

3. Provide back massage if it is comforting for patient.

4. Administer sedation promptly, as prescribed; avoid undersedation. During detoxification, the amount of benzodiazepine is usually increased.

Alteration in nutrition: Less than body requirements related to history of poor intake and malabsorption secondary to alcoholism

Desired outcome: Patient does not exhibit signs of malnutrition or weight loss.

1. Determine patient's food preferences that are congruent with dietary management; provide small, frequent feedings, including nighttime snacks.

2. Encourage SOs to bring in desirable, acceptable foods.

3. Provide encouragement during mealtimes.

4. Record food intake daily; record weight daily, or as indicated.

5. As needed, administer prescribed medications that decrease gastrointestinal distress: antacids, antiemetics, antidiarrheals, cathartics.

6. If indicated, obtain prescription for vitamin and mineral supplements.

7. If appropriate, arrange for dietitian to meet with patient and SOs.

Ineffective individual coping related to anger, denial, and poor self-esteem secondary to inability to manage stressors without alcohol

Desired outcomes: Patient does not exhibit signs of ineffective coping. Patient relates an increase in self-esteem, participates in choices related to care, and begins to set appropriate short-term goals.

1. Encourage patient to verbalize anxieties and ask questions about the disease.

2. Dispel common stereotypes about the disease such as moral weakness and skidrow personality. Avoid moralizing about the disease.

3. Provide reading material such as Alcoholics Anonymous (AA) publications and other relevant articles about the disease.

4. Emphasize patient's self-worth by providing choices related to his or her care where appropriate.

5. Assist patient with setting short-term goals.

6. Discourage patient from focusing on questions such as "Why me?" Encourage focusing on methods for staying sober instead.

7. Explore alternative methods for dealing with stress, including communications with others (such as AA members) and relaxation techniques.

8. Emphasize that prognosis is directly related to abstinence.

9. Provide positive reinforcement when changes are made.

10. Assess for suicidal ideation and institute suicide precautions (as prescribed by institution) when indicated.

See "Caring for Patients with Cancer and Other Life-Disrupting Illnesses" in "Appendix One" for the following: **Alteration in family processes**, p. 546.

E. Patient–Family Teaching and Discharge Planning

Provide patient and SOs with verbal and written information for the following:

1. Medications, including drug name, dosage, purpose, schedule, precautions, and potential side effects. For patient taking Antabuse, explain the necessity of avoiding "hidden" alcohol found in some foods and cosmetics, such as sauces, vinegars, cough mixtures, after-shave lotions, perfumes, mouthwashes, and astringents.

2. Appropriate referrals such as Alcoholics Anonymous, Al-anon, Al-a-teen, halfway houses, inpatient and outpatient treatment centers, community alcohol centers, and counseling services.

3. Prescribed diet.

4. Cross-tolerance to other drugs (CNS depressants) and the likelihood of becoming dependent on other mood-altering drugs.

5. Dry drunk syndrome: During sobriety, an alcoholic may think, act, and feel as though intoxicated, eg, by exhibiting grandiose, childish, or unrealistic behavior; a rigidly judgmental outlook; or tense impatience. Explain that this syndrome is common, and the patient should contact a support system such as AA if it occurs.

II. Sedative-Hypnotic Abuse (CNS Depressant)

Sedative-hypnotic agents are used clinically in lower doses to decrease anxiety and in higher doses to produce sleep. Barbiturates, which are used as sedatives, hypnotics, anesthetics, and anticonvulsants, can cause respiratory depression and are contraindicated in patients with pulmonary disease. Benzodiazepines are used to decrease anxiety, relax muscles, and produce anticonvulsant effects. There is a great potential for abuse with these drugs that can result in physiologic and psychologic dependence. Tolerance has occurred when greater doses are required to produce the initial effect. When any CNS depressant is taken in combination with others (eg, alcohol with diazepam), additive effects are often found and death can occur. This means that the combined effect of the drugs is greater than the summation of the single effects. Cross–tolerance to other CNS depressants such as sedative-hypnotics, alcohol, and anesthetics can be found in chronic users of benzodiazepines. Therefore, a patient who is tolerant to one will have a "built-in" tolerance to all.

Drug half-life: Withdrawal symptoms can be correlated with the half-life of the drug that was used (see Tables 4-3 and 4-4). Withdrawal from drugs with shorter half-lives produces intense symptoms that last for shorter periods of time, while withdrawal from drugs with longer half-lives produces less intense symptoms that can be

Table 4-3 Common Barbiturates

Generic Name	Common Brand Names	Half-Life (in hours)
amobarbital	Amytal	8–42
secobarbital	Seconal	19–34
pentobarbital	Nembutal	15–48
phenobarbital	Luminal and others	24–140
butabarbital	Butisol	34–42
secobarbital/ amobarbital	Tuinal	8–42

Table 4-4 Common Benzodiazepines

Generic Name	Common Brand Names	Half-Life (in hours)
chlordiazepoxide	Librium and others	7–28
diazepam	Valium and others	20–90
lorazepam	Ativan	10–20
oxazepam	Serax	3–21
prazepam	Centrax	24–200*
flurazepam	Dalmane	24–100*
chlorazepate	Tranxene, Azene	30–100
tenazepam	Restoril	9.5–12.4
clonazepam	Clonopin	18.5–50
alprazolam	Xanax	12–15
halazepam	Paxipam	14

*Includes half-life of major metabolites.

prolonged. Moreover, the severity of the withdrawal is directly related to the drug's dosage.

A. Assessment

Nursing history should include the following: Time of last drug; amount and type taken; length of time individual has used the drug; other drug/alcohol use; seizure history; and presence of other disease states.

Indicators of withdrawal: Anxiety, panic, weakness, tremors, tachycardia, hypertension, orthostatic hypotension, hyperreflexia, diaphoresis, hyperthermia, nausea, vomiting, malaise, sleep pattern disturbance, dysphoria, and irritability. Seizures and death can occur if the symptoms are severe. If the patient is not treated effectively, a psychosis similar to DTs can result, which manifests as disorientation, confusion, and auditory and/or visual hallucinations. Grand mal seizures may be seen 2–3 days into the withdrawal.

B. Diagnostic Tests

1. <u>Serum drug screen:</u> A quantitative and qualitative study that detects the presence of various drugs in the blood.

2. <u>Urine drug screen:</u> Can test a broad spectrum of drugs. Some urine drug screens are more sensitive than others. **Note:** Drugs can be excreted rapidly (within 24 hours as with alcohol), moderately (48–72 hours as with some barbiturates), or slowly (weeks or months as with PCP and marijuana) .

C. Medical Management

1. **Complete physical exam:** To detect co-existing health problems.

2. **Sedation:** Either phenobarbital or the drug from which the patient is withdrawing is administered in doses that are tapered daily to zero. Dosage may be increased if tapering appears to be too rapid and withdrawal symptoms are too uncomfortable. Tapering of hypnotics should be slower than that with alcohol. A "comedown" schedule should be set up in which the drug used is reduced by no more than 15%/day, even if symptoms disappear or are not obvious.

3. **Management of complications**

   □ *Delirium:* Increase the dosage and frequency of sedation.

   □ *Seizures:* Use of anticonvulsant agents is controversial. When a patient has a history of seizures, IV diazepam or other anticonvulsant agent may be administered to achieve a therapeutic level. If seizures occur, seizure management should reflect the institution's protocol.

D. Nursing Diagnoses and Interventions

Potential for injury related to tremors, disorientation, and hallucinations secondary to withdrawal from CNS depressant

Desired outcome: Patient does not exhibit signs of injury from withdrawal.

1. Monitor VS at frequent intervals to assess patient's degree of withdrawal. Be alert to the following indicators of increasing withdrawal: increased pulse rate, diaphoresis, tremors, anxiety, and nausea. Instruct patient about the potential for these symptoms.
2. Administer the prescribed sedative medication as indicated.
3. Institute seizure precautions.
4. Minimize environmental stimuli to help patient attain calmness.
5. Reorient patient to reality as necessary; do not support hallucinations.
6. Remove potentially harmful objects from patient.
7. Minimize the need for getting out of bed by keeping frequently used objects within patient's reach.

Alteration in comfort: Malaise and nausea related to withdrawal

Desired outcome: Patient relates a reduction in discomfort.

1. Administer prescribed sedatives promptly.
2. Speak with patient in a calm, unhurried manner.
3. Decrease environmental stimuli to promote a calm environment; be supportive of patient during withdrawal. Minimizing anxiety will enhance comfort.
4. Provide soft, relaxing music, and administer backrubs if they are comforting to patient.
5. Provide leisure or work activity to distract patient from focusing on physical symptoms.

See "Seizure Disorders" for the following: **Potential for injury** related to oral, musculoskeletal, and airway vulnerability secondary to seizure activity, p. 203. See "Alcohol Abuse" for the following: **Sleep pattern disturbance**, p. 209, **Alteration in nutrition:** Less than body requirements, p. 209, and **Ineffective individual coping**, p. 209. See "Caring for Patients with Cancer and Other Life-Disrupting Illnesses," Appendix One, for the following: **Alteration in family processes**, p. 546.

E. Patient–Family Teaching and Discharge Planning

Provide patient and SOs with verbal and written information for the following:

1. Referrals to outside agencies, including Narcotics Anonymous, halfway houses, inpatient and outpatient treatment centers, community drug abuse centers, and private and/or family counseling.
2. Importance of a direct transfer to a treatment program upon discharge. If the patient returns to his/her old environment, the potential for resuming drug use is great.
3. Prescribed diet.
4. Cross–tolerance to other CNS depressants, eg, alcohol.

III. Cocaine Abuse (CNS Stimulant)

Cocaine is an increasingly popular drug that produces euphoria without sedation, relieves fatigue, and enhances energy, confidence, and alertness. Because it is a short-acting stimulant, the effects of which last for only 5–15 minutes, it must be reintroduced every 15–30 minutes to produce a continued "high." A strong psychologic dependence can occur, but a well-defined physical dependency probably does not. In individuals with a psycho-physiologic predisposition (addictive personality), use of cocaine can become compulsive and continuous despite adverse consequences.

Most often, cocaine is inhaled (snorted), but it also can be injected IV, absorbed through buccal membranes, or smoked. A process known as free-basing removes all the water-soluble impurities, leaving pure cocaine, which is then smoked. The degree of CNS stimulation is directly related to the amount of cocaine used. With increasing doses, euphoria is supplanted by intense anxiety, repetitive motor behavior, and paranoid psychoses.

A. Assessment

Indicators of cocaine intoxication: Intense anxiety, psychomotor agitation, elation, grandiosity, loquacity, hypervigilance, tachycardia, mydriasis, hypertension, diaphoresis, chills, nausea, vomiting, violence, impaired judgment, delusions, hallucinations, and paranoia.

Indicators of cocaine withdrawal (seen in high-dose, chronic abusers): Prolonged sleep, lethargy, dysphoria or depression that can last up to several weeks, fatigue, strong craving for the drug, hyperphagia, cocaine psychosis, and anxiety.

Indicators of cocaine psychosis: Tactile and visual hallucinations and paranoia. Typically, treatment is that of psychosocial support; however, pharmacologic therapy with antipsychotic agents such as haloperidol or chlorpromazine may be instituted to diminish psychosis.

B. Diagnostic Tests

1. Urinalysis: To detect presence of the drug.
2. Hepatitis B surface antigen: Assessed for in IV drug users.

C. Medical Management

1. **Restriction of cocaine:** Unlike CNS depressants, which require tapering, cocaine can be stopped abruptly.
2. **Pharmacotherapy**

   □ *Antidepressants such as amitriptyline or other tricyclic antidepressant agents:* Can be used in severe depression when other treatment modalities fail. They should not be instituted before 3–4 weeks after cocaine use.

   □ *L-tryptophan:* An amino acid that may be given to promote sleep.
3. **Management of complications:** For example, hepatitis, septicemia, and endocarditis caused by unsterile IV administration; cardiovascular dysrhythmias; hypertension; seizures; perforated nasal septum (from inhaling the drug); pulmonary dysfunction (from free-basing); malnutrition; cocaine psychosis; and acute anxiety reactions.

D. Nursing Diagnoses and Interventions

Potential for violence related to hallucinations/paranoia secondary to cocaine use/withdrawal

Desired outcomes: Patient does not exhibit violent behavior. Patient can verbalize orientation to time, place, and person.

1. Because patient may be anxious and uncertain about unfamiliar actions, explain all procedures in a calm manner. Use simple language and speak softly and clearly.

2. Assess for hallucinations and psychosis. Orient patient to time, place, and person as needed; do not support hallucinations.

3. Assure patient that all information obtained is used for medical purposes only.

4. Remove potentially harmful objects from patient area.

5. Avoid moralizing or chastising patient about drug use.

6. To promote a calm, relaxed environment, minimize environmental stimuli.

7. Do not touch patient without first announcing your intention.

8. Visit patient at frequent intervals to provide reassurance and enhance patient's feelings of safety.

Ineffective individual coping related to dysphoria, poor self-esteem, and denial secondary to inability to manage stressors without cocaine

Desired outcomes: Patient does not exhibit signs of ineffective coping. Patient relates an increase in self-esteem and begins to plan appropriate short-term goals.

1. Discourage patient from focusing on "Why me?" Encourage patient to focus on ways to remain drug free, instead.

2. Avoid moralizing about drug use. Speak calmly and matter-of-factly.

3. Assist patient with formulating short-term goals.

4. Encourage patient to verbalize concerns; provide an atmosphere of acceptance.

5. Give positive reinforcement when changes are made.

6. Reassure patient that dysphoria will pass. Be supportive and gentle.

7. Be aware that craving cocaine is to be expected. Assist patient with talking through "drug hunger." If appropriate, arrange for individuals who also have experienced cocaine craving to speak with patient.

Alteration in nutrition: More than body requirements related to hyperphagia secondary to cocaine withdrawal

Desired outcome: Patient eats balanced meals and does not exhibit evidence of weight gain.

1. Note and record the amount of food patient consumes.

2. Teach patient to eat balanced meals for attaining optimal amounts of nutrients while avoiding overeating.

3. Have nutritious, low-calorie snacks available for patient.

4. Teach the importance of exercise, especially during the period of cocaine withdrawal, when rapid weight gain can occur.

5. Reassure patient that hyperphagia is related to withdrawal and that it will cease gradually along with the withdrawal.

See "Caring for Patients with Cancer and Other Life-Disrupting Illnesses" in "Appendix One" for the following: **Alteration in family processes**, p. 546.

E. Patient–Family Teaching and Discharge Planning

Provide patient and SOs with verbal and written information for the following:

1. Referrals to outside agencies such as Narcotics Anonymous, Cocaine Anonymous, halfway houses, inpatient or outpatient treatment centers, community drug abuse centers, and private and/or family counseling.

2. Importance of adequate nutrition with exercise program to promote optimal health and help prevent rapid weight gain.

IV. Opioid Abuse (CNS Depressant)

Opioids, sometimes known as narcotics, are the most effective drugs for pain relief. Opioids are either synthetic or nonsynthetic and all are compared to morphine, which is found in the opium poppy. Other opioids include codeine, heroin, oxymorphone (Numorphan), oxycodone (found in Percodan), hydromorphone (Dilaudid), diphenoxylate (found in Lomotil), meperidine (Demerol), alphaprodine (Nisentil), propoxyphene (Darvon), pentazocine (Talwin), butorphanol (Stadol), and nalbuphine (Nubain). Opioids differ slightly from one another in regard to duration of effects, severity of side effects, withdrawal symptoms, and absorption.

Opioids are either inhaled, smoked, swallowed, or injected. They produce physical dependence, and tolerance can occur along with cross-tolerance to other opioids. Tolerance seems to diminish after withdrawal has occurred. Additive effects can occur when taken with other drugs, and respiratory depression can result when they are mixed with alcohol or other CNS depressants.

A. Assessment

Indicators of adverse effects: Constipation, nausea, vomiting, orthostatic hypotension, rashes, delirium, endocarditis, hepatitis, muscle and joint problems, and respiratory infections from suppression of the cough reflex (especially with codeine).

Indicators of withdrawal (can be compared to symptoms of influenza): Lacrimation, rhinorrhea, mydriasis, piloerection, diaphoresis, diarrhea, yawning, mild hypertension, tachycardia, fever, insomnia, cold/hot flashes, twitching, tremors, muscle spasms, blurred vision, irritability, restlessness, increased anxiety, and aching of joints and muscles. Symptoms of opioid withdrawal occur approximately 8–12 hours after the last dose, intensify in 36–48 hours, and are generally complete in 10–14 days, although some symptoms can last up to 10 weeks. Withdrawal from opioids is not considered to be life threatening except in the elderly, severely debilitated patients, or newborns.

B. Diagnostic Tests

1. <u>Hematologic tests:</u> Total protein will be elevated, with globulin elevation greater than that of albumin. Levels of the following also will be elevated: SGOT (AST), SGPT (ALT), immunoglobulins, bilirubin, alkaline phosphatase, hepatitis A and hepatitis B antigens, lymphocytes, polymorphonuclear leukocytes, hemoglobin, and BUN.

2. <u>Serology test:</u> To rule out sexually transmitted diseases, which are often seen with drug addicts.

C. Medical Management

1. **Methadone substitution:** Implemented by physicians who are part of a licensed maintenance program. With this treatment, Methadone is withdrawn from the patient gradually.

2. **Adrenergic agonists such as clonidine:** May be used in place of Methadone. It is tapered off gradually. Clonidine lowers BP and pulse and can cause sedation.

3. **Pharmacologic treatment for symptomatic relief of discomfort:** For example, sedative-hypnotics for relief of anxiety and sleeplessness; mild anticholinergics for rhinorrhea.

4. **Follow-up care:** For example, counseling, long-term treatment, and rehabilitation.

D. Nursing Diagnoses and Interventions

Alteration in comfort: Malaise and other physiologic symptoms related to withdrawal from opioid substance

Desired outcome: Patient relates a reduction in discomfort and does not exhibit signs of malaise or other physiologic symptoms.

1. Monitor for indicators of withdrawal, including increases in pulse rate, BP, and temperature, as well as increasing anxiety, diaphoresis, and insomnia. Report significant findings to MD.
2. To help minimize patient's discomfort, promptly administer prescribed medications.
3. Reinforce that it is within patient's control for the detoxification program to occur only once.
4. Offer comfort measures such as backrubs, warm blankets, and soothing music if they are effective for the patient.
5. Ensure strict avoidance of narcotic antagonists, eg, pentazocine (Talwin), which can precipitate abrupt withdrawal.

Potential for infection related to increased susceptibility secondary to repeated IV drug injections and/or antitussive effects of opioids

Desired outcome: Patient does not exhibit signs of infection and can verbalize knowledge of preventive measures.

1. Inspect injection sites for evidence of infection such as redness, warmth, and purulent drainage. Notify MD of significant findings.
2. Institute measures that promote healing, such as cleansing the area and applying prescribed antibacterial ointment.
3. Instruct patient in the care of skin infections.
4. Teach patient about complications that can result from unsterile IV techniques.
5. Teach effective coughing techniques for patients who were users of opioids that have antitussive effects.
6. Monitor VS for general indicators of infection, such as an increase in temperature and rising pulse rate. Report significant findings to MD.

Ineffective individual coping related to denial, poor self-esteem, and depression secondary to inability to handle stressors without opioids

Desired outcomes: Patient does not exhibit ineffective coping mechanisms. Patient relates an increase in self-esteem, participates in self-care, and demonstrates efforts aimed at remaining drug free.

1. Encourage patient to verbalize anxieties and ask questions about the disorder.
2. Discourage patient from focusing on questions such as "Why me?" Encourage patient to focus on methods of remaining drug free, instead.
3. Provide positive reinforcement when changes are made.
4. Encourage patient to participate in self-care.
5. Avoid moralizing about drug use.
6. Do not hesitate to search visitors.

See "Alcohol Abuse" for the following: **Alteration in nutrition:** Less than body requirements, p. 209, and **Sleep pattern disturbance**, p. 209. See "Caring for Patients with Cancer and Other Life-Disrupting Illnesses" in "Appendix One" for the following: **Alteration in family processes**, p. 546.

E. Patient–Family Teaching and Discharge Planning

Provide patient and SOs with verbal and written information for the following:

1. Referrals to outside agencies such as Narcotics Anonymous, halfway houses, inpatient and outpatient treatment centers, community drug abuse centers, private and/or family counseling.

2. Importance of a direct transfer to a treatment program. Should the patient returns to his or her own environment, the potential for resumption of the drug is great.

3. Diet that provides optimal nutritional intake.

4. Cross-tolerance to other opioids.

▶ **Selected References**

Adams RD, Victor M: *Principles of Neurology*, 3rd ed. McGraw-Hill, 1985.

Bennet G et al (editors): *Substance Abuse: Pharmacologic, Developmental, and Clinical Perspectives*. Wiley, 1983.

Boss BJ: The nervous system. In: *The Handbook of Nursing*. Howe J et al (editors). Wiley, 1984.

Brodsley L: Avoiding a crisis: The assessment. *AJN* 1982; 82:1865–1871.

Burkhalter PK: *Nursing Care of the Alcoholic and Drug Abuser*. McGraw-Hill, 1975

Carpenito LJ: *Nursing Diagnosis: Application to Clinical Practice*. Lippincott, 1984.

Chatton MJ, Krupp, MA: *Current Medical Diagnosis and Treatment 1984*. Lange, 1984.

Di Dente P, McElmeel EF: Alcohol withdrawal. *Nurse Practitioner* Jan/Feb 1980; 5:18–26.

Estes NJ, et al: *Nursing Diagnosis of the Alcoholic Person*. Mosby, 1980.

Hickey JV: *The Clinical Practice of Neurological and Neurosurgical Nursing*. Lippincott, 1981.

Kramer J: *Intervertebral Disk Diseases: Causes, Diagnosis, Treatment, and Prophylaxis*. Yearbook, 1981.

Luckmann J, Sorensen K: *Medical-Surgical Nursing: A Psychophysiological Approach*, 2nd ed. Saunders, 1980.

Montgomery EB: Neurologic emergencies. In: *Manual of Medical Therapeutics*, 23rd ed. Freitag JJ, Miller LW (editors). Little, Brown, 1980.

Nursing Reference Library: *Diseases*. Intermed, 1981.

Nursing Reference Library: *Drugs*. Intermed, 1982.

Pajk M: Alzheimer's disease in patient care. *AJN* 1984; 84:216–224.

Pellino TA: Chymopapain: Alternatives to laminectomy for herniated lumbar disks. *Orthopaedic Nursing* March/April 1983; 2:14.

Reisberg B: Stages of cognitive decline. *AJN* 1984; 84:225–228.

Saxton DF et al: *The Addison-Wesley Manual of Nursing Practice*. Addison-Wesley, 1983.

Senay EC: *Substance Abuse Disorders in Clinical Practice*. John Wright—PSG, 1983.

The Saunders Health Care Directory, 84/85. Saunders, 1984.

Weinhouse I: Speaking to the needs of your aphasic patient. *Nursing 81* March 1981; 11:34–36.

5

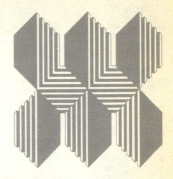

Endocrine Disorders

> ► Section One **Disorders of the Thyroid Gland**

The thyroid gland produces three hormones: thyroxine (T_4), triiodothyronine (T_3), and thyrocalcitonin (calcitonin). Secretion of T_3 and T_4 is regulated by the anterior pituitary gland via a negative feedback mechanism. When serum T_3 and T_4 levels decrease, thyroid-stimulating hormone (TSH) is released by the anterior pituitary. This stimulates the thyroid gland to secrete more hormones until normal levels are reached. T_3 and T_4 affect all body systems by regulating overall body metabolism, energy production, and fluid and electrolyte balance and controlling tissue utilization of fats, proteins, and carbohydrates. Thyrocalcitonin inhibits mobilization of calcium from bone and reduces blood calcium levels.

I. Hyperthyroidism

Hyperthyroidism is a clinical syndrome caused by excessive circulating thyroid hormone. Because thyroid activity affects all body systems, excessive thyroid hormone exaggerates normal body functions and produces a hypermetabolic state. Family history of hyperthyroidism is a significant factor for development of this disorder. Hyperthyroidism also can be caused by nodular toxic goiters in which one or more thyroid adenomas hyperfunction autonomously.

Graves' disease (diffuse toxic goiter) accounts for approximately 85% of reported cases of hyperthyroidism. It is characterized by spontaneous exacerbations and remissions that appear to be unaffected by therapy. The cause of Graves' disease is unknown, but recent advances in diagnostic techniques have isolated an immunoglobulin known as long-acting thyroid stimulator (LATS) in a majority of patients with this disorder, suggesting that Graves' disease is an autoimmune response.

The most severe form of hyperthyroidism is *thyrotoxic crisis* or *thyroid storm*, which results from a sudden surge of large amounts of thyroid hormones into the bloodstream, causing an even greater increase in body metabolism. This is a medical emergency. Precipitating factors include infection, trauma, and emotional stress, all of which place greater demands on body metabolism. Thyrotoxic crisis also can occur following subtotal thyroidectomy because of manipulation of the gland during surgery. Despite vigorous treatment, thyroid storm causes death in approximately 20% of affected patients.

A. Assessment

Signs and symptoms: Oligomenorrhea or amenorrhea; increased appetite with weight loss; diarrhea or frequent defecation; increased perspiration, especially on the palms of the hands; hyperglycemia; and generalized muscle weakness. In addition, heat intolerance, anxiety, excitability, restlessness, tremors, insomnia, and atrial fibrillation with congestive heart failure (CHF) are sometimes noted.

Physical exam: Tachycardia with irregular, bounding pulse; increased respirations; elevated temperature; enlargement of the thyroid gland 2–4 times greater than normal; bruit with auscultation over gland; atrophy of skeletal muscles; enlargement of the thymus and lymph nodes; hyperreflexia; and gynecomastia in males. In addition, these patients are usually thin and hyperkinetic with warm, moist skin and fine, silky hair that will not curl. A rare but positive diagnostic sign is the presence of Plummer's nails, in which the distal portion of the nail separates from the nailbed. Patients with Graves' disease may have exophthalmos and pretibial myxedema (nonpitting thickening of the skin over the front distal third of the leg).

Thyrotoxic crisis (thyroid storm): Severe tachycardia, high temperature, CNS irritability, and delirium.

B. Diagnostic Tests

1. <u>Serum thyroxine and triiodothyronine tests:</u> Will show elevation of T_3 and T_4 in the presence of disease.

2. <u>Thyroid stimulating hormone (TSH) test</u>: Decreased in the presence of disease.

3. <u>Free thyroxine index (FTI)</u>: Elevated in the presence of disease.

4. <u>Thyroid scanning</u>: Uses radionuclear scanning to determine function of thyroid gland and presence of nodules.

C. Medical Management and Surgical Interventions

1. Pharmacotherapy

□ *Propranolol (beta-adrenergic blocking agent):* To relieve tachycardia, anxiety, and heat intolerance. It is usually contraindicated in patients with CHF, but if the heart failure is specifically caused by hyperthyroidism and especially if the patient demonstrates atrial fibrillation, propranolol given in conjunction with digitalis may be of benefit.

□ *Antithyroid agents (thioamides), including propylthiouracil and methimazole:* To prevent the synthesis and release of thyroxine. Patients are continued on thioamides for a period that ranges from 6 months to several years. The relapse rate after discontinuation of therapy is high and drug reactions can be severe, including skin rash, fever, pharyngitis, granulocytopenia, arthralgia, myalgia, thrombocytopenia, alterations in taste, hair pigment changes, and lymphadenopathy. By far the most severe side effect is agranulocytosis (acute blood dyscrasia in which the WBC count drops to extremely low levels), which occurs in 0.5% of cases.

□ *Iodides:* May be given in conjunction with thioamides to inhibit thyroid hormone release. Adverse reactions include skin rash and fever. If used as the only drug to inhibit release of thyroid hormone in Graves' disease or multinodular toxic goiter, iodides must be given cautiously because normal inhibiting factors are absent and their administration can actually increase thyroxine production and release, potentially resulting in increased hyperthyroidism and thyroid storm.

□ *Radioactive iodide (sodium iodide ^{131}I):* Given orally, based on estimated weight of the gland and results of radioactive iodine uptake scan. The major complication is hypothyroidism, which occurs in 80% of patients receiving this type of therapy. Complications from the medication itself are rare, but a sore throat, swelling of the gland, radiation sickness, and transitory hypoparathyroidism do occur.

□ *Barbiturates and tranquilizers:* To minimize anxiety and promote rest.

□ *Antidiarrheals:* To decrease peristalsis and increase absorption of nutrients from the GI tract.

2. Diet: High in calories, protein, carbohydrates, and vitamins to restore a normal nutritional state.

3. Subtotal thyroidectomy: Surgical removal of part of the gland. To minimize postoperative complications, the patient is prepared with antithyroid (thioamide) agents for approximately 6 weeks until euthyroid. Nutritional status is maximized and approximately 2 weeks before surgery the patient is started on iodides to decrease vascularity of the gland and make it firmer, which facilitates removal. The most frequent postoperative complication is hemorrhage at the operative site. Damage to the laryngeal nerve occurs in 1–4% of cases. If this is unilateral, it will cause minimal voice changes, but if it is bilateral, nerve damage can cause upper airway obstruction. Thyroid storm and tetany occur rarely.

D. Nursing Diagnoses and Interventions

Sleep pattern disturbance related to agitation secondary to accelerated metabolism

Desired outcome: Patient relates the attainment of sufficient rest and sleep.

1. Adjust care activities to patient's tolerance.

2. Provide frequent rest periods. If possible, arrange for patient to have bed rest in a quiet, cool room with non-exertional activities such as reading, watching television, working crossword puzzles, or listening to soothing music.

3. As necessary, assist patient with walking up stairs or other exertional activities.

4. Administer tranquilizers and sedatives as prescribed to promote rest.

Anxiety related to untoward response secondary to sympathetic nervous system stimulation

Desired outcomes: Patient does not exhibit signs of harmful anxiety. Patient and SOs can verbalize knowledge of the causes of the patient's behavior.

1. Assess for signs of anxiety; administer tranquilizers and sedatives as prescribed.

2. Provide a quiet, stress-free environment away from loud noises or excessive activity.

3. Administer propranolol as prescribed to reduce symptoms of anxiety, tachycardia, and heat intolerance.

4. Reassure patient that anxiety symptoms are related to the disease process, and that treatment decreases their severity.

5. Inform SOs that patient's behavior is physiologic (a result of CNS irritability) and should not be taken personally.

6. Limit number of visitors and the amount of time they spend with patient. Advise SOs to avoid discussing stressful topics and refrain from arguing with patient.

Alteration in nutrition: Less than body requirements related to increased need secondary to hypermetabolic state

Desired outcomes: Patient does not exhibit signs of malnutrition or weight loss and can list the types of foods that are necessary to achieve optimal nutrition.

1. Provide a diet high in calories, protein, carbohydrates, and vitamins. Teach patient about foods that will provide optimal nutrients. To maximize patient's consumption, provide between-meal snacks.

2. Administer vitamin supplements as prescribed and explain their importance to the patient.

3. Administer prescribed antidiarrheal medications, which increase absorption of nutrients from the GI tract.

4. Weigh patient daily and report significant losses to MD.

Potential for injury related to risk of corneal damage secondary to exophthalmos

Desired outcomes: Patient does not exhibit signs of corneal injury and can verbalize measures to prevent it.

1. Teach patient to wear dark glasses to protect the cornea.

2. Administer eyedrops as prescribed to supplement lubrication and/or decrease sympathetic nervous system stimulation, which can cause lid retraction.

3. If appropriate, apply eye shields or tape the eyes shut at bedtime.

4. Administer thioamides as prescribed to maintain normal metabolic state and halt progression of exophthalmos.

Disturbance in self-concept related to altered body image secondary to exophthalmos and/or surgical scar

Desired outcome: Patient can verbalize measures for disguising exophthalmos and/or surgical scar and relates the attainment of self-acceptance.

1. Encourage patient to communicate feelings of frustration.

2. Advise patient to wear dark glasses to disguise exophthalmos.

3. Suggest that patient wear customized jewelery, high-necked clothing such as turtlenecks, or loose-fitting scarves to disguise the scar.

4. Suggest that after the incision has healed, patient use makeup in his or her skin tone to decrease visibility of the scar.

5. Caution patient that creams are contraindicated until the incision has healed completely, and even then there is little evidence that they minimize scarring. Patients are advised by some MDs to increase vitamin C intake to up to 1 g/day to promote healing. Some surgeons also advise against direct sunlight to the operative site for 6–12 months to avoid hyperpigmentation of the incision. Instruct patient accordingly.

Knowledge deficit: Potential for side effects from iodides or from taking or abruptly stopping thioamides

Desired outcomes: Patient can verbalize potential side effects of prescribed medications, signs and symptoms of hypothyroidism and hyperthyroidism, and the importance of following the prescribed medical regimen.

1. Explain the importance of taking antithyroid medications daily, in divided doses, and at regular intervals as prescribed.

2. Teach patient the indicators of hypothyroidism and the signs and symptoms that necessitate medical attention, including cold intolerance, fatigue, lethargy, and peripheral or periorbital edema.

3. Teach patient the side effects of thioamides and the symptoms that necessitate medical attention, including the appearance of a rash, fever, or pharyngitis, which can occur in the presence of agranulocytosis.

4. Alert patients taking iodides to signs of worsening hyperthyroidism, including high temperature, severe tachycardia, and CNS irritability with delirium.

Potential for injury related to risk of thyrotoxic crisis (thyroid storm) secondary to emotional stress, trauma, infection, or surgical manipulation of the gland

Desired outcomes: Patient does not exhibit signs of thyrotoxic crisis, or if they appear, they are detected and reported promptly, resulting in immediate treatment and absence of injury to patient.

1. Report rectal temperature >100 F, as this is often the first sign of impending thyroid storm.

2. Provide cool sponge baths or apply ice packs to patient's axilla and groin areas to decrease fever. If high temperature continues, obtain a prescription for a hypothermia blanket.

3. As prescribed, administer acetaminophen to decrease temperature. **Caution:** Aspirin is contraindicated because it releases thyroxine from protein-binding sites and increases free thyroxine levels.

4. Administer propylthiouracil as prescribed to prevent further synthesis and release of thyroid hormones.

5. Administer propranolol as prescribed to block sympathetic nervous system effects.

6. In unstable patients, monitor VS q15–30 min for evidence of hypotension and increasing tachycardia and fever.

7. Administer IV fluids as prescribed to provide adequate hydration and prevent vascular collapse. Carefully monitor I&O qh to prevent fluid overload or inadequate fluid replacement. Decreasing output with normal specific gravity may indicate decreased cardiac output, while decreasing ouput with increased specific gravity can signal dehydration.

8. Admininster sodium iodide as prescribed, 1 hour *after* administering propyl-

thiouracil. **Caution:** If given before propylthiouracil, sodium iodide can exacerbate symptoms in susceptible individuals.

9. Administer small doses of insulin as prescribed to control hyperglycemia.

10. Provide a cool, calm, protected environment to minimize emotional stress. Reassure patient and explain all procedures before performing them. Limit the number of visitors.

11. Ensure good handwashing and meticulous, aseptic technique for dressing changes and invasive procedures. Advise visitors who have contracted or been exposed to a communicable disease not to enter patient's room or to wear a surgical mask, if appropriate.

12. Because oxygen demands are increased as the metabolism increases, administer prescribed supplemental oxygen as necessary.

13. Monitor patient for signs of CHF, including jugular vein distention, crackles (rales), decrease in quality of peripheral pulses, peripheral edema, and hypotension. Immediately report any positive findings to MD and prepare to transfer patient to ICU if they are noted.

Alteration in comfort: Pain related to surgical procedure

Desired outcome: Patient relates a reduction in discomfort and does not exhibit signs of uncontrolled pain.

1. Inform patient that clasping the hands behind the neck when moving will minimize stress on the incision.

2. After MD has removed surgical clips and drain, teach patient to perform *gentle* ROM exercises for the neck.

3. For other interventions, see the same nursing diagnosis in "Appendix One," "Caring for Preoperative and Postoperative Patients," p. 528.

Potential alteration in respiratory function related to edema and/or laryngeal nerve damage secondary to surgical procedure

Desired outcome: Patient does not exhibit signs of respiratory dysfunction.

1. Monitor respiratory status for signs of edema (dyspnea, choking, inspiratory stridor, inability to swallow). Also assess patient's voice. Although slight hoarseness is normal following surgery, hoarseness that persists is indicative of laryngeal nerve damage and should be reported to MD promptly. If bilateral nerve damage has occurred, upper airway obstruction can occur.

2. Elevate HOB 30–45° to minimize edema and incisional stress. Support patient's head with flat or cervical pillows so that it is in a neutral position with the neck and does not flex or extend.

3. Keep tracheostomy set and oxygen equipment at bedside at all times. Suction upper airway as needed, using gentle suction to avoid stimulating laryngospasm.

4. To minimize pain and anxiety and enhance patient's ability to swallow, administer analgesics promptly and as prescribed.

See "Appendix One" for nursing diagnoses and interventions for the care of preoperative and postoperative patients, pp. 528–532.

E. Patient–Family Teaching and Discharge Planning

Provide patient and SOs with verbal and written information for the following:

1. Diet high in calories, protein, carbohydrates, and vitamins. Inform patient that as a normal metabolic state is attained, the diet may change.

2. Medications, including drug name, purpose, dosage, schedule, precautions, and potential side effects.

3. Changes that can occur as a result of therapy, including weight gain, normalized bowel function, increased strength of skeletal muscles, and a return to normal activity levels.

4. Importance of continued and frequent medical follow-up; confirm date and time of next appointment.

5. Indicators that necessitate medical attention, including fever, rash, or sore throat (side effects of thioamides), and symptoms of hypothyroidism or worsening hyperthyroidism.

6. For patients receiving radioactive iodine, the importance of not holding children to the chest for 72 hours following therapy. Explain that there is negligible risk for adults.

7. Importance of avoiding physical and emotional stress early in the recuperative stage and maximizing coping mechanisms for dealing with stress.

II. Hypothyroidism

Hypothyroidism is a condition in which there is an inadequate amount of circulating thyroid hormone, which causes a decrease in metabolic rate that affects all body systems.

Primary hypothyroidism accounts for more than 90% of cases of hypothyroidism and is caused by pathologic changes in the thyroid itself. There are several possible causes, including dietary iodine deficiency, thyroiditis, thyroid atrophy or fibrosis of unknown etiology, radiation therapy to the neck (such as with the treatment for hyperthyroidism), surgical removal of all or part of the gland, drugs that suppress thyroid activity including propylthiouracil and iodides, and a genetic dysfunction resulting in the inability to produce and secrete thyroid hormone. *Secondary hypothyroidism* is caused by dysfunction of the anterior pituitary gland, which results in decreased release of thyroid-stimulating hormone (TSH). It can be caused by pituitary tumors, postpartum necrosis of the pituitary gland, or hypophysectomy. *Tertiary hypothyroidism* is caused by a hypothalamic deficiency in the release of thyrotropin-releasing hormone (TRH).

When hypothyroidism is untreated or when a stressor such as infection affects an individual with hypothyroidism, a life-threatening condition known as *myxedema coma* can occur. The clinical picture of myxedema coma is that of exaggerated hypothyroidism, with dangerous hypoventilation, hypothermia, hypotension, and shock. Coma and seizures can occur as well. Myxedema coma usually develops slowly, has a >50% mortality rate, and requires prompt and aggressive treatment.

A. Assessment

Signs and symptoms can progress from mild early in onset to life-threatening.

Signs and symptoms: Early fatigue, weight gain, anorexia, constipation, menstrual irregularities, muscle cramps, lethargy, inability to concentrate, hair loss, cold intolerance, and hoarseness. Some usually placid patients may become depressed or extremely agitated.

Physical exam: Possible presence of goiter, cardiomegaly, bradycardia, hypothermia, peripheral nonpitting edema, and periorbital puffiness. Patients are often obese with cool, dry, yellowish skin. The voice is hoarse and the speech is frequently slurred. The hair is thin, coarse, and brittle and the tongue is enlarged. Slow mentation and reflexes are usually present.

Myxedema coma: Hypoventilation, hypoglycemia, hyponatremia, stupor, unresponsiveness, hypotension, and shock.

B. Diagnostic Tests

1. <u>Serum tests:</u> TSH will be elevated in the presence of primary hypothyroidism and low or normal in other forms of the disease. This is the most significant test for differentiating primary from secondary or tertiary hypothyroidism. Serum T_3 and T_4 will be decreased.

2. Iodine-131 uptake: Will be less than 10% in 24 hours. In secondary hypothyroidism, uptake increases with administration of exogenous TSH.

3. Thyroid antibody tests: Positive in primary hypothyroidism.

C. Medical Management

1. **Oral thyroid hormone:** Given early in treatment for primary hypothyroidism. To prevent hyperthyroidism caused by too much exogenous thyroid hormone, patients are started on low doses that are increased gradually, based on serial laboratory tests (T_3 and T_4) and the patient's response to medication. This therapy is continued for the patient's lifetime. For patients with secondary hypothyroidism, thyroid supplements can promote acute symptoms and are therefore contraindicated.

2. **Stool softeners:** To minimize constipation secondary to decreased gastric secretions and peristalsis.

3. **Diet:** High in roughage and protein to help prevent constipation; restriction of sodium to decrease edema; and reduction in calories to promote weight loss.

Treatment of myxedema coma:

1. **IV thyroid supplements:** Rapid IV administration of thyroid hormone can precipitate hyperadrenocorticism, but can be avoided by the concomitant administration of IV hydrocortisone.

2. **Intubation and mechanical ventilation:** To compensate for decreased ventilatory drive.

3. **Treat hyponatremia:** Restrict fluids and/or administer hypertonic (3%) saline.

4. **Treat associated illnesses such as infections.**

5. **Treat hypotension:** Administer IV isotonic fluids such as normal saline and lactated Ringer's solution. Hypotonic solutions such as 5% dextrose in water (D_5W) are contraindicated because they can further decrease serum sodium levels. Because of altered metabolism, these patients respond poorly to vasopressors.

6. **Treat hypoglycemia:** Administer IV glucose.

▶ **Caution:** Because of alterations in metabolism, patients do not tolerate barbiturates and sedatives, and therefore CNS depressants are contraindicated. Also, external warming measures are contraindicated for hypothermia because they can produce vasodilation and vascular collapse.

D. Nursing Diagnoses and Interventions

Alteration in bowel elimination: Constipation related to decreased peristalsis secondary to slowed metabolism

Desired outcome: Patient relates the attainment of a normal pattern of bowel elimination.

1. Query patient about current bowel function; document changes.

2. Be alert to decreasing bowel sounds and the presence of distention and increases in abdominal girth, which can occur with ileus or an obstructive process.

3. Encourage patient to maintain a diet with adequate roughage and fluids. Examples of foods high in bulk include fruits with skins, fruit juices, cooked fruits, vegetables, whole grain breads and cereals, and nuts. Ensure that fluid intake is at least 2–3 L/day.

4. Administer stool softeners and laxatives as prescribed. **Caution:** Suppositories are contraindicated because of the risk of stimulating the vagus nerve.

5. Advise patient to increase the amount of exercise to promote regularity.

Activity intolerance related to weakness and fatigue secondary to slowed metabolism and decreased cardiac output caused by pericardial effusions, atherosclerosis, and decreased adrenergic stimulation

Desired outcome: Patient exhibits increasing cardiac tolerance to activity.

1. Monitor VS and apical pulse at frequent intervals. Be alert to hypotension, slow pulse, dysrhythmias, complaints of chest pain or discomfort, decreasing urine output, and changes in mentation. Promptly report significant changes to MD.

2. Balance activity with adequate rest to decrease workload of the heart.

3. As prescribed, administer IV isotonic solutions such as normal saline to help prevent hypotension.

4. To prevent problems of immobility, assist patient with ROM and other in-bed exercises and consult with MD regarding the implementation of exercises that require greater cardiac tolerance to exercise. For detail, see **Potential impairment of physical mobility** related to inactivity, p. 535, in "Appendix One."

Potential alteration in respiratory function related to decreased ventilatory drive or upper airway obstruction secondary to myxedematous infiltration

Desired outcome: Patient does not exhibit signs of respiratory dysfunction.

1. Assess rate, depth, and quality of breath sounds and be alert to the presence of adventitious sounds (eg, from developing pleural effusion) or decreasing or crowing sounds (eg, from swollen tongue or glottis).

2. Teach patient coughing, deep breathing, and use of incentive spirometer. Suction upper airway prn.

3. Be alert to signs of inadequate ventilation, including changes in respiratory rate or pattern and circumoral or peripheral cyanosis. Immediately report significant findings to MD.

4. For a patient experiencing respiratory distress, be prepared to assist MD with intubation or tracheostomy and maintenance of mechanical ventilatory assistance and/or transfer patient to ICU.

Potential for infection related to increased susceptibility secondary to alterations in adrenal function

Desired outcome: Patient does not exhibit signs of infection.

1. Be alert to early indicators of infection, including fever, redness, swelling, or discharge from wounds or IV sites; urinary frequency, urgency, dysuria, cloudy or malodorous urine; presence of adventitious sounds on auscultation of lung fields and changes in color, consistency, and amount of sputum. Notify MD of significant findings.

2. Minimize the risk of UTI by providing meticulous care of indwelling catheters.

3. Use meticulous sterile technique when performing dressing changes and invasive procedures.

4. Because open sores are sites of ingress for bacteria, provide good skin care to maintain skin integrity and prevent decubitus ulcers.

5. Advise visitors who have contracted or been exposed to a communicable disease not to enter patient's room or to wear surgical mask, if appropriate.

Alteration in nutrition: More than body requirements of calories related to decreased need secondary to slowed metabolism

Desired outcomes: Patient does not experience weight gain. Patient can verbalize knowledge of the rationale and measures for the dietary regimen.

1. Provide a diet that is high in protein and low in calories. Restrict or limit sodium, as prescribed, to decrease edema. Teach patient about foods to augment and limit or omit.

2. Provide small, frequent meals of appropriate foods the patient particularly enjoys.

3. Encourage foods that are high in fiber content (eg, fruits with skins, vegetables, whole grain breads and cereals, nuts) to improve gastric motility and elimination.

4. Administer vitamin supplements as prescribed.

Sensory-perceptual alterations related to confusion secondary to cerebral retention of water

Desired outcome: Patient can verbalize orientation to person, place, and time.

1. Monitor patient's mental status at frequent intervals by assessing orientation to person, place, and time. Report increasing lethargy or confusion to MD, as these can signal onset of myxedema coma.

2. Reorient patient frequently. Have a clock and calendar visibile and use radio or television for orientation.

3. Clearly explain all procedures to patient before performing them. Allow adequate time for patient to ask questions.

4. If necessary, remind patient to complete ADLs such as bathing and brushing hair.

5. Encourage visitors to discuss topics of special interest to patient to enhance patient's alertness.

6. Administer thyroid replacement hormones as prescribed to increase metabolic rate, which in turn will enhance cerebral blood flow.

Fluid volume excess: Edema related to retention secondary to decreased metabolic rate and adrenal insufficiency

Desired outcome: Patient does not exhibit signs of fluid overload.

1. Restrict fluid and sodium intake as prescribed.

2. Administer IV fluids using a mechanical controller to prevent accidental fluid overload.

3. Monitor I&O qh for evidence of decreasing output.

4. Weigh patient at the same time every day, with the same clothing, and using the same scale. Report increasing weight gains to MD.

5. Monitor patient for signs of CHF: jugular vein distention, crackles (rales), SOB, dependent edema of extremities, and decreased peripheral pulses. Report significant findings to MD.

Potential for injury related to risk of myxedema coma secondary to inadequate response to treatment of hypothyroidism or stressors such as infection

Desired outcomes: Patient does not exhibit signs of myxedema coma, or if they appear they are detected and reported promptly, resulting in immediate treatment and absence of injury to the patient.

1. Monitor VS at frequent intervals and be alert to bradycardia, hypotension, or decrease in respiratory rate. Report systolic BP <90, pulse <60, or respiratory rate <10.

2. Monitor patient for signs of hypoxia (circumoral or peripheral cyanosis, decrease in LOC). Immediately report positive findings to MD.

3. Double check medication dosages carefully before administering, especially barbiturates and sedatives, which are not well tolerated by these patients. Ob-

serve for signs of toxicity such as decreased LOC and decreases in BP or ventilatory effort.

4. Monitor serum electrolytes and glucose levels. Be especially alert to decreasing sodium (<130 mEq/L) and glucose (<80 mg/100mL).

5. In the presence of myxedema coma, implement the following:

◻ Restrict fluids and/or administer hypertonic saline as prescribed to correct hyponatremia. Use an infusion control device to maintain accurate infusion rate of IV fluids.

◻ As prescribed, administer IV thyroid replacement hormones with IV hydrocortisone and IV glucose to treat hypoglycemia.

◻ Monitor patient for signs of CHF: jugular vein distention, crackles (rales), SOB, peripheral edema, weakening peripheral pulses, and hypotension. Notify MD of any significant findings.

◻ Prepare to transfer patient to ICU. Keep a bite block, oral airway, and manual rescusitator at the bedside in the event of seizure, coma, or the need for ventilatory assistance.

E. Patient–Family Teaching and Discharge Planning

Provide patient and SOs with verbal and written information for the following:

1. Medications, including drug name, purpose, dosage, schedule, precautions, and potential side effects. Remind patient that thioamides, iodides, and lithium are contraindicated because they decrease thyroid activity. Be sure that patient is aware that thyroid replacement medications are to be taken for life.

2. Dietary requirements and restrictions, which may change as hormone replacement therapy becomes more and more effective.

3. Expected changes that can occur with hormone replacement therapy: increased energy level, weight loss, and decreased peripheral edema. Neuromuscular problems should improve, as well.

4. Importance of continued, frequent medical follow-up; confirm date and time of next medical appointment.

5. Importance of avoiding physical and emotional stress, and ways for patient to maximize coping mechanisms for dealing with stress.

6. Signs and symptoms that necessitate medical attention, including fever or other symptoms of upper respiratory, urinary, or oral infections and signs and symptoms of hyperthyroidism, which may result from excessive hormone replacement.

▶ Section Two   **Disorders of the Parathyroid Glands**

The parathyroid glands regulate serum calcium and phosphorus levels via release of parathyroid hormone (PTH). This is accomplished by a negative-feedback mechanism: When serum calcium levels rise, PTH secretion is suppressed. PTH acts on bone to decrease calcium binding, and it stimulates the kidneys to increase resorption of calcium and excretion of phosphate. PTH is also involved in the synthesis of a renal enzyme that catalyzes the formation of vitamin D, which in conjunction with PTH, increases absorption of calcium from the GI tract.

I. Hyperparathyroidism

Hyperparathyroidism is a clinical syndrome in which there is excessive secretion of PTH. *Primary hyperparathyroidism* is caused by pathology of one or more of the parathyroid glands. Eighty percent of these cases are caused by a benign adenoma of one gland, another 10% by hyperplasia of all four glands, and in rare cases, by carcinoma. In this disorder, excessive PTH acts on the skeletal, renal, and GI systems, and the overall effect is that of increased serum calcium and decreased phosphate. It is the second most common cause of hypercalcemia. *Secondary hyperparathyroidism* is usually caused by renal insufficiency with decreased glomerular filtration. Although calcium and phosphorus are retained because of the lack of renal filtration, the high serum phosphate level depresses calcium concentration, which results in hypocalcemia. In turn, the resulting hypocalcemia stimulates the parathyroid glands to release PTH in an effort to increase serum calcium levels. Bone resorption occurs because of increased PTH, but absorption of calcium from the GI tract is depressed because of calcium binding with high-phosphate GI secretions. The overall effect is that of decreased calcium and increased phosphate levels. *Tertiary hyperparathyroidism* occurs when secondary hyperparathyroidism progresses to a state in which excessive PTH is released independent of serum calcium levels.

A. Assessment

Signs and symptoms: Muscular weakness, fatigue, personality disturbances, emotional lability, constipation, weight loss, renal calculi, nausea, vomiting, anorexia, polyuria, hematuria, drowsiness, stupor, and coma. In addition, the patient may have kidney infections, anemia, arthralgia, pancreatitis, peptic ulcers, and pathologic fractures, as well as heart disease caused by calcium deposits in the tissues.

Physical exam: Hypotonic muscles, enlarged parathyroid glands, hypertension. If the condition is severe, renal failure also may be present.

B. Diagnostic Tests

1. <u>Serum calcium:</u> Elevated in primary hyperparathyroidism and low in secondary hyperparathyroidism. This test is usually repeated at least three times to confirm the diagnosis. Venous blood is drawn in the morning after the patient has been in a fasting state. Because calcium is bound to protein, the test results must be "corrected," based on a simultaneous test for albumin level. Serum calcium will change by 0.8 mg/dL for each 1 g/dL change in albumin level above or below normal. This represents the circulating calcium available for use by body cells and is considered the "true" calcium level.

   ▶ **Note:** To avoid venous stasis, which can produce erroneously high results, care must be taken not to apply the tourniquet too tightly or occlude the vessel for longer than necessary.

2. <u>Serum PTH:</u> High or inappropriately high for serum calcium levels.

3. <u>Plasma phosphorus:</u> Decreased in primary hyperparathyroidism and elevated in secondary hyperparathyroidism.

4. <u>24-hour urine calcium:</u> Elevated in primary hyperparathyroidism. This test is often used to rule out other causes of hypercalcemia.

5. <u>Skeletal x-rays:</u> Will show diminution of bone mass in virtually all patients with hyperparathyroidism, as well as calcification of articular cartilage. X-rays of the hands will show subperiosteal resorption of the phalanges.

6. <u>EKG:</u> May show shortened Q–T interval, which is reflective of hypercalcemia.

C. Medical Management and Surgical Interventions

Surgical treatment for primary hyperparathyroidism: The most effective form of treatment for primary hyperparathyroidism is the surgical removal of one or more of the parathyroid glands (parathyroidectomy). The incision is somewhat wider than with a thyroidectomy, but the surgery is very similar. Only the affected gland(s) is removed, and in cases where all of the parathyroid glands are enlarged, 3½ of the glands are removed. The remaining tissue is enough to provide normal calcium regulation. In addition to the postoperative complications potentially found with a thyroidectomy, abnormalities in serum calcium levels also may be found.

Medical treatment for primary hyperparathyroidism: Reserved for patients who are poor surgical risks or who have only a mild form of the disease. The goals of treatment are to provide adequate hydration and reduce serum calcium levels. **Note:** Calcium levels >14 mg/dL are life-threatening and require vigorous and immediate treatment if the patient is to survive.

1. **Promote calcium excretion:** In the absence of congestive heart failure or renal insufficiency. This is accomplished by forcing fluids orally, or providing IV normal saline for patients who are stuporous or nauseated. Volumes up to 1000 mL/h may be given for short periods.

2. **Increase salt intake:** Either via diet or salt tablets. Because sodium competes with calcium for excretion by the kidneys, increased sodium levels will cause the kidneys to excrete more calcium.

3. **Diet:** Limit dietary calcium (eg, milk, many cheeses, cottage cheese, mustard greens, kale, broccoli) intake to one serving per day.

4. **Pharmacotherapy**

   □ *Diuretics:* To prevent volume overload and maintain brisk diuresis. Loop diuretics (furosemide and ethacrynate sodium) are preferred because they increase urinary calcium excretion. Thiazide diuretics are contraindicated because they decrease calcium excretion.

   □ *Oral phosphate supplements:* To decrease bone resorption of calcium and bind calcium in the intestine to limit calcium absorption. Because they may cause precipitation of insoluble calcium-phosphate complexes in the soft tissues of the kidneys, lungs, and heart conductive system, they are given only to patients with low serum phosphate or to those who have normal kidney function. Diarrhea is a common side effect. IV phosphates are avoided except for extreme emergency (calcium >14 mg/dL).

   □ *IM calcitonin:* To decrease bone resorption of calcium and increase renal clearance. This has limited use, however, because it is short acting and patients frequently become resistant.

   □ *IV mithramycin:* To inhibit bone resorption and lower serum and urine calcium levels. This is the drug of choice for treatment of *severe* hypercalcemia because it is more effective and works more rapidly than calcitonin. Effects are usually seen within 2 hours. Side effects include bleeding abnormalities and hypocalcemia.

   □ *Oral steroids:* For their calciuric effect and to decrease calcium absorption in the presence of vitamin D intoxication. To avoid the immunosuppressive effects of these drugs, they are given in as small a dose as it takes to achieve therapeutic effects.

5. **Hemodialysis in a low-calcium bath:** Sometimes prescribed for severe hypercalcemia.

Treatment for secondary hyperparathyroidism:

1. **Decrease dietary phosphorus:** For example, by limiting meat, poultry, fish, eggs, cheese, dried beans, and cereals.

2. **Oral calcium supplements:** To increase serum levels.

3. **Aluminum-containing antacids (eg, AlternaGel, Amphojel):** For patients with chronic renal failure to bind phosphorus in the intestine and prevent resorption.

4. **Oral vitamin D supplements:** To correct deficiency.

D. Nursing Diagnoses and Interventions

Activity intolerance related to neuromuscular weakness and joint pain secondary to increased serum calcium and altered phosphate levels

Desired outcome: Patient demonstrates progression to his or her highest level of mobility without evidence of weakness or joint pain.

1. Administer analgesics and anti-inflammatory agents as prescribed to minimize discomfort and enhance the effectiveness of prescribed or necessary activity. Time exercise/activity to coincide with the peak effectiveness of the medication.

2. Adjust activity to patient's tolerance and provide rest periods at frequent intervals. Discuss the importance of activity with the patient and set realistic short- and long-term goals in clearly understood, empirical terms (eg, "Ambulate the length of the ward three times.")

3. Assist with ambulation as necessary. Provide a walker or cane if appropriate.

4. Request PT and OT consultations for gradually increasing muscular strength and endurance.

Fluid volume deficit related to abnormal loss secondary to osmotic diuresis, vomiting, or diarrhea caused by oral phosphate supplements

Desired outcome: Patient does not exhibit signs of dehydration.

1. Monitor and document I&O. Be alert to indications of dehydration, including dry mucous membranes, poor skin turgor, thirst, furrowed tongue.

2. Unless patient has coexisting renal or cardiac disease, encourage oral fluids to 3 L/day.

3. Rehydrate with IV fluids (typically normal saline) if prescribed.

4. Administer prescribed medications (eg, calcitonin, mithramycin) to decrease hypercalcemia and medications (eg, loop diuretics, steroids) to increase urinary calcium excretion.

5. Monitor serum calcium levels. Decreasing levels signal correction of the dehydration.

6. Be alert to the presence of hypotension, which can be further potentiated by phosphates.

Potential for injury related to risk of tetany, thyroid storm, and hypercalemia secondary to surgical procedure and/or manipulation of the gland

Desired outcome: Patient does not exhibit signs of hyperalcemia, tetany, or thyroid storm, or if they occur, they are detected and reported promptly, resulting in immediate treatment and absence of injury to the patient.

1. Be alert to the presence of hypercalcemia, which can be caused by an increased release of PTH secondary to surgical manipulation of the gland. Signs include nausea, vomiting, anorexia, abdominal pain, weakness, thirst, dyspnea, and coma.

2. Monitor patient for numbness and tingling around the mouth, an early sign of hypocalcemia. Also be alert to indicators of tetany: muscle twitching, painful tonic muscle spasms, and grimacing facial spasms. Two tests for assessing for tetany include Chvostek's and Trousseau's signs. Chvostek's sign is elicited by tapping the face just below the temple where the facial nerve emerges. The sign is positive if twitching occurs along the nose, lip, or side of the face. Trousseau's sign is tested by applying a BP cuff to the arm and inflating it to slightly higher than the systolic BP and leaving it inflated for 1–4 minutes. Carpopedal spasms are indicative of hypocalemia. Report significant findings to MD.

3. Keep IV calcium at the bedside for prescribed treatment.

4. Be alert to indicators of thyroid storm, including tachycardia, agitation, and hyperpyrexia. Immediately report the presence of these signs to MD. Although thyroid storm occurs rarely, it can be caused by a sudden release of excessive amounts of thyroid hormone into the bloodstream from manipulation of the gland during surgery.

Alteration in bowel elimination: Constipation related to decreased peristalsis secondary to increased serum calcium level

Desired outcomes: Patient can verbalize knowledge of measures that promote bowel elimination and relates bowel elimination within normal pattern.

1. Inform patient that increasing fluid intake to 3 L/day will help promote bowel elimination.
2. Teach patient to increase dietary fiber by adding dried fruits, whole-grain cereals, nuts, fresh fruits, and vegetables to the diet.
3. Administer stool softeners and laxatives as prescribed.
4. Encourage as much activity as tolerated.

Potential for injury related to risk of pathologic fractures secondary to bone demineralization

Desired outcome: Patient does not exhibit signs of pathologic fractures.

1. Minimize the risk of pathologic fractures from falling by keeping the bed in its lowest position, keeping walkway free of clutter, and assisting patient with ambulation or any strenuous activity. Instruct unstable patient to request help when getting out of bed, promote the use of a cane and/or walker, and keep call light within patient's reach.
2. Pad the siderails for patients with severe bone pathology.
3. Apply chest or wrist restraints for patients who are severely confused and may attempt to leave the bed, or arrange for SO to sit with patient.
4. Notify MD of patient complaints of back or chest pain, which may signal vertebral or rib fracture.

Alteration in comfort: Pain/arthralgia related to bone demineralization and/or surgery

Desired outcome: Patient relates a reduction in discomfort and does not exhibit signs of uncontrolled pain.

1. Advise patient to notify staff as soon as discomfort occurs so that analgesics can be administered before pain becomes too severe.
2. Administer analgesics as prescribed and document their effectiveness.
3. Administer analgesics 30–60 minutes before scheduled activities such as turning or ambulation.
4. Teach patient to clasp hands behind the neck during postoperative moving to minimize stress on the incision.
5. Teach gentle ROM exercises for the neck, as well as assisted or active ROM for painful joints.
6. Provide comfort measures such as an eggcrate mattress and a foot cradle to minimize pressure on the extremities.
7. Provide backrubs, especially at bedtime, to reduce discomfort from prolonged bed rest and enhance relaxation.

Knowledge deficit: Potential for negative side effects from steroids, phosphate supplements, and mithramycin

Desired outcome: Patient can verbalize knowledge of side effects of prescribed medications and the importance of notifying MD should they occur.

1. Teach patient the importance of monitoring for side effects of steroids. This includes frequent BP checks for hypertension, assessment for mental changes, and blood tests for the presence of hyperglycemia.

2. For patient taking phosphate supplements, explain that diarrhea is a common side effect.

3. Teach patient to be alert to the following side effects of mithramycin: lower-extremity petechiae, which signal thrombocytopenia; jaundice, which signals hepatocellular necrosis; and tetany, which occurs with hypocalcemia. Explain that urinalysis results must be monitored for evidence of proteinuria.

4. Explain the importance of notifying MD promptly should side effects occur.

See "Hyperthyroidism" for the following: **Potential alteration in respiratory function** related to edema and/or laryngeal nerve damage secondary to surgical procedure, p. 224. See "Renal Calculi," p. 101, in Chapter 3 for nursing diagnoses and interventions for the care of patients with renal calculi. See "Appendix One," pp. 528–532, for the care of preoperative and postoperative patients.

E. Patient–Family Teaching and Discharge Planning

Provide patient and SOs with verbal and written information for the following:

1. Diet, including the foods to limit or restrict. As appropriate, arrange for a dietary consult to help patient with meal planning and integration of individual restrictions into family meals.

2. Importance of continued medical follow-up; confirm date and time of next medical appointment.

3. Signs and symptoms of hypocalcemia and hypercalcemia, which necessitate medical attention if they occur.

4. Medications to be taken at home, including drug name, purpose, dosage, schedule, precautions, and potential side effects.

5. If surgery was performed, the indications of wound infection (eg, redness, local warmth, swelling, discharge, pain, or fever).

II. Hypoparathyroidism

Hypoparathyroidism is a condition in which there is decreased production of parathyroid hormone (PTH). Most commonly, this disorder is iatrogenic, caused by damage to or accidental removal of the parathyroid glands during thyroid surgery or radioactive iodine treatment for hyperthyroidism. Damage can be temporary or permanent. If injury occurs in the absence of gland removal, the tissue generally recovers within a period of months and returns to normal function. Familial or autoimmune factors also can be significant in the development of hypoparathyroidism. Because the function of PTH is the regulation of serum calcium levels, symptoms relate to tissue response to hypocalcemia.

A. Assessment

Signs and symptoms: Numbness and tingling around the mouth, fingertips, and sometimes in the feet; painful contractions or twitching of skeletal muscles; clonic and tonic spasms; grand mal seizures; laryngeal spasms; carpopedal spasm; nausea; vomiting; dysrhythmias; heart failure; cataracts (from calcium deposits); conjunctivitis; and photophobia.

Physical exam: Dry, scaly skin with increased pigmentation; thinning of scalp hair; loss of hair in axilla and pubic areas, eyebrows, and eyelashes; brittle fingernails and toenails, which may be deformed with horizontal ridges; and positive Chvostek's and Trousseau's signs.

B. Diagnostic Tests

1. <u>Serum tests:</u> Levels of calcium will be decreased; phosphate will be increased; and plasma PTH will be decreased.

2. <u>Skull and skeletal x-rays:</u> May show evidence of increased density and calcification of basal ganglia.

C. Medical Management

1. **Calcium supplements:** For cases of severe hypocalcemia, given either orally (route of choice) or IV.

2. **Parathyroid hormone injections:** To replace lost PTH.

3. **Vitamin D preparations:** To facilitate absorption of calcium from the GI tract.

4. **Sedatives (phenobarbital) and magnesium sulfate:** To minimize tetany and seizures. **Phenytoin** may be given to control seizures.

5. **Aluminum hydroxide gels (eg, AlternaGel, Amphojel):** To bind phosphorus in the intestines and decrease serum phosphate levels.

6. **Diet:** High in calcium (1 quart milk/day) and low in phosphorus (limit meat, poultry, fish, eggs, cheese, dried beans, and cereals). If hyperphosphatemia persists, it may be necessary to restrict dairy products and egg yolks and provide oral calcium supplements. Foods high in oxalate, which binds to calcium, also should be avoided. These include beets, figs, nuts, spinach, black tea, and chocolate.

D. Nursing Diagnoses and Interventions

Activity intolerance related to weakness and fatigue secondary to decreased cardiac contractility

Desired outcome: Patient is able to achieve activities at his or her highest level without evidence of cardiac intolerance.

1. Monitor patient for indicators of increasing cardiac failure, including hypotension, weak and thready pulse, tachycardia, SOB, pallor, or cyanosis. Report significant findings to MD.

2. Provide adequate rest periods.

3. Administer oral or IV calcium supplements as prescribed.

4. Assist patient with ROM and other in-bed exercises to help prevent complications of inactivity. Consult with MD regarding exercises that require increased cardiac tolerance. For guidelines, see **Potential impairment of physical mobility** related to prolonged inactivity, p. 535, in "Appendix One."

Potential for injury related to risk of seizures, tetany, and respiratory distress secondary to hypocalcemia

Desired outcome: Patient does not exhibit signs of injury due to hypocalcemia.

1. Observe for early signs of hypocalcemia, such as tingling around the mouth and in the hands. Be alert to indicators of tetany, including muscle twitching, painful tonic muscle spasms, grimacing facial spasms, and positive Chvostek's and Trousseau's signs. Report significant findings to MD.

2. Monitor for evidence of respiratory distress, including stridor, wheezing, and dyspnea; report significant findings to MD immediately.

3. Monitor serum calcium levels, noting whether levels are increased or decreased. Either extreme will require a change in calcium therapy. Serum calcium levels <7mg/dL or >14 mg/dL (after being "corrected" with albumin level) are life-threatening. If they occur, notify MD immediately.

4. Provide a restful, quiet environment away from loud noises and bright lights.

5. Administer sedatives and anticonvulsant medications as prescribed.

6. Pad siderails and keep them up at all times; keep padded tongue blade at bedside.

7. Keep tracheostomy set, oxygen equipment, and IV calcium at the bedside.

E. Patient—Family Teaching and Discharge Planning

Provide patient and SOs with verbal and written information for the following:

1. Diet, including foods to increase or limit. As appropriate, arrange for a dietary consult so that patient's requirements and restrictions can be integrated into family meal planning.

2. Medications, including drug name, purpose, dosage, schedule, precautions, and potential side effects.

3. Signs and symptoms necessitating medical attention, including signs of worsening hypocalcemia (such as tetany) or signs of hypercalcemia, including weakness, fatigue, constipation, polyuria, and renal calculi.

4. Importance of continued medical follow-up; confirm date and time of next appointment.

► Section Three   **Disorders of the Adrenal Gland**

Each of the two adrenal glands is composed of two distinct parts: the adrenal cortex and the medulla. Adrenocortical hormones include glucocorticoids (cortisol is the primary glucocorticoid), which are responsible for regulation of protein, fat, and carbohydrate metabolism and affect the immunologic and inflammatory responses; mineralocorticoids (aldosterone), which affect salt and water metabolism; and androgens, which affect sexual development. These hormones are released in response to serum levels of adrenocorticotropic hormone (ACTH), which functions via a negative-feedback mechanism: When serum cortisol levels decrease, ACTH release increases. The medulla secretes the catecholamines epinephrine and norepinephrine, which are released in response to sympathetic nervous system stimulation.

I. Addison's Disease

Addison's disease is a deficiency of adrenocortical hormones following destruction of the adrenal cortex, which can occur suddenly as a result of stress such as trauma, infection, or surgery. More commonly, however, the process occurs gradually. Eighty percent of reported cases involve an autoimmune factor. *Primary Addison's disease* is a pathology of the adrenal glands themselves; *secondary Addison's disease* results from impaired functioning of the pituitary gland, which causes decreased levels of ACTH.

The presence of acute symptoms in response to stressors is called *adrenal* or *Addisonian crisis.* It can be precipitated by any emotional stressor, simple infection, minor surgery, or trauma. Abrupt withdrawal of exogenous steroids also can precipitate a crisis. Unless treated rapidly and aggressively, this condition can lead to death within hours.

A. Assessment

Signs and symptoms: Apprehension, headache, nausea, anorexia, abdominal pain, diarrhea, confusion, and restlessness. In addition, patients may have muscular weakness that becomes progressively worse throughout the day, fatigue, weight loss, postural hypotension, and emotional instability.

Physical exam: Possible presence of cyanosis, fever, pallor, weak pulse, and tachypnea. Often, there is emaciation with dehydration, generalized dark pigmentation of the skin with brown or black freckles, hypotension, and a small heart size.

Addisonian crisis: Headache, nausea, vomiting, fever, intractable abdominal pain, and severe hypotension, which can lead to vascular collapse and shock.

History of: Familial tendency, bilateral adrenalectomy, tuberculosis, any kind of trauma or infection, damage to the pituitary gland.

B. Diagnostic Tests

1. Blood cortisol levels: Drawn at 8 AM, 4 PM, and 12 midnight. In normal individuals, blood cortisol levels are highest in the morning and gradually decrease until they reach their lowest level at 12 midnight. Patients with Addison's disease do not show this variation.

2. Other blood studies: Will reveal elevated potassium and BUN; decreased plasma aldosterone, sodium, and chloride levels; and decreased blood sugar. Serum ACTH will be increased in primary Addison's disease and decreased in secondary Addison's disease.

3. Urine sodium: Increased.

4. IM ACTH stimulation test: Involves drawing a fasting blood sample for blood cortisol levels, giving 25 units of ACTH IM, and drawing blood for cortisol levels after 30 and 60 minutes. If the cortisol level does not rise by at least 10 μg/100 mL, the test is positive for Addison's disesase.

5. IV ACTH stimulation test: On the first day, the patient is given 25 units of ACTH IV in 500 mL 5% dextrose and normal saline (D_5NS) between 8 AM and 4 PM. After the infusion, blood cortisol levels are drawn at 12 midnight, 8 AM, and 4 PM. This procedure is repeated on the second day. If there is no increase in blood cortisol levels, the patient has primary Addison's disease. If the cortisol levels show a gradual increase over several days, the patient has secondary Addison's disease.

C. Medical Management and Surgical Interventions

1. **Pharmacotherapy**

   □ *Antibiotics or antituberculosis therapy:* If infection or tuberculosis is the cause.

   □ *Maintenance doses of mineralocorticoids; oral supplementary sodium; and oral corticosteroids:* Exogenous steroids must be increased before and immediately after surgery, during times of stress, or in the presence of infection, because these conditions deplete adrenocortical hormones and place greater demands on body tissue. Patients must take hormone replacements for life.

2. **Diet:** High in calories, carbohydrates, proteins, and vitamins, provided in small, frequent feedings to enhance nutritional state for these patients, who tend to be anorexic.

For adrenal crisis:

1. **Replace fluids:** To correct severe dehydration. 1–2 L D_5NS is given over a brief period of time, eg, 2 hours.

2. **Hydrocortisone sodium succinate:** To replace decreased cortisol. It is given 100 mg IV immediately and then q6h via infusion drip.

3. **Vasopressors:** To maintain adequate BP.

4. **Continuous cardiac monitoring:** For prompt identification of life-threatening dysrhythmias.

D. Nursing Diagnoses and Interventions

Potential for infection related to lowered resistance secondary to decreased adrenal function

Desired outcome: Patient does not exhibit signs of infection.

1. Monitor for and report early signs of infection including fever; leukocytosis; frequency, urgency, dysuria, and cloudy or malodorous urine; persistent redness, pain, swelling, or discharge from wounds or the IV site; complaints of sore throat and pharyngitis. As directed, culture any drainage. Teach patient these signs and symptoms and the importance of reporting them to MD or staff promptly should they occur.

2. Monitor temperature q2–4h and report significant elevation to MD.

3. Use meticulous aseptic technique for all invasive procedures or when changing dressings. Ensure meticulous indwelling catheter care to help prevent UTI. Perform stringent handwashing techniques before caring for these patients.

4. Caution visitors who have contracted or been exposed to a communicable disease not to enter room (or to wear surgical masks when visiting patient).

Potential for injury related to risk of Addisonian crisis or side effects from the drug therapy used to treat it

Desired outcomes: Patient does not exhibit signs of Addisonian crisis or side effects from drug therapy, or if they occur, they are detected and treated promptly, resulting in absence of injury to the patient.

1. Place patient in a quiet room away from loud noises and excessive activity. Caution staff and visitors not to discuss stress-provoking topics with patient.

2. As prescribed, administer corticosteroids and prophylactic antibiotics.

3. If Addisonian crisis is diagnosed, implement the following:

   □ As prescribed, administer vasopressors to maintain BP and hydrocortisone sodium succinate to replace cortisol.

   □ Administer IV fluids as prescribed to prevent circulatory collapse.

   □ Monitor VS q15min until stable, then as prescribed. Report significant changes in BP, heart rate, or respiratory rate or pattern to MD.

   □ Administer oxygen as prescribed.

   □ Usually, a continuous cardiac monitor is used if Addisonian crisis is diagnosed. Monitor for signs of hypokalemia (increased PVCs, depressed T waves) or hyperkalemia (peaked T waves).

4. Monitor for and report signs of sodium retention and fluid volume excess (peripheral, pulmonary, and cerebral edema) caused by excessive doses of corticosteroids, sodium, and fluids. For example, be alert to dependent edema, crackles (rales), weight gain, severe headache, irritability, and confusion. Teach these symptoms to the patient and stress the importance of reporting them promptly to MD or staff.

Activity intolerance related to fatigue and weakness secondary to decreased cardiac output

Desired outcome: Patient achieves his or her highest activity level without evidence of cardiac intolerance.

1. Monitor VS at frequent intervals. Observe for and report indicators of impending circulatory collapse such as hypotension, tachycardia, weak and thready pulse, pallor, and/or cyanosis.

2. Gear activities to patient's tolerance. Provide for frequent rest periods.

3. To prevent complications of immobility, assist patient with ROM and other in-bed exercises. For details, see **Potential impairment of physical mobility**, p. 535, in "Appendix One."

Fluid volume deficit related to abnormal loss secondary to diuresis

Desired outcome: Patient does not exhibit signs of dehydration.

1. Monitor I&O and be alert to indicators of fluid volume deficit, including thirst, poor skin turgor, and furrowed tongue.

2. If deficit is noted, encourage oral fluids.

3. Administer maintenance doses of mineralocorticoids as prescribed to promote salt and water retention.

4. If prescribed, administer supplementary sodium to correct hyponatremia. As appropriate, advise patient to add salt to foods or eat foods relatively high in sodium, such as meat, fish, poultry, eggs, and milk.

▶ If patient experiences Addisonian crisis, see "Appendix One" for nursing diagnoses and interventions for the care of patients with life-disrupting illnesses, pp. 544–546.

E. Patient–Family Teaching and Discharge Planning

Provide patient and SOs with verbal and written information for the following:

1. Medications, including drug name, purpose, dosage, schedule, precautions, and potential side effects. Ensure that patient understands the necessity of lifetime hormone replacement.

2. Diet, for example, foods to increase such as those high in sodium.

3. Relationship between hormonal levels and stress. Instruct patient to seek medical help during periods of emotional or physical stress so that medication dosages can be adjusted accordingly.

4. Signs and symptoms that necessitate medical attention. These include indicators of excessive adrenal hormones (eg, weight gain, moon face, dependent edema, headache, weakness, irritability), adrenal insufficiency (eg, progressive fatigue, nausea, vomiting, weakness, and postural hypotension), and infections (eg, URI, wound, UTI, and oral).

5. Methods for maximizing coping mechanisms to deal with stress, such as diversional activities and relaxation exercises. Explain the importance of avoiding physical or emotional stress.

6. Need for continued medical follow-up.

7. Obtaining a Medic-Alert bracelet and identification card outlining the diagnosis and emergency treatment.

In addition:

8. Prepare an emergency kit, including alcohol sponges and syringes with 100 mg hydrocortisone to be carried and used in the event of Addisonian crisis. Teach technique for IM administration of the medication to patient and SOs.

II. Cushing's Disease

Cushing's disease is a spectrum of symptoms associated with prolonged elevated plasma concentration of adrenal steroids. Basically, there are two mechanisms by which this can occur. In normal individuals, the pituitary gland secretes adrenocorticotropic hormone (ACTH), which stimulates the adrenal glands to release the adrenal steroid hormones. This is regulated by a negative-feedback mechanism in which increasing levels of plasma cortisol suppress ACTH. In cases of pituitary pathology, this mechanism does not function and the pituitary gland continues to secrete excessive amounts of ACTH, with resultant abnormally high levels of adrenocorticol hormones. This accounts for approximately 70% of reported cases and is termed *Cushing's disease.*

Cushing's syndrome, on the other hand, is caused by pathology of the adrenal glands themselves, from ectopic ACTH-secreting tumors or from iatrogenic causes such as excessive ingestion of cortisol or ACTH.

A. Assessment

Signs and symptoms: Weight gain; muscle weakness; kyphosis and back pain; generalized osteoporosis, especially in the vertebrae; pathologic fractures of the long bones; mental and emotional disturbances; easy bruising; arteriosclerotic changes in the heart, brain, and kidney; renal calculi; thirst and polyuria; menstrual changes; and impotence.

Physical exam: Patients exhibit "central obesity" with pendulous abdomens and thin legs and arms; moon face; fat deposits on the neck and supraclavicular area (buffalo obesity); edema; hypertension; and thin, transparent skin with multiple ecchymoses. Androgen excess is most noticeable in females, as evidenced by changes in menstruation, as well as virilism and hirsutism. Patients frequently have stretch marks with red and purple striae showing through the stretched skin. Patients with Cushing's syndrome have hyperpigmentation of facial skin secondary to ectopic ACTH-secreting tumors.

History of: Excessive exogenous steroid ingestion, pituitary tumor.

B. Diagnostic Tests

1. <u>Blood cortisol:</u> Elevated at least part of the day. Normally, cortisol levels fluctuate throughout the day, with the highest level in the morning and a gradual decline until the lowest level is reached about midnight. Therefore, early-morning samples can be misleading, and several specimens are usually drawn throughout the day.

2. <u>Serum ACTH:</u> Measured in the same way as blood cortisol and will be abnormally high at least part of the day.

3. <u>Overnight dexamethasone suppression test:</u> Will show absence of suppression in patients with Cushing's syndrome. At exactly 11 PM the patient is given 1 mg of dexamethasone, which is enough to suppress adrenal production of cortisol in patients with normal adrenal function. At the same time, 100 mg of pentobarbital is administered to ensure an unstressed night's sleep. In the morning, a fasting cortisol level is drawn. In patients with Cushing's syndrome, it will not be suppressed lower than 10 μg/100 mL. Women using birth control pills should have baseline levels of cortisol drawn before this test so that results can be adjusted to avoid false positives.

4. <u>Other blood tests:</u> Will reveal elevated postprandial blood sugar in 80–90% of patients with Cushing's disease and decreased serum potassium.

5. <u>24-hour urinary free cortisol:</u> Will be elevated. Cushing's syndrome is confirmed if the test is elevated in a patient with no cortisol suppression.

6. <u>High-dose dexamethasone test:</u> Patient is given 8 mg dexamethasone orally over a 24-hour period. A 24-hour urine analysis for 17-hydroxycorticosteroid (17-OHCS) is obtained and the results are interpreted as follows:

   □ High ACTH with no 17-OHCS suppression indicates an ectopic source of ACTH production.

   □ Low ACTH with no 17-OHCS suppression indicates an adrenal tumor.

   □ Normal to high ACTH with suppression of 17-OHCS indicates Cushing's disease.

C. Medical Management and Surgical Interventions

1. **Adrenocortical inhibitors:** Include metapyrone, aminoglutethimide, and cyproheptadine. Exogenous steroids also may be given in conjunction with the adrenocortical inhibitors to prevent hypocortisolism. Adrenocortical inhibi-◀

tors are used only short-term, however, because increased ACTH production quickly overcomes their effect.

2. **Irradiation of the pituitary gland:** To decrease pituitary production of ACTH. It is used for patients with a mild form of the disease or those who are poor surgical risks.

3. **Diet:** Low in calories and carbohydrates to reduce hyperglycemia. Salt is restricted to reduce BP; and foods high in potassium, including bananas, apricots, figs, dried peaches and prunes, oranges, and tomatoes are given to raise serum potassium levels.

4. **Transphenoidal hypophysectomy:** May be performed if the pathology involves the pituitary gland. Patients return from this surgery with nasal packing and nasopharyngeal airways in place. Potential complications of this surgery include transient diabetes indipidus and CSF leakage. See "Pituitary Tumors," p. 245, for more information about this procedure.

5. **Adrenalectomy, either bilateral or unilateral:** May be performed, depending on the extent of involvement. Potential complications of this surgery include splenic injury, retroperitoneal hemorrhage, pancreatitis, infection, and wound dehiscence. Hemorrhage, infection, and wound dehiscence are especially prevalent because of abnormal cortisol levels, which can cause thinning of the skin and poor wound healing.

D. Nursing Diagnoses and Interventions

Disturbances in self-concept related to alteration in body image secondary to physical changes associated with increased ACTH production

Desired outcomes: Patient relates the attainment of self-acceptance and verbalizes knowledge that symptoms will abate with treatment.

1. Encourage patient to verbalize feelings and frustrations.

2. Reassure patient that symptoms should subside with adequate treatment of the disorder.

3. Assist patient with measures to improve appearance, such as keeping hair well groomed, wearing own gown or pajamas if possible, and performing personal hygiene such as bathing and brushing of teeth. Encourage women to apply makeup and perfume, if appropriate.

4. Provide privacy, if indicated.

Potential impairment of skin integrity related to vulnerability secondary to thinning of skin and of fragility of capillaries

Desired outcome: Patient does not exhibit signs of irritation or skin breakdown.

1. Ensure that patient on bed rest turns q2h. Establish and post a turning schedule. Provide gentle massage with lotions to help prevent decubitus ulcers.

2. Place alternating air pressure mattress or other pressure-relief mattress or pad on the bed.

3. Position foot cradle over the bed to prevent pressure areas on lower extremities by keeping bed linen off the feet.

4. To protect the skin of confused patients, pad the siderails of the bed.

See "Hyperparathyroidism" for the following: **Potential for injury** (risk of pathologic fractures), p. 233. See "Addison's Disease" for the following: **Potential for infection**, p. 237. See "Pituitary Tumors" for the following: **Potential for injury** related to risk of increased ICP, CSF leak, and diabetes insipidus secondary to transphenoidal hypophysectomy, p. 246. See "Appendix One" for nursing diagnoses and interventions for the care of preoperative and postoperative patients, pp. 528–532, and care of patients with life-disrupting illnesses, pp. 544–546.

E. Patient–Family Teaching and Discharge Planning

Provide patient and SOs with verbal and written information for the following:

1. Diet, including foods to increase, such as those high in potassium, and foods to restrict, including those that are high in sodium or carbohydrates. Arrange for a dietary consult to help patient with meal planning and integration of individual restrictions into family diet.

2. Medications, including drug name, purpose, dosage, schedule, precautions, and potential side effects. Advise patient with bilateral adrenalectomy of the necessity for lifetime hormone replacement therapy.

3. Importance of continued medical follow-up; confirm date and time of next medical appointment.

4. Relationship between hormone levels and stress. Advise patient to seek medical assistance during periods of emotional or physical stress so that medications can be adjusted accordingly. Provide suggestions for patient to maximize coping mechanisms such as relaxation exercises or diversional activities.

5. Indicators of *excessive adrenal hormone:* weight gain, thirst, polyuria, easy bruising, and muscle weakness; or of *adrenal insufficiency:* easy fatiguability, weight loss, and abdominal pain, any of which necessitate medical attention.

6. Signs and symptoms of UTI, URI, wound, and oral infections and the importance of seeking medical care should they occur.

7. Importance of wearing a Medic-Alert bracelet and carrying an identification card to describe the disease and the necessary emergency measures.

In addition:

8. For patients with bilateral adrenalectomy, provide an emergency kit with alcohol sponges and syringes filled with 100 mg of hydrocortisone for episodes of acute adrenal insufficiency. Teach patient and SOs the technique for IM administration of the medication for emergency treatment.

▶ Section Four **Disorders of the Pituitary Gland**

The pituitary (hypophysis) is composed of two lobes: the anterior pituitary (adenohypophysis) and posterior pituitary (neurohypophysis). The anterior lobe is larger and its secretory activities are controlled by tropic hormones produced by and transmitted from the hypothalamus in response to negative feedback mechanisms. It secretes seven of the nine pituitary hormones. These include (1) adrenocorticotropic hormone (ACTH), which stimulates adrenal cortical growth and secretion of adrenocortical hormones; (2) thyrotropic hormone (TSH), which stimulates thyroid growth and secretion of thyroid hormones; (3) follicle-stimulating hormone (FSH), which stimulates ovulation in females and the production of sperm in males; (4) luteinizing hormone (LH), called the interstitial cell-stimulating hormone (ICSH) in males, in whom it stimulates production of testosterone, and in females stimulates ovulation and development of ovarian follicles; (5) melanocyte-stimulating hormone (MSH), which causes pigmentation; (6) luteotropic hormone (LTH), also called prolactin, which stimulates secretion of milk in females; and (7) growth hormone (GH) or somatotropic hormone (STH), which accelerates body growth.

Posterior pituitary secretion is regulated by nerve impulses originating in the hypothalamus in response to stimuli from other parts of the body. It produces two hormones: antidiuretic hormone (ADH) or vasopressin, which acts on the renal tubules to increase reabsorption of water; and oxytocin, which stimulates milk "letdown" and contraction of the uterus.

I. Diabetes Insipidus

Diabetes insipidus results from a defect in the release or synthesis of ADH from the hypothalamus, or a defect in renal tubular response to ADH causing impaired renal conservation of water. The onset is usually insidious, with progressively increasing polydipsia and polyuria, but it can develop rapidly following an injury or infectious disease. Depending on the degree of injury, the condition can be either temporary or permanent.

There are three phases associated with diabetes insipidus. The first phase of polydipsia and polyuria immediately follows the injury and lasts 4–5 days. In the second phase, which lasts about 6 days, the symptoms disappear; and in the third phase, the patient experiences permanent polydipsia and polyuria. The chief danger to these patients is dehydration from the inability to take in adequate fluids to balance the excessive output of urine.

A. Assessment

Signs and symptoms: Polydipsia, polyuria with dilute urine.

Physical exam: Usually within normal limits; however, patient may show signs of dehydration if fluid intake is inadequate.

History of: Cranial injury, especially basilar skull fracture; meningitis; primary or metastatic brain tumor; surgery in the pituitary area; cerebral hemorrhage; encephalitis; syphilis; or tuberculosis. Familial incidence is rarely a factor.

B. Diagnostic Tests

1. Urine osmolality: Decreased (50–200 mOsm/kg) in the presence of disease.
2. Specific gravity: Decreased (1.000–1.005) in the presence of disease.
3. Serum osmolality: Increased in the presence of disease.
4. Water deprivation test: Baseline measurements of body weight, serum and urine osmolalities, and urine specific gravity are obtained. Fluids are not permitted and the above measurements are repeated hourly. The test is terminated when urine specific gravity exceeds 1.020 and osmolality exceeds 800 mOsm/kg, a normal response; or when 5% of body weight is lost. The latter is, in itself, an abnormal resonse and the corresponding urine osmolality will be less than 400 mOsm/kg, which is diagnostic of diabetes insipidus. Because the most serious side effect of this test is severe dehydration, the test should be performed early in the day so the patient can be more closely monitored. Before a firm diagnosis of diabetes insipidus can be made from an abnormal water deprivation test, it is also necessary to demonstrate that the kidneys can respond to vasopressin (see next paragraph).
5. Vasopressin (exogenous antidiuretic hormone): Given SC, followed by urine collections q15min for 2 hours. Quantity and specific gravity are then measured. The normal individual will show a concentration of urine, but not as pronounced as that for the person with diabetes insipidus; while a person with kidney disease will have a lesser response to vasopressin. **Note:** One serious side effect of this test is the precipitation of CHF in susceptible individuals.

C. Medical Management

1. **Administer exogenous vasopressin (Pitressin):** Replacement therapy for ADH. There are several preparations available, and it is important to read

the package insert carefully to ensure proper administration. Potential side effects include hypertension secondary to vasoconstriction, myocardial infarction secondary to constriction of coronary vessels, uterine cramps, and increased peristalsis of the GI tract.

2. Achieve a mild antidiuretic effect: For example, with chlorpropamide.

D. Nursing Diagnoses and Interventions

Fluid volume deficit related to abnormal loss secondary to polyuria

Desired outcome: Patient can verbalize knowledge of the importance of fluid intake and does not exhibit signs of dehydration.

1. Provide unrestricted fluids. Keep water pitcher full and within easy reach of patient. Explain the importance of consuming as much fluid as can be tolerated.

2. Administer vasopressin and antidiuretic agents as prescribed.

3. For unconscious patient, administer IV fluids as prescribed. Unless otherwise directed, for every mL of urine output deliver 1 mL of IV fluid.

4. Monitor I&O, daily weights, and VS closely. Be alert to evidence of hypovolemia, including weight loss, inadequate fluid intake to balance output, thirst, poor skin turgor, furrowed tongue, hypotension, and tachycardia. If prescribed, monitor CVP for evidence of hypotension.

Potential for injury related to negative side effects of vasopressin

Desired outcome: Negative side effects of vasopressin, if they occur, are detected and treated promptly, resulting in absence of injury to the patient.

1. Monitor VS, especially BP, and report significant changes such as systolic BP elevated >20 mm Hg or pulse increased >20 over baseline.

2. For the elderly or patients with vascular disease, keep prescribed coronary vasodilators such as amyl nitrate or nitroglycerine at the bedside for use should angina occur. Teach patient and SOs how to administer these medications.

3. Be alert to indicators of water intoxication, including changes in LOC, confusion, weight gain, headache, convulsions, and coma. If these develop, stop the medication, restrict fluids, and notify MD. Institute safety precautions accordingly.

E. Patient—Family Teaching and Discharge Planning

Provide patient and SOs with verbal and written information for the following:

1. Importance of continued medical follow-up; confirm date and time of next appointment.

2. Indicators that necessitate medical attention, for example, signs of dehydration or water intoxification

II. Pituitary Tumors

Pituitary adenomas account for approximately 10% of intracranial tumors and constitute the most frequent cause of pituitary dysfunction. These tumors are almost always benign and easily treated if discovered early. Ninty percent of pituitary tumors produce no hormones, but if they are allowed to grow, they will compress the rest of the gland, ultimately leading to pituitary destruction with resultant hypopituitarism. This will decrease the levels of all the hormones produced by the pituitary gland. Usually, gonadotropic hormones are suppressed first; and eventually, signs of hypothyroidism and adrenocortical insufficiency will appear, as discussed earlier in this chapter. Of the remaining 10% of pituitary tumors that do produce hormones, 60% secrete excessive prolactin and 20% secrete excess growth hormone (GH). Another 10% secrete excess ACTH (see "Cushing's Disease," p. 239).

A. Assessment

Hypopituitarism: Weakness, easy fatigue, myxedema coma (see "Hypothyroidism," p. 225), or Addisonian crisis (see "Addison's Disease," p. 236). Patients also may have atrophy of external genitalia; amenorrhea and vaginal mucosal atrophy; impotence and/or loss of libido; minimal perspiration; and lessening of resistance to colds, stress, and infections. Patients often present with extreme pallor; sallow complexion; visual deficits; thinning of eyebrows and hair; dry skin with thin-lined wrinkling of the face; sparse pubic, axillary, and facial hair; hypotension; and/or orthostatic hypotension.

Excessive growth hormone (acromegaly): Hoarseness, headache, diplopia, hemianopsia (blindness in half the field of vision, either unilateral or bilateral), papilledema, lethargy, amenorrhea, loss of libido, impotence, and weight gain. Patients often present with coarse facial features and enlargement of hands and feet, wide-spaced teeth, thickening of skin and nails, skeletal enlargement (can be 7–8 feet tall) with protusion of the lower jaw, joint deformities, arthritis, and multiple fleshy tumors on the skin, especially the scalp.

Excessive prolactin: Weight gain, fluid retention, irritability, and hirsutism and decrease in vaginal lubrication in females. Males often present with impotence or decreased libido; females often have galactorrhea and amenorrhea.

Excessive ACTH: See "Cushing's Disease," p. 240.

B. Diagostic Tests

General:

1. <u>X-ray of skull:</u> Will show enlarged pituitary gland, thickened skull, and distorted, enlarged pituitary fossa.

2. <u>Skeletal x-rays:</u> Will show thickening of long bones.

3. <u>Pneumoencephalogram:</u> Will reveal extension of pituitary tumor above the sella turcica.

4. <u>Serum tests (in hyperpituitarism):</u> Elevated phosphate and postprandial blood glucose will be present.

5. <u>Urinary calcium (in hyperpituitarism):</u> Increased secondary to increased production of calcitonin from the thyroid.

6. <u>Growth hormone and basal prolactin:</u> Increased.

For hypopituitarism:

1. <u>Urinary 17-ketosteroids, 17-hydroxycorticosteroids, and plasma cortisol:</u> Decreased, but will rise slowly after administration of ACTH. See "Addison's Disease," p. 237.

2. <u>Urinary and serum gonadotropins:</u> Decreased.

3. <u>Plasma testosterone and estradiol:</u> Decreased.

4. <u>Serum levels of ACTH, thyroid-stimulating hormone (TSH), luteinizing hormone (LH), follicle-stimulating hormone (FSH), and growth hormone (GH):</u> Decreased.

C. Medical Management and Surgical Interventions

1. **Exogenous hormone replacements:** As appropriate for syndromes of insufficiency secondary to hypopituitarism.

2. **X-ray and heavy-particle radiation therapy:** For hormone-secreting tumors. Typically, the response with a return to normal is slow, but tumor progression is halted in most patients. Side effects can include malaise, nausea, serous otitis media, and hypopituitarism.

3. **Transphenoidal hypophysectomy:** Treatment of choice because it offers a more rapid cure with a low morbidity rate. The surgeon makes an incision in

the inner aspect of the upper lip and enters the sella turcica through the sphenoid process. Because an opening is created between the nose and upper airway, the patient is at increased risk for postoperative infection, so nasal antibiotics are frequently used preoperatively. In addition, the patient will have two black eyes after surgery. The pituitary is a highly vascularized gland; and therefore, hemorrhage at the operative site is another potential risk. Diabetes insipidus can result from pituitary destruction and removal. For larger tumors, a frontal craniotomy may be necessary. (See "Brain Tumors" in Chapter Four, "Neurologic Disorders," p. 183.)

D. Nursing Diagnoses and Interventions

Potential for injury related to risk of increased intracranial pressure (ICP), cerebrospinal fluid (CSF) leak, hemorrhage, infection, and/or diabetes insipidus secondary to transphenoidal hypophysectomy

Desired outcomes: Patient does not exhibit signs of injury from complications of surgery. If signs and symptoms of complications occur, they are detected and reported promptly, resulting in immediate treatment and absence of injury to patient. Patient can verbalize knowledge of actions that can result in increased ICP or disruption in the integrity of the operative site.

1. Elevate the HOB 30° to decrease ICP and swelling.

2. Be alert to indicators of increasing ICP such as a change in LOC, sluggish or unequal pupils, and changes in respiratory rate or pattern. Report significant findings to MD.

3. Inspect nasal packing at frequent intervals for the presence of frank bleeding and/or CSF leakage. After nasal packing is removed, test *non*sanguineous drainage for CSF fluid with a glucose reagent strip. If the drainage contains CSF, the test will be positive for the presence of glucose. **Note:** Because the presence of CSF represents a serious breach in the integrity of the cranium, elevate the HOB to minimize the potential for bacteria entering the brain and immediately report any suspicious drainage.

4. Explain to patient that coughing, sneezing, and other Valsalva-type maneuvers must be avoided because these actions can stress the operative site and increase ICP, causing CSF leakage. If coughing or sneezing is unavoidable, tell patient to do so with an opened mouth. If indicated, obtain a prescription for a mild cathartic or stool softener to prevent straining with bowel movements.

5. To prevent disturbance in the integrity of the operative site, do not allow patient to brush teeth. Provide mouthwash and/or glycerine swabs for oral hygiene.

6. Measure accurate I&O qh for 24 hours and monitor urine specific gravity. Output >200 mL/h for 2 consecutive hours or a total of 500 mL/h should be reported. Specific gravity <1.007 is found with diabetes insipidus. Monitor weight daily for evidence of loss. Report significant findings to MD.

Sexual dysfunction related to physiologic limitations secondary to abnormal hormone levels

Desired outcome: Patient relates the attainment of satisfying sexual activity.

1. Encourage patient to express feelings of anger and frustration and to communicate feelings to SO.

2. If appropriate, suggest alternatives other than sexual intercourse for pleasuring partner and self.

3. Administer testosterone or estrogens as prescribed.

4. Support MD's referral or suggest referral for psychotherapy related to loss of libido, sterility, impotence, and/or loss of self-esteem.

See "Appendix One" for nursing diagnoses and interventions for the care of preoperative and postoperative patients, pp. 528–532.

E. Patient–Family Teaching and Discharge Planning

Provide patient and SOs with verbal and written information for the following:

1. Medications, including drug name, purpose, dosage, schedule, precautions, and potential side effects. Reinforce that following hypophysectomy, patient will be on lifetime hormone replacement therapy.

2. Relationship between hormone levels and stress. Advise patient to seek medical help during times of emotional or physical stress so that dosages of medications can be adjusted accordingly.

3. Measures for maximizing coping mechanisms to deal with stress, such as relaxation tapes, meditation, diversional activities.

4. Importance of continued medical follow-up; confirm time and date of next appointment.

5. Indicators of *adrenal hormone excess:* weight gain, easy bruising, muscle weakness, moon face, thirst, and polyuria; of *adrenal hormone insufficiency:* weight loss, easy fatigue, and adominal pain; of *hypothyroidism:* weight gain, anorexia, apathy, slowed mentation, and cold intolerance; and of *hyperthyroidism:* tachycardia, diaphoresis, and heat intolerance. All of these signs and symptoms necessitate medical attention.

6. Importance of obtaining a Medic-Alert bracelet and identification card outlining diagnosis and emergency treatment.

For patients who have had a transphenoidal hypophysectomy:

7. Importance of avoiding bending or straining until after postoperative follow-up and clearance by MD.

8. Not brushing front teeth until the incision is healed (about 10 days). Recommend use of mouthwash and gentle use of glycerine swabs instead.

9. Signs and symptoms of infection that necessitate medical attention, eg, fever, nuchal rigidity, headache, photophobia.

▶ Section Five   **Disorders of the Pancreas**

The pancreas serves both exocrine (nonhormonal) and endocrine functions. The exocrine portion comprises 98% of tissue mass. Its function is the secretion of potent enzymes that act to reduce proteins, fats, and carbohydrates into simpler chemical substances. Pancreatic lipase acts on fats to produce glycerides, fatty acids, and glycerol; pancreatic amylase acts on starch to produce disaccharides. The pancreas also secretes sodium bicarbonate to neutralize the strongly acidic gastric contents as they enter the duodenum. The resultant mixture of acids and bases provides an optimal pH for the activation of pancreatic enzymes.

I. Pancreatitis

Pancreatitis can involve edema, hemorrhage, or necrosis of the pancreas and its blood supply. It is characterized by varying degrees of pancreatic insufficiency, which results in decreased production of enzymes and bicarbonate and malabsorption of fats and proteins. The digestion of fat is affected most severely. As a result, a high fat content in the bowel stimulates water and electrolyte secretion, which produces diarrhea. The action of bacteria on fecal fat produces flatus, steatorrhea, and abdominal cramps. Autodigestion, the activation of pancreatic enzymes within the pancreas, is the pathologic process in pancreatitis. It destroys pancreatic tissues, causes vascular permeability, and results in edema and pain. Although the cause of this process is unknown, the backflow of pancreatic secretions into the biliary and pancreatic ducts is a response to high pressure within the ducts, such as that caused by a gallstone or cancer of the pancreatic head. Diabetes mellitus often occurs as a result of chronic pancreatitis because of damage to the beta cells, which results in alterations in insulin production.

A. Assessment

Acute pancreatitis: Sudden onset of severe epigastric pain following a large meal or alcohol intake. The pain radiates to the back and is unrelieved by vomiting. The patient also may have persistent vomiting, extreme malaise, restlessness, cold and sweaty extremities, dehydration, left pleural effusion, adult respiratory distress syndrome (ARDS), and jaundice.

Physical exam: Diminished or absent bowel sounds, suggesting presence of ileus; crackles (rales) at the lung bases related to persistent hypoventilation associated with splinting and guarding with pain. In addition, edema in and around the pancreas impinges on the diaphragm and prevents full expansion of the lungs with inspiration. Patients also may have low-grade fever (100–102F) and an abdominal mass.

Chronic pancreatitis: Constant, dull epigastric pain; steatorrhea (foamy, foul-smelling stools) resulting from malabsorption of fats and protein; severe weight loss; and onset of symptoms of diabetes mellitus: polydipsia, polyuria, polyphagia. In addition, chemical addiction is often seen because of the chronic pain.

History of: Biliary tract disease, chronic excessive alcohol consumption, duodenal ulcer, coxsackie virus, mumps, hypothermia, and use of estrogen-containing oral contraceptives, glucocorticoids, sulfonamides, chlorothiazides, and azothioprine.

B. Diagnostic Tests

1. Serum amylase: When significantly elevated (>500 U/100 mL), rules out acute abdomen conditions such as cholecystitis, appendicitis, bowel infarction/obstruction, and perforated peptic ulcer and confirms presence of pancreatitis. These levels return to normal 48–72 hours after the onset of acute symptoms, even though clinical indicators may continue.

2. Serum lipase: Levels rise more slowly than serum amylase, and therefore this test is useful only in late diagnosis of pancreatitis. Both lipase and amylase levels reflect the degree of necrotic pancreatic tissue.

3. Serum calcium and magnesium: Levels may be lower than normal. On EKG, hypocalcemia is evidenced by prolonged QT segment with a normal T wave.

4. CBC: Elevated WBCs and polymorphonuclear (PMN) bodies if bacterial peritonitis is present secondary to duodenal rupture.

5. Urinalysis: May show presence of glycosuria, which may signal the onset of diabetes mellitus. Elevated urine amylase levels are useful diagnostically when serum levels have dropped off. An elevated specific gravity reflects the presence of dehydration.

6. Hyperglycemia: Occurs because of interference with beta-cell function. It is transient with acute pancreatitis but common with chronic pancreatitis, during which diabetes mellitus is likely to develop.

7. Abdominal x-rays: May show dilation of the small or large bowel and presence of pancreatic calcification in chronic pancreatitis.

8. GI x-rays: May reveal an edematous pancreatic head that exerts pressure on the duodenum or stomach.

9. Percutaneous transhepatic cholangiogram (PTHC): To rule out obstructive versus non-obstructive jaundice.

10. Endoscopic retrocholangiopancreatography (ERCP): A combined endoscopic-radiographic tool that is used to study the degree of pancreatic disease via assessment of biliary-pancreatic ductal systems. It allows direct visualization of the ampulla of Vater, diagnoses biliary stones and duct stenosis, and distinguishes cancer of the pancreas from pancreatic calculi. This test is also used for patients with bleeding tendencies for whom PTHC is contraindicated; it is not performed until the acute episode has subsided.

C. Medical Management and Surgical Interventions

Medical goals are to reduce stimuli for pancreatic secretion and rehydrate with fluids.

For acute pancreatitis:

1. **Fluid and electrolyte replacement:** To maintain adequate circulating blood volume. For example, protein solutions that do not stimulate the pancreas, such as glucose or free amino acids, and blood volume expanders such as plasma and albumin.

2. **Bed rest:** To reduce metabolic demands on the body and thereby minimize need for pancreatic activity.

3. **Pharmacotherapy**

   □ *Meperidine:* For pain. **Note:** Both morphine and meperidine may cause spasms at the sphincter of Odi. Atropine is often given to prevent this from occurring.

   □ *Broad spectrum antibiotics:* For infection, if present.

   □ *Steroids:* To reduce inflammation.

   □ *Anticholinergics:* To impede impulses that stimulate pancreatic secretions.

4. **NPO status and NG suction:** To decrease stimulus for pancreatic secretions and alleviate pressure in the GI tract.

5. **Rule out underlying factors such as hyperparathyroidism and hyperlipoproteinemia:** Can contribute to the development of pancreatitis.

6. **Surgery:** May be performed for biliary pancreatitis or acute necrotizing hemorrhagic pancreatitis. (See "Surgical Interventions" in this section.)

For chronic pancreatitis:

1. **For exacerbations:** See treatment for acute pancreatitis.

2. **Alcohol rehabilitation:** If alcoholism is the cause of pancreatitis.

3. **Long-term pain management:** With analgesics or the lowest effective dose of meperidine.

4. **Oral enzyme supplements such as pancreatin and pancrelipase:** To treat malabsorption.

5. **Diet:** High in carbohydrates and protein and low in fat.

6. **Insulin therapy:** May be required to ensure adequate carbohydrate metabolism if endocrine function is impaired. Lab values of fasting blood sugar and bedside monitoring of blood glucose will reveal abnormalities in blood glucose levels and direct the appropriate insulin therapy. (See "Diabetes Mellitus," p. 257, for more information.)

7. **Surgical interventions:** Often indicated when pancreatitis is due to an obstructive process such as gallstone formation or cancer. When gallstones are the cause of the pancreatitis, surgical removal of the stone(s) and usually the gallbladder is performed (see "Cholelithiasis/Cholecystitis" in Chapter 6, "Gastrointestinal Disorders," p. 335). The surgery is performed when the acute symptoms of pancreatitis have abated or if there is no improvement after 48 hours. A common bile duct exploration may be done at the time of surgery to uncover and retrieve all stones. See "Pancreatic Tumors," p. 252,

for a discussion of total pancreatectomy or other surgical procedures performed if cancer of the pancreatic head is present.

D. Nursing Diagnoses and Interventions

Fluid volume deficit related to abnormal loss secondary to NG suctioning, vomiting, diaphoresis, or pooling of fluids in the abdomen and retroperitoneum

Desired outcome: Patient does not exhibit signs of dehydration.

1. Monitor VS at q2–4h and be alert to falling BP and increasing tachycardia, which can occur with moderate to severe fluid loss.
2. Measure I&O and, if appropriate, CVP. Because fluid loss requires immediate replacement to prevent shock and circulatory collapse, be alert to and report I&O imbalances. CVP <2mL H_2O can occur with volume-related hypotension.
3. Administer plasma volume expanders as prescribed. For high volumes, use volume control pump to prevent sudden fluid shifts caused by excessive osmotic pressure, which can result in fluid overload.
4. Administer electrolytes (potassium, calcium) as prescribed to prevent cardiac dysrhythmias and tetany.
5. Be alert to indicators of hypocalcemia such as muscle twitching, tetany, or irritability, which can occur with electrolyte loss.
6. Monitor lab values such as hematocrit, hemoglobin, calcium, glucose, BUN, and potassium.

Alteration in comfort: Pain related to inflammatory process of the pancreas

Desired outcome: Patient relates a reduction in discomfort and does not exhibit signs of uncontrolled pain.

1. To minimize pancreatic secretions and pain and to maximize needed rest, ensure that patient maintains bed rest.
2. Maintain NPO status to minimize stimulation of pancreatic secretions.
3. Administer analgesics, steroids, and anticholinergics as prescribed; be alert to patient's response to medications. If analgesia is ineffective, notify MD because patient may require surgical intervention.
4. Assist patient with attaining position of comfort. A supine position with knees flexed often helps to relax abdominal muscles.
5. Emphasize nonpharmacologic pain interventions (eg, relaxation techniques, distraction, guided imagery, massage). This is especially important for patients who develop chronic pancreatitis and are prone to chemical dependence.

Alteration in nutrition: Less than body requirements related to decreased intake secondary to anorexia and dietary restrictions; and increased need secondary to digestive dysfunction

Desired outcomes: Patient can verbalize knowledge of the prescribed dietary regimen. Patient does not exhibit signs of malnutrition or weight loss.

1. When NG tube is removed, provide diet as prescribed, for example, small high-carbohydrate meals at frequent intervals (eg, 6/day) and adding protein to patient's tolerance. Keep diet bland to minimize pancreatic stimulation and instruct patient to avoid stimulants that increase enzyme secretion, such as coffee, tea, alcohol, and nicotine.
2. Provide oral hygiene at frequent intervals to enhance appetite and minimize nausea.
3. Monitor blood sugar levels for presence of hyperglycemia and be alert to dysphagia, polydipsia, and polyuria, which occur with diabetes mellitus. These indicators reflect the need for medical evaluation and intervention to ensure proper metabolism of carbohydrates.

4. Weigh patient daily to assess gain or loss. Weight loss may signal the need to change the diet and/or provide enzyme replacement therapy.

5. Note amount and degree of steatorrhea as an indicator of fat intolerance. As prescribed, adminster pancreatic enzyme supplements, which are given before introducing fat into the diet.

6. If prescribed, administer other dietary supplements that support nutrition and caloric intake. These may include products that consist of medium-chain triglycerides (MCTs) such as Isocal or MCT oil. Their advantage is that they do not require pancreatic enzymes for absorption.

7. Avoid administering pancreatin with hot foods or drinks, which will deactivate enzyme activity.

8. To help alleviate the bloating, nausea, and cramps experienced by some patients, provide meals in small feedings throughout the day.

See "Appendix One" for nursing diagnoses and interventions for the care of preoperative and postoperative patients, pp. 528–532.

E. Patient–Family Teaching and Discharge Planning

Provide patient and SOs with verbal and written information for the following:

1. Cause for current episode of pancreatitis, if known, so that recurrence may be avoided.

2. Alcohol consumption, which can cause and/or exacerbate chronic pancreatitis.

3. Availability of chemical dependency programs to prevent/treat drug dependence, which is a common occurrence with chronic pancreatitis; or to treat alcoholism.

4. Diet: frequent small meals that are high in carbohydrates and protein. Food should be bland until gradual return to normal diet is prescribed. Remind patient to avoid enzyme stimulants such as coffee, tea, nicotine, and alcohol.

5. Medications, including drug name, purpose, dosage, schedule, precautions, and potential side effects.

6. Signs and symptoms of diabetes mellitus, including fatigue, weight loss, polydipsia, polyuria, and polyphagia.

7. Necessity of medical follow-up; confirm time and date of next medical appointment.

8. Potential for recurrence of steatorrhea as evidenced by foamy, foul-smelling stools that are high in fat content. Steatorrhea can indicate recurrence of disease process or ineffectiveness of drug therapy and should be reported to MD.

9. Weighing daily at home; importance of reporting weight loss to MD.

10. If surgery was performed, the indicators of wound infection: redness, swelling, discharge, fever, pain, or local warmth.

II. Pancreatic Tumors

Pancreatic tumors, either benign (adenoma) or malignant (carcinoma), can develop anywhere within the pancreas. A tumor that develops at the islet cells is called an insulinoma and is characterized by hypersecretion of insulin. Usually it is treated surgically with a subtotal pancreatectomy. The most frequent site for pancreatic tumors is the pancreatic head, particularly in the region around the ampulla of Vater. These are malignant tumors (adenocarcinomas), for which detection is difficult and the prognosis poor. Because of vague, ill-defined symptoms that appear early in the disease process with pancreatic cancer, metastasis often occurs before a diagnosis can be made.

A. Assessment

Signs and symptoms: Progressive, unexplained, rapid weight loss; upper or mid-abdominal pain that radiates to the back, can be aggravated by eating, and is not related to posture or activity. The patient also may have clay-colored stools, dark urine, pruritus, anorexia, nausea, vomiting, steatorrhea caused by fat and protein malabsorption, bleeding tendency from vitamin K deficiency, malnutrition, and electrolyte disturbances. In addition, diabetes mellitus symptoms often appear as early indicators of the disorder. (See "Diabetes Mellitus," p. 255.)

Physical exam: Jaundice caused by obstruction of the flow of bile from the liver. The patient also may have generalized weakness and poor skin turgor.

B. Diagnostic Tests

1. <u>Serum alkaline phosphatase:</u> Elevated with obstructive bile duct disease.

2. <u>Serum bilirubin:</u> Elevated if the pancreatic tumor obstructs the flow of bile from the liver. Levels >3 mg/100 mL will result in jaundice; levels >25 mg/100 mL are common with this condition.

3. <u>Prothrombin time (PT):</u> Prolonged because of vitamin K deficiency. Vitamin K is required for synthesis of prothrombin in the liver, and it is absorbed poorly in the presence of pancreatic insufficiency because it is a fat-soluble vitamin.

4. <u>GI x-rays:</u> May show displacement of visceral organs by the enlarged pancreatic tumor.

5. <u>Percutaneous transhepatic cholangiogram (PTHC):</u> To determine the level of biliary obstruction and confirm the presence of cholelithiasis.

6. <u>Endoscopic retrocholangiopancreatography (ERCP):</u> Permits direct visualization of the ampulla of Vater via injection of a radiopaque dye into the pancreatic and biliary ducts. In patients with marked bleeding tendencies, neither ERCP nor PTHC is performed.

7. <u>Five-hour glucose tolerance test:</u> Helps confirm diagnosis of insulinoma.

8. <u>CT scan of pancreas:</u> To delineate pancreatic mass.

9. <u>Cytologic examination of duodenal contents:</u> Reveals malignant cells, if present.

10. <u>Ultrasound:</u> To rule out presence of cystic lesions and metastases.

11. <u>Fine-needle aspiration biopsy:</u> To confirm diagnosis.

C. Surgical Interventions

Pancreatic cancer frequently results from metastasis, and even when the pancreas is the primary site, diagnosis and interventions are thwarted by the vague symptomatology and insidious onset of this disease. The medical and surgical approaches will vary depending on the status of the tumor found with the initial exploratory surgery (exploratory laparotomy).

1. **Whipple procedure (pancreatoduodenectomy):** A surgical attempt to cure cancer of the pancreatic head when the tumor is judged to be resectable, for example, if it has not metastasized and is not interfering with major blood vessels. This extensive surgery involves resection of the head of the pancreas and duodenum and three anastomoses of the following: common bile duct to the jejunum (choledochojejunostomy); the remainder of the pancreas to the jejunum (pancreaticojejunostomy); and the stomach to the jejunum (gastrojejunostomy).

2. **Vagotomy (dividing the vagus nerve branches to the stomach):** May be done in addition to the Whipple procedure to minimize gastric secretions.

3. **Total pancreatectomy:** May be performed for patients with chronic pancreatitis or cancer of the pancreatic head. The location of the surgical incision

will vary with the extent of the surgery; however, whether it is vertical or oblique, the incision usually extends high into the abdomen. The patient will have one or two drains, depending on the extensiveness of the surgery. A Penrose drain may exit from the abdomen; a T-tube, sump tube, or portable wound drainage system also may be present. For patients who have undergone a total pancreatectomy, the resultant pancreatic endocrine and exocrine deficiency requires treatment with insulin, pancreatic enzymes, and a diabetic diet that is low in fat.

4. **Palliative measures:** Initiated when the tumor is not resectable (90% of the cases). Although the tumor is left intact, the gallbladder may be anastomosed to the duodenum to permit bile from the liver to bypass the tumor and flow directly into the duodenum. Another approach is the percutaneous biliary drain, which is used for inoperable liver, pancreatic, or bile duct carcinoma. This tube or catheter, which is perforated with holes at the distal end, is inserted percutaneously through the liver, past the obstructed common bile and pancreatic ducts, and into the duodenum. The catheter collects fluid from the surrounding tissues and permits their passage into the duodenum for excretion. It is a palliative measure to prolong life and minimize discomfort. The catheter must be changed q6–8 weeks and flushed qod with small amounts of saline to maintain patency.

5. **Postoperative chemotherapy:** Sometimes used for further palliation after patient has recovered from surgery.

▶ **Note:** Postoperative prognosis is extremely poor: Patients usually survive <1 year, and the 5-year survival rate is 2%.

D. Nursing Diagnoses and Interventions

Potential fluid volume deficit related to loss secondary to postsurgical hemorrhage and/or fluid shift to interstitial compartments

Desired outcome: Patient does not exhibit signs of hemorrhage or dehydration.

1. Monitor BP, pulse, and respirations, and check capillary refill in nail beds at frequent intervals. Tachycardia, hypotension, increased respirations, and slow capillary refill can signal the presence of dehydration and hypovolemia, which can lead to shock. Also be alert to cool, clammy skin, which can occur with hemorrhage, and a low urinary output (<30–40 mL/h for 2 consecutive hours). Report significant findings to MD.

2. Prevent increased pressure on suture lines by keeping all tubes patent and free of kinks. *Gently* irrigate NG tube with air or saline q4h or as needed. Keep gravity drains dependent to the wound site and secure all connections with tape.

3. Note and document the amount and character of drainage from the tubes. Persistent, bloody drainage in steady or increasing amounts is indicative of active bleeding. Report significant findings to MD.

4. Monitor blood study results, including PT for clotting factor and CVP and hemoglobin, which can fall with blood loss.

5. Monitor serum protein levels and be alert to weight gain, which may signal interstitial spacing of fluids. Monitor I&O and note occurrence of intake exceeding output. Preoperatively, most of these patients are protein deficient. Low serum protein alters serum colloid osmotic pressure, resulting in fluid shift from intravascular to interstitial compartments. **Note:** Intravascular fluid loss can occur despite adequate fluid replacement.

6. Monitor lab study results for evidence of electrolyte imbalances, especially potassium and sodium.

Potential impairment of skin integrity related to irritation secondary to wound drainage and/or pressure on incision

Desired outcome: Patient does not exhibit signs of skin irritation or impaired wound healing.

1. Promote adequate drainage from drainage tubes to prevent pressure from fluid collection around wound site.

2. Assess and document condition of incision and quality/quantity of wound drainage. Fistula formation is a major complication of the Whipple procedure, so it is important to monitor peri-incisional skin carefully for signs of irritation. If irritation occurs or a fistula does form, cover site with a pectin wafer skin barrier (and stoma pouch for fistula).

3. Keep patient in semi-Fowler's position to minimize pressure on incision. Use alternating pressure mattress to minimize potential for skin breakdown.

4. When regular diet is resumed after surgery, provide small, frequent meals that are high in protein, vitamins, and calories, and low in fat. Administer pancreatic enzyme replacements and insulin, as prescribed, for patient who has had a total pancreatectomy. These interventions will help ensure optimal tissue repair, as well.

Alteration in comfort: Pain related to major abdominal surgery

Desired outcome: Patient relates a reduction in discomfort and does not exhibit signs of uncontrolled pain.

1. Because physical dependence on narcotics is of minimal importance in patients who are terminally ill, administer analgesics liberally, but use caution to prevent respiratory depression.

2. Because peritonitis and pancreatitis are potential postoperative complications, note and report patient's failure to respond to analgesics.

3. Because intra-abdominal pressure may be a source of the patient's discomfort, ensure proper drainage from tubes.

4. Minimize anxiety, which can compound the intensity of pain, by explaining all procedures, keeping call light within patient's reach, and including SOs in patient care.

5. Augment pharmacologic analgesia with nonpharmacologic interventions: rhythmic breathing, relaxation, massage, distraction, guided imagery.

Ineffective breathing patterns related to hypoventilation secondary to respiratory depression with use of narcotics and/or guarding secondary to painful abdominal incision

Desired outcome: Patient's respiratory rate and depth are within acceptable limits.

1. Assess rate and character of respirations q2–4h. Be alert to shallow, rapid, or depressed respirations, which can prevent adequate gas exchange.

2. Teach patient to deep-breathe, cough, and use incentive spirometer qh while awake. Use pillows to splint wound and assist patient into semi- to high Fowler's position for optimal lung expansion. Assist patient with turning and positioning q2h.

3. Administer analgesics at frequent intervals for patient comfort and to ensure optimal coughing and moving. Because narcotics depress the respiratory center, administer the lowest effective doses.

4. Because backed-up fluid in the abdomen creates pressure on the diaphragm, ensure patency of drains.

5. If patient exhibits or reports presence of dyspnea, consult with MD about obtaining ABG levels.

6. Encourage oral fluids (at least 2–3 L/day), when appropriate, to liquify pulmonary secretions and facilitate their expulsion.

See "Hepatitis" in "Gastrointestinal Disorders," for the following: **Impairment of skin integrity** related to pruritus, p. 328, **Potential for injury** related to bleeding tendency secondary to decreased vitamin K absorption, p. 328, and **Disturbance in self-concept** related to alteration in body image secondary to jaundice, p. 328. See "Appendix One" for nursing diagnoses and interventions for the care of preoperative and postoperative patients, pp. 528–532, and the care of patients with cancer and other life-disrupting illnesses, pp. 544–551.

E. Patient–Family Teaching and Discharge Planning

Provide patient and SOs with verbal and written information for the following:

1. For patients who are diabetic, a review of insulin action, dosage, and administration; diabetic diet; and signs and symptoms of hyperglycemia and hypoglycemia.

2. Wound care, such as cleansing, dressing changes, and care of drains if patient is discharged with them; indicators of wound infection, such as drainage, warmth along incision line, persistent incisional redness, swelling, fever, and pain.

3. Medications, including drug name, purpose, dosage, schedule, precautions, and potential side effects.

4. Arrangements for community services in home care such as Visiting Nurse Association, or placement in hospice facility.

▶ Section Six **Diabetes Mellitus**

I. General Discussion

Normal physiology maintains a range of blood glucose (60–120 mg/dL) to provide a source of energy for cellular metabolism. An increase in blood glucose from any source (food intake, glycogen breakdown, gluconeogenesis) triggers the insulin response. The healthy individual produces an appropriate amount of insulin that parallels the level of glucose and permits glucose utilization, with an eventual return of blood glucose values to normal levels. Diabetes mellitus (DM) is a chronic, progressive, metabolic disorder characterized by various degrees of glucose intolerance stemming from the complete (type I) or relative (type II) lack of insulin. DM may be precipitated by any of the following factors: genetics, autoimmune defect, obesity, stress, pregnancy, or medications.

Type I diabetes: Also known as insulin-dependent diabetes mellitus (IDDM) or juvenile DM, it most commonly develops in childhood or adolescence. Onset is sudden, with possible ketoacidosis when untreated. Type I diabetes accounts for 10% of cases of diabetes. These diabetics lack endogenous insulin because of the absence of beta-cell function and require exogenous insulin to meet the demands of glucose metabolism and normal physiologic function. Type I diabetics are totally dependent on insulin for survival.

Type II diabetes: Also known as non-insulin-dependent diabetes mellitus (NIDDM) or adult-onset diabetes, it most commonly begins after age 40. Normal or above-normal quantities of insulin are present in the body fluids. It is ketosis-resistant because the presence of insulin prevents lipolysis. These diabetics may require insulin during times of stress, including surgery and infection, or when diet and oral hypoglycemic medications fail to control hyperglycemia. Ninty percent of type II diabetics are obese at the time of diagnosis. Their glucose intolerance relates to the failure of their bodies to use the normal, and sometimes above-normal, levels of insulin properly. Type II diabetics may become insulin-dependent when diet or diet plus oral hypoglycemic medications fail to maintain normoglycemia.

DM affects all body systems. Patient involvement in self-management is crucial for maintaining normoglycemia and delaying long-term complications.

A. Assessment

Early indicators

□ *Type I:* Fatigue, weakness, nocturnal enuresis, weight loss, and the cardinal symptoms of hyperglycemia: polyuria, polydipsia, and polyphagia.

□ *Type II:* Peripheral neuropathy, fatigue, polyuria, polydipsia.

Late indicators

□ *Type I:* Dehydration, electrolyte imbalance, possible hypovolemic shock, changes in mentation, possible coma, Kussmaul's respirations, acetone breath, weak and rapid pulse, hypotension, hyperglycemia.

□ *Type II:* Marked dehydration, hypovolemic shock, obtundation, shallow respirations, gross hyperglycemia. There is absence of ketosis.

B. Complications

1. **Potential acute complications:** *For type I* include diabetic ketoacidosis (DKA) and hypoglycemia; *for type II* include hyperosmolar hyperglycemic nonketotic coma (HHNC) and hypoglycemia. These complications are usually preventable. Each is discussed later in this section.

2. **Long-term complications:** The most important factor in prevention is the maintenance of consistent, stable blood glucose levels within normal physiologic range. The following describe the levels of vascular pathology.

   □ *Microangiopathy:* Thickening of the basement membrane of the capillaries. Diabetic microangiopathy is manifested by retinopathy, nephropathy, and neuropathy. It compounds the effects of macroangiopathy.

   □ *Macroangiopathy:* Affects the larger vessels of the brain, heart, and lower extremities, resulting in cerebrovascular, cardiovascular, and peripheral vascular disease. The risk factors are hyperglycemia, hypertension, hypercholesterolemia, smoking, aging, and extended duration of DM.

C. Diagnostic Tests

1. Fasting blood sugar (FBS): A value >140 mg/dL is indicative of glucose intolerance.

2. Oral glucose tolerance test (OGTT): When two or more values of glucose are >200 mg/dL for 0–2 hours, glucose intolerance is present. It is sometimes used concurrently with serum insulin values by radioimmunoassay (RIA). The presence of insulin can help distinguish between type II and type I diabetics.

3. Two-hour postprandial blood glucose (2-hour PPG): Can be diagnostic if a standard glucose load (1.75 g/kg body wt) is administered with the meal. A blood glucose level of 180 mg/dL or higher in an individual for whom there is no other cause for impaired carbohydrate intolerance is significant.

4. Urinalysis for glycosuria and/or ketonuria: By itself is a poor diagnostic tool, but it is reflective of the renal threshold for glucose when used in addition to the above tests. Glycosuria is usually present when blood glucose exceeds 170 mg/dL. The renal threshold for glucose is elevated in the elderly. Ketonuria will be present in type I diabetes in the presence of ketosis.

5. Glycosylated hemoglobin: Measured to assess diabetic control over a preced-

ing 2–3 month period. The larger the percentage of glycosylated hemoglobin, the poorer the diabetic control. Normal range = 3.5–8.5%. Diabetics often have values between 8 and 20%.

D. Medical Interventions

1. **Diet:** The exchange programs of the American Diabetes and American Dietetic Associations are the most commonly used methods of diet calculation and patient education. Dietary management is individually based on ideal body weight and adjusted to metabolic and activity needs. The ratio of carbohydrates to proteins to fats is approximately 2 : 1 : 1. The focus on weight reduction for type II diabetics necessitates significant carbohydrate restriction for the type II diabetic treated by diet alone. When treatment also includes oral hypoglycemic medications or insulin, increased amounts of carbohydrates are required to offset the hypoglycemic effects of these medications. Type I diabetics require day-to-day consistency in diet and exercise to prevent hypoglycemia. Typically, three daily meals and an evening snack are prescribed. Some fat and protein should be present in all meals and snacks to slow down the elevation of postprandial blood glucose. Added fiber will slow the digestion of monosaccharides and disaccharides. For both types of diabetics, refined and simple sugars must be avoided. Various artificial sweeteners are used in "diet" products. Some contribute calories, which must be accounted for in a calorie-restricted diet.

2. **Oral hypoglycemic medications (sulfonylureas):** Used in symptomatic type II diabetics for whom diet alone cannot control hyperglycemia. Their primary action is to increase insulin production by affecting existing beta-cell function. The most serious side effect is hypoglycemia, particularly with chlorpropamide (Diabenese), which has a 72-hour duration and an average half-life of 36 hours. Hypoglycemia involving the oral hypoglycemics can be severe and persistent. Nursing monitoring needs to be diligent. Oral hypoglycemics should be omitted several days before planned surgery. Any condition, situation, or medication that enhances the hypoglycemic effects of these drugs requires close monitoring of blood glucose when symptoms of hypoglycemia arise. Fasting for diagnostic purposes, malnourishment related to illness or nausea and vomiting, and other medication therapy, any of which adds to the hypoglycemic action of the oral hypoglycemics, are common factors in the development of hypoglycemia.

3. **Insulin:** Examples of short-, intermediate-, and long-acting insulins are shown in Table 5-1.

Table 5-1 Types of Insulin

Insulin Type		Onset of Action (After Subcutaneous Injection)*	Peak Action*
Rapid-acting	Regular	0.5–1 hour	2–5 hours
	Semilente	0.5–1 hour	4–6 hours
☐ Human	Actrapid	0.5 hour	4 hours
	Humulin	0.5 hour	4 hours
Intermediate-acting	NPH	0.5–3 hours	6–12 hours
	Lente	1–3 hours	6–12 hours
☐ Human	Monotard	May be slower than	May be faster than
	Humulin N	nonhuman insulin	nonhuman insulin
Long-acting	Ultralente	2–6 hours	18–24 hours

*Action times may vary slightly.

□ A split-dose regimen of insulin adminstration is preferred because it allows for a higher level of blood glucose control. Daily insulin therapy usually consists of administering two-thirds of the total daily intermediate-acting insulin dose in the morning, with the remaining dose given in the evening. A rapid-acting insulin might be added to either or both doses. This regimen precludes the use of the longer-acting insulins, which are rarely used in a single dose because of the risk of nocturnal hypoglycemia.

□ Multidose therapy permits better control of blood glucose for some individuals. Alteration in the quantity of food and timing of meals is a benefit to the patient who values flexibilty. For the self-motivated diabetic who has control difficulties in spite of multidose therapy, portable insulin pumps can be helpful.

□ The degree to which bovine and porcine sources of insulin deviate from the protein structure of human insulin relates to the extent of their antigenic properties. Purified forms of insulin are less immunogenic and are used for patients who demonstrate insulin resistance as an allergic response. The recently developed biosynthetic and semisynthetic human insulins are the least immunogenic and are used for patients who have allergies to animal insulins.

4. **Portable insulin pumps:** Devices that deliver a constant basal rate of insulin throughout the day and night with the capability of delivering a bolus of insulin at mealtime. The needle, which attaches to a syringe via a long strip of plastic tubing, remains indwelling in the subcutaneous tissue of the abdomen. Patients program their own pumps to deliver the optimal amount of insulin, based on self-monitoring of blood glucose.

5. **Patient teaching about drugs that potentiate hyperglycemia:** These include estrogens, corticosteroids, thyroid preparations, diuretics, phenytoin, glucagon, and medications that contain sugar, such as cough syrup.

6. **Patient teaching about drugs that potentiate hypoglycemia:** These include salicylates, sulfonamides, methyldopa, anabolic steroids, acetaminophen, ethanol, haloperidol, marijuana. Propranolol masks the signs of and inhibits recovery from hypoglycemia.

7. **Exercise:** As important as diet and insulin in treating DM. It lowers blood glucose levels, helps maintain normal cholesterol levels, and increases circulation. These effects increase the body's ability to metabolize glucose and help reduce the therapeutic dose of insulin in most patients. The exercise program must be consistent and individualized (especially for type I diabetics). Patients should be given a complete physical exam and encouraged to incorporate acceptable activities as part of their daily routine.

E. Nursing Diagnoses and Interventions

Alteration in tissue perfusion: Peripheral, cardiopulmonary, renal, cerebral, and gastrointestinal related to impaired circulation and sensation secondary to development and progression of macroangiopathy and microangiopathy

Desired outcome: Patient complies with the therapeutic regimen and exhibits physical findings within acceptable limits.

1. Check blood glucose before meals and at bedtime. Encourage patient to perform regular home blood-glucose monitoring. Urine testing is less reliable and should not be used by patients with reduced renal function.

2. Hypertension is a common complication of diabetes. Careful control of BP is critical in preventing or limiting the development of heart disease, retinopathy, or nephropathy. Check BP q4h. Alert MD to values outside of the patient's norm. Administer antihypertensive agents as prescribed and document the response.

3. Patients may experience decreased sensation in the extremities because of pe-

ripheral neuropathy. Protect patients from injury from sharp objects or heat. For example, avoid the use of heating pads.

4. Provide a safe environment for patients with diminished eyesight secondary to diabetic retinopathy. Orient patient to the location of items such as water, tissues, glasses, and call light.

5. Approximately half of all type I diabetics develop chronic renal failure (CRF) and end-stage renal disease (ESRD). Monitor patients for changes in renal function, for example, increases in BUN and creatinine and altered urine output. Proteinuria is an early indicator of developing CRF. Diabetics with reduced renal function are at significant risk for developing acute renal failure after exposure to contrast media. Observe these patients for indicators of acute renal failure. (See "Acute Renal Failure," p. 106, and "Chronic Renal Failure," p. 111, in Chapter 3 for further information.) Insulin dosages will decrease as renal function decreases. Also be alert to indicators of hypoglycemia. See Table 5-2, p. 262, for clinical indicators and treatment.

6. Diabetics may experience multiple problems secondary to autonomic neuropathy such as the following:

   □ *Orthostatic hypotension:* Assist patients when getting up suddenly or after prolonged recumbency. Check BP while patient is lying down, sitting, and then standing to document presence of orthostatic hypotension. Alert MD to significant findings.

   □ *Impaired gastric emptying with nausea, vomiting, and diarrhea:* Administer metoclopramide before meals, if prescribed. Keep a record of all stools. Nausea, vomiting, and anorexia can be indicative of developing uremia in patients with progressive renal failure.

   □ *Neurogenic bladder:* Encourage patients to void q3−4h during the day, utilizing manual pressure (Credé's maneuver) if necessary. Intermittent catheterization may be necessary in severe cases. Avoid the use of indwelling urinary catheters because of the high risk of infection.

Potential for infection related to increased susceptibility secondary to disease process (eg, hyperglycemia, neurogenic bladder, poor circulation)

Desired outcome: Patient does not exhibit signs of infection.

▶ **Note:** Infection is the most common cause of diabetic ketoacidosis (DKA).

1. Monitor temperature q4h. Alert MD to elevations.

2. Maintain meticulous sterile technique when changing dressings, performing invasive procedure, or manipulating indwelling catheters.

3. Monitor for indicators of infection: dysuria, urgency, frequency, cloudy and/or foul-smelling urine; redness, local warmth, swelling, discharge, and pain from skin wounds or lesions; complaints of sore throat and swollen glands and inflamed pharynx; changes in the color, amount, or consistency of sputum; chest pain and SOB; fever; leukocytosis.

4. Consult MD about obtaining cultures for blood, sputum, and urine during temperature spikes or for wounds that produce purulent drainage.

Potential impairment of skin integrity related to increased susceptibility secondary to peripheral neuropathy and vascular pathology

Desired outcomes: Patient's skin remains intact. Patient can verbalize and demonstrate knowledge of proper foot care.

1. Assess integrity of the skin and evaluate reflexes of the lower extremities by checking knee and ankle deep tendon reflexes (DTRs), proprioceptive sensa-

tions, and vibration sensation (using a tuning fork on the medial malleolus). If sensations are impaired, anticipate patient's inability to respond appropriately to harmful stimuli. Monitor peripheral pulses, comparing the quality bilaterally.

2. Use foot cradle on bed, spaceboots for ulcerated heels, elbow protectors, and alternating air pressure mattress to prevent pressure points and promote patient comfort.

3. To alleviate acute discomfort yet prevent hemostasis, minimize patient activities and incorporate progressive passive and active exercises into daily routine. Discourage extended rest periods in the same position.

4. Teach patient the following steps for foot care:

   ☐ Wash feet daily with mild soap and warm water; check water temperature with water thermometer or elbow.

   ☐ Inspect feet daily for the presence of redness or trauma, using mirrors as necessary for adequate visualization.

   ☐ Alternate between at least two pairs of properly fitted shoes to avoid potential for pressure points that can occur by wearing one pair only.

   ☐ Prevent infection from moisture or dirt by changing socks or stockings daily and wearing cotton or wool blends.

   ☐ Prevent ingrown toenails by cutting toenails straight across after softening them during bath.

   ☐ Do not self-treat corns or calluses; visit podiatrist regularly.

   ☐ Attend to any foot injury immediately, and seek medical attention to avoid any potential complication.

Knowledge deficit: Procedure for insulin administration

Desired outcome: Patient can demonstrate procedure for administration of insulin.

1. Teach patient to check expiration date on insulin vial and to avoid using it if outdated.

2. Explain that intermediate- and long-acting insulins require mixing. Demonstrate rolling the insulin vial between the palms to mix the contents. Caution patient that vigorous shaking produces air bubbles that can interfere with accurate dosage measurement.

3. Explain that insulin should be injected 30 minutes before mealtime.

4. Explain that either making a change in insulin type or withholding a dose of insulin may be required for the following: when fasting for studies or surgery, when not eating because of nausea/vomiting, or when hypoglycemic. Adjustments are always individually based and require clarification with patient's MD.

5. Provide patient with a chart that depicts rotation of the injection sites. Explain that injection sites should be at least 1 inch apart.

As appropriate, see "Atherosclerotic Arterial Occlusive Disease" in Chapter 2, "Cardiovascular Disorders," p. 77, and "Amputation" in Chapter 8, "Musculoskeletal Disorders," p. 404. See "Appendix One" for nursing diagnoses and interventions for the care of patients with life-disrupting illnesses, pp. 544–546.

F. Patient–Family Teaching and Discharge Planning

Provide patient and SOs with verbal and written information for the following:

1. Importance of carrying a diabetic identification card and wearing Medic-Alert bracelet or necklace.

2. Recognizing warning signs of both hyperglycemia and hypoglycemia and factors that contribute to both conditions. Remind patient that stress from illness or infection can increase insulin requirements (or necessitate insulin therapy for one who is normally controlled with oral hypoglycemics) and that increased exercise will necessitate additional food intake to prevent hypoglycemia when there is no change made in insulin dosage.

3. Home monitoring of blood glucose using commercial kits and/or daily urine testing for glucose and ketones, which provides ongoing data reflecting the degree of control and may identify necessary changes in diet and/or medication before severe metabolic changes occur. These tests also provide a means for patient's self-control and psychologic security. Stress the need for careful control of blood glucose as a means of preventing long-term complications of DM.

4. Importance of daily exercise, good blood-glucose control, maintenance of normal body weight, and yearly medical evaluation, including visits to a podiatrist and ophthalmologist.

5. Diet that is low in fat and high in fiber as an effective means of controlling blood fats, especially cholesterol and triglycerides. Stress that diet is the sole method of control for many type II diabetics. The importance of adequate nutrition and controlled calories is essential in maintaining normoglycemia in these diabetics.

6. Necessity for type I diabetics to use U-100 syringes with U-100 insulin and U-40 syringes with U-40 strength insulin. Stress that using an insulin strength that does not correspond to the calibrated syringe sets up a condition for dangerous under- or over-dosage.

7. Availability of syringe magnifiers that can be used for patients with poor visual acuity. Other products that permit safe and accurate filling of syringes are also available.

8. Necessity of rotating injection sites and injecting insulin at room temperature. Provide a chart showing possible injection sites and describe the system for rotating the sites.

9. Importance of good foot care.

10. Importance of annual eye examinations for early detection and treatment of retinopathy.

In addition:

11. Explain the importance of inserting the needle perpendicular to the skin rather than at an angle to ensure deep subcutaneous administration of insulin.

12. Assist patient with identifying available resources for ongoing assistance and information, including nurses, dietitian, patient's MD, and other diabetics in the patient care unit. Other resources include the local chapter of American Diabetes Association (ADA), subscription to *ADA Forecast* (a publication of ADA), and local library for free access to current materials on diabetes.

13. For any supplemental medications used, patient should be taught the name, purpose, dosage, schedule, precautions, and potential side effects.

II. Diabetic Ketoacidosis

Diabetic ketoacidosis (DKA), a catabolic state, reflects glucose and ketone production from the breakdown of fats and protein acids. Hyperglycemia leads to osmotic diuresis with the loss of fluid and electrolytes. As ketones accumulate and bicarbonate excretion occurs, ketoacidosis develops. Coma and death will ensue if the condition remains untreated. Stress (eg, infection) is the most common precipitating cause of DKA.

Table 5-2 Quick Comparison of Acute Diabetic Complications*

	DKA	HHNC**	Hypoglycemia
Clinical Indicators	Alteration in mentation: confusion, emotional irritability; acetone breath; flushed face; Kussmaul's respirations; blurred vision; nausea, vomiting; abdominal cramps; tachycardia; hypotension	Alteration in mentation/coma (can be mistaken for CVA); obtundation; marked dehydration; marked hyperglycemia; tachycardia; hypotension; hypovolemic shock. **Note:** Acetone breath, Kussmaul's respirations, or GI symptoms found with DKA will be absent	Mentation changes: apprehension, erratic behavior; trembling; slurred speech; staggering gait; pounding tachycardia; cool, clammy skin; pallor; possible seizure activity
Blood Glucose Levels	Usually >300 mg/dL, <800 mg/dL	Usually >500 mg/dL; can be as high as 2000 mg/dL or more	<50 mg/dl
Onset	Slow (can take hours to days)	Slow	Rapid (minutes to an hour)
Precipitating Factors	Physical stress (infectious process) or emotional upset; omitting insulin; excessive food intake; undiagnosed type I diabetic; drug interactions	Undiagnosed type II diabetic; acute infection; intake of medications that potentiate hyperglycemia (thyroid preparations, diuretics, phenytoin, corticosteroids); TPN	Vomiting; missing meals; relative excess in insulin; increased exercise; alcohol intake; drug interactions
Interventions	Initially, continuous low-dose regular insulin drip in hypotonic IV solution. IV solutions include some dextrose once blood glucose reaches 350 mg/dL. Potassium replacement (in the presence of good renal function); ABGs to assess degree of acidosis; bicarbonate replacement if pH <7.1	Massive fluid replacement (up to 20 L/48 hr); CVP monitoring to evaluate fluid load on cardiovascular system; potassium replacement	If patient is alert, promptly give absorbable glucose orally (eg, 2 packets sugar in orange juice). If patient cannot take oral glucose, administer glucagon IM or 1 ampule of 50% (50 mL) IV dextrose. Consciousness should return within minutes

*Usually, a combination of factors precipitates acute complications.
**Hyperosmolar hyperglycemic nonketotic coma.

A. Assessment

See Table 5-2.

B. Diagnostic Tests

1. <u>Serial measurement of plasma glucose and electrolytes:</u> A widening anion gap $[Na^+ - (Cl^- + HCO_3^-)]$ is an indicator of acid concentration—the wider the gap, the higher the concentration. Normal gap = 12.

2. <u>Urine tests:</u> Evaluate for the presence of glucose and ketones, but are less reliable than plasma values.

3. <u>Other studies:</u> Include ABGs to obtain arterial pH and document degree of acidosis; EKG and cardiac enzymes to rule out myocardial infarction (MI); chest x-ray and urine and blood cultures to detect possible infections; plasma creatinine and BUN to assess renal function; and plasma osmolality to determine type of fluid replacement needed. In addition, serum amylase is drawn to rule out pancreatitis.

C. Medical Management

1. **IV fluids:** To restore intravascular fluid and prevent hypovolemic shock.

2. **Insulin administration:** To correct hyperglycemia, usually via IV bolus and then by continuous low-dose IV infusion. Only regular insulin should be used.

3. **Bicarbonate administration:** If arterial pH is <7.1 (or <7.2 in the presence of hypotension or shock) or when CO_2 level falls to 8 mEq/L.

4. **Potassium replacement:** To compensate for potassium depletion secondary to osmotic diuresis. PO_4 replacement also may be necessary.

5. **Identification of precipitating cause:** Such as infection, failure to take insulin, MI, pancreatitis, stroke, trauma, or surgery.

D. Nursing Diagnoses and Interventions

Fluid volume deficit related to abnormal loss secondary to osmotic diuresis

Desired outcome: Patient does not exhibit signs of dehydration or hypovolemic shock.

1. Accurately monitor I&O qh to evaluate renal perfusion. Because decreasing urinary output precedes hypovolemic shock, report urine output <30 mL/h for 2 consecutive hours. **Note:** Some patients may have pre-existing renal disease secondary to DM.

2. Monitor for poor skin turgor, weight loss, and cracked lips as indicators of dehydration.

3. Monitor peripheral pulses, BP, and respirations q30–60 min until stable. With developing hypovolemic shock, the patient will have hypotension, tachycardia, and diminished or absent peripheral pulses.

4. Monitor hematocrit, serum osmolality, creatinine, and BUN; their increase occurs with dehydration and hemoconcentration. Elevation of both BUN and creatinine lab values over time is indicative of impaired renal function.

5. If dehydration is severe, it may be necessary to administer prescribed IV fluids rapidly. Observe for the following indicators of fluid overload: tachycardia, crackles (rales), rhonchi, and SOB.

▶ **Note:** Death in DKA is often the result of dehydration and electrolyte imbalance.

Potential for injury related to risk of complications secondary to hyperglycemia and acid–base imbalance

Desired outcome: Hyperglycemia and acid–base imbalance, if they occur, are detected and treated promptly and correctly, resulting in absence of injury to the patient.

1. Administer regular insulin as prescribed. Monitor blood glucose q1–2h until it is stable. Blood sugar should decrease slowly over several hours. Too rapid a correction of hyperglycemia can lead to a sudden drop in serum osmolality or dangerous hypokalemia secondary to the sudden shift of potassium into the cells.

2. Administer dextrose-free IV fluids as prescribed. When blood glucose drops to the range of 200–300 mg/dL, dextrose should be added to the IV solution (eg, D_5NS). Keep MD informed of glucose levels.

3. Monitor baseline and serial ABG values to define the degree of acidosis and compensation. When the pH value is within normal limits, physiologic compensation is occurring; a below-normal pH value reflects inadequate compensation, and medical intervention is warranted.

4. Set up a bedside chart showing serial values of blood glucose and electrolytes. An increasing anion gap $[Na^+ - (Cl^- + HCO_3^-)]$ is indicative of metabolic acidosis. If patient is "shocky," lactic acidosis also may be present.

5. Monitor the respiratory pattern. Kussmaul's respirations and acetone breath reflect ketoacidosis. With resolving acidosis, acetone breath disappears. Shallow respirations in the comatose patient suggest severe acidosis with respiratory depression. Notify MD of significant findings.

6. Administer IV $NaHCO_3$ as prescribed. *Sudden* increases in serum pH can cause potassium to shift into the cells. Watch for hypokalemia (see item 3 below).

Potential alterations in cardiac output: Decreased: Fluid loss and serum electrolyte imbalance secondary to osmotic diuresis associated with hyperglycemia

Desired outcome: Patient's VS and physical findings are within acceptable limits.

1. Monitor BP and pulse at frequent intervals. Tachycardia often reflects the heart's effort to maintain adequate cardiac output. Notify MD of changes in heart rate or rhythm.

2. Monitor I&O and electrolyte values, especially potassium. Acidosis and insulin deficiency may lead to temporary hyperkalemia due to the movement of potassium out of the cells. Loss of potassium from polyuria, administration of insulin, and correction of acidosis may result in hypokalemia. Be alert to potassium >6 mEq/L or <3.5 mEq/L, which can lead to cardiac compromise.

3. If continuous cardiac monitoring is prescribed, monitor EKG at frequent intervals for evidence of hyperkalemia or hypokalemia. A depressed S–T segment and flattened T wave are indicative of hypokalemia. Premature ventricular contractions also occur frequently with hypokalemia. For that reason, alert the MD to the development of an irregular pulse. A tall and tented T wave, prolonged P–R interval, and widened QRS complex occur with hyperkalemia. If continuous monitoring is unavailable, the patient may require a transfer to ICU or other area in which monitoring is available.

See "General Discussion," p. 258, for nursing diagnoses and interventions for the care of patients with diabetes mellitus.

E. Patient–Family Teaching and Discharge Planning

See "General Discussion," p. 260.

III. Hyperosmolar Hyperglycemic Nonketotic Coma

Hyperosmolar hyperglycemic nonketotic coma (HHNC), also known as hyperosmolar hyperglycemic nonketotic dehydration (HHND), is characterized by marked hyperglycemia, osmotic diuresis, dehydration, hyperosmolality of serum, and azotemia. Unlike DKA, there is no ketosis, and insulin deficiency is mild. Frequently, these patients are undiagnosed type II diabetics, often with some degree of renal failure. HHNC can develop slowly and insidiously, and is common in patients with existing dehydration. A gram-negative infection is another common cause of HHNC. Typically, patients are obtunded, with shallow respirations and no acetone breath. The patient's age, presenting symptoms, and previously negative history for diabetes sometimes lead to a misdiagnosis of cerebrovascular accident (CVA). Prevention and early detection are critical in reducing the high mortality rate in these patients.

A. Assessment

See Table 5-2, p. 262.

B. Diagnostic Tests and Medical Interventions

▶ **Note:** Medical diagnostics and interventions are very similar to those with DKA. However, with HHNC, dehydration and electrolyte imbalances tend to be more severe. Because HHNC occurs more frequently in the elderly, CVP monitoring and pulmonary artery pressures are required for close management of fluid volume. Typically, ketoacidosis is not present, and therefore the patient will not have Kussmaul's respirations or acetone breath. Because ketosis is not present, large doses of insulin are not needed, and should not be used even in the presence of massive hyperglycemia.

C. Nursing Diagnoses and Interventions

Potential alterations in cardiac output: Decreased: Fluid loss and serum electrolyte imbalance secondary to osmotic diuresis associated with hyperglycemia

Desired outcome: Patient's VS and physical findings are within acceptable limits.

1. Assess LOC; color, turgor, and temperature of skin; peripheral pulses; and I&O q1–2h as indicators of the degree of hydration, tissue perfusion, and cardiac output.

2. Monitor apical pulse, BP, and respirations q1–2h until stable, noting changes from patient's baseline, for indicators of impaired cardiac status and dangerous dysrhythmias.

3. Monitor electrolyte values, especially potassium. Be alert to potassium <3.5 mEq/L, which can lead to cardiac compromise.

4. If continuous cardiac monitoring is prescribed, monitor EKG at frequent intervals to alert you to the presence of hypokalemia, as evidenced by a depressed S–T segment and flattened T wave. In addition, premature ventricular contractions also can occur with hypokalemia. For that reason, alert MD to the development of an irregular pulse.

See "General Discussion," p. 258, for nursing diagnoses and interventions for the care of patients with diabetes mellitus. See "Diabetic Ketoacidosis" (DKA) for the following: **Fluid volume deficit** related to abnormal loss secondary to osmotic diuresis, p. 263. **Caution:** Because most patients with HHNC are elderly and dehydration is often severe, careful fluid replacement is crucial.

D. Patient–Family Teaching and Discharge Planning

See "General Discussion," p. 260.

IV. Hypoglycemia

Hypoglycemia is a lowering of blood glucose caused by an overdose of insulin, skipping meals, or too much exercise without a concomitant increase in food intake. Unlike DKA and HHNC, hypoglycemia can have a sudden onset, and its course is precipitous if it is left untreated. Typically, hypoglycemia occurs during the time of the peak action of the hypoglycemic medication or at night when the patient is fasting.

The patient usually becomes symptomatic when blood glucose is less than 50 mg/dL or there is a significant relative drop in blood glucose, for example, when an elderly patient's blood glucose drops to 90 mg/dL from 180–200 mg/dL. Alcohol consumption also can cause hypoglycemia because it depletes glycogen stores, resulting in increased insulin levels.

▶ **Note:** Mentation changes caused by severe hypoglycemia can be indistinguishable from those caused by alcoholic stupor. If hypoglycemic symptoms are misdiagnosed as alcoholic stupor and a hypoglycemic diabetic is left to "sleep it off," death can ensue.

A. Assessment

See Table 5-2, p. 262.

B. Nursing Diagnoses and Interventions

Potential for injury related to risk of complications secondary to hypoglycemia

Desired outcome: Hypoglycemia, if it occurs, is detected and treated promptly, resulting in absence of injury to the patient.

▶ **Caution:** Hypoglycemia requires immediate intervention because it can lead to brain damage and death if it is severe. When in doubt as to the cause of coma in a diabetic patient, draw a stat blood glucose and prepare to administer 50% IV glucose.

---

1. Administer a fast-acting carbohydrate: 4 ounces orange or apple juice, 2½ tsp sugar, 3 ounces nondiet soda, or 5–7 Lifesavers. Notify MD if patient is incoherent, unresponsive, or incapable of taking carbohydrates by mouth. If any of these indicators occur, an IV access is required and you should prepare to administer prescribed 50 mL 50% dextrose by IV push. Consciousness should be restored within 10 minutes.

2. Using an appropriate reagent strip, continue to monitor blood glucose level q30–60 min to identify recurrence of hypoglycemia.

3. Once patient is alert, question patient about recent intake or absence of food. Any situation preventing food intake, such as nausea, vomiting, dislike of hospital food related to cultural preferences, or fasting for a scheduled test, should be determined and addressed immediately.

4. If food intake has been adequate, consult with MD regarding a reduction in patient's daily dose of antihyperglycemic medication.

▶ **Note:** Sometimes hypoglycemia leads to rebound hyperglycemia (Somogyi effect). If hypoglycemia goes undetected, the rebound hyperglycemia may be inappropriately treated with increased insulin. Suspect the Somogyi effect if there are wide fluctuations in blood glucose over a few hours, or if urine tests change from negative to positive too quickly after insulin administration. Notify MD if these changes are observed or if the patient is experiencing nocturnal hypoglycemia.

Potential for injury related to alterations in LOC and risk of seizures secondary to hypoglycemia

Desired outcome: Patient does not experience injury caused by seizures or alterations in LOC.

1. Monitor LOC at frequent intervals. Anticipate seizure potential in presence of severe hypoglycemia and have airway, protective padding, padded tongue blade, and suction equipment at bedside. Keep all siderails up.

2. Notify MD of any seizure activity; do not leave patient unattended if it occurs.

3. Place call light within patient's reach and have patient demonstrate its proper use q shift. Inability to use the call light properly necessitates checking on the patient at least q30 min. If necessary, consider moving patient to a room next to the nurses' station for close monitoring.

4. Keep all potentially harmful objects such as knives, forks, and hot beverages out of patient's reach.

5. If necessary to prevent patient from wandering and causing self-injury, obtain a prescription for soft restraints. Explain these safety precautions to patient and SOs.

6. For other information, see "Seizure Disorders" in Chapter 4, "Neurologic Disorders," p. 201.

Knowledge deficit: Disease process, diagnostic testing, indicators of hypoglycemia, and therapeutic regimen

Desired outcome: Patient can verbalize knowledge of DM, including testing and management, the indicators of hypoglycemia, and the therapeutic regimen.

1. Assess patient's knowledge of DM, including diagnostic testing and management. Provide information or clarify as appropriate.

2. Review the indicators and immediate interventions for hypoglycemia with the patient.

3. Evaluate current diet for adequate nutritional requirements, calorie content, and patient satisfaction. Assist patient with making acceptable and realistic changes. Take into account patient's activity level and need for changes to achieve normoglycemia. Refer patient and SOs to dietitian as needed.

4. Review with patient the onset, peak action, and duration of the hypoglycemic medication. Advise patient to avoid drugs that contribute to hypoglycemia (see p. 258).

5. Stress the importance of testing blood glucose at the time symptoms of hypoglycemia occur.

6. Explain that injection of insulin into a site that is about to be exercised heavily, for example, the thigh of a jogger, will result in quicker absorption of the insulin and possible hypoglycemia.

7. Inform patient that a change in the type of medication may require a change in dosage to prevent hypoglycemia. Caution patient about the need to follow prescription directions precisely.

See "General Discussion," p. 258, for nursing diagnoses and interventions for the care of patients with diabetes mellitus.

C. Patient–Family Teaching and Discharge Planning

See "General Discussion," p. 260–261.

▶ **Selected References**

Brunner LS, Suddarth DS: *Textbook of Medical-Surgical Nursing*, 5th ed. Lippincott, 1984.

Burch WM: *Endocrinology for the House Officer*. Williams & Wilkins, 1984.

Campbell RK (editor): Human insulin. *Pharmacology Update* 8:66.

Campbell WJ, Frisse M (editors): *Manual of Medical Therapeutics*, 24th ed. Little, Brown, 1983.

Carpenito LJ: *Handbook of Nursing Diagnosis*. Lippincott, 1984.

Cavalier JP: Crucial decisions in diabetic emergencies. *RN* 1980; 43:32–37.

Conn HF (editor): *Current Therapy*. Saunders, 1983.

Daggett P: *Clinical Endocrinology: Physiological Principles in Medicine*. University Park Press, 1981.

De Vita TV, Hellman S, Rosenberg SA (editors): *Cancer: Principles and Practice of Oncology*. Lippincott, 1982.

Doenges ME, Jeffries MF, Moorhouse MF: *Nursing Care Plans: Nursing Diagnoses in Planning Patient Care*. F A Davis, 1984.

Duncan TG: *The Diabetes Fact Book: A Guide to Understanding, Controlling, and Living with Diabetes*. Charles Scribner's Sons, 1982.

Friesen SR, Bolinger RE (editors): *Surgical Endocrinology: Clinical Syndromes*. Lippincott, 1978.

Garafano CD: Helping diabetics live with their neuropathies. *Nursing 80* 1980; 10:42–44.

Gotch PM: Are you ready for a total pancreatectomy patient? *RN* 1981; 44:54–57.

Gramse CA: Pancreatitis: Review what pancreatitis is and how to help patients who have this disease. *Nursing 82* 1982; 12.

Greenspan FS, Forsham PH (editors): *Basic and Clinical Endocrinology*. Lange, 1983.

Guthrie DW: Helping the diabetic manage his self-care. *Nursing 80* 1980; 10:57–64.

Guthrie DW, Guthrie RA: The disease process of diabetes mellitus: Definitions, characteristics, trends, and developments. *Nurs Clin North Am* 1983; 18:617–630.

Guthrie DW, Guthrie RA: *Nursing Management of Diabetes Mellitus*, 2nd ed. Mosby, 1982.

Krieger DT, Hughes JC (editors): *Neuroendocrinology*. Sinauer Associates, 1980.

Levine CD: Preventing complications in the pancreatoduodenectomy patient. *Dimensions of Critical Care Nursing* 1983; 2:90–97.

Lueg MC: Asymptomatic primary hyperparathyroidism. *Hospital Practice* 1982; 17:29–30.

Moorman NH: Acute complications of hyperglycemia and hypoglycemia. *Nurs Clin North Am* 1983; 18:707–719.

Muthe NC: *Endocrinology, a Nursing Approach*. Little, Brown, 1981.

Nurses Clinical Library: *Endocrine Disorders*. Springhouse, 1984.

Osborne S: Total pancreatectomy and splenectomy for a patient with chronic pancreatitis. *Nursing Times* 1980; 76:1836–1840.

Pagana K, Pagana T: *Diagnostic Testing and Nursing Implications*, 2nd ed. Mosby, 1985.

Payloyan E et al: Subtotal parathyroidectomy for primary hyperparathyroidism: Long-term results in 292 patients. *Arch Surg* (April) 1983; 118:425–431.

Popkess-Vawter S: The adult living with diabetes mellitus. *Nurs Clin North Am* 1983; 18:777.

Price MJ: Insulin and oral hypoglycemic agents. *Nurs Clin North Am* 1983; 18: 687–706.

Ramsey JM: *Basic Pathophysiology: Modern Stress and the Disease Process*. Addison-Wesley, 1982.

Saxton DE et al: *The Addison-Wesley Manual of Nursing Practice*. Addison-Wesley, 1983.

Schrock TR: *Handbook of Surgery*, 7th ed. Jones Medical Publications, 1982.

Smith J, Davis B: An inside view. *Nursing Mirror* 1983; 157:30–33.

Spies ME: Vascular complications associated with diabetes mellitus. *Nurs Clin North Am* 1983; 18:721–731.

Stiklorius C: Two diagnostic procedures that demand your all-out care. *RN* 1982; 45:64–65.

Streck WF, Lockwood DH (editors): *Endocrine Diagnosis: Clinical and Laboratory Approach*. Little, Brown, 1983.

Valente CL: Urine testing and home blood-glucose monitoring. *Nurs Clin North Am* 1983; 18:645–659.

Widmann FK: *Clinical Interpretation of Laboratory Tests*, 9th ed. F A Davis, 1983.

Wills MR, Harvard B: *Laboratory Investigation of Endocrine Disorders*, 2nd ed. Butterworth, 1983.

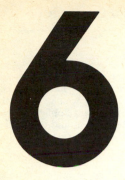

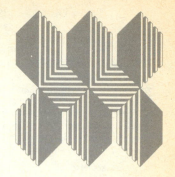

Gastrointestinal Disorders

► Section One **Disorders of the Mouth and Esophagus**

I. Stomatitis

Inflammatory and infectious diseases of the mouth are commonly overlooked in the debilitated hospitalized patient. Typically, they occur secondary to systemic disease and infection, nutritional and fluid deficiencies, poorly fitting dentures, and neglect of oral hygiene, and as side effects of irritants and drugs. Stomatitis (inflammation of the mouth and mucous membrane) is the term generally applied to a variety of mouth disorders characterized by mucosal cell destruction and disruption of the mucosal lining. It is one of the major side effects of cancer chemotherapy, occurring in over 30% of this population.

A. Assessment

Signs and symptoms: Oral pain; sensitivity to hot, spicy foods; foul taste; oral bleeding or drainage; fever; xerostomia (dry mouth); difficulty chewing or swallowing; poorly fitting dentures.

Physical exam: The oral mucosa will appear swollen, red, and ulcerated; the lymph glands may be swollen; and the breath is often foul-smelling. The lips may have cracks, fissures, blisters, ulcers, and lesions; the tongue may appear dry, cracked, and contain masses, lesions, or exudate.

B. Diagnostic Tests

In most incidences, diagnosis of the offending organism is made by physical exam. However, the following may be used in selected patients:

1. <u>Culture:</u> May be taken of the lesion or drainage to identify the offending organism, if appropriate.
2. <u>Platelet count:</u> Taken if bleeding is present in the immunosuppressed patient.

C. Medical Management

The treatment varies, depending on the type of impairment and its cause.

1. **Identify and/or attempt to control or remove causative factor(s):** If appropriate.
2. **Oral hygiene/mouth irrigations.**
3. **Pharmacotherapy**
   □ *Local/systemic analgesics and local anesthetics:* For relief of pain.
   □ *Topical/systemic steroids:* To reduce inflammation and promote healing.
   □ *Antibiotics, antifungals, and antiviral agents:* To combat infection.
   □ *Vitamins:* To correct deficiencies (eg, vitamin C to strengthen connective tissue in the gums, and niacin and riboflavin to promote efficient cellular growth).
   □ *Artificial saliva products:* To maintain a normal fluid and electrolyte environment in the mouth.
4. **Dietary management:** Typically, high in protein to promote wound healing, high in calories for protein sparing, and high in vitamins to correct the specific deficiency. Usually, hot and spicy foods are restricted, and the consistency of the food ranges from liquid to regular, as tolerated. Fluids are encouraged.
5. **Cauterization of ulcerations:** If required.
6. **Dental restoration and repair:** If needed.
7. **Adequate rest:** For optimal tissue repair.

D. Nursing Diagnoses and Interventions

Alterations in oral mucous membrane related to stomatitis

Desired outcomes: Patient demonstrates knowledge of oral hygiene interventions and complies with the therapeutic regimen. Patient's physical findings are within acceptable limits.

1. Administer analgesics, corticosteroids, anesthetics, and mouthwashes as pre-scribed. For moderate stomatitis, provide mouth care q4h; for severe sto-matitis, provide mouth care q2h or even hourly if indicated.

2. If mouthwashes/irrigations are not prescribed, prepare a solution containing equal parts of mouthwash, hydrogen peroxide, and water. Instruct patient to rinse the mouth with this solution at least q4h during the day to provide local relief and promote healing.

3. Instruct the patient to brush teeth after meals and at hs, using a soft-bristled toothbrush and nonabrasive toothpaste. Patients with severe stomatitis who have dentures should remove them until the oral mucosa has healed. Dietary alterations may be necessary, for example, changing to a full liquid or pureed diet.

4. Advise patient to floss teeth gently qd, using unwaxed floss.

5. Keep the lips moist with emollients such as lanolin or petroleum jelly.

6. Advise patient to avoid irritants, including smoking and foods that are hot, spicy, and rough in texture.

7. Offer ice or Popsicles to help anesthetize the mouth.

8. Inspect the mouth tid for inflammation, lesions, and bleeding. Record observations and report significant findings to MD.

Self-care deficit: Inability to perform oral hygiene related to sensorimotor deficit or decreased LOC

Desired outcomes: Patient does not exhibit signs of poor oral hygiene. Patient or SO demonstrates ability to perform oral care.

1. Assess patient's ability to perform mouth care. Identify performance barriers such as sensorimotor or cognitive deficits.

2. If the patient has decreased LOC and/or is at risk for aspiration, remove dentures and store them in a water-filled denture cup.

3. If the patient cannot perform mouth care, cleanse the teeth, tongue, and mouth at least bid with a soft-bristled toothbrush and nonabrasive toothpaste. If the patient is unconscious or at risk for aspiration, turn the patient into a side-lying position. Swab the mouth and teeth with a gauze pad or swab moistened with a 4:1 solution of water and hydrogen peroxide, and irrigate the mouth with a syringe. If the patient cannot self-manage the secretions, use only a small amount of liquid at a time, using a suction catheter to remove the secretions. This regimen should be performed at least q4h. As appropriate, teach the procedure to SOs.

4. For patients with physical disabilities, the following toothbrush adaptations can be made:

   □ *For patients with limited hand mobility:* Enlarge the toothbrush handle by covering it with a sponge hair roller or aluminum foil, attaching either with an elastic band; or by attaching a bicycle handle grip with plaster of Paris.

   □ *For patients with limited arm mobility:* Extend the toothbrush handle by overlapping another handle or rod over it and taping them together.

Knowledge deficit: Disease process, treatment, and factors that potentiate bleeding

Desired outcome: Patient can verbalize knowledge of the cause, preventive measures, and treatment of stomatitis and the factors that potentiate bleeding.

1. Describe the causes of the patient's stomatitis and remind patient that the best treatment is prevention.

2. Explain the importance of meticulous, frequent oral hygiene and periodic dental exams.

3. Advise patient to avoid irritating foods and substances (eg, alcohol, tobacco, and hot, spicy, and rough foods).

4. Teach the importance of discontinuing flossing when the platelet count drops to below 15,000; and discontinuing brushing when the count drops to below 10,000 to avoid possible bleeding. Instead, instruct patient to perform oral hygiene using mouthwash, irrigations, or swabs or gauze pads moistened in these solutions.

Alteration in nutrition: Less than body requirements related to decreased intake secondary to discomfort with chewing and swallowing

Desired outcome: Patient does not exhibit signs of malnutrition or weight loss.

1. Assess the patient's ability to chew and swallow.

2. Monitor I&O. Unless contraindicated, ensure that patient has optimal hydration (at least 2–3 L/day) and a diet that is high in protein, calories, and essential vitamins and minerals. Alert MD if the need for IV or NG tube feedings becomes apparent.

3. Provide any special equipment that will facilitate ingestion, such as straws, nipples, syringes.

4. If the mouth is very painful, encourage intake of soft foods (eg, cooked cereals, soups, gelatin, ice cream). Drinks that are high in calories and protein are especially helpful. Consider adding polycose to beverages and powdered milk or protein powder to food preparations.

E. Patient–Family Teaching and Discharge Planning

Provide patient and SOs with verbal and written information for the following:

1. Essentials of diet, medications, and oral hygiene; adaptations that may be required at home.

2. Importance of notifying MD if any of the following recur or worsen: oral pain, fever, drainage, continuous bleeding, or inability to eat or drink.

3. Necessity of follow-up care; reconfirm date and time of next medical appointment.

4. Importance of visiting the dentist at least twice a year.

II. Hiatal Hernia and Reflux Esophagitis

A hiatal hernia occurs when there is a weakening of the muscular collar around the esophageal and diaphragmatic junction, permitting a portion of the lower esophagus and stomach to rise up into the chest during an increase in intra-abdominal pressure. Causative factors include degenerative changes (aging), trauma, esophageal neoplasms, kyphoscoliosis (a curvature of the spine), and surgery. Increased intra-abdominal pressure can occur with coughing, straining, bending, vomiting, obesity, pregnancy, trauma, constricting clothing, ascites, and severe physical exertion. The incidence of hiatal hernia increases with age, and women and obese individuals are more often affected. Complications of hiatal hernia include pulmonary aspiration of reflux contents, ulceration, hemorrhage, stenosis, obstruction, and gastritis. The most common complication of hiatal hernia is gastroesophageal reflux, the result of an incompetent lower cardiac sphincter that allows regurgitation of acidic gastric contents into the esophagus.

The most common type of hiatal hernia is the *sliding hernia*, which accounts for 90% of adult hiatal hernias. It is characterized by the upper portion of the stomach and esophageal junction sliding up into the chest when the individual assumes a supine position, and sliding back into the abdominal cavity when sitting or standing.

A. Assessment

Many patients are asymptomatic unless esophageal reflux is also present.

Signs and symptoms: Reflux esophagitis 1–4 hours after eating, possibly aggravated by reclining, stress, and increased intra-abdominal pressure. Heartburn, belching, regurgitation, vomiting, retrosternal or substernal chest pain (dull, full, heavy), hiccups, mild or occult bleeding found in vomitus or stools, mild anemia, and dysphagia also can occur. Elderly individuals may have symptoms of pneumonitis caused by aspiration of reflux contents into the pulmonary system.

Physical exam: Auscultation of peristaltic sounds in the chest, presence of palpitations, abdominal distention.

B. Diagnostic Tests

1. Chest x-ray: May reveal a large hernia, and infiltrates will be seen in the lower lobes of the lungs if aspiration has occurred.

2. Barium swallow: Will reveal gastroesophageal and diaphragmatic abnormalities. With fluoroscopy, a hernia will appear as a barium-containing outpouching at the lower end of the esophagus, and gastric barium will move into the esophagus with reflux . Sometimes it is necessary for the patient to be in Trendelenburg's position for the hernia to appear on x-ray.

3. Esophagoscopy and biopsy: Aid in differentiating between hiatal hernia, varices, and gastroesophageal lesions; determine the extent of esophagitis or ulceration; detect organic stenosis; rule out malignancies.

4. Esophageal function studies (EFS): Identify primary and secondary motor dysfunction before surgical repair of the hernia is performed. Included are manometry, which graphically records swallowing waves; pH probe, which will be low (acidic) in the presence of gastroesophageal reflux; and Bernstein test (acid perfusion), which attempts to reproduce the symptoms of reflux by instilling hydrochloric acid into the esophagus. If the patient has pain from the acid, the patient has gastroesophageal reflux.

5. Gastric analysis: To assess for bleeding, which can occur if ulceration is present.

6. CBC: May reveal an anemic condition if bleeding ulcers are present.

7. Stool guaiac test: Will be positive if bleeding has occurred.

8. EKG: To rule out cardiac origin of pain.

C. Medical Management and Surgical Interventions

Conservative management, which is successful in 90% of the cases, is preferred over surgical intervention. The goals are to prevent or reduce gastric reflux caused by increased intraabdominal pressure and increased gastric acid production.

1. **Encourage limitation of activities that increase intra-abdominal pressure:** For example, coughing, bending, straining, and physical exertion.

2. **Restrict or limit gastric acid stimulants:** For example, caffeine and nicotine.

3. **Dietary management:** Small, frequent meals; bland foods; weight reduction for obese patients; food restriction 2–3 hours before reclining.

4. **Elevate HOB:** Using 6–10 inch blocks to prevent postural reflux at night.

5. **Restrict tight, waist-constricting clothing.**

6. **Pharmacotherapy**

   □ *Antiemetics, cough suppressants, and stool softeners:* To prevent increased intra-abdominal pressure from vomiting, coughing, and straining with bowel movements; *antacids* to neutralize gastric acid.

    □ *Cholinergics:* To promote motility and prevent reflux.

    □ *Histamine H₂ receptor blockers:* To suppress acid secretion.

    □ *Gastrointestinal stimulators:* To augment gastric emptying and increase lower esophageal sphincter (LES) pressure.

7. Surgery: To restore gastroesophageal integrity and prevent reflux if symptoms do not resolve and complications (obstruction, bleeding, aspiration) occur. The most common procedure is a fundoplication, in which a portion of the upper stomach is wrapped around the distal esophagus and sutured to itself to prevent reflux from recurring. Typically, an abdominal rather than a thoracic approach is used.

8. Postsurgical management: Includes chest physiotherapy to prevent respiratory complications, administration of IV fluids and electrolytes until bowel sounds are present, a gradual increase in diet as tolerated after the return of peristalsis, and in some cases, gastric tubes for decompression and feeding.

D. Nursing Diagnoses and Interventions

Knowledge deficit: Disease process and treatment for hiatal hernia and reflux esophagitis

Desired outcome: Patient can verbalize knowledge of the cause and therapeutic regimen for hiatal hernia and reflux esophagitis.

    1. Assess the patient's knowledge of the disorder, its treatment, and the methods used to prevent symptoms and their complications. Provide instructions as appropriate.

    2. Explain the following methods of dietary management: eating a low-fat, high-protein diet; eating small, frequent meals; eating slowly; chewing well to avoid reflux; avoiding extremely hot or cold foods; limiting stimulants of gastric acid such as alcohol, caffeine, chocolate, spices, fruit juices, nicotine, and stress; and losing weight, if appropriate.

    3. Advise the patient to drink water after eating to cleanse the esophagus of residual food, which can be irritating to the esophageal lining.

    4. Explain the following alterations in body positions and activities: avoiding the supine position 2–3 h after eating; sleeping on the right side with the HOB elevated on 6–10 inch blocks to promote gastric emptying; and avoiding bending, coughing, lifting heavy objects, straining with bowel movements, strenuous exercise, and clothing that is too tight around the waist.

Alterations in comfort: Pain, nausea, and feeling of fullness related to gastroesophageal reflux and increase in intra-abdominal pressure

Desired outcome: Patient relates a reduction in discomfort and does not exhibit signs of uncontrolled pain.

    1. Assess and document the amount and character of the discomfort.

    2. Administer medications as prescribed.

    3. Encourage the patient to follow dietary and activity restrictions.

    4. If prescribed, insert a nasogastric tube and connect it to suction to reduce pressure on the diaphragm and relieve vomiting.

Ineffective breathing pattern related to guarding secondary to pain of thoracic incision and/or chest tube insertion

Desired outcome: Patient's respiratory rate and depth are within acceptable range.

    1. If a thoracic rather than an abdominal approach was used, chest tubes may be present. Assess the insertion site and suction apparatus for integrity, patency, function, and character of drainage. **Caution:** Be alert to the following indications of a pneumothorax: dyspnea, cyanosis, sharp chest pain. (See

"Hemothorax," p. 10–12 in Chapter 1 ("Respiratory Disorders"), for care of the patient with a chest tube.)

2. Encourage and assist patient with coughing, deep breathing, and turning q2–4h, and note quality of breath sounds, cough, and sputum.

3. Facilitate coughing and deep breathing by teaching patient how to splint incision with hands or pillow.

4. To enhance compliance with the postoperative routine, medicate patient about a half-hour prior to major moves such as ambulation and turning. Be aware that narcotics will depress respirations.

5. Reassure patient that sutures will not break and tubes will not fall out with coughing and deep breathing.

Potential for injury related to risk of gastrointestinal complications (obstruction, recurring reflux, esophageal tear, or perforation) secondary to surgery

Desired outcomes: Patient does not exhibit signs of postoperative gastrointestinal complications; or, if they do occur, they are detected and treated promptly, resulting in absence of injury. Patient can verbalize knowledge of the signs and symptoms of complications and the importance of reporting them promptly should they occur.

1. Assess the abdomen for the presence of distention, tenderness, and bowel sounds; document all findings. Bowel sounds normally reappear within 24–72 hours.

2. Instruct the patient to report reflux, a symptom that should *not* be present after fundoplication, and which may signal that the surgical wraparound is too loose. Also have the patient alert you to difficulty with swallowing, which may be indicative of a wraparound that is too tight and may lead to obstruction.

3. Patient will have an NG tube after surgery, and often it will remain in place until the esophagus has healed. Assess for patency at frequent intervals. **Caution:** Do not attempt to replace or manipulate the NG tube because esophageal perforation can occur.

4. Take measures to decrease intra-abdominal pressure, which may cause disruption of the suture line: Control nausea and/or vomiting; prohibit the use of straws, which can cause aerophagia; and introduce food and/or fluids gradually and in small amounts because the stomach will have a decreased storage capacity. When fluids are allowed, administer them in amounts < 60 mL/h, and be alert to indicators of esophageal tear (see below).

5. An esophageal tear or perforation can be a complication of the surgery. Be alert to and report the following indicators: severe midsternal pain, a drop in BP, and increases in TPR.

6. Teach the patient the signs and symptoms of the potential complications, and stress the importance of reporting them to the staff promptly should they occur.

See "Providing Nutritional Therapy" in Chapter 11 ("Metabolic Disorders"), p. 520, for nursing diagnoses and interventions for administering NG tube feedings. See "Appendix One" for nursing diagnoses and interventions for the care of preoperative and postoperative patients, pp. 528–532.

E. Patient–Family Teaching and Discharge Planning

Provide patient and SOs with verbal and written information for the following:

1. Importance of dietary management and activity restrictions.

2. Medications, including drug name, dosage, schedule, purpose, precautions, and potential side effects.

3. Indicators that signal recurrence of hernia and/or of reflux (which happens only rarely following surgery): dysphagia, hematemesis, and increased pain.

4. Importance of follow-up care; reconfirm date and time of next medical appointment.

5. Care of incision, including dressing changes. Ensure that the patient can verbalize indicators of infection, eg, increasing pain, local warmth, fever, purulent drainage, swelling, and foul odor.

6. Procedure for enteral feedings and care of tubes, if appropriate.

III. Achalasia

Achalasia (cardiospasm) is a chronic, progressive motor disorder that affects the lower two-thirds of the esophagus. It is characterized by ineffective peristalsis, a hypertonic lower esophageal sphincter (LES) that does not relax in response to swallowing, and esophageal dilation. The exact cause of achalasia is unknown, but evidence indicates there is an impairment in the innervative response of the esophagus to parasympathetic activity. Complications of achalasia include esophagitis with edema and hemorrhage, respiratory complications caused by aspiration of esophageal contents, malnutrition, and a predisposition for esophageal carcinoma. Symptoms can be potentiated by pregnancy, emotional stress, and URIs.

A. Assessment

As the disease progresses, symptoms increase in severity and frequency.

Signs and symptoms: Dysphagia, especially with cold liquids; halitosis; feeling of fullness in the chest; weight loss; and retrosternal pain during or after meals that radiates to the back, neck, and arms. In addition, regurgitation of esophageal contents can occur when the patient is horizontal, and nocturnal choking can occur during the later stages of the disorder.

B. Diagnostic Tests

Barium swallow, esophageal function studies, esophagoscopy, and biopsy may be performed.

See "Hiatal Hernia and Reflux Esophagitis," p. 275, for a description of these tests.

C. Medical Management and Surgical Interventions:

Medical management strives toward relieving symptoms caused by the LES obstruction and emptying esophageal contents.

1. **Activity/positional alterations:** Patient is instructed to remain upright after meals, wait 2–4 hours after a meal before lying down, and sleep with the HOB elevated or raised on 6–10 in. blocks. In addition, to help increase hydrostatic pressure and thereby facilitate swallowing, patients are taught to arch their back, flex the chin toward the chest, and strain (Valsalva maneuver) while swallowing.

2. **Dietary management:** Small, frequent meals. The patient is taught to eat and drink slowly in a relaxed environment; avoid rough foods and foods that can cause discomfort, such as spices, stimulants, and cold fluids; and drink fluids with meals to enhance movement of food into the stomach.

3. **Pharmacotherapy:** Steroids and non-steroidal anti-inflammatory agents are contraindicated because they can cause ulceration.

   ☐ *Vitamins and iron supplements:* To treat malnutrition and anemia.

   ☐ *Antacids:* To reduce the amount of gastric acid and relieve pain.

   ☐ *Local anesthetics/analgesics:* Before meals to minimize discomfort and promote esophageal relaxation.

4. **Mechanical esophageal dilation:** Achieved by the insertion of a graduated instrument or inflatable tube into the esophagus. This treatment provides temporary symptomatic relief of dysphagia and facilitates emptying of the esophagus.

5. **Presurgical interventions:** To correct pre-existing conditions such as anemia, malnutrition, and fluid and electrolyte disturbances. Esophageal lavage may be necessary to remove food residue in preparation for surgery.

6. **Surgical interventions:** Required in approximately 20–25% of cases. The most common procedure is an esophagomyotomy or cardiomyotomy, in which an incision is made through the muscle fibers that surround the narrowed area of the esophagus. This enables the mucosa under the muscular layers to expand and allow food to pass into the stomach unobstructed. Often, a pyloroplasty (enlargement of the pyloric sphincter) is performed in combination with the myotomy to allow rapid emptying and prevent reflux.

D. Nursing Diagnoses and Interventions

Alterations in nutrition: Less than body requirements related to decreased intake secondary to dysphagia and/or surgery

Desired outcome: Patient does not exhibit signs of malnutrition or weight loss.

1. Monitor I&O; document weight daily.
2. Administer local anesthetics/analgesics before meals as prescribed to relax the esophagus and aid ingestion.
3. Monitor for and document substances patient can and cannot swallow.
4. Provide oral hygiene before and after meals and at bedtime.
5. During the non-acute phase, provide foods that increase LES pressure, for example, proteins and complex carbohydrates.
6. Restrict or limit (as prescribed) foods and substances that decrease LES pressure, such as fats and refined carbohydrates, as well as stimulants such as chocolate, peppermint, alcohol, and tobacco.
7. Restrict or limit (as prescribed) foods that can irritate the esophageal lining, for example, coffee, citrus juices, and tomato juice, as well as all other foods known to cause patient distress.
8. Administer vitamin and iron supplements if prescribed.
9. If advised by MD, have the patient drink large amounts of water and perform the Valsalva maneuver with swallowing to promote ingestion.

Knowledge deficit: Disease process and therapeutic regimen for achalasia

Desired outcome: Patient can verbalize knowledge of the disease process and therapeutic regimen for achalasia.

1. Assess the patient's knowledge of the disorder, its treatment, and the measures used to prevent symptoms and complications. Provide information as appropriate.
2. Instruct the patient to avoid or limit the intake of foods and substances that decrease LES pressure, irritate the esophageal lining, and cause distress. Provide patient with lists of foods to eat and foods to restrict or limit.
3. Advise the patient to avoid smoking and constrictive clothing.
4. Emphasize the importance of increased nutritional intake and the precautions to take while eating. Teach the patient to eat small, frequent meals; chew thoroughly; eat slowly; and dine in a relaxed atmosphere.
5. Instruct the patient to remain upright after meals, wait 2–4 hours after meals before reclining, and sleep with the HOB elevated.
6. Provide information about how stress can precipitate the symptoms and measures that can be taken to reduce stress.

7. See **Alterations in nutrition**, p. 279, for additional information.

See "Appendix One" for nursing diagnoses and interventions for the care of preoperative and postoperative patients, pp. 528–532.

E. Patient–Family Teaching and Discharge Planning

Provide patient and SOs with verbal and written information for the following:

1. Prescribed alterations in dietary patterns.
2. Activity restrictions/precautions.
3. Medications, including drug name, dosage, schedule, purpose, precautions, and potential side effects.
4. Need for follow-up care; confirm date and time of next medical appointment.

▶ Section Two **Disorders of the Stomach and Intestines**

I. Peptic Ulcers

Peptic ulcer is an erosion of the stomach (gastric ulcer) or duodenum (duodenal ulcer). Erosions can penetrate deeply into the mucosal layers and become a chronic problem; or they can be more superficial and manifest as a more acute problem as a result of severe physiologic or psychologic trauma, infection, or shock (stress ulceration of the stomach or duodenum). Both duodenal and gastric ulcers can occur in association with high-stress lifestyle, smoking, use of irritating drugs, and secondary to other disease states. Ulceration commonly occurs as a part of Zollinger-Ellison syndrome, in which gastrinomas (gastrin-secreting tumors) of the pancreas and/or other organs develop. Gastric acid hypersecretion and ulceration subsequently occur.

Up to 25% of individuals afflicted with peptic ulcers develop complications such as hemorrhage, gastrointestinal obstruction, perforation, or intractable ulcer. With treatment, ulcer healing occurs within 4–6 weeks, but there is potential for recurrence in the same or another site.

A. Assessment

Signs and symptoms: Postprandial epigastric pain (eg, burning, gnawing, dull ache), often relieved with ingestion of food or fluids; GI bleeding, as evidenced by hematemesis or melena.

Physical exam: Tenderness over the involved area of the abdomen.

History of: Chronic or acute stress; use of irritating drugs such as caffeine, alcohol, steroids, salicylates, reserpine, indomethacin, or phenylbutazone; disorders of the endocrine glands, pancreas, or liver; and Zollinger-Ellison syndrome.

B. Diagnostic Tests

1. <u>Barium swallow (upper GI series, small bowel series):</u> Uses contrast agent (usually barium) to detect abnormalities. Patient should be kept NPO and not smoke for at least 8 hours before the test. Post-procedure care involves administration of prescribed laxatives and/or enemas to facilitate passage of the barium and prevent constipation and fecal impaction.
2. <u>Endoscopy:</u> Allows visualization of the stomach (gastroscopy), duodenum (duodenoscopy), or both (gastroduodenoscopy). Patient is kept NPO 8–12 hours before the procedure and given sedatives and anticholinergics to de-

crease GI secretions. If a local anesthetic was used, perform post-procedure assessment of the return of the gag reflex before allowing patient to eat.

3. Gastric secretion analysis: Helpful in differentiating gastric ulcer from gastric cancer. If an NG tube is passed, the stomach contents are aspirated and analyzed for the presence of blood and free hydrochloric acid. Achlorhydria (absence of free hydrochloric acid) is suggestive of gastric cancer, while mildly elevated levels suggest gastric ulcer. Excessive elevation of free hydrochloric acid occurs with Zollinger-Ellison syndrome. A tubeless gastric analysis involves administration of a gastric stimulant followed by a resin dye. A urine specimen is obtained 2 hours later and analyzed for the presence of dye. Absence of dye indicates achlorhydria. The patient is kept NPO for at least 8 hours before either test.

4. CBC: Reveals a decrease in hemoglobin and hematocrit when acute or chronic blood loss accompanies ulceration.

5. Stool guaiac test: Positive if bleeding is present.

C. Medical Management and Surgical Interventions

Conservative management is preferred over surgical intervention, with the therapy aimed at decreasing hyperacidity, healing the ulcer, relieving symptoms, and preventing complications.

1. **Activity as tolerated with adequate rest:** So that tissue repair can occur. The patient who is anemic from bleeding ulcers will require activity limitations and more assistance with ADLs.

2. **Dietary management:** Well-balanced diet with avoidance of foods that are not tolerated. A bland diet that limits spicy, irritating foods might be prescribed. Smaller, more frequent meals help to prevent symptoms. For acute episodes of upper GI hemorrhage, the patient will be NPO and given IV fluid and electrolyte replacement, with foods and fluids introduced orally as bleeding subsides.

3. **Pharmacotherapy (generally short-term and given in combination)**

   □ *Antacids:* Administered po or through an NG tube to provide symptomatic relief, facilitate ulcer healing, and prevent further ulceration; or they might be administered prophylactically in patients who are especially prone to ulceration. They are administered after meals and at bedtime, or are given periodically (q1–6h) via NG tube for patients who are intubated.

   □ *Histamine H_2 receptor antagonists:* Administered po or IV to suppress secretion of gastric acid and facilitate ulcer healing. They also can be used prophylactically for limited periods of time, especially in patients susceptible to stress ulceration.

   □ *Anticholinergics:* To suppress gastric acid secretion (not as effective as H_2 receptor antagonists).

   □ *Sucralfate:* An antiulcer agent used to treat duodenal ulcers. This drug coats the ulcer with a protective barrier so that healing can occur.

4. **NG tube with iced saline lavage:** For acute, severe GI bleeding to diminish bleeding and prevent accumulation of clotted blood.

5. **Surgical interventions:** Indicated for hemorrhage, intractable ulcers, GI obstruction, and perforation. Common surgical procedures include the following, singly or in combination:

   □ *Pyloroplasty:* Enlargement of the pyloric opening to relieve obstruction.

   □ *Vagotomy:* Severing of the branches of the vagus nerve to inhibit gastric acid secretion.

   □ *Subtotal gastrectomy:* Removal of part of the stomach with anastomosis to the duodenum (Billroth I for gastric ulcer) or removal of part of the stomach and the duodenum with anastomosis to the jejunum (Billroth II for duodenal ulcer). Vagotomy may accompany subtotal gastrectomy.

  □ *Total gastrectomy:* Removal of the entire stomach (rarely performed).

6. **Postsurgical care for gastrectomy or subtotal gastrectomy:** Involves temporary GI decompression with NG tube; analgesics for pain; temporary IV fluid and electrolyte replacement; symptomatic relief of dumping syndrome (rapid gastric emptying characterized by abdominal fullness, weakness, diaphoresis) with a low-carbohydrate, high-fat, high-protein diet, small meals without liquids, and supine position after meals; treatment of pernicious anemia (decreased production of intrinsic factor secondary to removal of part of the stomach) with B_{12} injections; and treatment with iron supplements for iron-deficiency anemia (which might occur secondary to loss of blood or iron-absorbing surface in the GI tract).

7. **Lifestyle alterations:** Such as smoking cessation, avoidance of irritating drugs, and stress reduction therapies.

See "Obstructive Processes," p. 289, for treatment of GI obstruction secondary to inflammatory edema or scar tissue formation with ulcer healing. See "Peritonitis," p. 293, for care of the patient with peritonitis due to perforation.

D. Nursing Diagnoses and Interventions

Alteration in comfort: Acute epigastric pain related to ulcerations

Desired outcomes: Patient verbalizes a reduction in discomfort and does not exhibit signs of uncontrolled pain. Patient can verbalize knowledge of foods to avoid and the importance of eating smaller, more frequent meals.

1. Assess for and document presence of pain, including its severity, character, location, duration, precipitating factors, and methods of relief.

2. Administer antacids, histamine H_2-receptor antagonists, and/or sucralfate as prescribed.

3. Advise patient to avoid irritating foods and drugs, especially those associated with the symptoms.

4. Advise patient to eat smaller, more frequent meals.

5. Provide comfort measures such as distraction, verbal interaction to allow expression of feelings and reduction of anxiety, backrubs, and stress reduction techniques.

Potential for injury related to risk of gastrointestinal complications (bleeding, obstruction, and perforation) secondary to ulcerative process

Desired outcomes: Patient does not exhibit signs of gastrointestinal complications; or, if they occur, they are detected and treated promptly, resulting in absence of injury. Patient can verbalize knowledge of necessary lifestyle alterations and demonstrates compliance with the medical therapy.

1. Teach the patient the rationale for lifestyle alterations and compliance with medical therapy to prevent exacerbation of the condition. Examples include smoking cessation, stress reduction, and avoidance of irritating foods and drugs.

2. Assess for indicators of bleeding, including hematemesis, melena, and occult blood in stool. Administer iced saline lavage as prescribed, if necessary.

3. Monitor patient for indicators of obstruction, including abdominal pain, distention, nausea and vomiting, and the inability to pass stool or flatus.

4. Be alert to indicators of peritonitis such as abdominal pain, distention and abdominal rigidity, anorexia, nausea, and vomiting.

5. Teach the patient the signs and symptoms of GI complications and the importance of reporting them promptly to the staff or MD should they occur. Notify MD of significant findings.

Alteration in comfort: Abdominal fullness, weakness, and diaphoresis related to postgastrectomy dumping syndrome

Desired outcomes: Patient relates the relief of discomfort and does not exhibit signs of uncontrolled pain. Patient can verbalize preventive measures for discomfort.

1. Advise the patient to avoid high-carbohydrate meals, which precipitate an osmotic pull of fluids into the GI tract and contribute to symptoms.

2. Advise the patient to avoid taking liquids with meals and to lie supine after meals to discourage rapid gastric emptying.

See "Appendix One" for nursing diagnoses and interventions for the care of preoperative and postoperative patients, pp. 528–532.

E. Patient–Family Teaching and Discharge Planning

Provide patient and SOs with verbal and written information for the following:

1. Importance of following the prescribed diet to facilitate ulcer healing, prevent exacerbation or recurrence, or control postsurgical dumping syndrome. If appropriate, arrange a consultation with a dietician.

2. Medications, including drug name, rationale, dosage, schedule, precautions, and potential side effects.

3. Signs and symptoms of exacerbation or recurrence, and of potential complications.

4. Care of the incision line and dressing change technique, as necessary. Teach patient about the signs of wound infection, including persistent redness, swelling, purulent drainage, local warmth, fever, and foul odor.

5. Role of lifestyle alterations in preventing exacerbation or recurrence of ulcer, including smoking cessation, stress reduction, and avoidance of irritating foods and drugs.

II. Gastric Neoplasm

The incidence of cancerous lesions of the stomach has declined in the United States (except in Hawaii) in recent years, although it continues to be a significant problem in Japan, Central and South America, Mexico, Malaysia, and parts of eastern Europe. Its incidence has been associated with dietary intake and a history of various disease processes. Because of the late appearance of the symptoms, detection is often delayed until the disease process is well advanced. Prognosis is grave, especially with late detection. Complications can include bleeding and subsequent anemia, pernicious anemia, GI obstruction, or perforation with peritonitis. Metastases can occur in the liver, bones, and lungs.

A. Assessment

Signs and symptoms: Epigastric discomfort, anorexia, bloating, nausea, vomiting, and weight loss.

Physical exam: A mass might be palpated in some patients.

History of: Excessive intake of starches, smoked foods, preservatives; chronic gastritis; adenomatous gastric polyps; pernicious anemia; surgical repair of peptic ulcer.

B. Diagnostic Tests

1. Barium swallow, gastroscopy, and gastric secretion analysis: See discussion in "Peptic Ulcers," p. 280.

2. <u>CBC:</u> Will reveal decreased hemoglobin and hematocrit when acute or chronic blood loss accompanies the neoplastic process.

3. <u>Biopsy/cytology:</u> Performed in conjunction with gastroscopy or the insertion of a gastric tube. Post-procedure care involves monitoring for bleeding by noting presence of signs such as hematemesis and melena.

C. Medical Management and Surgical Interventions

1. **Activity as tolerated.**

2. **Nutritional support:** With oral supplements, if possible, to maintain patient's weight. With significant weight loss or patient's inability to take oral feedings, parenteral nutrition might be administered. See "Providing Nutritional Therapy," p. 522, in Chapter 11.

3. **IV fluid replacement:** As necessary.

4. **If GI obstruction occurs:** Care of the patient with an obstructive process will apply. See "Obstructive Processes," p. 289.

5. **NG tube with iced saline lavage:** For acute, severe GI bleeding.

6. **NPO status:** If indicated; IV fluid and electrolyte/blood replacement therapy as necessary.

7. **Chemotherapy:** Fluorouracil, doxorubicin, and mitomycin C, which might promote tumor regression in a small percentage of patients.

8. **Radiation:** May be used to control bleeding or alleviate pain associated with bone metastasis.

9. **Analgesics** to relieve pain; **antiemetics** for symptomatic relief of nausea and vomiting.

10. **Total or subtotal gastrectomy:** Offers the best choice of cure. See description in "Peptic Ulcers," pp. 281–282.

D. Nursing Diagnoses and Interventions

Alteration in nutrition: Less than body requirements related to decreased intake secondary to nausea, vomiting, bloating, and anorexia

Desired outcome: Patient does not exhibit signs of malnutrition or weight loss.

1. Encourage smaller, more frequent feedings in a conducive environment that is free of odors.

2. Determine and offer the patient's diet preferences.

3. Administer prescribed antiemetic agents as indicated.

4. Administer prescribed IV fluids and/or nutrients (see "Providing Nutritional Therapy," p. 522, in Chapter 11).

5. Monitor and record daily weight and I&O.

See "Peptic Ulcers" for the following: **Potential for injury** related to risk of gastrointestinal complications, p. 282, and **Alteration in comfort** (related to postgastrectomy dumping syndrome), p. 283. See "Appendix One" for nursing diagnoses and interventions for the care of preoperative and postoperative patients, pp. 528–532, and for the care of patients with cancer and other life-disrupting illnesses, pp. 544–551.

E. Patient–Family Teaching and Discharge Planning

Provide patient and SOs with verbal and written information for the following:

1. Measures for symptomatic relief of pain, anorexia, nausea, vomiting, and bloating. Include appropriate use of medications, such as drug name, purpose, dosage, route, schedule, precautions, and potential side effects.

2. Indicators of complications that necessitate medical attention, including bleeding, obstruction, perforation, and exacerbation of the symptoms.

3. Care of incision line and dressing change technique, as necessary. Patient should be able to describe indicators of wound infection, including persistent redness, swelling, pain, purulent drainage, and foul odor.

4. Measures to prevent/alleviate complications of radiation and chemotherapy as necessary.

5. Referral to support person/group as indicated.

6. As appropriate, referrals to visiting nurse association (VNA), community health nurses, and hospice.

III. Malabsorption/Maldigestion

Malabsorption or maldigestion refers to a condition in which a specific nutrient or a variety of nutrients is inadequately digested and/or absorbed from the GI tract. The causes of malabsorption are varied and can include the following:

Inadequate presence of digestive substances in the GI tract. Examples are lactase enzyme deficiency, which is characterized by an inability to digest and absorb lactose, a disaccharide found in milk and dairy products; bile deficiency secondary to liver and/or gallbladder disease and/or biliary tract obstruction, which is characterized by inability to digest and absorb fats and fat-soluble vitamins; and pancreatic secretion deficiency secondary to pancreatic insufficiency or obstruction to the flow of pancreatic secretions as seen with pancreatic disorders or cystic fibrosis.

Inadequate absorptive space in the the GI tract secondary to GI surgery (especially ileal resection) and characterized by general nutrient malabsorption.

Mucosal lesions that impair absorption. Mucosal changes occur secondary to intestinal invasion of micro-organisms endemic to tropical islands (tropical sprue) or ingestion of gluten in the diet (celiac disease, nontropical sprue, gluten-induced enteropathy). Gluten-containing foods include malt, rye, barley, oats, and wheat. With Whipple's disease, which is a rare disorder, a small bowel lipodystrophy occurs, resulting in impaired absorption.

Inflammatory conditions of the GI tract such as ulcerative colitis and Crohn's disease, which involve significant diarrhea and malabsorption and deficiencies of various nutrients.

Overgrowth of microbes in the GI tract secondary to diverticula (outpouching) of the small intestine, inadequate gastric acid secretion (eg, secondary to total/partial gastrectomy), immunologic defects, gastroenteritis, blind loop syndrome, and intestinal obstruction.

Excessive use of enemas or cathartics. Complications can include specific or generalized malnutrition, fluid and electrolyte imbalances, and acid-base imbalances, any of which might require hospitalization.

A. Assessment

Signs and symptoms: Symptoms will vary, depending on the specific nutrients that are not absorbed. Patient might have unexplained weight loss with muscle atrophy, despite normal or increased appetite; diarrhea; steatorrhea (greasy, pale, foul-smelling stools); bloating; excessive flatus; abdominal cramping; and signs and symptoms of specific nutrient deficiencies (eg, anemia with iron or B_{12} deficiency, tetany with calcium deficiency, bleeding or easy bruising with calcium or vitamin K deficiency).

History of: GI surgery; excessive use of enemas or cathartics; diseases that cause diarrhea; immunologic defects; diverticulosis; liver, pancreatic, or gallbladder disease; inflammatory/infectious disorders of the intestinal tract.

B. Diagnostic Tests

1. <u>72-hour fecal fat test:</u> Increased when steatorrhea characterizes malabsorption.

2. <u>Stool culture:</u> May be diagnostic of bacterial overgrowth.

3. <u>Schilling's test:</u> Analysis of a 24-hour urine specimen collected after ingestion of radioactive B_{12} will reveal below-normal levels of vitamin B_{12}.

4. <u>D-xylose tolerance test:</u> Will show inadequate presence of xylose (an easily absorbed monosaccharide) in a 5-hour collection of urine after oral administration.

5. <u>Serum tests:</u> Will show depressed levels of carotene, calcium, magnesium, and other electrolytes and minerals.

6. <u>Lactose tolerance test:</u> Will show failure of fasting blood glucose levels to rise and the presence of abdominal symptoms after ingestion of lactose. These signs are diagnostic of lactase deficiency (lactose intolerance).

7. <u>Hydrogen breath test:</u> Will show an increase in hydrogen after ingestion of lactose. Because unabsorbed lactose is converted to hydrogen, this test is diagnostic of lactase deficiency.

8. <u>Lactulose breath test:</u> Assesses for presence of bacterial overgrowth. Nonabsorbent lactulose is administered and the breath is tested for hydrogen. With the abnormal presence of bacteria in the proximal intestine, lactulose is hydrolyzed earlier than normal.

9. <u>Barium swallow:</u> Facilitates diagnosis of the specific etiology of malabsorption. For a description, see "Peptic Ulcers," p. 280.

10. <u>Abdominal x-ray:</u> Facilitates diagnosis of the specific etiology of malabsorption; for example, pancreatic calcifications might be noted, which are suggestive of pancreatic etiology.

11. <u>Ultrasound of the abdomen:</u> Facilitates diagnosis of the specific etiology of malabsorption; for example, abnormalities of specific organs might be noted. Patient usually is NPO 8–12 hours before the procedure.

12. <u>CT scan of the abdomen:</u> Facilitates diagnosis, especially for pancreatic involvement. Patients are NPO 3–4 hours before the procedure and should be assessed ahead of time for allergy to iodine (as well as to shellfish if patient is not knowledgeable about iodine allergy). For this procedure an iodine dye is injected, and scanning is done over a 1–1½ hour period. A warm flushed feeling or burning sensation and nausea may be felt with administration of the dye, and patients are required to hold several deep breaths during scanning. Written consent of the patient is required prior to performing a CT scan.

13. <u>Small bowel biopsy:</u> For diagnosis of mucosal lesions.

14. <u>Endoscopic retrograde cholangiopancreatography (ERCP):</u> Involves the passage of an endoscope into the duodenum to the ampulla of Vater (distal end of the pancreatic and common bile duct drainage system) for visualization. A contrast medium is injected into the scope and x-rays are taken. This test is diagnostic for pancreatic disease. Patient is NPO for 8–12 hours before the test and must be assessed for allergies to iodine (and/or to shellfish) before undergoing the test. Written consent is required.

15. <u>Hormonal stimulation test:</u> Checks for pancreatic insufficiency. A collecting tube is passed into the duodenum of the NPO patient. IV secretin and/or cholecystokinin is given and the duodenal secretions are collected and analyzed for bicarbonate and trypsin levels, which are decreased with pancreatic insufficiency. Written consent is required.

Table 6-1 Sample Diet Plans

Low-Residue Diet	High-Residue Diet
Encourage intake of enriched/refined breads and cereals; rice and pasta dishes. Avoid fruits, vegetables, whole wheat products (cereals and breads).	Encourage intake of fruits, vegetables, large amounts of fluid, whole grain breads and cereals. Avoid highly refined cereals and pasta (eg, white rice, white bread, spaghetti noodles) and ice cream.

Gluten-Free Diet	
Avoid cereals and bakery products made from wheat, barley, rye, and oats. In addition, avoid the following if they contain any of the above grain products: coffee substitutes, sauces, commercially prepared luncheon meats, gravies, noodles, macaroni, spaghetti, flour tortillas, crackers, cakes, cookies, pastries, puddings, commercial ice cream and alcoholic beverages.	Use the following (if allowed): rice, corn, eggs, potatoes; breads made from rice flours, cornmeal, soybean flour, gluten-free wheat starch, and potato starch; cereals made from corn or rice (grits, corn meal mush, cooked Cream of Rice, puffed rice, rice flakes); pasta made from corn flour; homemade ice cream; tapioca pudding.

C. Medical Management and Surgical Interventions

Management will vary, depending on the specific etiology of malabsorption and the nutrient deficiencies that are exhibited.

1. **Activity as tolerated:** Patient may be fatigued and require limited activity as a consequence of diarrhea and malnutrition.

2. **Dietary management:** Will vary, depending on the specific disorder that is precipitating the malabsorption. A *low-residue diet* may be useful for controlling diarrhea. For lactase deficiency, a *low-lactose diet* (avoidance of milk and milk products) is prescribed and for nontropical sprue, a *gluten-free diet* is prescribed (see Table 6–1). Until specific problems (such as liver or gallbladder disorders) are corrected, offending foods such as fats are avoided. Any specific nutrient deficiencies are corrected. For the seriously malnourished patient, parenteral nutrition may be necessary (see "Providing Nutritional Therapy," p. 522, in Chapter 11).

3. **Pharmacotherapy:** Will vary, depending on the specific disorder that has precipitated malabsorption and the specific nutrient deficiencies.

   □ *Mineral, vitamin, and electrolyte supplements:* To correct specific deficiencies.

   □ *Antibiotics:* For treatment of bacterial overgrowth.

   □ *Cholestyramine (an antihyperlipidemic agent):* May be given to control diarrhea when it is associated with ileal resection.

4. **IV fluids and electrolytes:** As necessary to correct imbalances.

5. **Surgical intervention:** May be necessary to correct specific disorders that precipitate malabsorption, such as biliary tract obstruction.

D. Nursing Diagnoses and Interventions

Alteration in bowel elimination: Diarrhea, bloating, excessive flatus, and abdominal cramping related to specific malabsorption disorder

Desired outcome: Patient can verbalize knowledge of precipitating factors and preventive measures and relates a reduction in symptoms.

1. Assess and document presence of GI discomfort and symptoms, including the onset and duration of symptoms and the precipitating and palliative factors. Instruct patient to avoid foods associated with symptoms.

2. Teach the patient about the importance of dietary compliance in the treatment for some malabsorptive disorders. For example, dietary restriction (eg, low-lactose diet with lactase intolerance or gluten-free diet with nontropical sprue) may be necessary to prevent symptoms.

Fluid volume deficit related to increased need secondary to impaired absorption and/or abnormal loss secondary to diarrhea

Desired outcomes: Patient does not exhibit signs of dehydration. Patient demonstrates compliance with the prescribed dietary regimen.

1. Assess patient for evidence of fluid volume deficit: weight loss, hypotension, poor skin turgor, dry skin and mucous membranes, and thirst.

2. Ensure precise maintenance and assessment of fluid I&O records.

3. Administer IV fluids and parenteral nutrients appropriately and at prescribed rate.

4. Encourage prescribed dietary compliance for relief of symptomatic diarrhea.

5. Administer medications and/or teach patient self-administration of medications to control diarrhea and/or treat underlying condition.

▶ **Note:** For assessment of nutrient deficiencies, dehydration, and acid–base imbalances and nursing diagnoses and interventions for delivering parenteral nutrition, see Chapter 11, "Metabolic Disorders," p. 498.

E. Patient–Family Teaching and Discharge Planning

Provide patient and SOs with verbal and written information for the following:

1. Use of medications (vitamins, antibiotics), including drug name, purpose, dosage, schedule, precautions, and potential side effects.

2. Prescribed dietary replacement of deficient nutrients and/or dietary management of symptoms, if appropriate.

3. Problems that necessitate medical attention: nutrient deficiencies, dehydration, acid–base imbalances. (Review Chapter 11, "Metabolic Disorders," p. 513, for guidelines.)

IV. Obstructive Processes

Obstruction of the GI tract is a condition in which the normal peristaltic transport of GI contents does not take place. Therefore, digestion and absorption of foods and fluids and the elimination of wastes are impaired or totally blocked. Furthermore, GI fluids become hypertonic, precipitating osmotic fluid loss from the body into the GI lumen. Subsequently, nutritional and fluid and electrolyte status are compromised and distention occurs. Increased pressure in the GI tract also can result in perforation and/or peritonitis and/or strangulation with necrosis. Obstruction can occur anywhere along the GI tract, but most commonly it occurs at the pyloric area of the stomach or in the small or large intestine. Obstruction can occur as a result of the inflammation and edema that accompany GI disease (peptic ulcers, diverticulitis, colitis, gastroenteritis, trauma); GI surgery with subsequent edema and possibly adhesions (gastrectomy, appendectomy, colon resection); growths (polyps, tumors); adynamic (paralytic) ileus secondary to peritoneal insult such as surgery or peritonitis; volvulus; or incarcerated hernia.

A. Assessment

Signs and symptoms: Abdominal pain and distention, nausea and vomiting, hiccoughs, and inability to pass stool or flatus. With partial obstruction, however, diarrhea might be present.

Physical exam: Distention, poor skin turgor, dry skin and mucous membranes; and borborygmus with peristaltic rushes (periodic loud bursts of noise) noted on auscultation of abdomen. With paralytic ileus, bowel sounds will be absent or diminished.

History of: Abdominal hernia, recent or past abdominal surgery, GI inflammation or perforation secondary to various disease processes (see above).

B. Diagnostic Tests

1. <u>WBC count:</u> Usually elevated in the presence of strangulation.

2. <u>X-ray of abdomen:</u> Will reveal distention of bowel loops, with air and fluid proximal to the obstruction.

3. <u>Barium swallow/barium enema:</u> Used with caution in selected cases to facilitate diagnosis. (See "Peptic Ulcers," p. 280.)

C. Medical Management and Surgical Interventions

Management is supportive and aimed at identifying specific cause of obstruction so that appropriate treatment can be instituted.

1. **Activity as tolerated:** With paralytic ileus, the patient is encouraged to ambulate to enhance return of peristalsis.

2. **GI decompression:** Accomplished with NG or intestinal tube, depending on site of obstruction. The tube is usually attached to intermittent, low suction and the patient is NPO.

3. **IV fluid and electrolyte support.**

4. **Pharmacotherapy:** May include the following:

   □ *Antibiotics:* To prevent infection.

   □ *Analgesics:* For pain relief. However, they can mask symptoms and interfere with diagnosis.

   □ *Antiemetic agents:* For relief of nausea and vomiting.

5. **Surgical intervention:** Indicated for obstruction that does not subside. In some cases, inflammatory processes subside and obstruction resolves without surgery. Paralytic ileus generally resolves in 2–3 days without any treatment. In most cases, surgery is indicated to identify and/or relieve the source of obstruction. Exploratory laparatomy is performed when diagnosis is uncertain. When diagnosis is known, the indicated surgery is performed, for example, pyloroplasty or colon resection with removal of tumor or adhesions.

D. Nursing Diagnoses and Interventions

Alteration in comfort: Nausea, distention, and pain related to abdominal visceral disorder and gastrointestinal obstructive process

Desired outcome: Patient relates a reduction in discomfort and does not exhibit signs of uncontrolled pain.

1. Implement comfort measures to provide pain relief: distraction, backrubs, conversation, relaxation therapy.

2. Administer prescribed analgesics and antiemetic agents as indicated.

3. Maintain patency and proper functioning of the gastric tube.

Fluid volume deficit related to abnormal losses secondary to vomiting and/or gastric decompression of large volumes of GI fluids and decreased intake secondary to fluid restrictions

Desired outcome: Patient does not exhibit signs of dehydration.

1. Ensure precise measurement and assessment of fluid I&O records. Take special note of the amount of GI aspirate.
2. Administer appropriate IV fluids at the prescribed rate. Replace volume of GI fluids aspirated by suction, if prescribed.
3. For other interventions, see the same nursing diagnosis in "Appendix One," "Caring for Preoperative and Postoperative Patients," p. 529.

For nursing diagnoses and interventions for the delivery of enteral and parenteral nutrition, see "Providing Nutritional Therapy" in Chapter 11, "Metabolic Disorders," p. 520. If surgery is performed, see "Appendix One," "Caring for Preoperative and Postoperative Patients," pp. 528–532.

E. Patient–Family Teaching and Discharge Planning

Provide patient and SOs with verbal and written information for the following:

1. Specific disease process that precipitated the obstruction and methods to prevent recurrence, such as compliance with prescribed therapies.
2. Symptoms of obstruction to report to MD.
3. Medications, including drug name, purpose, dosage, schedule, precautions, and potential side effects.

V. Hernia

A hernia is a protrusion of the intestine through the abdominal wall. Although a hernia can occur secondary to a congenital weakness in the abdominal wall, most commonly it occurs as a consequence of disease, old age, increased abdominal pressure, or disruption of the abdominal wall secondary to trauma or surgery (incisional hernia). Hernias can develop at the umbilicus, inguinal opening (most common), femoral ring, or at a previous surgical or trauma site. They can be precipitated or aggravated by those factors related to an increase in intra-abdominal pressure such as lifting, sneezing, coughing, straining at stool, pregnancy, and obesity. Potential complications include strangulation of the protruding bowel, which can result in necrosis and/or infection; and incarceration, with subsequent intestinal obstruction.

A. Assessment

Signs and symptoms: Tenderness and bulging at herniation site; pain with straining.

Physical exam: Bulge with straining will be noted on inspection; palpation of herniation site will reveal a soft and tender mass or bulge. In men, the scrotum should be examined whenever a hernia is diagosed or suspected because herniation at the inguinal area can cause herniation of bowel into the scrotum.

B. Diagnostic Test

X-ray: May reveal presence of a hernia or incarceration. However, diagnosis is made primarily through physical exam.

C. Medical Management and Surgical Interventions

Management is aimed at reduction of the hernia (placement of herniated area back through the abdominal wall) and prevention of strangulation and incarceration.

1. **Activity as tolerated:** With restriction of stretching and straining, and emphasis on proper body mechanics.
2. **Manual reduction:** Placement of the herniated area back to its anatomically correct position. The patient is usually placed in Trendelenburg's position and given sedatives/relaxants to facilitate the procedure.
3. **Truss (firm support):** Might be prescribed for applying pressure to the herniated area to maintain correct anatomic position.

4. **High-residue diet:** To prevent constipation and straining with stools.
5. **Stool softeners and cathartics:** May be prescribed to prevent constipation and straining.
6. **Antibiotics:** Usually prescribed in the presence of strangulation and infection.
7. **With incarceration:** Care of the patient with an obstructive process will apply (see p. 289).
8. **Herniorrhaphy:** Surgery performed when the hernia is irreducible by other means, or when strangulation or incarceration occurs. It is performed under general or regional anesthesia, and often is done on an outpatient basis. Minimal dietary and activity restrictions are necessary.

D. Nursing Diagnoses and Interventions

Alteration in comfort: Pain (especially with straining) related to hernia condition and/or surgical intervention

Desired outcomes: Patient relates a reduction in discomfort and does not exhibit signs of uncontrolled pain. Patient can verbalize knowledge of activities that can worsen the condition and demonstrates splinting of the incision, use of a truss, and application of scrotal support or ice packs, if appropriate.

1. Assess and document presence of pain: severity, character, location, duration, precipitating factors, and methods of relief. Report presence of severe, persistent pain, which can signal complications.
2. Advise patient to avoid straining, stretching, coughing, and heavy lifting. Teach patient to splint incision manually or with a pillow during coughing episodes. This is especially important during the early postoperative period and for up to six weeks after surgery.
3. Teach patient the use of a truss, if prescribed, and advise its use as much as possible, especially when out of bed.
4. Apply or teach patient application of scrotal support or ice packs, which are often prescribed to limit edema and control pain after inguinal hernia repair.
5. Administer prescribed analgesics as indicated, especially before postoperative activities. Use comfort measures as well: distraction, verbal interaction to enhance expressions of feelings and reduction of anxiety, backrubs, and stress reduction techniques such as relaxation exercises.

Knowledge deficit: Potential for gastrointestinal complications and measures that can prevent their occurrence

Desired outcome: Patient can verbalize knowledge of the signs and symptoms of gastrointestinal complications and complies with the prescribed measures for prevention.

1. Teach patient to be alert to and report severe and persistent pain, nausea and vomiting, fever, and abdominal distention, which can herald onset of incarceration or strangulation.
2. Encourage patient to comply with medical regimen: use of a truss or other support and avoidance of straining, stretching, constipation, and heavy lifting.
3. Teach the patient to consume a high-residue diet to prevent constipation (see Table 6–1, p. 287). Encourage the intake of at least 2–3 L/day of fluids to promote soft consistency of stools.

See "Appendix One" for nursing diagnoses and interventions for the care of preoperative and postoperative patients, pp. 528–532.

E. Patient–Family Teaching and Discharge Planning

Provide patient and SOs with verbal and written information for the following:

1. Care of incision and dressing change technique, if appropriate. Teach patient the signs of infection at the incision site that require medical intervention: persistent redness, swelling, local warmth, tenderness, purulent drainage, and foul odor.

2. Symptoms of hernia recurrence and postsurgical complications.

3. Postsurgical activity limitations as directed: usually heavy lifting (>5 lb) and straining are contraindicated for about 6 weeks.

4. Importance of proper body mechanics to prevent recurrence, especially when lifting and moving.

5. Prevention of constipation and straining with stools, for example, by following a high-residue diet and using stool softeners and cathartics when needed.

6. Medications, including drug name, purpose, dosage, schedule, precautions, and potential side effects.

VI. Peritonitis

Peritonitis is the inflammatory response of the peritoneum to offending chemical and bacterial agents invading the peritoneal cavity. The inflammatory process can be local or generalized and acute or chronic, depending on the etiology and pathogenesis of the inflammation. Common causes include intraoperative and abdominal trauma; postoperative leakage into the peritoneal cavity; ischemia; ruptured or inflamed organs; poor aseptic techniques, for example, with peritoneal dialysis; and direct contamination of the bloodstream. The peritoneum responds to invasive agents by attempting to localize the infection, which results in tissue edema, the development of fibrinous exudate, and hypermotility of the intestinal tract. As the disease progresses, paralytic ileus occurs, and intestinal fluid, which then cannot be reabsorbed, leaks into the peritoneal cavity. As a result of the fluid shift, cardiac output and tissue perfusion are reduced, and this leads to hypoxia and sepsis. If the infection continues, respiratory failure and shock can ensue. Peritonitis is frequently progressive and can be fatal. It is the most common cause of death following abdominal surgery.

A. Assessment

Signs and symptoms: Abdominal pain, nausea, vomiting, fever, malaise, weakness, prostration, hiccoughs, diaphoresis.

Physical exam: Presence of tachycardia, hypotension, and shallow and rapid respirations caused by abdominal distention and discomfort. Often, the patient assumes a supine position with the knees flexed. On abdominal exam, palpation usually reveals distention and abdominal rigidity with general or localized tenderness (often rebound). Auscultation findings include hyperactive bowel sounds during the gradual development of the peritonitis and an absence of bowel sounds during later stages if paralytic ileus occurs.

History of: Abdominal illness, trauma, surgery, peritoneal dialysis.

B. Diagnostic Tests

1. Serum tests: May reveal the presence of leukocytosis, hemoconcentration, and electrolyte imbalance.

2. ABGs: May reveal the presence of hypoxemia.

3. Urinalysis: Often performed to rule out genitourinary involvement.

4. Peritoneal aspiration with culture and sensitivity: May be performed to determine the presence of blood, bacteria, bile, pus, and amylase content and identify the causative organism.

5. <u>Abdominal x-rays:</u> May be performed to determine the presence of abnormal levels of fluid and gas, which usually collect in the large and small bowels.

C. Medical Management and Surgical Interventions

1. **Bed rest:** With patient in semi- or high Fowler's position to enhance fluid shift to the lower abdomen, which will reduce pressure on the diaphragm and allow for deeper and easier respirations.

2. **NG or intestinal tube:** Inserted to reduce or prevent gastrointestinal distention or ileus and promote intestinal function.

3. **IV fluids, electrolyte therapy, and parenteral feedings:** To correct fluid, electrolyte, and nutritional disorders. Daily measurements of serum electrolytes and calculations of fluid volume are performed to determine the necessary types of fluids and electrolyte replacement. Plasma, protein, and blood may be administered to correct hypovolemia, hypoproteinemia, and anemia. Patient is NPO during the acute phase, and oral fluids are not resumed until the patient has passed flatus and the gastric tube has been removed.

4. **CVP catheter:** May be inserted to monitor circulatory status in the critically ill patient.

5. **Parenteral antibiotic therapy.**

6. **Oxygen:** Often prescribed to treat hypoxia and intestinal anoxia.

7. **Narcotics and sedatives:** To relieve severe pain and discomfort once the diagnosis has been confirmed.

8. **Surgical intervention:** May be required to remove the source of infection or drain the abscess and accumulated fluids. This can include the removal of an organ such as the appendix or gallbladder. Drains are usually inserted to remove purulent drainage and excessive fluids. Intestinal decompression may be employed to decrease massive abdominal distention. Intraoperative and postoperative irrigation may be indicated if there has been gross contamination of the peritoneal cavity with bowel contents.

D. Nursing Diagnoses and Interventions

Alterations in comfort: Pain, abdominal distention, and nausea related to the inflammatory process

Desired outcome: Patient relates a reduction in discomfort and does not exhibit signs of uncontrolled pain.

1. Assess and document character and severity of the pain.

2. Once the diagnosis has been made, administer narcotics, analgesics, and sedatives as prescribed to promote comfort and rest.

3. Keep patient on bed rest to minimize pain, which can be aggravated by activity; provide a restful and quiet environment.

4. Explain all procedures to patient to help minimize anxiety, which can augment discomfort.

5. Offer mouth care and lip moisturizers at frequent intervals to help relieve discomfort/nausea from continuous suction, dehydration, and NPO status.

Alteration in respiratory function related to diminished oxygen transport secondary to loss of circulating volume and/or guarding secondary to severe abdominal pain

Desired outcome: Patient does not exhibit signs of respiratory dysfunction.

1. Monitor ABG results and be alert to indicators of hypoxemia, including low PaO_2 and to the following clinical signs: hypotension, tachycardia, hyperventilation, restlessness, CNS depression, and possibly cyanosis.

2. Auscultate lung fields to assess ventilation and detect pulmonary complications. Note and document the presence of adventitious sounds.

3. Keep patient in semi- or high Fowler's position to aid respiratory effort; encourage deep breathing to enhance oxygenation.

4. Administer oxygen as prescribed.

Potential for injury related to risk of GI complications secondary to inflammatory process

Desired outcome: A worsening condition is detected promptly, resulting in immediate medical treatment and absence of injury to the patient.

1. Assess the abdomen q1–2h during the acute phase and q4h once the patient is stabilized. Monitor for increasing distention by measuring abdominal girth. Auscultate bowel sounds to assess motility. They are often frequent during the beginning phase of peritonitis, but are absent in the presence of paralytic ileus. *Lightly* palpate the abdomen for evidence of increasing rigidity and/or tenderness, which is indicative of disease progression. Notify MD of significant findings.

2. If prescribed, insert NG tube and connect it to suction to prevent or decrease distention.

Alteration in nutrition: Less than body requirements related to losses secondary to vomiting and intestinal suctioning and increased need secondary to GI dysfunction (septic peritonitis)

Desired outcomes: Patient does not exhibit signs of malnutrition. Patient demonstrates adequate oral intake of nutrients once gastric motility has returned.

1. Keep patient NPO as prescribed during acute phase of the disorder. Reintroduce oral fluids gradually once motility has returned, as evidenced by presence of bowel sounds, decreased distention, and passing of flatus.

2. Administer replacement fluids, electrolytes, vitamins, and protein as prescribed.

Potential for injury related to risk of septic shock secondary to infectious process

Desired outcomes: Patient does not exhibit signs of septic shock; or, if they appear, they are detected promptly, resulting in immediate treatment and absence of injury.

1. Perform comprehensive physical assessments at frequent intervals. Monitor VS (at least q4h, and more frequently if patient's condition is unstable), and be alert to elevated temperature, hypotension, tachycardia, and shallow and rapid respirations, which can occur with sepsis. Also evaluate circulatory status. In the early stages of shock, the skin is usually warm, pink, and dry because of peripheral venous pooling. In later stages, the BP and CVP start to drop and the extremities become cold and pale because of the lack of tissue perfusion.

2. Administer antibiotics promptly as prescribed.

3. Monitor CBC for for an increase in WBC count, which occurs with infection; and for hemoconcentration, which occurs with a decrease in plasma volume. Notify MD of all significant findings.

4. If abdominal surgery has been performed, maintain sterile technique with dressing changes and all invasive procedures.

See "Appendix One" for nursing diagnoses and interventions for the care of preoperative and postoperative patients, pp. 528–532. See "Providing Nutritional Therapy" in Chapter 11, "Metabolic Disorders," p. 520, for the care of patients on tube or parenteral feedings.

E. Patient–Family Teaching and Discharge Planning

Provide patient and SOs with verbal and written information for the following:

1. Medications, including the drug name, dosage, schedule, purpose, precautions, and potential side effects.

2. Activity precautions as prescribed by MD, such as avoiding heavy lifting (>5 lb), resting after periods of fatigue, getting maximum amounts of rest, gradually increasing activities to tolerance.

3. Notifying MD of the following indicators of recurrence: fever, chills, abdominal pain, vomiting, abdominal distention.

4. If patient has undergone surgery, the indicators of wound infection: fever, pain, chills, incisional swelling, persistent redness, purulent drainage.

5. Importance of follow-up medical care; confirm date and time of next medical appointment.

VII. Appendicitis

Appendicitis is the most commonly occurring inflammatory lesion of the bowel and one of the most frequent reasons for abdominal surgery. The appendix is a blind, narrow tube that extends from the inferior portion of the cecum and does not serve any useful function. Appendicitis is usually caused by obstruction of the appendiceal lumen by a fecalith (hardened bit of fecal material), inflammation, a foreign body, or a neoplasm. Obstruction prevents drainage of secretions that are produced by epithelial cells in the lumen, thereby increasing intraluminal pressure and compressing mucosal blood vessels. This tension causes impaired viability, which can lead to necrosis and perforation. Inflammation and infection result from normal bacteria invading the devitalized wall. Mild cases of appendicitis can heal spontaneously, but severe inflammation can lead to a ruptured appendix, which can cause local or generalized peritonitis (see "Peritonitis," p. 292).

A. Assessment

Signs and symptoms: Vary because of differences in anatomy, size, and age.

□ *Early stage:* Abdominal pain (either epigastric or umbilical) that is vague and diffuse and later becomes generalized; nausea and vomiting.

□ *Intermediate, "acute" stage:* Pain that shifts from epigastrium to RLQ at McBurney's point (halfway between umbilicus and right iliac crest) and is aggravated by walking or coughing. Anorexia, malaise, constipation (or occasionally, diarrhea), and diminished or absent peristalsis also can occur.

□ *Acute appendicitis with perforation:* Increasing, generalized pain; recurrence of vomiting.

Physical exam

□ *Intermediate, "acute" stage:* Pain in RLQ elicited by light palpation of abdomen; presence of rebound tenderness; RLQ guarding, rigidity, and muscle spasms; tachycardia; fever; absent or diminished bowel sounds; pain elicited with rectal exam. A palpable, tender mass may be felt in the peritoneal pouch if the appendix lies within the pelvis.

□ *Acute appendicitis with perforation:* Increasing fever; generalized abdominal rigidity. Typically, patient remains still or rigid in either a side-lying or supine position with flexed knees. Presence of abscess can result in a tender, palpable mass.

B. Diagnostic Tests

1. <u>WBC with differential:</u> Will reveal presence of leukocytosis and an increase in neutrophils.

2. <u>Urinalysis:</u> To rule out genitourinary conditions mimicking appendicitis; may reveal microscopic hematuria and pyuria.

3. <u>Abdominal x-ray:</u> May reveal presence of a fecalith.

4. <u>IVP:</u> May be performed to rule out ureteral stone or pyelitis.

C. Medical Management and Surgical Interventions

Preoperative care:

1. **Bed rest:** For observation.

2. **NPO status:** Parenteral fluids are begun if surgery is imminent.

3. **Pharmacologic therapy:** Narcotics are avoided until diagnosis is certain because they mask clinical signs and symptoms.

   □ *Antibiotics:* To prevent systemic infection.

   □ *Tranquilizing agents:* For sedation.

4. **Ice packs:** May be used for some patients to help relieve pain and decrease blood flow to the area, impeding inflammatory response. **Note:** Local applications of heat are contraindicated because heat can cause the appendix to rupture.

5. **NG tube:** Inserted for gastric suction and lavage, if needed. **Note:** Cathartics and enemas are contraindicated because they increase peristalsis and can cause perforation.

Surgery:

6. **Appendectomy:** Performed as soon as the diagnosis is confirmed and fluid imbalance and systemic reactions have been controlled. The appendix is removed through an incision made over McBurney's point or through a right paramedial incision. In the presence of abscess, rupture, or peritonitis, an incisional drain is inserted.

Postoperative care:

7. **Activities:** Ambulation begins either the day of surgery, or the first postoperative day; normal activities are resumed 2–3 weeks after surgery.

8. **Diet:** Advances from clear liquids to soft solids during the second through fifth postoperative day; parenteral fluids are continued if required.

9. **Pharmacotherapy**

   □ *Antibiotics:* Continued in the presence of infection.

   □ *Mild laxatives:* Given, if necessary; but enemas continue to be contraindicated during the first few postoperative weeks until adequate healing has occurred and bowel function has been restored.

   □ *Analgesics:* For postoperative pain.

D. Nursing Diagnoses and Interventions

Potential for infection related to risk of rupture, peritonitis, and abscess formation secondary to inflammatory process

Desired outcomes: Patient does not exhibit signs of infection; or, if they appear, they are detected and reported promptly, resulting in immediate treatment. Patient can verbalize the rationale for not administering enemas or laxatives preoperatively and enemas postoperatively, and demonstrates compliance with the therapeutic regimen.

1. Assess and document quality, location, and duration of pain. Be alert to pain that becomes accentuated and generalized or to the presence of recurrent vomiting, and note whether patient assumes side-lying or supine position with flexed knees. Any of these can signal impending rupture.

2. Monitor VS for elevated temperature, increased pulse rate, hypotension, and shallow/rapid respirations; and assess the abdomen for presence of rigidity, distention, and decreased or absent bowel sounds, any of which can occur with rupture. Report significant findings to MD.

3. Caution patient about the danger of preoperative self-treatment with enemas and laxatives because they increase peristalsis, which increases the risk of perforation. If constipation occurs postoperatively, MD may prescribe hs laxatives/stool softeners after the third day. Remind patient that enemas should be avoided until approved by MD (usually several weeks after surgery).

See "Peritonitis," p. 292, for more information.

Alteration in comfort: Acute pain and nausea related to the inflammatory process

Desired outcome: Patient verbalizes a reduction in discomfort and does not exhibit signs of uncontrolled pain.

1. Assess and document quality, location, and duration of pain.

2. Medicate patient with antiemetics, sedatives, and analgesics as prescribed; evaluate and document response.

3. Preoperatively, apply ice packs to RLQ as prescribed.

4. Keep patient NPO before surgery; after surgery, nausea and vomiting usually disappear. If prescribed, insert NG tube for decompression.

5. Teach technique for slow, diaphragmatic breathing to reduce stress and help relax tense muscles.

See "Appendix One" for nursing diagnoses and interventions for the care of preoperative and postoperative patients, pp. 528–532.

E. Patient—Family Teaching and Discharge Planning

Provide patient and SOs with verbal and written information for the following:

1. Medications, including drug name, dosage, purpose, schedule, precautions, and potential side effects.

2. Care of incision, including dressing changes and bathing restrictions, if appropriate.

3. Indicators of infection: fever, chills, incisional pain, redness, swelling, and purulent drainage.

4. Postsurgical activity precautions: Avoid lifting heavy objects (>5 lb) for the first six weeks or as directed, be alert to and rest after symptoms of fatigue, get maximum rest, gradually increase activities to tolerance.

5. Importance of avoiding enemas for the first few postoperative weeks.

VIII. Hemorrhoids

Hemorrhoids are distended, tortuous veins found in the rectum and anus. Internal hemorrhoids are found proximal to the anal sphincter and are not visible unless they become large enough to protrude through the anus. External hemorrhoids are distal to the anal sphincter and can become thrombosed if the vein ruptures. Hemorrhoids are caused by conditions that precipitate increased intra-abdominal pressure and/or obstruct venous return, for example, pregnancy, chronic constipation, portal hypertension, infiltrating carcinoma, physical exertion, infection, and ulcerative colitis.

A. Assessment

Internal hemorrhoids: Bleeding with defecation, anemia if blood loss occurs over an extended period of time, narrowing of stool, mucus discharge. Discomfort is minimal.

External hemorrhoids: Perianal pain and itching, bleeding, and intense pain if a vein ruptures and thromboses.

Physical exam: Detection of internal hemorrhoids with proctoscopy and digital palpation; grapelike appearance of external hemorrhoids on inspection.

Risk factors: Diet low in fiber, obesity, long-term constipation and straining, lifestyle or career that requires constant sitting or standing.

B. Diagnostic Tests

1. Stool guaiac test: To assess for the presence of blood.
2. CBC: To assess for anemia from chronic blood loss.

C. Medical Management and Surgical Interventions

1. **Regulation of bowel movements:** Bulk cathartic, stool softener, high-fiber diet, exercise, augmenting fluid intake.
2. **Treat pain and itching:** Warm or cold compresses and warm sitz baths.
3. **Pharmacotherapy:** *Topical anesthetics* such as dibucaine hydrochloride (Nupercainal) ointment, *astringents* such as witch Hazel (Tucks) pads, and *anti-inflammatory preparations* such as hydrocortisone ointment to relieve pain and itching and shrink mucous membranes.
4. **Manual reduction of prolapsed and strangulated hemorrhoids:** Returning hemorrhoid to rectum with a lubricated, gloved finger.
5. **Sclerosing agent:** Injection into the submucosal tissue surrounding the hemorrhoids to produce an inflammatory response, which leads to tissue shrinkage. This is a palliative and temporary measure.
6. **Rubber band ligation:** Nonsurgical method of constricting the circulation of the hemorrhoid and causing tissue necrosis, separation, and sloughing to occur.
7. **Incision and drainage:** To remove clots from thrombosed hemorrhoids. This is performed on an outpatient basis, using a local anesthetic.
8. **Hemorrhoidectomy:** Removal by cautery, clamp, or excision, of hemorrhoids that do not respond to the above therapies.

D. Nursing Diagnoses and Interventions

Alteration in comfort: Postoperative pain and itching

Desired outcome: Patient relates a reduction in discomfort and does not exhibit signs of uncontrolled pain.

1. Administer topical anesthetics, astringents, and anti-inflammatory preparations as prescribed.
2. Administer cold or warm compresses to rectal area. Provide warm sitz baths 3–4 times a day, or as prescribed. **Caution:** Be alert to hypotension, which can be caused by the dilation of pelvic blood vessels.
3. Administer narcotics for severe postoperative pain as prescribed.
4. Ensure that the patient takes stool softeners during the early postoperative period in preparation for the first bowel movement; administer oil-retention enema if prescribed.
5. If indicated, position a flotation pad under the buttocks for comfort.

Doughnut-shaped cushions are contraindicated because they can increase rather than decrease pressure at the operative site.

6. Provide warm sitz baths after each bowel movement to minimize discomfort and promote healing.

Alteration in bowel elimination: Constipation related to fear of pain with postoperative defecation

Desired outcomes: Patient has bowel movements without straining during the early postoperative period. Patient can verbalize the rationale for the importance of postoperative bowel movements and complies with the therapeutic regimen.

1. Explain to patient that discomfort is common with the first bowel movements after surgery.

2. Administer stool softeners and bulk cathartics as prescribed. Administer analgesic ½–1 hour before the patient attempts defecation.

3. Encourage ambulation the day of surgery or first postoperative day to enhance peristalsis.

4. In nonrestricted patients encourage fluid intake of at least 2–3 L/day to help soften stools and promote elimination.

5. Document the first bowel movement, which should occur by the third or fourth postoperative day. Stay with the patient or stand just outside the bathroom door because dizziness and fainting are common at this time due to dilation of the pelvic blood vessels. Record the amount and character of the stool and the patient's response.

6. If the patient avoids having a bowel movement after surgery because of anticipated pain, explain that a normal postsurgical bowel movement will prevent complications such as constriction of the anal lumen.

Alteration in pattern of urinary elimination: Anuria or dysuria related to local swelling and/or presence of rectal packing secondary to hemorrhoidectomy

Desired outcome: Patient relates the resumption of the normal pattern of voiding.

1. If patient has difficulty voiding in the early postoperative period because of local swelling and/or rectal packing, encourage patient to get out of bed to void.

2. Encourage sitz baths or warm showers, which stimulate the voiding reflex.

Potential fluid volume deficit related to abnormal blood loss secondary to slipped ligatures

Desired outcomes: Patient can verbalize knowledge of the therapeutic and preventive measures for healing of the operative site and does not exhibit signs of abnormal bleeding or hypovolemia.

1. Hemorrhage can result from a slipped ligature, yet the bleeding can easily go undetected. Be alert to the presence of pallor, diaphoresis, hypotension, and increasing pulse and respiration rates. If bleeding does occur, be prepared to assist MD with insertion of a Foley catheter into the rectum and inflation of balloon to provide pressure to bleeding site.

2. Assess for rectal bleeding. After surgery and into the first or second postoperative day, the patient will have rectal packing. Inspect the perianal area for evidence of fresh bleeding. After MD removes the packing, replace the perianal dressing (typically a sanitary napkin) as necessary. Be alert to excess bleeding, as evidenced by >2 saturated pads in 8 hours. Query patient about the presence of a frequent, unrelieved urge to defecate, which can signal sequestered hemorrhage.

3. Advise patient to avoid straining or sitting on the toilet longer than necessary.

4. Instruct patient to keep perianal area clean but to avoid vigorous wiping after bowel movement. *Moist* perineal wipes should be used to cleanse the area. Encourage sitz baths after every bowel movement to cleanse the rectal area and relieve local irritation. Be alert to hypotension, which can be caused by dilation of pelvic blood vessels.

5. As appropriate, advise the patient to abstain from anal intercourse until proper healing has taken place and it is approved by MD.

6. Explain to patient that some bleeding can be expected about 8–12 days postoperatively when the sutures begin to dissolve.

Knowledge deficit: Potential for recurrence of hemorrhoids and measures that help prevent it

Desired outcome: Patient can verbalize knowledge of the potential for recurrence and can list preventive measures.

1. Advise patient to use mild, bulk cathartics and/or stool softeners if constipation recurs and to avoid straining with defecation.

2. Encourage a diet high in fiber content such as whole grain products (breads, cooked grains, and cereals), apples, peas, and kidney and other dried beans.

3. For nonrestricted patients, explain that a minimum fluid intake of 2–3 L/day is necessary to soften the stool and promote elimination.

4. Encourage daily exercise, which enhances peristalsis and promotes elimination. Advise patient to avoid prolonged standing and sitting.

See "Appendix One" for nursing diagnoses and interventions for the care of preoperative and postoperative patients, pp. 528–532.

E. Patient–Family Teaching and Discharge Planning

Provide patient and SOs with verbal and written information for the following:

1. Medications, including drug name, dosage, schedule, purpose, precautions, and potential side effects.

2. Methods for preventing constipation such as exercise, diet high in fiber content, augmenting fluid intake, and taking stool softeners or mild, bulk cathartics if necessary.

3. Postoperative activity precautions as directed: Avoid fatigue, get maximum rest, gradually increase activities to tolerance.

4. Awareness that some bleeding can occur about 8–12 days postoperatively, when sutures begin to dissolve.

▶ Section Three   **Intestinal Neoplasms and Inflammatory Processes**

I. Diverticulosis/Diverticulitis

Diverticulosis is acquired small pouches or sacs (diverticula) in the colon formed by the herniation of mucosal and submucosal linings through the muscular layers of the intestine. Although diverticula can be found anywhere in the colon, they are seen most frequently in the sigmoid colon. It is theorized that diverticula develop secondary to a low-residue diet and increased intracolonic pressure, such as that created with straining to have a bowel movement.

Diverticulitis is a complication of diverticulosis, and it occurs when one or more diverticula perforate through the bowel wall, resulting in inflammation and infection, which can include peritonitis. If untreated, death can ensue.

A. Assessment

Diverticulosis: Lower GI bleeding and/or symptoms of irritable bowel syndrome such as steady or crampy abdominal pain in the LLQ, associated with constipation or diarrhea and increased flatulence. The patient may be asymptomatic.

Diverticulitis: See the above indicators. In addition, fever, nausea, vomiting, and obstipation can be present if obstruction and/or peritonitis occur. Fistulas to the bladder, vagina, or skin, and gas or stool elimination from the involved site also may be present.

Physical exam: Presence of tender, palpable mass, usually in the LLQ; rebound tenderness secondary to infection and/or abscess formation; abdominal distention, hypoactive or hyperactive bowel sounds; and possibly, absence of stool felt on rectal examination. Tachycardia, hypotension, and shallow respirations can be present if there is severe abdominal discomfort. Often the patient assumes a side-lying position with the knees flexed to relieve pain.

B. Diagnostic Tests

Diverticulosis:

1. Barium enema: To determine presence and number of diverticula.
2. CBC: To determine if anemia is present.
3. Sigmoidoscopy: To reveal presence of diverticula and thickening of bowel wall.

Diverticulitis:

1. Abdominal x-rays: To determine presence of abnormal levels of gas and fluid, which collect in the intestine above the affected area of the colon.
2. WBC with differential: Usually reveals leukocytosis and an increase in neutrophils, indicating presence of infection.
3. Hemogram: May reveal presence of anemia if bleeding has occurred.
4. Urinalysis: To rule out bladder involvement.

C. Medical Management and Surgical Interventions

Diverticulosis:

1. **High-residue diet:** Including fruits and vegetables and the use of wheat bran in the form of 100% bran cereal or 2 tbs/day of unprocessed bran to increase moisture content of the stool, thus softening it to enhance elimination and reduce intracolonic pressure.
2. **Pharmacotherapy:** Commercial *bulk laxative*, eg, psyllium (Metamucil) 1−2 tsp po bid, which can replace bran in the diet.

Diverticulitis:

1. **Emergency diverting colostomy** with or without resection of the affected bowel segment. This is the therapy of choice for most surgeons. Once inflammation has subsided (after approximately 6 weeks), the affected bowel segment is surgically resected if this was not done with the surgery creating the colostomy. After surgical anastomoses have healed, as documented by x-ray (3−6 weeks later), a third surgery is performed. The colostomy is taken down and the continuity of the GI tract is restored.

D. Nursing Diagnoses and Interventions

For diverticulitis treated by emergency surgical intervention with diverting temporary colostomy:

See "Appendix One" for nursing diagnoses and interventions for the care of pre-operative and postoperative patients, pp. 528–532, and the care of patients with cancer and other life-disrupting illnesses, pp. 544–551. See "Fecal Diversions" for the following: **Alteration in bowel elimination**, p. 316, **Disturbance in self-concept**, p. 317, and **Potential impairment of skin integrity**: Stoma and peristomal area, p. 315.

E. Patient–Family Teaching and Discharge Planning

Provide patient and SOs with verbal and written information for the following:

1. Medications, including the name, rationale, dosage, schedule, precautions, and potential side effects.

2. Signs and symptoms that necessitate medical attention, including fever; nausea or vomiting; cloudly or malodorous urine; diarrhea or constipation; change in stoma color from the normal bright and shiny red; peristomal skin irritation; and incisional pain, drainage, swelling, or redness.

3. Importance of a normal diet that includes all four food groups (meat, eggs and fish; fruits and vegetables; milk and cheese; cereal and breads) and drinking adequate fluids (at least 2–3 L/day).

4. Gradual resumption of ADLs, excluding heavy lifting (>5 lb), pushing, or pulling for 6 weeks to prevent development of incisional herniation.

5. Care of incision, dressing changes, and permission to take baths or showers once sutures/drains are removed.

6. Care of stoma and peristomal skin; use of ostomy skin barriers, pouches, and accessory equipment; and method for obtaining supplies.

7. Referral to community resources, including enterostomal therapy (ET) nurse, home health care agency, and the United Ostomy Association (UOA).

8. Importance of follow-up care with MD or ET nurse; confirm date and time of next appointment.

II. Colorectal Cancer

Colorectal cancer is second only to lung cancer and nonmelanoma skin cancer in the annual number of newly diagnosed cancer cases. Over 90% of colorectal cancers are adenocarcinomas, of which 50% are located in the rectum, 20% in the sigmoid colon, 6% in the descending colon, 8% in the transverse colon, and 16% in the cecum and ascending colon. Many arise from malignant degeneration of benign adenomatous polyps. Metastatic disease occurs through lymph nodes, direct extension to adjacent tissues, and the bloodstream.

The cause of colorectal cancer is unknown, but risk factors include family history of colorectal cancer, familial polyposis coli, ulcerative colitis and/or granulomatous colitis, and the presence of adenomatous colon polyps.

A. Assessment

Right colon cancer: Vague, dull abdominal pain. The patient may be asymptomatic.

Physical exam: Possible presence of a palpable mass in the RLQ, black or dark-red stools, and presence of abdominal distention.

Left colon cancer: Increasing abdominal cramping ("gas pains"), change in bowel elimination patterns, decrease in caliber of stools, constipation, vomiting, obstipation, and acute large bowel obstruction causing progressive increase in abdominal pain. Patient may be asymptomatic.

Physical exam: Possible absence of stool felt on rectal examination, presence of bright red blood coating the surface of the stool, and abdominal distention.

Rectal cancer: Sense of incomplete evacuation, tenesmus, and pain (a late manifestation). Patient may be asymptomatic.

Physical exam: Potential presence of palpable mass; bright red blood coating surface of the stool.

History of (for all types of colorectal cancer): Blood on or in stools, change in stool elimination pattern, vague abdominal discomfort or pain.

B. Diagnostic Tests

1. Occult blood test of three serial stool specimens: To detect presence of blood associated with tumor mass bleeding.

2. Proctosigmoidoscopy and/or colonoscopy: To examine areas of intestine visually.

3. Biopsy: To confirm diagnosis.

4. Barium enema with air contrast: To detect colon irregularities suspicious of tumor.

5. Carcinoembryonic antigen (CEA): Serum elevation can be indicative of intestinal tumor.

C. Medical Management and Surgical Interventions

1. **Surgery:** Resection of tumor mass and lymph nodes that drain the area, with reanastomosis of colon. If bowel ends cannot be reanastomosed, a colostomy is created.

2. **Radiation therapy:** To eliminate cancer cells, reduce tumor mass, and/or decrease pain from advanced disease.

3. **Chemotherapy:** For advanced disease, usually fluorouracil (5-FU), alone or in combination with other agents to eliminate cancer cells and provide relief from pain with advanced disease.

4. **Nutritional management:** May include elemental fluid supplements and/or parenteral nutrition if oral intake is inadequate. For further details, see "Providing Nutritional Therapy," p. 513, in Chapter 11.

D. Nursing Diagnoses and Interventions

See "Appendix One" for nursing diagnoses and interventions for the care of preoperative and postoperative patients, pp. 528–532, and the care of patients with cancer and other life-disrupting illnesses, pp. 544–551. See "Fecal Diversions" for the following: **Alteration in bowel elimination**, p. 316, **Disturbance in self-concept**, p. 317, **Potential impairment of skin integrity:** Stoma and peristomal area, p. 315, and **Knowledge deficit:** Colostomy irrigation procedure, p. 318.

E. Patient–Family Teaching and Discharge Planning

Provide patient and SOs with verbal and written information for the following:

1. Medications, including drug name, rationale, dosage, schedule, precautions, and potential side effects.

2. Signs and symptoms that necessitate medical attention, including fever, nausea and/or vomiting, diarrhea, or constipation.

3. If an intestinal stoma is present, the importance of reporting change in stoma color from the normal bright and shiny red; presence of peristomal skin irritation; and incisional pain, drainage, swelling, or redness.

4. Importance of a normal diet that includes all four food groups (meat, eggs and fish; fruits and vegetables; milk and cheese; cereal and breads) and drinking adequate fluids (at least 2–3 L/day).

5. Enteral or parenteral feeding instructions if patient is to supplement diet or is NPO.

6. Gradual resumption of ADLs, excluding heavy lifting (>5 lb), pushing, or pulling for 6 weeks to prevent incisional herniation.

7. Care of incision and perianal wounds, including dressing changes, and bathing once sutures/drains are removed. Sitz baths may be recommended for perianal wound.

8. If stoma is present, care of stoma and peristomal skin; use of ostomy skin barriers, pouches, and accessory equipment; and method for obtaining supplies.

9. Referral to community resources, including home health care agency, American Cancer Society (ACS) and, if appropriate, to enterostomal therapy (ET) nurse and United Ostomy Association (UOA).

10. Importance of follow-up care with MD (or ET nurse if appropriate); confirm date and time of next appointment.

III. Polyps/Familial Polyposis

Of the single, multiple, sessile, and pedunculated polypoid colon tumors, the adematous polyp is the most common. The practical significance of these polyps is their tendency to become malignant (see "Colorectal Cancer," p. 302). *Familial polyposis* is characterized by, but distinct from, frequent colon polyp formation. This disorder is also known as multiple familial adenomatosis, adenomatosis coli, and hereditary multiple polyposis. In this disorder the glandular epithelia of the colon and rectum undergo excessive proliferation throughout the mucous membranes, which leads to the formation of sessile or pedunculated polyps. These are soft and red or purplish-red in color, vary in size from a few millimeters to several centimeters, and range in number from a few to several thousand. They can be found anywhere along the entire length of the colon, but the rectum is almost always involved. Every individual with untreated familial polyposis will develop cancer, because at some point in time, one or more of these polyps will undergo malignant degeneration. This is a hereditary disease passed from generation to generation as an autosomal dominant trait and it appears most often during late childhood through the early thirties.

A. Assessment

Familial polyposis: Mild, early symptoms such as diarrhea or melena, although many patients remain asymptomatic for years. Once malignant degeneration has begun, these symptoms become more pronounced and there can be intermittent or constant colicky pain. Tenesmus and a frequent urge to defecate also can be present. If blood loss is significant, anemia, weight loss, loss of appetite, and fatigue can occur.

Physical exam: In the presence of a well-developed malignant growth, a mass can be palpated on abdominal exam. Digital rectal examination may detect presence of polyps.

History of: Familial polyposis, mild colicky abdominal discomfort with or without diarrhea, presence of blood in stools.

B. Diagnostic Tests

1. Proctosigmoidoscopy and/or colonoscopy: For visualization of polyposis.

2. Biopsy: To confirm diagnosis.

3. X-ray examination with barium enema and air contrast: To determine extent of the disease.

4. CBC: To detect presence of anemia.

C. Medical Management and Surgical Interventions

1. **Proctocolectomy:** Surgical cure via removal of colon and rectum with continent (Kock) ileostomy, conventional (Brooke) ileostomy, or ileoanal reservoir for fecal diversion (see "Fecal Diversions," p. 314).

2. **Colectomy with preservation of rectum and ileorectal anastomosis:** After this procedure, follow-up proctoscopies are necessary at frequent intervals to assess the rectum for further evidence of the disease or malignant changes.

3. **Radiation and/or chemotherapy:** May be indicated as adjuvant therapy or for advanced malignant disease.

D. Nursing Diagnoses and Interventions

See "Fecal Diversions" for the following: **Alteration in bowel elimination**, p. 316, **Disturbance in self-concept**, p. 317, and **Potential impairment of skin integrity:** Stoma and peristomal area, p. 315. See "Appendix One" for nursing diagnoses and interventions for the care of preoperative and postoperative patients, pp. 528–532, and patients with cancer and other life-disrupting illnesses, pp. 544–551.

E. Patient–Family Teaching and Discharge Planning

Provide patient and SOs with verbal and written information for the following:

1. Importance of informing all close members of the family that because familial polyposis is inherited, periodic examinations of the rectum and/or colon are essential.

2. For other guidelines, see Section E in "Colorectal Cancer," p. 303.

IV. Ulcerative Colitis

Ulcerative colitis is a nonspecific, chronic, inflammatory disease of the mucosa and submucosa of the colon. Generally, the disease begins in the rectum and sigmoid colon, but it can extend proximally and uninterrupted as far as the cecum. In some instances, a few centimeters of distal ileum are affected. This is sometimes referred to as "backwash ileitis," and it occurs in only about 10% of the patients with ulcerative colitis involving the entire colon. The etiology of ulcerative colitis is unknown, but theories include infection, allergy, immunologic abnormalities, psychosomatic factors, and heredity. Individuals with ulcerative colitis develop colonic adenocarcinomas at ten times the rate of the general population.

A. Assessment

Signs and symptoms: Bloody diarrhea (the cardinal symptom). The clinical picture can vary, from acute episodes with frequent discharge of watery stools mixed with blood, pus, and mucus accompanied by fever, abdominal pain, rectal urgency, and tenesmus, to loose or frequent stools, to formed stools coated with a little blood. However, nearly two-thirds of patients have cramping abdominal pain and varying degrees of fever, vomiting, anorexia, weight loss, and dehydration. Remissions and exacerbations are common. Extracolonic manifestations also can occur, including polyarthritis, skin lesions (erythema nodosum, pyoderma gangrenosum), liver impairment, and ophthalmic complications (iritis, uveitis).

Physical exam: With severe disease, the abdomen will be tender, especially in the LLQ; and distention and a tender and spastic anus also may be present. With rectal examination, the mucosa might feel gritty, and the examining gloved finger may be covered with blood, mucus, or pus.

Risk factors: Duration of active disease greater than 10 years, pancolitis, and family history of colonic cancer.

B. Diagnostic Tests

1. <u>Stool examination:</u> Reveals the presence of frank and/or occult blood. Stool cultures and smears rule out bacterial and parasitic disorders. **Note:** Collect specimens *before* barium enema is performed.

2. <u>Sigmoidoscopy:</u> Reveals red, granular, hyperemic, and extremely friable mucosa; strips of inflamed mucosa undermined by surrounding ulcerations, which form pseudopolyps; and thick exudate composed of blood, pus, and mucus. **Note:** Enemas should not be given before the examination because they can produce hyperemia and edema and may cause exacerbation of the disease.

3. <u>Colonoscopy:</u> Will help determine the extent of the disease and differentiate ulcerative colitis from Crohn's disease. **Note:** This test may be contraindicated in patients with acute disease because of the risk of perforation.

4. <u>Rectal biopsy:</u> Will aid in differentiating ulcerative colitis from carcinoma and other inflammatory processes.

5. <u>Barium enema:</u> Reveals mucosal irregularity from fine serrations to ragged ulcerations, narrowing and shortening of the colon, presence of pseudopolyps, loss of haustral markings, and the presence of spasms and irritability.

6. <u>Blood tests:</u> Anemia is common because of iron deficiency and chronic inflammation; leukocytosis and elevated sedimentation rate are common, and hypoalbuminemia and electrolyte disturbances are often found.

C. Medical Management and Surgical Interventions

Medical therapy is symptomatic. The goals are to terminate the acute attack, reduce symptoms, and prevent recurrences.

1. **Parenteral replacement of fluids, electrolytes, and blood products:** To maintain acutely ill patient, as indicated by laboratory test results.

2. **Physical and emotional rest:** Including bed rest and limitation of visitors.

3. **Pharmacotherapy**

   □ *Sedatives and tranquilizers:* To promote rest and reduce anxiety.

   □ *Hydrophilic colloids* (eg, kaolin and pectin mixture) and *anticholinergics and antidiarrheal preparations* (eg, tinctures of belladonna and opium, diphenoxylate hydrochloride, loperamide, and codeine phosphate): To relieve cramping and diarrhea.

   □ *Anti-inflammatory agents:* Corticosteroids to reduce mucosal inflammation.

   □ *Sulfasalazine:* To help maintain remissions.

   □ *Immunosuppressive agents:* To reduce inflammation in patients not responding to steroids and sulfasalazine and who are unwilling or unable to undergo colectomy.

   □ *Antibiotics:* To limit secondary infection.

4. **Nutritional management:** Varies with the patient's condition. In severely ill patients, TPN along with NPO status is prescribed to replace nutritional deficits while allowing complete bowel rest and improving patient's nutritional status before surgery. For less severely ill patients, low-residue elemental diet provides good nutrition with low fecal volume to allow bowel rest. A bland, high-protein, high-calorie, low-residue diet with vitamin and mineral supplements and excluding raw fruits and vegetables provides good nutrition and decreases diarrhea. Milk and wheat products are restricted to reduce cramping and diarrhea in patients with lactose and gluten intolerances.

5. **Referral to mental health practitioner:** As indicated for supportive psychotherapy for patient who has difficulty dealing with any type of chronic or disabling illness.

6. **Surgical interventions:** Indicated only when the disease is intractable to medical management or when the patient develops a disabling complication. *Total proctocolectomy* cures ulcerative colitis and results in construction of a permanent fecal diversion such as Brooke ileostomy, continent (Kock pouch) ileostomy, or ileoanal reservoir. See "Fecal Diversions," p. 314, for additional details.

Postoperative management includes routine chest physiotherapy to prevent respiratory complications; IV fluid and electrolyte replacement or TPN as the patient's condition warrants; NG tube for decompression until bowel sounds are present and the patient is eliminating flatus or stool; gradual resumption of diet as tolerated following NG tube removal and return of bowel function; aseptic incisional care to prevent infection; and fecal diversion care and teaching.

D. Nursing Diagnoses and Interventions

Alteration in comfort: Pain, abdominal cramping, and nausea related to inflammatory process of the intestines

Desired outcome: Patient relates a reduction in discomfort and does not exhibit signs of uncontrolled pain, abdominal cramping, and/or nausea.

1. Monitor and document characteristics of pain, and assess whether it is associated with ingestion of certain foods or medications or with emotional stress. Eliminate foods that cause cramping and discomfort.
2. As prescribed, maintain patient on NPO and/or TPN to provide bowel rest.
3. Provide nasal and oral care at frequent intervals to lessen discomfort from NPO status or presence of NG tube.
4. Keep patient's environment quiet and plan nursing care to provide maximum periods of rest.
5. Administer sedatives and tranquilizers as prescribed to promote rest and reduce anxiety.
6. Administer hydrophilic colloids, anticholinergics, and antidiarrheals as prescribed to relieve cramping and diarrhea.
7. Observe for intensification of symptoms, which can indicate the presence of complications. Notify MD of significant findings.

Potential for injury related to risk of complications secondary to intestinal inflammatory disorder

Desired outcome: If signs of complications appear, they are detected promptly, resulting in immediate medical intervention and absence of injury to the patient.

1. Monitor patient for fever, chills, diaphoresis, and increased abdominal discomfort, which can occur with perforation of the colon and potentially result in localized abscess or generalized fecal peritonitis. **Note:** Systemic therapy with corticosteroids and antibiotics can mask the development of this complication.
2. Report any evidence of sudden abdominal distention associated with the above symptoms, since they can signal toxic megacolon. Factors contributing to the development of this complication include hypokalemia, barium enema examinations, and use of opiates and anticholinergics.
3. Monitor patient for signs of hemorrhage: hypotension, increased pulse and respiratory rate, pallor, diaphoresis, and restlessness. Assess stool for quality (eg, is it grossly bloody and liquid secondary to large amount of bleeding from mucosa?) and quantity (eg, is it mostly blood or mostly stool?). Report significant findings to MD.

Alterations in bowel elimination: Diarrhea related to intestinal inflammatory process

Desired outcome: Patient experiences fewer episodes of diarrhea.

1. Provide covered bedpan, commode, or bathroom that is easily accessible and ready to use at all times.

2. Empty bedpan and commode promptly to control odor and decrease patient anxiety and self-consciousness.

3. Administer hydrophilic colloids, anticholinergics, and antidiarrheals as prescribed to decrease fluidity and number of stools.

4. Administer topical corticosteroid preparations and antibiotics via retention enema, as prescribed, to relieve local inflammation. If patient has difficulty retaining the enema for the prescribed amount of time, consult with MD regarding the use of corticosteroid foam, which is easier to retain and administer.

Potential impairment of skin integrity: Perineal/perianal area related to irritation secondary to persistent diarrhea

Desired outcome: Patient's perineal/perianal skin remains intact.

1. Provide materials or assist patient with cleansing and drying of perineal/perianal area after each bowel movement.

2. Apply protective skin care products, such as skin preparations, gels, or barrier films, *only* to normal, unbroken skin. Petrolatum emollients, moisture barrier ointments, and vanishing creams also can be used to prevent irritation from frequent liquid stools.

3. Administer hydrophilic colloids, anticholinergics, and antidiarrheals as prescribed to decrease fluidity and number of stools.

Fluid volume deficit related to abnormal loss secondary to diarrhea

Desired outcome: Patient does not exhibit signs of dehydration.

1. If the patient is acutely ill, maintain parenteral replacement of fluids, electrolytes, and vitamins as prescribed.

2. Administer blood products and iron as prescribed to correct existing anemia.

3. Monitor I&O; weigh patient daily; and monitor laboratory values to evaluate fluid and electrolyte status.

4. Monitor frequency and consistency of stool. Assess and record presence of blood, mucus, fat, or undigested food.

5. Monitor patient for indicators of dehydration: thirst, poor skin turgor, dryness of mucous membranes, fever, and concentrated and decreased urinary output.

6. When patient is taking food by mouth, provide bland, high-protein, high-calorie, and low-residue diet, as prescribed. Assess tolerance to diet by determining incidence of cramping, diarrhea, and flatulence.

If surgery is performed, see "Appendix One" for nursing diagnoses and interventions for the care of preoperative and postoperative patients, pp. 528–532, and the care of patients with cancer and other life-disrupting illnesses, pp. 544–551. See "Fecal Diversions" for the following: **Alteration in bowel elimination,** p. 316, **Disturbance in self-concept,** p. 317, and **Potential impairment of skin integrity:** Stoma and peristomal area, p. 315.

E. Patient—Family Teaching and Discharge Planning

Provide patient and SOs with verbal and written information for the following:

1. Medications, including name, rationale, dosage, schedule, route of administration, precautions, and potential side effects.

2. Signs and symptoms that necessitate medical attention, including fever, nausea and/or vomiting, diarrhea or constipation, and any significant change in appearance and frequency of stools, any of which can signal exacerbation of the disease.

3. Dietary management to promote nutritional and fluid maintenance and prevent abdominal cramping, discomfort, and diarrhea.

4. Importance of perineal/perianal skin care after bowel movements.

5. Enteral or parenteral feeding instructions if patient is to supplement diet or is NPO.

6. Referral to community resources including National Foundation for Ileitis and Colitis.

7. Importance of follow-up medical care, particularly in patients with long-standing disease, since so many of them develop colonic adenocarcinoma.

8. Referral to a mental health specialist if recommended by MD.

In addition, if patient has a fecal diversion:

9. Care of incision, dressing changes, and permission to take baths or showers once sutures/drains are removed.

10. Care of stoma, peristomal/perianal skin, or perineal wound; use of ostomy equipment; and method for obtaining supplies. Sitz baths may be indicated for perineal wound.

11. Medications that are contraindicated (eg, laxatives) or that may not be well tolerated or absorbed (eg, antibiotics, enteric-coated tablets, or long-acting tablets).

12. Gradual resumption of ADLs, excluding heavy lifting (>5 lb), pushing, or pulling for 6–8 weeks to prevent incisional herniation.

13. Referral to community resources, including home health care agency, enterostomal therapy (ET) nurse, and the local chapter of United Ostomy Association (UOA).

14. Importance of reporting signs and symptoms that require medical attention, such as change in stoma color from the normal bright and shiny red; peristomal or perineal/perianal skin irritation; diarrhea; incisional pain, drainage, swelling, or redness; signs and symptoms of fluid and electrolyte imbalance; and signs and symptoms of mechanical or functional obstruction.

V. Crohn's Disease

Crohn's disease, also known as regional enteritis, granulomatous colitis, or transmural colitis, is a chronic inflammatory disease, which can involve any part of the GI tract from the mouth to the anus. Usually the disease occurs segmentally, demonstrating discontinuous areas of disease with segments of normal bowel in between. The terminal ileum is the most frequent site of involvement, followed by the colon. The disease affects all layers of the bowel: the mucosa, submucosa, circular and longitudinal muscles, and serosa. A family history of this disease or ulcerative colitis occurs in 15–20% of affected patients. The cause is unknown, but theories include infection, immunologic factors, environmental factors, and genetic predisposition.

A. Assessment

Signs and symptoms: Clinical presentation varies as a direct reflection of the location of the inflammatory process, its extent, severity, and relationship to contiguous structures. Sometimes the onset is abrupt and the patient can appear to have appendicitis, ulcerative colitis, intestinal obstruction, or a fever of obscure origin. Acute symptoms include RLQ pain, tenderness, spasm, flatulence, nausea, fever, and diarrhea. A more typical picture is insidious onset with more persistent but less severe symptoms, such as vague abdominal pain, unexplained anemia, and/or fever. Diarrhea—liquid, soft, or mushy stools—is the most common symptom. The presence of gross blood is rare. Abdominal pain is a freqent symptom, and it may be colicky or crampy, initiated by meals, centered in the lower abdomen, and relieved by defecation because of the chronic partial obstruction of the small intestine, colon, or both. As the disease progresses, anorexia, malnutrition, weight loss, anemia, lassitude, malaise, and fever can occur in addition to fluid, electrolyte, and metabolic disturbances.

Physical exam: In the early stages the exam is often normal, but might demonstrate mild tenderness in the abdomen over the affected bowel. In more advanced disease, a palpable mass might be present, especially in the RLQ, with terminal ileum involvement. Persistent rectal fissure, large ulcers, perirectal abscess, or rectal fistula is the first indication of disease in 15−25% of patients with small bowel involvement and in 50−75% of patients with colonic involvement. Rectovaginal, abdominal, and enterovesical fistulas also can occur. Extraintestinal manifestations characteristic of ulcerative colitis do occur, but less frequently (10−20%).

B. Diagnostic Tests

1. Stool examination: Usually reveals the presence of occult blood; frank blood may be noted in stools of patients with colonic involvement or with ulcerations and fistulas of the rectum. A few patients present with bloody diarrhea. Stool cultures and smears rule out bacterial and parasitic disorders. Specimens are also examined for presence of fecal fat.

2. Sigmoidoscopy: To evaluate possible colonic involvement.

3. Colonoscopy: May help differentiate Crohn's disease from ulcerative colitis. Characteristic patchy inflammation (skip lesions) rules out ulcerative colitis.

4. Rectal biopsy: Often reveals granulomas, which confirm Crohn's disease.

5. Barium enema and upper GI series with small bowel follow through: Contribute to the diagnosis of Crohn's disease. Involvement of only the terminal ileum or segmental involvement of the colon and/or small intestine is almost always indicative of Crohn's disease. Thickened bowel wall with stricture (string sign) separated by segments of normal bowel, cobblestone appearance, and presence of fistulas and skip lesions are common findings.

6. Blood tests: Are nonspecific and can reveal presence of anemia, elevated WBC count, increased sedimentation rate, hypoalbuminemia, prolonged prothrombin time, and fluid and electrolyte imbalance.

7. Other laboratory tests: Include D-xylose tolerance test (upper jejunal involvement); bile acid breath test (ileal involvement or bacterial overgrowth), and Schilling's test (ileal involvement).

C. Medical Management and Surgical Intervention

The initial treatment is nonoperative, and it is individualized and based on symptomatic relief. Medical treatment is more likely to be successful early in the course of the disease, before permanent structural changes have occurred.

1. **Parenteral replacement of fluids, electrolytes, and blood products:** Maintenance therapy for acute exacerbation as indicated by laboratory test results.

2. **Physical and emotional rest:** Complete bed rest, with assistance with ADLs during acute phases.

3. **Pharmacotherapy:** It has not been proven that drugs, singly or in combination, can prolong remission and prevent relapse of Crohn's disease.

   □ *Sedatives and tranquilizers:* To promote rest and reduce anxiety.

□ *Anticholinergics and antidiarrheals:* To decrease diarrhea and cramping.

□ *Hydrophilic colloids:* To decrease fluidity and number of stools.

□ *Sulfasalazine:* To treat acute exacerbations of colonic and ileocolonic disease.

□ *Corticosteroids:* To reduce the active inflammatory response, decrease edema, and control exacerbations.

□ *Topical corticosteroids:* To reduce inflammation and edema with anorectal involvement.

□ *Immunosuppressive agents:* To reduce inflammation when corticosteroids have failed, or in combination with corticosteroids to allow dosage reduction of corticosteroids.

□ *Antibiotics:* To control suppurative complications.

4. **Nutritional management:** A major component of therapy. During acute exacerbations TPN and NPO status can be used to replace nutritional deficits and allow complete bowel rest. Elemental diets that are free of bulk and residue, low in fat, and digested in the upper jejunum provide good nutrution with low fecal volume to allow bowel rest in select patients. Bland diets low in residue, roughage, and fat but high in protein, calories, carbohydrates, and vitamins provide good nutrition and reduce excessive stimulation of the bowel. A diet free of milk, milk products, gas-forming foods, alcohol, and iced beverages reduces cramping and diarrhea. When remission occurs, a less restricted diet can be tailored to the individual patient, excluding foods known to precipitate symptoms. Patients with involvement of the small intestine frequently require supplementation of vitamins and minerals, especially calcium, iron, folate, and magnesium secondary to malabsorption or to compensate for foods excluded from the diet. Patients with extensive ileal disease or resection frequently require vitamin B_{12} replacement and, if bile salt deficiency exists, cholestyramine and medium-chain triglycerides might be needed to control diarrhea and reduce fat malabsorption and steatorrhea.

5. **Referral to mental health practitioner for supportive psychotherapy:** If indicated, because of the chronic and progressive nature of Crohn's disease.

6. **Surgical management:** Because surgery is not a cure for Crohn's disease, it is reserved for complications rather than used as a primary form of therapy. Common indications for surgery include bowel obstruction, internal and enterocutaneous fistulas, intra-abdominal abscesses, and perianal disease. Conservative resection of the affected bowel segments with restoration of bowel continuity, preserving as much of the intestine as possible, is the preferred surgical approach. If fecal diversion using an ostomy is required, the type of diversion used will depend on the location and amount of intestinal segment(s) to be resected. (For details, see "Fecal Diversions," p. 314.)

D. Nursing Diagnoses and Interventions

Alteration in comfort: Pain, abdominal cramping, and nausea related to intestinal inflammatory process

Desired outcome: Patient relates a reduction in discomfort and does not exhibit signs of uncontrolled pain, cramping, or nausea.

1. Monitor and document characteristics of pain, and assess whether it is associated with ingestion of certain foods or with emotional stress. Eliminate foods that cause cramping and discomfort.

2. As prescribed, keep patient NPO and provide parenteral nutrition to provide bowel rest.

3. Administer analgesics as prescribed to reduce abdominal discomfort.

4. Provide nasal and oral care at frequent intervals to lessen discomfort from NPO status and presence of NG tube.

5. Administer antiemetic medications before meals to enhance appetite when nausea is a problem.

6. As prescribed, administer anticholinergics before meals to decrease diarrhea and cramping.

Activity intolerance related to weakness and fatigue secondary to intestinal inflammatory process

Desired outcome: Patient adheres to prescribed rest regimen. Patient sets appropriate goals for self-care as the condition improves.

1. Keep patient's environment quiet to allow rest.

2. Because adequate rest is necessary to sustain remission, assist patient with ADLs and plan nursing care to provide maximum rest periods.

3. As prescribed, administer sedatives and tranquilizers to promote rest and reduce anxiety.

4. As the the patient's physical condition improves, encourage self-care to the greatest extent possible, and assist patient with setting realistic, attainable goals.

Potential for injury related to negative side effects of pharmacotherapy

Desired outcomes: Patient does not experience side effects of pharmacotherapy; or, if they do occur, they are detected promptly, resulting in immediate medical intervention and absence of injury.

1. In patients receiving corticosteroids, monitor for signs of GI bleeding, electrolyte imbalances, fluid retention, and emotional changes.

2. Administer prescribed antacids during steroid therapy to help prevent gastric ulceration.

3. Monitor patient for signs of intestinal obstruction, including abdominal ridigity and increased nausea and vomiting. Contributory factors to development of this complication include use of opiates and anticholinergics and the prolonged use of antidiarrheals and hydrophilic colloids.

4. Report significant findings to MD.

Alterations in bowel elimination: Diarrhea related to intestinal inflammatory process and/or malabsorption

Desired outcome: Patient experiences fewer episodes of diarrhea.

1. If the patient is experiencing frequent and urgent passage of loose stools, provide covered bedpan or commode, or be sure the bathroom is easily accessible and ready to use at all times.

2. Empty the bedpan and commode promptly to control odor and decrease patient anxiety and self-consciousness.

3. Administer hydrophilic colloids, anticholinergics, and antidiarrheals as prescribed to decrease fluidity and number of stools.

4. If bile salt deficiency (because of ileal disease or resection) is contributing to diarrhea, administer cholestyramine as prescribed to control diarrhea.

5. Eliminate or decrease fat content in the diet because it can increase diarrhea.

Fluid volume deficit related to abnormal loss secondary to diarrhea and/or GI fistula

Desired outcome: Patient does not exhibit signs of dehydration.

1. Maintain patient on parenteral replacement of fluids, electrolytes, and vitamins as prescribed to promote anabolism and healing.

2. Monitor I&O; weigh patient daily; and monitor laboratory values to evaluate fluid and electrolyte status.

3. Monitor frequency and consistency of stools. Assess and record presence of blood, mucus, fat, or undigested food.

4. Monitor patient for indicators of dehydration: thirst, poor skin turgor, dryness of mucous membranes, fever, and concentrated and decreased urinary output.

5. When the patient is taking food by mouth, provide bland, high-protein, high-calorie, and low-residue diet, as prescribed. Assess tolerance to diet by determining incidence of cramping, diarrhea, and flatulence. Modify diet plan accordingly.

If surgery is performed, see "Appendix One" for nursing diagnoses and interventions for the care of preoperative and postoperative patients, pp. 528–532, and care of the patients with cancer and other life-disrupting illnesses, pp. 544–551. See "Fecal Diversions" for the following: **Alteration in bowel elimination,** p. 316, **Disturbance in self-concept,** p. 317, and **Potential impairment of skin integrity:** Stoma and peristomal area, p. 315.

E. Patient–Family Teaching and Discharge Planning

Provide patient and SOs with verbal and written information for the following:

1. Medications, including name, rationale, dosage, schedule, route of administration, precautions, and potential side effects.

2. Signs and symptoms that necessitate medical attention, including fever, nausea and/or vomiting, abdominal discomfort, any significant change in appearance and frequency of stools, passage of stool through the vagina, or stool mixed with urine, any of which can signal recurrence or complications of Crohn's disease.

3. Importance of dietary management to promote nutritional and fluid maintenance and prevent abdominal cramping, discomfort, and diarrhea.

4. Importance of perineal/perianal skin care after bowel movements.

5. Importance of balancing activities with rest periods, even during remission, because adequate rest is necessary to sustain remission.

6. Referral to community resources, including National Foundation for Ileitis and Colitis.

7. Importance of follow-up medical care, including supportive psychotherapy, because of the chronic and progressive nature of Crohn's disease.

In addition, if the patient has a fecal diversion:

8. Care of incision, dressing changes, and bathing.

9. Care of stoma and peristomal skin, use of ostomy equipment, and method for obtaining supplies.

10. Gradual resumption of ADLs, excluding heavy lifting (>5 lb), pushing, or pulling for 6–8 weeks to prevent incisional herniation.

11. Referral to community resources, including home health care agency, enterostomal therapy (ET) nurse, and local chapter of United Ostomy Association (UOA).

12. Importance of reporting signs and symptoms that require medical attention, such as change in stoma color from the normal bright and shiny red; lesions on stomal mucosa, which may indicate recurrence of the disease; peristomal skin irritation; diarrhea or constipation, fever, chills, abdominal pain, distention, nausea, and vomiting; and incisional pain, drainage, swelling, or redness.

VI. Fecal Diversions

For a discussion of diverticulitis, see p. 300; colorectal cancer, see p. 302; polyps/familial polyposis, see p. 304; ulcerative colitis, see p. 305; and Crohn's disease, see p. 309.

A. Surgical Interventions

It is sometimes necessary to interrupt the continuity of the bowel because of intestinal disease and/or its complications. The resulting fecal diversion can be located anywhere along the bowel, depending on the location of the diseased and/or injured portion; and it can be permanent or temporary. The most common sites for fecal diversion are the colon and ileum.

1. **Colostomy:** Created when the surgeon brings a portion of the colon to the abdominal skin surface. An opening in the exteriorized colon permits elimination of flatus and stool through the stoma. The continuity of the colon can be interrupted anywhere along its length.

   □ *Cecostomy or ascending colostomy:* Uncommon. The procedure done most often is a temporary diverting stoma, which eliminates unformed soft or liquid stool unpredictably. Surgical intervention is similar to that with transverse colostomies.

   □ *Transverse colostomy:* This is the most frequently created stoma to divert the fecal stream on a temporary basis. Surgical indications include relief of bowel obstruction before definitive surgery for tumors or diverticulitis and colon perforation secondary to trauma. Stool is usually soft, unformed, and eliminated unpredictably. A temporary colostomy might be double-barrelled, with a proximal stoma through which stool is eliminated and a distal stoma adjacent to the proximal stoma called a mucous fistula. More commonly, a loop colostomy is created with a supporting rod placed beneath it until the exteriorized loop of colon becomes affixed to the skin.

   □ *Descending or sigmoid colostomy:* This is usually a permanent fecal diversion. Cancer of the rectum is the most common cause for surgical intervention. Stool is usually formed and some individuals might have stool elimination at predictable times. In a permanent colostomy, the surgeon brings the severed end of the colon to the abdominal skin surface. To mature the stoma, the colon above the skin surface is cuffed back on itself and sutured to the skin so that the mucosal surface of the intestine is exposed.

2. **Ileostomy:**

   □ *Conventional (Brooke) ileostomy:* Created by bringing a distal portion of the ileum up and out onto the surface of the skin of the abdominal wall. A permanent ileostomy is matured by the same procedure discussed with a permanent colostomy. Surgical indications include ulcerative colitis, Crohn's disease, and familial polyposis requiring excision of the entire colon and rectum.

   □ *Temporary ileostomy:* Usually a loop stoma with a supporting rod in place beneath the loop of the ileum until the exteriorized loop of ileum becomes affixed to the skin. The purpose is to divert the fecal stream away from a more distal anastomosis site or fistula repair site until healing has occurred. Output is usually liquid or pastelike, contains digestive enzymes, and is eliminated continually. A collection pouch is worn over the stoma on the abdomen to collect gas and fecal discharge.

   □ *Continent (Kock pouch) ileostomy:* An intra-abdominal pouch constructed from approximately 30 cm of distal ileum. A 10-cm portion of ileum is intussuscepted to form an outlet valve from the pouch to the skin of the abdomen, where a stoma is constructed flush with the skin. The intra-abdominal pouch is continent for gas and fecal discharge and is emptied approximately qid by inserting a catheter through the stoma. No external pouch is needed and a Band-Aid or small dressing is worn over the stoma to collect mucus. Surgical indications include ulcerative colitis and familial polyposis requiring removal of the colon and rectum. Crohn's disease is generally a contraindication for this procedure because the disease can recur in the pouch, necessitating its removal.

3. **Ileoanal reservoir:** A two-stage surgical procedure developed to preserve fecal continence and avoid the need for a permanent ileostomy. During the first stage following total colectomy and removal of the rectal mucosa, an ileal reservoir is constructed just above the junction of the ileum and anal canal; the ileal outlet from the reservoir is brought down through the cuff of the rectal muscle and anastomosed to the anal canal. The anal sphincter is preserved and the resulting ileal reservoir provides a storage place for feces. A temporary diverting ileostomy is required for 2–3 months to allow healing of the anastomosis. The second stage occurs when the diverting ileostomy is taken down and fecal continuity is restored. Initially, the patient experiences fecal incontinence and 10 or more bowel movements a day. After 3–6 months, the patient experiences a decrease in urgency and frequency with 4–8 bowel movements per day. This procedure is an option for patients requiring colectomy for ulcerative colitis or familial polyposis. It is contraindicated in patients with Crohn's disease and incontinence problems.

B. Nursing Diagnoses and Interventions

Potential impairment of skin integrity: Stoma and peristomal area related to erythema, improper appliance, or sensitivity to appliance material

Desired outcome: Patient's stoma and peristomal skin remain intact.

After colostomy or conventional ileostomy (permanent or temporary):

1. Apply a pectin, methylcellulose-based, solid-form skin barrier around the stoma to protect the peristomal skin from contact with stool, which would cause irritation.

   □ Cut an opening in the skin barrier the exact circumference of the stoma, remove the release paper, and apply the sticky surface directly to the peristomal skin.

   □ Remove the skin barrier and inspect the skin q2–3 days to assess its condition. Peristomal skin should look like other abdominal skin. Changes such as erythema, erosion, serous drainage, bleeding, or induration signal the presence of infection, irritation, or sensitivity to materials placed on the skin and should be documented and reported to the MD because topical medication might be required. Irritating materials should be discontinued and other materials substituted. Patch-test the patient's abdominal skin to determine sensitivity to suspected materials.

   □ Because stomas will lose surgically induced edema for some weeks following surgery, the opening in the skin barrier must be recalibrated each time it is changed so that it is always the exact circumference of the stoma to prevent contact of stool with the skin.

2. Apply a two-piece pouch system or a pouch with access cap so that the stoma can be inspected for viability q12–24h. A matured stoma will be red in color, with overlying mucus. A nonmatured stoma will be red and moist where the mucous membrane is exposed, but can be a darker, mottled, grayish-red with a transparent or translucent film of serosa elsewhere.

3. When removing the skin barrier and pouch for routine care, cleanse the patient's skin with mild soap and water, rinse well, and dry it so that the skin will retain its normal integrity and the skin barrier and pouch materials will adhere well to the skin.

4. To maintain a secure pouch seal, empty the pouch when it is a third to a half full of stool and/or gas.

After a continent ileostomy (Kock pouch):

1. A catheter is inserted through the stoma and into the pouch and sutured to the peristomal skin. Avoid stress on the suture and monitor for erythema, induration, drainage, or erosion. Report significant findings to MD. As prescribed, maintain catheter on low continuous suction or gravity to prevent stress on the nipple valve, and maintain pouch decompression so that suture lines are allowed to heal without stress or tension.

2. Check the catheter q2h for patency and irrigate with sterile saline (30 mL) to prevent obstruction. Notify MD if unable to instill solution, if there are no returns per suction catheter, or if leakage of irrigating solution or pouch contents appears around the catheter.

3. To prevent peristomal skin irritation, change 4x4 dressing around the stoma q2h or as often as it becomes wet. The drainage will be serosanguinous at first and mixed with mucus. Report presence of frank bleeding to MD.

4. Assess stoma for viability with each dressing change. It should be red in color and wet and shiny with mucus. A stoma that is pale or dark purple to black and/or dull in appearance can indicate circulatory impairment and should be reported to MD immediately and documented.

After ileoanal reservoir:

1. Perform routine care for the diverting ileostomy (see "continent ileostomy," above).

2. After the first stage of the operation, patient may have incontinence of mucus. Maintain perineal/perianal skin integrity by irrigating the mucus out of the reservoir qd with 60 mL water or gently cleanse the area with water and cotton balls. Soap should be avoided because it can cause itching or irritation. Use 4x4 gauze at night to absorb incontinence of mucus.

3. After the second stage of operation (when the ileostomy is taken down), expect the patient to experience frequency and urgency of defecation.

4. Wash perineal/perianal area with water or Domeboro solution, using a squeeze bottle or cotton balls. Do not use toilet paper because it can cause irritation. If desired, dry the area wtih a hair dryer on a cool setting.

5. Provide sitz baths to increase patient comfort and help clean the perineal/perianal area.

6. Apply protective skin sealants or ointments. Skin sealants should not be used on irritated or eroded skin because of the high alcohol content, which would cause a painful burning sensation.

Alteration in bowel elimination related to disruption of normal function secondary to fecal diversion

Desired outcomes: Complications specific to the fecal diversion are detected and treated promptly. Patient can verbalize knowledge of measures that will prevent output problems and demonstrate care techniques specific to the fecal diversion.

After colostomy and conventional ileostomy (permanent and temporary):

1. Empty stool from the bottom opening of the pouch and assess the quality and quantity of stool to document return of normal bowel function.

2. If the colostomy is not eliminating stool after 3−4 days and bowel sounds have returned, gently insert a gloved, lubricated finger into the stoma to determine presence of stricture at the skin or fascial levels and note presence of any stool within reach of the examining finger. To stimulate elimination of gas and stool, MD might prescribe a colostomy irrigation. (For procedure, see **Knowledge deficit:** Colostomy irrigation procedure, p. 318.)

After continent ileostomy (Kock pouch):

1. Monitor I&O, and record color and consistency of output.

2. Expect aspiration of bright red blood or serosanguinous liquid drainage from the Kock pouch during the early postoperative period.

3. As GI function returns after 3−4 days, expect the drainage to change in color from blood-tinged to greenish-brown liquid. When ileal output appears, suction is discontinued and the pouch catheter is placed to gravity drainage.

4. As the patient's diet progresses from clear liquids to solid food, the ileal output thickens. Check and irrigate the catheter q2h and as needed to maintain patency. If the patient reports abdominal fullness in the area of the pouch along with decreased fecal output, check placement and patency of the catheter.

5. When the patient is alert and taking food by mouth, teach catheter irrigation procedure, which should be performed q2h; and demonstrate how to empty the pouch contents through the catheter into the toilet.

6. Before hospital discharge, teach the patient how to remove and reinsert the catheter.

After ileoanal reservoir:

1. Monitor I&O, observing quantity, quality, and consistency of output from diverting ileostomy and reservoir. Monitor patient for elevation of temperature accompanied by perianal pain and discharge of purulent, bloody mucus from drains and/or anal orifice. Report significant findings to MD.

2. Irrigate drains as prescribed to maintain patency, decrease stress on suture lines, and decrease incidence of infection.

3. After the first stage of the operation, patient might experience incontinence of mucus. Advise patient to wear small pad to avoid soiling of outer garments.

4. After the second stage of the operation, expect incontinence and 15−20 bowel movements per day with urgency when patient is on a clear-liquid diet. Assist patient with perianal care and apply protective skin care products. To decrease incontinence at night, the catheter can be placed in the reservoir and connected to gravity drainage bag.

5. Expect the number of bowel movements to decrease to 6−12/day and the consistency to thicken when the patient is on solid foods.

6. Administer hydrophilic colloids and antidiarrheals as prescribed to decrease frequency and fluidity of stools.

7. Provide diet consultation so that patient will be able to avoid foods that cause liquid stools (spinach, raw fruits, highly seasoned foods, green beans, broccoli) and increase intake of foods that cause thick stools (cheese, ripe bananas, apples, jello, pasta).

8. Reassure patient that frequency and urgency are temporary and that as the reservoir expands and absorbs fluid, bowel movements should become thicker and less frequent.

Disturbance in self-concept related to alteration in body image secondary to fecal diversion

Desired outcomes: Patient does not exhibit discomfort with verbalizing feelings and fears. Patient demonstrates actions that reflect beginning acceptance of the fecal diversion.

1. Expect the following fears, which may be expressed by patients experiencing a fecal diversion: Physical, work, and social activities will be curtailed seriously; rejection, isolation, and feelings of uncleanliness will occur; everyone will know about the altered pattern of fecal elimination; and loss of voluntary control might occur (many patients view incontinence as a return to infancy).

2. Encourage patient to discuss feelings and fears; clarify any misconceptions. Involve family members in the discussions because they, too, might have anxieties and misconceptions.

3. Provide a calm and quiet environment for patient and SOs to discuss the surgery. Initiate an open and honest discussion. Monitor carefully for and listen closely to expressed or nonverbalized needs, since each patient will react differently to the surgical procedure.

4. Encourage acceptance of fecal diversion by having patient participate in care. Assure patient that education offers a means of control.

5. Assure patient that physical, social, and work activities will not be affected by the presence of a fecal diversion.

6. Expect the patient to have fears regarding sexual acceptance, although usually they are not expressed overtly. Concerns center on: change in body image; fears about odor and the ostomy appliance interfering with intercourse; conception, pregnancy, and discomfort from perineal wound and scar in women; and impotence and failure to ejaculate in men, especially after more radical dissection of the pelvis in the patient with cancer. If you are uncomfortable talking about sexuality with patients, be aware of these potential concerns and arrange for a consultation with someone who can speak openly and honestly about these problems.

7. Consult with patient's surgeon regarding a visit by another ostomate. Patients gain reassurance and build positive attitudes by seeing a healthy, active individual who has undergone the same type of surgery.

Knowledge deficit: Colostomy irrigation procedure

Desired outcome: Patient can demonstrate proficiency with the procedure for colostomy irrigation before hospital discharge.

▶ **Note:** Teach prescribed colostomy irrigation to patient with permanent descending or sigmoid colostomy. Colostomy irrigation is performed qd or qod so that wearing a pouch becomes unnecessary. An appropriate candidate is a patient who has 1–2 formed stools each day at predictable times (same as normal stool elimination pattern before illness). In addition, the patient must be able to manipulate the equipment, remember the technique, and be willing to spend approximately an hour a day performing the procedure. It may take 4–6 weeks for the patient to have stool elimination regulated with irrigation.

Instruct patient in the following steps:

1. Position an irrigating sleeve over the colostomy and hold it in place with an adhesive disk or belt. Place the distal end in the toilet.

2. Fill an enema container with 800–1000 mL warm water. Flush the tubing with the water to remove the air from the tubing. Allow the water to slowly enter the colostomy from the container through tubing that has either a lubricated cone attachment or a shield on a lubricated catheter, which keeps the irrigating water in the colostomy. Hold the cone snugly against the stoma. It should take 3–5 minutes for fluid to enter the colon.

3. After water has entered the colon, advise the patient to remove the cone and wait 30–40 minutes for the water to be eliminated along with the stool in the colon.

4. Remove the irrigation sleeve and cleanse and dry the peristomal area.

5. Apply a small dressing or security pouch over the colostomy between irrigations.

See "Appendix One" for nursing diagnoses and interventions for the care of preoperative and postoperative patients, pp. 528–532, and care of patients with cancer and other life-disrupting illnesses, pp. 544–551.

E. Patient–Family Teaching and Discharge Planning

Provide patient and SOs with verbal and written information for the following:

1. Medications, including name, rationale, dosage, schedule, route of administration, precautions, and potential side effects.

2. Importance of dietary management to promote nutritional and fluid maintenance.

3. Care of incision, dressing changes, and permission to take baths or showers once sutures/drains are removed.

4. Care of stoma, peristomal, and/or perianal skin; use of ostomy equipment; and method for obtaining supplies.

5. Gradual resumption of ADLs, excluding heavy lifting (>5 lb), pushing, or pulling for 6–8 weeks to prevent development of incisional herniation.

6. Referral to community resources, including home health care agency, enterostomal therapy (ET) nurse, and local chapter of United Ostomy Association (UOA).

7. Importance of follow-up care with MD and ET nurse; confirm date and time of next appointment.

8. Importance of reporting signs and symptoms that require medical attention such as change in stoma color from the normal bright and shiny red; peristomal and/or perianal skin irritation; any significant changes in appearance, frequency, and consistency of stools; fever, chills, abdominal pain, or distention; and incisional pain, drainage, swelling, or redness.

▶ Section Four   **Obesity**

Obesity is excessive body fat. Although overeating is the primary cause, other factors can predispose an individual to obesity, including genetics, the environment, inactivity, endocrine disorders, and excessive weight gain during pregnancy. *Juvenile-onset (hyperplastic/developmental) obesity* is characterized by a marked increase in the number of adipose tissue cells (hyperplasia) and triggered by increased caloric intake during infancy and early childhood. Hyperplasia occurs rapidly in the early years and continues (with excess caloric intake) until growth and development are completed. The fat cells do not disappear, and the number remains constant. Eighty percent of obese children become obese adults. *Adult-onset (hypertrophic/mature/reactive) obesity* is characterized by enlargement of individual adipose cells; the total number remains constant. Adult-onset obesity is not as severe as juvenile obesity, and weight loss is usually more successful. This type of obesity often occurs in response to traumatic or stressful life events.

Obesity affects multiple organ systems and is a major contributing factor to male premature death, fatal myocardial infarctions in males under age 40, coronary artery disease in males and females over age 40, hypertension and hyperlipidemia, cerebrovascular accidents, gynecologic irregularities, toxemia during pregnancy, postoperative complications, orthopedic problems in the lower extremities and spine, and peripheral vascular disorders. Mortality rate is higher for obese individuals, and most morbidly obese people live to less than age 50. Obesity can precipitate diabetes mellitus, and the majority of diabetics over age 40 are obese when the disorder is diagnosed. Obese individuals also can suffer social and emotional problems associated with their weight problems.

A. Assessment

Overweight: Weight that is greater than the average (ideal) weight given in insurance tables for given sex and height in the United States. See Table 11-2, p. 518.

Obesity: Weight >20% over ideal body weight.

Morbid obesity: Weight >45 kg (100 lb) above normal weight for 3 or more years.

B. Diagnostic Tests

There are no tests specific for obesity. Obtaining weight, height, and anthropometric measurements in conjunction with weight and diet history provides evidence for the diagnosis of obesity. (For guidelines, see "Providing Nutritional Therapy," p. 513, in Chapter 11.) If an endocrine disorder is suspected as being a factor in the patient's obesity, specific diagnostic tests should be performed to confirm or deny endocrinopathy.

C. Medical Management and Surgical Interventions

1. **Diet:** The cornerstone of obesity therapy. The caloric intake must be lowered below the caloric expenditure. A calorie deficit of 3500 kcal is required to lose one pound. Diet education is crucial to diet therapy because new eating habits must be formed before therapy can be successful on a long-term basis. Starvation/semistarvation is not a diet of choice because lean body mass is lost to a significant extent rather than adipose tissue.

2. **Exercise:** Integral part of weight loss/maintenance program. It increases caloric expenditure, keeps tissues firm, and aids circulation and digestion. It must be coupled with diet to afford significant weight reduction.

3. **Pharmacotherapy:** Used only as an adjunct to diet and exercise.

   ☐ *Anorexiant agent:* Temporary use can aid in "reprogramming" eating habits.

   ☐ *Thyroid hormones:* Used if there is evidence of hypometabolism.

   ☐ *Maintenance vitamin supplements:* Often indicated, especially if the patient reports use of "fad" diets. Amphetamines are avoided.

4. **Psychotherapy:** Often helpful in conjunction with diet and exercise therapy program. Examples include group therapy as found in Weight Watchers, Take Off Pounds Sensibly (TOPS), and Overeaters Anonymous; all can help to reinforce motivation. Diets approved by these groups have been proven to be nutritionally sound. Behavior modification is frequently used with encouraging results.

5. **Surgical treatment (bariatric operations):** Used as a last resort when all medical therapies for successful weight loss have failed. Usually, it is reserved for individuals who are morbidly obese.

   ☐ *Jejunoileal bypass* (JIB): Approximately 90% of the small bowel is bypassed. Weight loss results from malabsorption of food. Complications can include diarrhea, liver pathology, renal calculi, osteoporosis, mineral deficiencies, and abdominal distention and cramping. Because of the multiple, serious complications, this surgery is rarely performed.

   ☐ *Gastric bypass-loop gastrojejunostomy* (GB-L): Creation of a very small functioning stomach (approximately 25 mL) and a small opening for food to pass into the jejunum. The lower (larger) part of the stomach is bypassed rather than removed. Weight loss results from reduced calorie intake because of early satiety. Complications are similar to those with JIB.

   ☐ *Gastric bypass-Roux-en-Y gastrojejunostomy* (GB-RY): Creation of a small stomach pouch with a small opening into the jejunum. The lower stomach is bypassed and the jejunum is divided. A foot-long segment is attached to the small pouch and the other end is attached to the jejunum. Weight loss results from early satiety and decreased calorie intake. There is less chance of afferent limb obstruction and anastomotic leak. Complications can include "dumping syndrome," obstruction, and gastric leak.

☐ *Greater curvature gastroplasty* (GCG) *and gastrogastrostomy* (GG): A modified gastric bypass. The upper portion of the stomach is partitioned to form a small pouch and a 1/2-inch opening is made between the upper and lower stomach partitions. There is no change in the patient's ability to absorb and utilize food. Weight loss results from early satiety, leading to decreased calorie intake. Complications can include greater curvature obstruction, leak at staples, and nausea and vomiting if patient overeats. Diarrhea does not occur.

☐ *Vertical banded gastroplasty* (VBGP): Vertical partitioning of the stomach is made with staples (pouch size is approximately 25 mL). A 1/2-inch opening is made into the lower stomach partition and is reinforced with a Marlex band to prevent stretching. Weight loss results from early satiety. This type of surgery has the lowest complication rate. Nausea and vomiting can occur if patient overeats.

D. Nursing Diagnoses and Interventions

Knowledge deficit: Healthy dietary behaviors and patterns

Desired outcome: Patient can verbalize knowledge of healthy dietary behaviors and patterns.

1. Instruct patient to record typical 24-hour dietary intake, including the time, amount, type of food, and feelings prior to eating. This will help patient determine whether the eating response is stimulated by internal or external factors.

2. Reinforce for patient and SOs that food is not a reward or solace and that being overweight is not a sign of happiness or prosperity.

3. Provide lists of low-calorie nutritious foods for snacks, if they are allowed (see Table 6-2).

4. Promote exercise (unless contraindicated) as an adjunct to diet therapy.

5. Review diet plan with patient and SOs and answer questions.

Potential for noncompliance related to reluctance secondary to need for major lifestyle change and disappointment secondary to slow weight loss

Desired outcome: Patient complies with the prescribed dietary regimen, as evidenced by steady progress toward the weight loss goal.

1. Because weight may show daily fluctuations due to water loss/retention, weigh patient no more than once or twice a week. Ensure a consistent schedule, however.

2. Discourage SOs from bringing in food to the patient. A thorough explanation of the diet often alleviates this problem.

3. Assess cultural and economic influences of family diet. Formulating a diet regimen based on realistic family information leads to best results.

Table 6-2 Suggested Low-Calorie Snacks

any fresh fruit (bananas and kiwi fruit are acceptable in small quantities)	rice cake
	bouillon (1 cup)
raw vegetables: carrots, broccoli, celery, cauliflower, snowpeas, tomatoes	skim milk (½ cup)
	dill pickles
plain yogurt	sugar-free beverages
plain herb tea	sugar-free gelatins
plain coffee	angel food cake (1 slice)
low-fat cottage cheese (½ cup)	graham crackers (2)

4. Explain dietary exchange items if allowed, so that patients feel they have some control in the diet regimen and preferences can be satisfied.

5. Encourage exercise, which can elevate patient's mood and enhance compliance.

6. Recognize and provide positive reinforcement for patient compliance with the dietary regimen and concomitant weight loss.

7. Provide emotional support for patient and SOs. Encourage patient to verbalize feelings concerning body image and expected body changes.

8. Encourage patient to join group therapy such as that provided in the following: TOPS, Weight Watchers, and Overeaters Anonymous.

Potential alterations in nutrition and fluid volume related to decreased intake secondary to dietary restrictions and/or postsurgical regimen

Desired outcome: Patient does not exhibit signs of malnutrition, fluid overload, or dehydration.

1. Encourage prescribed diet and oral intake to ensure that the patient attains adequate nutrients and hydration.

2. Maintain accurate I&O records. Administer and record prescribed IV fluids, assessing for indicators of overhydration (edema, hypertension) or dehydration (decreased urinary output and/or high specific gravity, hypotension, poor skin turgor, dry skin and mucous membranes); report significant findings to MD.

3. Once oral fluids are allowed after surgery, provide small amounts at frequent intervals (for example, 30 mL q30min) for specified total. Small amounts of fluid will not overdistend the small stomach pouch.

4. Because obese individuals often have insulin resistance with altered diet, hypoglycemia can occur. Test urine for acetone and observe for indicators of hypoglycemia, including headaches, weakness, syncope, diaphoresis, or VS changes.

5. Administer multivitamin supplements as prescribed.

6. After patient has recovered from surgery, and as directed by MD, encourage intake of 6 cups of fluid per day, consumed between meals. Explain that adequate fluid intake will enhance hydration to help prevent constipation, especially in the presence of decreased dietary intake.

Potential for injury related to risk of gastrointestinal complications secondary to bariatric surgery

Desired outcomes: If gastrointestinal complications occur, they are detected promptly, resulting in immediate treatment and absence of injury to the patient. Patient can verbalize knowledge of indicators of bariatric surgical complications and is aware of the need to report them immediately.

1. Monitor patient for pain, including its focus and character, and auscultate abdomen for bowel sounds. Be alert to absence of sounds or high-pitched "tinkling" sounds, and monitor for GI disturbances, including nausea, vomiting, distention, and a stabbing or constant, dull pain. Guaiac-test suspicious NG drainage, aspirate, or stool, and notify MD of positive results. Early detection of the above indicators can alert MD to complications such as volvulus, stomal obstruction, subphrenic abscess, iatrogenic vagotomy, and stomal ulcer.

2. Monitor for the following indicators of gastric leak: gastric fluid on dressings, increasing drainage output, and absence of stool.

3. Assess for indicators of dumping syndrome, including diaphoresis, tachycardia, abdominal cramping, weakness, and diarrhea.

4. Report significant findings to MD, and instruct patient to alert the staff should any of the above indicators occur.

Ineffective breathing patterns related to decreased inspiratory depth secondary to anesthesia and/or guarding from painful abdominal incision

Desired outcome: Patient demonstrates compliance with deep-breathing and coughing regimen and does not exhibit signs of pulmonary dysfunction.

1. Because obese patients are frequently respiratorily compromised before surgery, assess respiratory status at frequent intervals after surgery. Monitor respiratory rate q15–30min until patient stabilizes and then as prescribed unless respiratory distress is noted. Be alert to the following indicators of hypoxia: SOB, mentation changes, pallor, increased respiratory rate, and anxiety.

2. Assist patient into positions that facilitate breathing, typically reverse Trendelenberg's, and encourage deep breathing (and coughing as indicated) at frequent intervals to help prevent atelectasis and pneumonia.

Potential impairment of skin integrity (with concomitant risk of poor wound healing) related to vulnerability secondary to sedentary lifestyle

Desired outcome: Patient does not exhibit signs of impaired skin integrity or wound healing.

1. Poor skin integrity can be present before surgery because of the sedentary lifestyle associated with many obese individuals. Maintain skin integrity before and after surgery by using sheepskin, air, or eggcrate mattress. Monitor skin for redness or irritation, especially in areas prone to breakdown, such as the sacrum, iliac crests, elbows, heels, and greater trochanters.

2. Inspect dressing for wound drainage or blood. Circle the amount with a pen, and record the amount and character. Notify MD of copious drainage. Change dressings as prescribed, using aseptic technique.

3. Be alert to signs of poor wound healing. For details, see nursing diagnoses and interventions in "Managing Wound Care," p. 483+, in Chapter 10, "Sensory Disorders."

Alteration in comfort: Pain and nausea related to surgical procedure

Desired outcome: Patient relates a reduction in discomfort and does not exhibit signs of uncontrolled pain or nausea.

1. When oral fluids are allowed, provide small quantities at frequent intervals (30 mL q30min) for the specified total. This will minimize nausea and prevent distention to promote comfort.

2. For other interventions, see the same nursing diagnosis in "Appendix One," "Caring for Preoperative and Postoperative Patients," p. 528.

Knowledge deficit: Dietary regimen after bariatric surgery

Desired outcome: Patient can verbalize knowledge of the postsurgical diet and demonstrates compliance with the prescribed regimen.

1. Assess patient and SOs for knowledge of bariatric surgery and the dietary program. Provide or clarify information as appropriate.

2. Explain that the new stomach is egg-sized (approximately one-fourth cup). Stress the importance of not eating once the sensation of fullness occurs, as signaled by nausea, pain referred to the left shoulder, and/or pressure in the center of the abdomen.

3. Advise patient to allow 30 minutes to eat each meal and take small bites of food, chewing each bite 20–30 times to prevent food from occluding the small stomach opening into the intestine. Suggest that the patient use the increased chewing time to note the flavor, texture, and consistency of the food.

4. Instruct patient to eat only three meals a day and to avoid snacking, which would result in less weight loss.

5. Inform patient that drinking liquids with meals should be avoided because the small stomach does not allow room for food *and* fluid and this would result in distention and pain.

6. Advise patient to drink 6 cups of liquids per day, consumed between meals, and to sip them slowly. Explain that adequate fluid intake will help prevent constipation.

7. Explain that alcoholic beverages are contraindicated because they are high in calories and often stimulate the appetite.

8. Inform patient that the diet is composed of lean proteins and low amounts of carbohydrates. Exchanges are possible when the stomach and intestine adapt to the surgical changes. The average gastric bypass diet supplies 700–800 kcal and 50 g of protein/day.

9. Stress the importance of supplementing the diet with multivitamins as directed by MD.

10. If constipation becomes a problem, advise patient to increase daily fluid intake and/or add prune juice or fruit to the diet.

11. Reinforce the importance of complementing the diet with exercise, including stretching and brisk walking.

For patients who have undergone bariatric surgery, see additional nursing diagnoses and interventions for the care of preoperative and postoperative patients, pp. 528–532 in "Appendix One."

E. Patient–Family Teaching and Discharge Planning

Provide patient and SOs with verbal and written information for the following:

1. Importance of weight loss, including health-related problems that can ensue if obesity continues or recurs.

2. Importance of responding to internal stimuli (gastric motility, hypoglycemia, hunger) rather than external stimuli (time of day and the availability, sight, taste, and advertisements for food) for eating.

3. Names and addresses of commercial weight loss programs such as TOPS, Weight Watchers, and Overeaters Anonymous.

4. Importance of coupling exercise with diet for significant weight reduction.

5. Nutritious foods that make healthful snacks.

6. Importance of reporting symptoms of hypoglycemia to MD, including headaches, weakness, syncope, diaphoresis.

7. Medications (typically multivitamins), including drug name, purpose, dosage, schedule, precautions, and potential side effects.

In addition, for patients who have had bariatric surgery:

8. See **Knowledge deficit:** Dietary regimen after bariatric surgery, above. Explain that overeating will stretch the stomach over time.

9. Explain that there will be mandatory clinic follow-ups at 1, 3, 6, and 12 months and then annually.

▶ Section Five **Hepatic and Biliary Disorders**

The liver lies directly beneath the diaphragm and occupies most of the right upper quadrant of the abdomen. It governs the formation and secretion of bile. The gallbladder, which lies directly beneath the right lobe of the liver, and the hepatic, cystic, and common bile ducts comprise the biliary system. The biliary duct system transports bile from the liver to the gallbladder. Bile is concentrated and stored in the gallbladder and released to the small intestine (duodenum), where it facilitates the absorption of fats, fat-soluble vitamins, and certain minerals, and also activates the release of pancreatic enzymes. If an obstructive lesion is present in the biliary ducts, the flow of bile is blocked, resulting in hemoconcentration. When this occurs, a variety of clinical manifestations can surface, including obstructive jaundice, dark-amber urine, and clay-colored stools. Pruritus occurs because of the deposition of bile salts in skin tissue. Steatorrhea and bleeding tendencies result from the inability of the duodenum to absorb fats and fat-soluble vitamins A, D, E, and K. Vitamin K is necessary for adequate clotting of the blood. **Note:** Pancreatic problems are discussed in Chapter 5, "Endocrine Disorders," p. 247–255.

I. Hepatitis

Viral hepatitis is caused by one of the hepatitis viruses: A, B, non-A or non-B. Although symptomatology is similar, immunologic and epidemiologic characteristics are different (see Table 6–3, next page). When hepatocytes are damaged, necrosis and autolysis can occur, which in turn lead to abnormal liver functioning. Generally, these changes are completely reversible after the acute phase. In some cases, however, massive necrosis can lead to liver failure and death.

Jaundice may be seen in any patient with decreased hepatic function. It is classifed as prehepatic (hemolytic), caused by increased production of bilirubin; hepatic (hepatocellular), which is caused by the dysfunction of the liver cells; or posthepatic (obstructive), caused by an obstruction of the flow of bile out of the liver.

A. Assessment

Signs and symptoms: Nausea, vomiting, anorexia, signs of URI, fatigue, irritability, distaste for cigarettes in smokers, slight to moderate temperature increases, epigastric discomfort, dark urine, clay-colored stools, pruritus.

Physical exam: Inspection of the skin, mucous membranes, and sclera may reveal yellow coloration; palpation of lymph nodes and abdomen may reveal lymphadenopathy, hepatomegaly, and splenomegaly.

History of: Blood dyscrasias, multiple blood transfusions, alcohol or drug abuse, exposure to hepatotoxic chemicals.

B. Diagnostic Tests

1. <u>Hematologic tests:</u> Anti-HAV IgM will be present with hepatitis A, as will HBsAg with hepatitis B. SGOT (frequently called serum aspartate transaminase, AST) and SGPT initially will be elevated and then drop. Total bilirubin will be elevated and the PT will be prolonged. Differential WBC count will reveal leukocytosis, monocytosis, atypical lymphocytes, and plasma cells.

2. <u>Bromsulphalein (BSP) excretion test:</u> Dye is injected intravenously. In a normal liver it is almost completely cleared from the blood; in hepatitis the blood level is elevated. Because excretion is more rapid after eating because of the increased blood flow, the patient must be NPO 8–12 hours before and during the test. Weigh patient prior to test because the amount of dye injected is proportionate to body weight. Usually this is a 24-hour test, but a 2-hour test of a single specimen also may be ordered. **Note:** Collect the 2-hour specimen from between 1 and 4 pm, the hours of peak excretion.

3. <u>Urine tests:</u> Will reveal elevation of urobilinogen.

C. Medical Management

1. **Bed rest:** During acute phase and when patient is fatigued.

2. **Diet:** No alcohol for 6 months. Parenteral and/or enteral nutrition may be initiated if anorexia is severe. Vitamins are usually given.

Table 6-3 Comparison of Characteristics of Types of Viral Hepatitis

	Type A	Type B	Non-A Non-B
Mode of Transmission	Fecal—oral route; large-scale outbreaks caused by contamination of food or water	Percutaneous inoculation (needle stick); usually through blood, but may result from saliva or semen	Usually blood; also semen and saliva
Population Affected	More common in children and in overcrowded areas with poor sanitation	All ages. Drug addicts, male homosexuals and sexual partners of infected individuals. Patients and staff in hemodialysis units are at high risk.	All ages. Highest risk in recipients of blood transfusions. Also at risk are drug addicts and hemodialysis patients. Nosocomial spread possible
Diagnosis of Acute Disease	Anti-hepatitis A virus (IgM) antibody in serum (anti-HAV IgM)	Hepatitis B surface antigen in serum (HBsAg)	When causes of type A and type B are ruled out
Incubation Period	2–6 weeks	6 weeks–6 months	2 weeks–6 months
Carrier State	No	Yes	Yes
Chronicity	No	Yes	Yes
Measures for Reducing Exposure	Handwashing; stool precautions first 2–3 weeks	Handwashing; wearing gloves when handling body fluids and masks when fluids may splatter; using care when discarding needles and syringes; autoclaving all nondisposable items. Patient can never become a blood donor	Same as for type B
Prophylaxis	IG (immune globulin) before or within 1–2 weeks after exposure	HBIG (hepatitis B immune globulin) within 24 hours after exposure and 1 month later. Hepatitis B vaccine recommended for medical and laboratory personnel, male homosexuals, neonates of infected mothers, and sexual partners of chronic HBsAg carriers	Still controversial, but currently a single dose of IG is recommended

Table 6-4 Hepatotoxic Drugs

Generic/Category Name	Common Trade Names
acetaminophen	Tylenol
acetylsalicylic acid	Aspirin
chlorpromazine	Thorazine
dantrolene sodium	Dantrium
isoniazid	Isotamine
methyldopa	Aldomet
nitrofurantoin macrocrystals	Macrodantin
phenytoin sodium	Dilantin
propylthiouracil (PTU)	Propyl-Thyracil
sulfonamides	Bactrim, Septra, Gantrisin

3. **Manage pruritis:** Restrict alkaline soaps; prescribe emollients. Antihistamines and tranquilizers, if used, are administered with caution and in low doses, because they are metabolized by the liver. See Table 6-4, which lists hepatotoxic drugs.

4. **Pharmacotherapy**

   □ *Parenteral vitamin K:* For those patients with prolonged PT.

   □ *Antiemetics:* For patients with nausea.

5. **Restrict hepatotoxic drugs:** See Table 6-4.

D. Nursing Diagnoses and Interventions

Sleep pattern disturbance related to agitation secondary to hepatic dysfunction (faulty absorption, metabolism, and storage of nutrients)

Desired outcome: Patient relates the attainment of adequate sleep and rest.

1. Provide rest periods before and after activities and treatments.

2. Keep frequently used objects within easy reach.

3. Promote rest and sleep by decreasing environmental stimuli, providing back massage and/or relaxation tapes, speaking with patient in short, simple terms.

Knowledge deficit: Causes of hepatitis and modes of transmission

Desired outcome: Patient can verbalize knowledge of the causes of hepatitis and measures that help prevent transmission.

1. Assess patient's knowledge of the disease process and educate as necessary. Make sure patient knows you are not making moral decisions regarding alcohol/drug use and/or sexual behavior.

2. Teach patient and SOs the importance of good handwashing.

3. If appropriate, advise patients with hepatitis A that crowded living conditions with poor sanitation should be avoided to prevent recurrence.

4. Remind patients with hepatitis B and non-A non-B hepatitis that sexual relations should be avoided, as directed by MD. Explain that blood donation is no longer possible.

5. Advise patients with hepatitis B that their sexual partners should receive hepatitis B vaccine.

6. Refer patient to alcohol/drug treatment programs as necessary.

7. See Table 6-3 for other data.

Alteration in nutrition: Less than body requirements related to decreased intake secondary to anorexia, nausea, and gastric distress

Desired outcome: Patient does not exhibit signs of malnutrition or weight loss.

1. Take a diet history to determine food preferences.
2. Monitor and record intake.
3. Offer mouth care prior to meals to alleviate unpleasant taste and thereby enhance appetite.
4. Encourage small, frequent feedings and provide emotional support during meals.
5. Obtain prescription for vitamin and mineral supplements, if appropriate.
6. Administer antacids, antiemetics, antidiarrheals, and cathartics as prescribed to minimize gastric distress.
7. Encourage SOs to bring in desirable foods, if permitted.

Impairment of skin integrity related to pruritus secondary to hepatic dysfunction

Desired outcome: Patient's skin remains intact.

1. Keep skin moist by using tepid water or emollient baths, avoiding soap, and applying emollient lotions at frequent intervals.
2. Encourage patient not to scratch skin and to keep nails short and smooth. Suggest the use of the knuckles if patient must scratch. Wrap or place gloves on patient's hands (especially comatose patients).
3. To prevent infection, treat any skin lesion promptly.
4. Encourage patient to wear loose, soft clothing; provide soft linens (cotton is best).
5. Keep the environment cool.
6. Change wet linen often.

Disturbance in self-concept related to alteration in body image secondary to jaundice

Desired outcomes: Patient verbalizes feelings and concerns. Patient can verbalize knowledge of measures for enhancing appearance and demonstrates an interest in daily grooming.

1. Encourage patient and SOs to verbalize feelings, concerns.
2. Encourage patient to maintain daily grooming.
3. Explain that wearing yellow and green intensifies yellow skin tone. Suggest wearing bright reds and blues or black instead.
4. Provide privacy as necessary.

Potential for injury related to increased risk of bleeding secondary to decreased vitamin-K absorption

Desired outcomes: Patient does not exhibit signs of bleeding due to handling, invasive procedures, or sharp objects. If bleeding does occur, it is detected promptly, resulting in immediate treatment and absence of injury to the patient.

1. Monitor PT levels daily.
2. Handle patient gently (eg, when turning or transferring).
3. Minimize IM injections. Rotate sites, and use small-gauge needles. Apply moderate pressure after an injection, but do not massage the site.
4. Observe for ecchymotic areas. Inspect the gums and test the urine and feces for the presence of bleeding. Report significant findings to MD.
5. Teach patient to use electric razor and soft-bristled toothbrush.
6. Administer vitamin K as prescribed.

E. Patient–Family Teaching and Discharge Planning

Provide patient and SOs with verbal and written information for the following:

1. Importance of rest and getting adequate nutrition.
2. Hepatotoxic agents, especially OTC drugs.
3. Prescribed medications, eg, multivitamins, including the name, purpose, dosage, schedule, potential side effects, and precautions.
4. Potential complications, including delayed healing, skin injury, and bleeding tendencies.
5. Referral to alcohol/drug treatment programs as appropriate.

II. Cirrhosis

Cirrhosis is a chronic, serious disease in which there are structural changes in the liver. Although pathologic changes do not occur for many years, structural changes gradually lead to total liver dysfunction. Complications include portal hypertension, ascites, esophageal varices, hemorrhoids, splenomegaly, bleeding tendencies, jaundice, hepatorenal syndrome, and hepatic encephalopathy (hepatic coma).

Laennec's (alcoholic/portal) cirrhosis: Associated with chronic alcohol abuse and accounts for 50% of all cases. Half survive for 2 years and 35% survive for 5 years. The major survival factor is the cessation of alcohol intake. Portal hypertension and liver failure will result if alcoholic intake is continued.

Postnecrotic cirrhosis: Associated with history of viral hepatitis or hepatic damage from industrial chemicals; accounts for 20% of all cases. Three-fourths die within 1–5 years. This type appears to predispose the patient to the development of a hepatoma.

Biliary cirrhosis: Associated with post-hepatic biliary obstruction and accounts for 15% of all cases.

A. Assessment

Chronic indicators: Lassitude, anorexia, nausea, vomiting (especially early in the morning), dyspepsia, flatulence, change in bowel habits, slight weight loss, discomfort in epigastric area or RUQ.

Acute indicators: Hepatocellular failure resulting in jaundice, peripheral edema, fetor hepaticus (a musty, sweetish odor on the breath), hepatic encephalopathy (can progress from slight changes in personality and behavior to coma); hematologic disorders, including bleeding tendencies, anemia, leukopenia, thrombocytopenia; excess circulating estrogen as evidenced by spider angiomas, testicular atrophy, gynecomastia, pectoral and axillary alopecia, palmar erythema; and portal hypertension complications, including splenomegaly, esophageal and gastric varices, hemorrhoids, and ascites.

History of: Exposure to hepatotoxic agents, viral hepatitis, alcoholism, poor nutrition.

B. Diagnostic Tests

1. <u>Hematologic tests:</u> SGOT (AST) and SGPT will be elevated. Alkaline phosphatase will rise in the presence of biliary obstruction because it cannot be excreted. Direct and total bilirubin will be elevated and BUN will be decreased with liver failure and increased with GI bleeding. Uric acid will be increased in the presence of alcholism. PT will be prolonged. Ammonia will be increased in hepatic coma. WBCs will be decreased with hypersplenism and increased with infection. RBCs will be decreased in hypersplenism and hemorrhage. Creatinine will be increased. Sodium will be decreased and potassium will be increased. **Note:** Keep patient NPO except for water for 8

hours before the drawing of the ammonia level. Notify the lab of all antibiotics taken by patient as these will lower the ammonia level.

2. <u>Bromsulphalein (BSP) test:</u> Usually elevated. (For details, see "Hepatitis," p. 325.)

3. <u>Urine tests:</u> Urine bilirubin will be increased; urobilinogen will be normal or increased.

4. <u>Liver biopsy:</u> Provides a microscopic picture of hepatocytes and aids in confirming a diagnosis. It is contraindicated in patients with clotting abnormalities, in cases of obstructive jaundice, or in the presence of local infection at biopsy site or ascites. **Note:** After the biopsy, monitor VS and check site at frequent intervals. Be alert to presence of respiratory distress and to indicators of peritonitis, including severe abdominal pain, nausea, vomiting, rising temperature, tachycardia, pallor, and rigid abdomen.

5. <u>Barium swallow:</u> Verifies the presence of esophageal or gastric varices. **Note:** Keep patient NPO from 12 midnight until completion of the test. Check subsequent stools to determine complete evacuation of barium.

6. <u>Radiologic studies:</u> Ultrasound differentiates hemolytic and hepatocellular jaundice from obstructive jaundice (see "Hepatitis," p. 325) and shows hepatomegaly and intrahepatic tumors. CT scans show fine density differences. Percutaneous trans-hepatic cholangiography reveals the extent of obstruction via contrast dye. Endoscopic retrograde cholangiopancreatography is a fiber-optic technique used to show pancreatic causes of jaundice. Liver scans allow visualization of the spleen and liver via injection of radioisotopes. **Note:** After injection of the dye, the patient may experience nausea, vomiting, and transient elevated temperature.

7. <u>Esophagoscopy:</u> A fiberoptic technique used to verify presence of esophageal varices and/or bleeding.

C. Medical Management and Surgical Interventions

1. **Identify and treat underlying causes:** For example, exposure to hepatotoxins, use of alcohol, biliary obstruction.

2. **Pharmacotherapy**

   □ *Diuretics:* To reduce edema.

   □ *Antibiotics:* To control intestinal flora.

   □ *Hematinics:* To control anemia.

   □ *Blood coagulants and vasopressors:* To control bleeding.

   □ *Laxatives and stool softeners:* To prevent straining.

   □ *Antidiarrheals:* As necessary to control diarrhea.

   □ *Antipruritics:* For pruritus.

   □ *Topical anesthetics:* For hemorrhoids.

   □ *Supplemental vitamins and minerals:* Such as folic acid for macrocytic anemia and vitamin K for prolonged PT.

▶ **Note:** Narcotics and sedatives, which are metabolized by the liver, are contraindicated. Small doses of IV diazepam may be administered if absolutely necessary. See Table 6-4, p. 327, for a list of hepatotoxic drugs.

---

3. **Dietary management:** With fluid retention and ascites, sodium and fluids are restricted. Usually, half the calories are supplied as carbohydrates. Protein is restricted in hepatic coma or precoma. Parenteral or enteral nutrition is administered in the presence of bleeding or coma.

4. **Bed rest:** In the presence of fever, infection.

5. Treatment of complications

□ *Hemorrhage from esophageal varices:* Usually, a 4-lumen Minnesota sump tube or 3-lumen Sengstaken-Blakemore tube is used for tamponade, and surgical management includes a portocaval shunt (anastomosis of portal vein and vena cava) or a splenorenal shunt (anastomosis of splenic vein and left renal vein). Both shunts divert blood from the portal system to the vena cava. Shunts, however, are usually not successful for prolonging life.

□ *Ascites:* Dietary management may include sodium and fluid restrictions. Diuretics, usually aldosterone antagonists, are often given to minimize fluid collection. If indicated, surgical management includes a peritoneovenous shunt (LeVeen or Denver) to shunt portal bloodflow to renal bloodflow. Paracentesis is usually not indicated unless there is severe respiratory distress or discomfort or if it is essential for diagnosis of a tumor or bacterial peritonitis.

□ *Hepatic encephalopathy (hepatic coma):* Dietary management includes restriction of protein from the diet, giving sweetened fruit juices, and administering parenteral/enteral nutrition if the patient is comatose. Pharmacologic management includes antibiotics to inhibit intestinal bacteria and magnesium sulfate or enemas to cleanse the intestines after GI bleeding. The following drugs are contraindicated: barbiturates, narcotics, potassium-depleting diuretics, and ammonia-containing medications.

D. Nursing Diagnoses and Interventions

Alteration in nutrition: Less than body requirements related to decreased intake secondary to anorexia and nausea

Desired outcomes: Patient does not exhibit signs of malnutrition or weight loss. Patient can verbalize knowledge of foods that are permitted and restricted.

1. Encourage foods that are permitted within patient's dietary restrictions. Remember that sodium and/or fluids are restricted, and if the ammonia level rises, protein also will be restricted. Explain dietary restrictions to the patient.

2. Encourage small, frequent meals to ensure adequate nutrition.

3. Encourage SOs to bring in desirable foods as permitted.

4. Have nourishing foods available to patient at night.

5. Administer vitamin and mineral supplements, as prescribed.

6. Administer the following medications, as prescribed, to decrease gastric distress: antacids, antiemetics, antidiarrheals, cathartics.

7. Monitor I&O; weigh patient daily.

8. Promote bed rest to reduce metabolic demands on the liver.

9. Provide soft diet if patient has esophageal varices, or discuss need for tube feedings with MD if appropriate.

Impaired gas exchange related to decreased lung expansion secondary to pressure on the diaphragm caused by ascites

Desired outcome: Patient's ABG values and physical findings are within acceptable range.

1. During complaints of dyspnea or orthopnea, assist patient into semi- or high Fowler's position to enhance gas exchange.

2. Administer oxygen as prescribed.

3. Monitor ABG values; notify MD of significant findings.

4. Encourage patient to change positions and deep-breathe at frequent intervals to enhance gas exchange. If secretions are present, ensure that the patient coughs frequently.

5. Notify MD of indicators of respiratory infection such as spiking temperatures, chills, diaphoresis, and adventitious breath sounds.

6. Obtain baseline abdominal girth measurement, and then measure girth either daily or q shift. Measure around the same circumferential area each time; mark the site with indelible ink.

Potential for injury related to increased risk of bleeding secondary to altered clotting factors and portal hypertension

Desired outcomes: Patient does not exhibit signs of bleeding due to irritating foods, actions that increase intra-abdominothoracic pressure, or defecation. Patient can verbalize knowledge of actions or foods that can cause bleeding.

1. Instruct patient to avoid swallowing foods that are chemically or mechanically irritating (eg, rough or spicy foods, hot foods, hot liquids).

2. Advise patient to avoid actions that increase intra-abdominothoracic pressure, such as coughing, sneezing, lifting, or vomiting.

3. Administer stool softeners, as prescribed, to help prevent patient from straining with defecation.

4. Inspect stools for presence of occult blood; perform a guaiac test as indicated.

5. As appropriate, instruct patient about alcohol's role in causing esophageal varices.

6. See **Potential for injury** in "Hepatitis," p. 328, for other interventions.

Potential for injury related to risk of hepatic coma secondary to cerebral accumulation of ammonia and/or GI bleeding

Desired outcome: Potentially precipitating causes of hepatic coma, if they occur, are detected and reported promptly, resulting in immediate treatment and absence of injury to the patient.

1. Perform a baseline assessment of patient's personality characteristics. Enlist the aid of SOs to help determine slight changes in personality or behavior.

2. Have patient demonstrate his or her signature daily. If the writing deteriorates, ammonia levels may be increasing. Be alert to generalized muscle twitching and asterixis (flapping tremor induced by dorsiflexion of wrist and extension of fingers). Report significant findings to MD.

3. Remind patient to avoid protein and foods high in ammonia, such as gelatin, onions, and strong cheeses. The diseased liver is unable to convert ammonia to urea and the buildup of ammonia adds to the progression of hepatic encephalopathy.

4. Observe for indicators of GI bleeding, including melena or hematemesis. GI bleeding can precipitate hepatic coma. Report bleeding to MD promptly and obtain prescription for cleansing enemas.

5. Protect patient against injury that can be precipitated by confused state.

Fluid volume excess: Edema and ascites related to retention secondary to portal hypertension and hepatocellular failure

Desired outcomes: Patient can verbalize knowledge of food and nonfood items that increase swelling and exhibits physical findings and laboratory values within acceptable range.

1. Obtain baseline abdominal girth measurement. Mark abdomen with indelible ink to ensure serial measurements from the same circumferential site. Measure girth daily or q shift as appropriate.

2. Monitor I&O; weigh patient daily. Notify MD of significant findings.

3. Give frequent mouth care and provide ice chips to help minimize thirst.

4. Monitor electrolyte values and report abnormalities to MD.

5. Remind patient to avoid food and nonfood items that contain sodium (eg, antacids, baking soda, and some mouthwashes).

Knowledge deficit: Factors that precipitate or aggravate cirrhosis

Desired outcome: Patient can verbalize knowledge of factors that can aggravate or precipitate cirrhosis.

1. Determine patient's pattern of alcohol use. Inform patient that a major survival factor is cessation of alcohol.

2. If appropriate, refer patient to an alcohol treatment program and/or Alcoholics Anonymous.

3. Refer family members to Al-Anon and Alateen.

4. Assure patient that you are not making a moral decision about his or her drinking, if this is a factor. Acknowledge that alcoholism is a disease, not a moral weakness.

5. Assist patient with identifying hepatotoxins other than alcohol (see Table 6-4, p. 327).

6. Encourage patient to adhere to medical regimen, including dietary restrictions and pharmacologic management.

See "Hepatitis" for the following: **Disturbance in self-concept**, p. 328.

E. Patient–Family Teaching and Discharge Planning

Provide patient and SOs with verbal and written information for the following:

1. Medications, including drug name, purpose, dosage, schedule, precautions, and potential side effects.

2. Dietary restrictions.

3. Potential need for lifestyle changes, including cessation of alcohol. Include appropriate referrals.

4. Awareness of hepatotoxic agents, especially OTC drugs.

III. Cholelithiasis and Cholecystitis

Cholelithiasis is a condition characterized by the presence of stones in the gallbladder and/or the biliary ducts. Gallstones can be composed of cholesterol, calcium bilirubinate, or calcium carbonate. Precipitating factors include disturbances in metabolism, biliary stasis, obstruction, and infection. Gallstones are especially prevalent in women who are multiparous, on estrogen therapy, or who use oral contraceptives. Other risk factors include obesity, dietary intake of fats, sedentary lifestyle, and familial tendencies. The incidence increases with age, and it is estimated that one out of every three persons who reach age 75 has gallstones. Cholelithiasis is frequently seen in disease states such as diabetes mellitus, regional enteritis, inflammatory disease of the terminal ileum, and certain blood dyscrasias. Usually, cholelithiasis is asymptomatic until a stone becomes lodged in the biliary tract. If the obstruction is unrelieved, biliary colic and cholecystitis can ensue.

Cholecystitis is most commonly associated with bile duct obstructions. Acute cholecystitis is typically caused by a gallstone that obstructs the cystic duct. With obstruction, structural changes can occur such as hypertrophy of the gallbladder and a swelling and thickening of the gallbladder walls. If the edema is prolonged, the walls become scarred and fibrosed, and the constant presence of bile can lead to mucosal irritation. As a complication of the impaired circulation and edema, pressure ischemia and necrosis can develop, resulting in gangrene or perforation. With chronic cholecystitis, stones almost always are present, and the gallbladder walls are thickened and fibrosed.

A. Assessment

Cholelithiasis: History of intolerance to fats and occasional discomfort after eating. As the stone moves through the duct or becomes lodged, a sudden onset of mild, aching pain will occur in the midepigastrium after eating and increase in intensity during a colic attack, potentially radiating to the RUQ and right subscapular region. Nausea, vomiting, tachycardia, and diaphoresis also can occur. This condition may also be asymptomatic.

Cholecystitis: History of intolerance to fats and discomfort after eating, including regurgitation, flatulence, belching, epigastric heaviness, indigestion, heartburn, chronic upper abdominal pain, and nausea. Amber-colored urine, clay-colored stools, pruritus, jaundice, steatorrhea, and bleeding tendencies can be present if there is bile obstruction. Symptoms may be vague.

Physical exam

□ *Cholelithiasis:* Palpation of RUQ will reveal a rigid abdomen during colic attack, with flaccidity between pains.

□ *Cholecystitis:* Palpation will elicit tenderness localized behind the inferior margin of the liver. With progressive symptoms, a tender, globular mass might be palpated behind the lower border of the liver.

B. Diagnostic Tests

1. <u>Radiologic studies:</u> Oral cholangiogram, IV cholangiogram, and percutaneous trans-hepatic cholangiogram assess the patency of the gallbladder and biliary ducts and help to rule out other conditions that mimic cholelithiasis or cholecystitis. Chest, abdominal, upper GI, and barium enema x-rays are often used to rule out pulmonary or other GI disorders.

2. <u>EKG:</u> To rule out cardiac disease.

3. <u>Ultrasonography of the gallbladder and biliary tract</u>: To detect gallstones and tumors and help distinguish between intrahepatic and extrahepatic jaundice.

4. <u>CT scan:</u> To detect dilated bile ducts and the presence of gallbladder cysts.

5. <u>Endoscopic retrograde cholangiopancreatography:</u> To visualize and evaluate the biliary tree.

6. <u>CBC:</u> To assess for presence of infection and/or blood loss.

7. <u>PT:</u> To assess for a prolonged clotting time secondary to faulty vitamin K absorption.

8. <u>Bilirubin tests (serum and urine) and urobilinogen tests (urine and fecal):</u> To differentiate between hemolytic disorders, hepatocellular disease, and obstructive disease. Usually there is an increase of bilirubin in the plasma and urine with biliary disease.

9. <u>Serum liver enzyme test:</u> Will show a small elevation in SGOT, SGPT, and LDH. With biliary obstruction, the alkaline phosphatase and 5 nucleotidase will have values ten times normal.

C. Medical Management and Surgical Interventions

1. Pharmacologic therapy

□ *Analgesics and antacids:* For pain.

□ *Anticholinergics:* To prevent smooth muscle contraction.

□ *Antispasmodics:* To relieve spasms.

□ *Antibiotics:* For infection.

□ *Antiemetics:* For nausea and vomiting.

□ *Bile salts:* To facilitate absorption of fats and fat-soluble vitamins.

□ *Fat-soluble vitamins such as A, D, E, and K:* Replacement is necessary because of faulty vitamin absorption in the small intestine.

□ *Hyperlipidemic agents:* Bind with bile salts in the intestine to facilitate excretion, and may be given to provide relief from pruritus.

2. **Chemical dissolution of cholesterol gallstones with a solvent:** May be used in patients with a functioning gallbladder and an unobstructed biliary tract. The solvent is infused via a T-tube. An oral preparation of bile salts, eg, chenodeoxycholic acid, may be administered to dissolve cholesterol stones.

3. **Dietary management:** Varies according to the patient's condition. During an acute attack, NPO with IV fluids may be instituted. With severe nausea and vomiting, an NG tube is inserted and attached to low, intermittent suction. Diet advances to patient's tolerance and small, frequent feedings of a low-fat diet are recommended for both the acute and chronic conditions.

4. **Non-operative biliary stone removal:** One method of stone extraction, which is performed under fluoroscopy in the radiology department. The stone is removed with a basket that is inserted via a catheter or T-tube through the sinus tract into the common duct. If this technique is unsuccessful, forceps are used to manipulate the stone. A cholangiogram is done before and after the procedure. If the x-ray is normal after the procedure, the T-tube is removed; if the stones are still present, a new T-tube or catheter is inserted and the patient returns the following day for the same procedure.

5. **Surgical interventions:** Usually required for relief of long-term symptoms of cholelithiasis and acute cholecystitis. The type of surgery depends on the severity and length of illness and site of obstruction. The following procedures may be performed:

   □ *Cholecystostomy:* Opening and draining the gallbladder of gallstones.

   □ *Choledochotomy:* Opening the common bile duct to remove stones.

   □ *Choledochoduodenostomy:* Anastomosis of the common bile duct to the duodenum.

   □ *Choledochojejunostomy:* Anastomosis of the common bile duct to the jejunum.

6. **Cholecystectomy (removal of the gallbladder):** The most commonly performed procedure for biliary disease, which accounts for one-third of all surgical procedures that are performed. A right subcostal incision is made, allowing exploration of the common duct. The stones are removed and a T-tube is often inserted to maintain patency of the common duct and drain bile. The gallbladder is then excised from the liver; the cystic duct, vein, and artery are ligated; and a drain (usually Penrose) is inserted and brought out through a stab wound for drainage of blood, serum, and bile.

D. Nursing Diagnoses and Interventions

Alteration in comfort: Pain, spasms, nausea, and itching related to obstructive and/ or inflammatory process

Desired outcome: Patient verbalizes a reduction in discomfort and does not exhibit signs of uncontrolled pain, spasms, nausea, and itching.

1. Explain to patient that a low Fowler's position will minimize pressure in the RUQ.

2. Teach patient to avoid fatty and rough/fibrous foods to prevent nausea and spasms.

3. Administer hyperlipidemic agent (eg, cholestyramine) as prescribed for itching.

4. Help control itching by providing Alpha-Keri baths and using soft linens on the bed.

5. For other interventions, see **Alteration in comfort** in "Appendix One," "Caring for Preoperative and Postoperative Patients," p. 528.

Potential for injury related to risk of complications secondary to surgical procedure, use of T-tube, and/or recurrence of biliary obstruction

Desired outcomes: Patient does not exhibit signs of complications; or, if they occur, they are detected and reported promptly, resulting in immediate treatment and absence of injury to the patient.

1. When the patient returns from surgery, mark the T-tube at the skin line with a narrow strip of sterile tape to provide a baseline for position assessment.

2. Tape the tube securely to the abdomen with adhesive tape, avoiding any tension on the tube.

3. Note and record the color, amount, odor, and consistency of drainage q2h on the day of surgery and at least q shift thereafter. Initially the drainage will be dark brown with small amounts of blood and can amount to 500–1000 mL/day. Report greater amounts of blood and/or drainage to MD. The amount should subside gradually as the swelling diminishes in the common duct and drainage into the duodenum normalizes. Typically, the tube is removed within 6 days of surgery.

4. Be alert to abdominal distention, rigidity, and complaints of diaphragmatic irritation along with a cessation or significant decrease in the amount of drainage. If these occur, notify MD immediately and anticipate tube replacement with a number 14 F catheter.

5. When the patient ambulates with a T-tube, attach a small drainage collection container to the distal end, position it in a robe pocket, and ensure that it is below the level of the common duct to prevent reflux.

6. Monitor the color of the skin, sclera, urine, and stool. If obstruction recurs and bile is forced back into the bloodstream, jaundice will be present, the urine will be amber, and the stools will be clay-colored. (Clay color is normal if bile is drained via the tubes.) The brown color should return to the stools once bile begins to drain normally into the duodenum.

See "Providing Nutritional Therapy" in Chapter 11, "Metabolic Disorders," p. 520, for nursing diagnoses and interventions for the care of patients with tube feedings. See "Appendix One" for nursing diagnoses and interventions for the care of preoperative and postoperative patients, pp. 528–532. See "Hepatitis" for the following: **Impairment of skin integrity** related to pruritus, p. 328.

E. Patient–Family Teaching and Discharge Planning

Provide patient and SOs with verbal and written information for the following:

1. Notifying MD if the following indicators of recurrent biliary obstruction occur: dark urine, pruritus, jaundice, clay-colored stools. Inform patient that loose stools may occur for several months as the body adjusts to the continuous flow of bile.

2. Medications, including drug name, dosage, schedule, purpose, precautions, and potential side effects.

3. Care of dressings and tubes if patient is discharged with them and monitoring the incision and drain sites for signs of infection, for example, persistent redness, pain, purulent discharge, swelling, and local warmth.

4. Importance of maintaining a diet low in fat and eating frequent, small meals.

5. Importance of follow-up appointments with MD; reconfirm time and date of next appointment.

6. Avoiding alcoholic beverages during the first 2 postoperative months to minimize the risk of pancreatic involvement.

7. Necessity of postsurgical activity precautions: Avoid lifting heavy objects (>5 lb) for the first 4–6 weeks or as directed, rest after periods of fatigue, get maximum amounts of rest, and gradually increase activities to tolerance.

▶ Selected References

Broadwell DC, Jackson BS (editors): *Principles of Ostomy Care*. Mosby, 1982.

Brunner LS, Suddarth DS: *The Lippincott Manual of Nursing Practice*, 3rd ed. Lippincott, 1982.

Brunner LS, Suddarth DS: *Textbook of Medical-Surgical Nursing*, 5th ed. Lippincott, 1984.

Buckwalter JA, Herbst CA: *Surgery for Morbid Obesity*. North Carolina Memorial Press, 1983.

Campbell JW, Frisse M (editors): *Manual of Medical Therapeutics*, 24th ed. Little, Brown, 1983.

Carpenito LJ: *Handbook of Nursing Diagnosis*. Lippincott, 1984.

Carpenito LJ: *Nursing Diagnosis: Application to Clinical Practice*. Lippincott, 1983.

Chatton MJ, Krupp MA: *Current Medical Diagnosis and Treatment*. Lange, 1984.

CME at "The Brigham": Differentiating malabsorption causes. *Patient Care* 1983; 17:96.

CME at "The Brigham": Infectious diarrhea. What's the cause? *Patient Care* 1983; 17:79.

CME at "The Brigham": Simplifying diagnosis of malabsorption. *Patient Care* 1981; 15:128.

Edwards GB, Fox FA: *El Camino Hospital Laboratory Guide*. El Camino Hospital, 1980.

Farmer RG, Achkar E, Fleshler B: *Clinical Gastroenterology*. Raven Press, 1983.

Fredette SL: When the liver fails. *AJN* 1984; 84:64–67.

Galambos JT, Hirsh T: *Digestive Diseases*. Butterworth, 1983.

Gannon RB, Pickett K: Jaundice. *AJN* 1983; 83:404–407.

Given BA, Simmons SJ: *Gastroenterology in Clinical Nursing*, 4th ed. Mosby, 1984.

Greenberger NJ: *Gastrointestinal Disorders*, 2nd ed. Yearbook Medical Publishers, 1981.

Greenberger NJ, Isselbacher KJ: Disorders of absorption. In: *Harrison's Principles of Internal Medicine*, 10th ed., Petersdorf RG et al (editors). McGraw-Hill, 1983.

Gurevich I: Viral hepatitis. *AJN* 1983; 83:571–586.

Halpern SL: *Quick Reference to Clinical Nutrition*. Lippincott, 1979.

Hirsch J, Hannock L (editors): *Mosby's Manual of Clinical Nursing Procedures*. Mosby, 1981.

Kee JL: *Laboratory and Diagnostic Tests with Nursing Implications*. Appleton-Century-Crofts, 1983.

Leffall LD, Stearns MW: *Early Diagnosis of Colorectal Cancer*. American Cancer Society, 1981.

Lerner AM: Enteric viruses. In: *Harrison's Principles of Internal Medicine*, 10th ed. Petersdorf RG et al (editors). McGraw-Hill, 1983.

Lewis SM, Collier IC: *Medical-Surgical Nursing: Assessment and Management of Clinical Problems*. McGraw-Hill, 1983.

McGuigan JE: Peptic ulcer. In: *Harrison's Principles of Internal Medicine*, 10th ed. Petersdorf RG et al (editors). McGraw-Hill, 1983.

Pagana KD, Pagana TJ: *Diagnostic Testing and Nursing Implications*, 2nd ed. Mosby, 1986.

Petersdorf RG et al (editors): *Harrison's Principles of Internal Medicine*, 10th ed. McGraw-Hill, 1983.

Phipps WJ, Long BC, Woods NF (editors): *Medical-Surgical Nursing: Concepts and Clinical Practice*, 2nd ed. Mosby, 1983.

Price SA, Wilson LM: *Pathophysiology—Clinical Concepts of Disease Processes*. McGraw-Hill, 1982.

Rubin P (editor): *Clinical Oncology*. American Cancer Society, 1983.

Saxton DF, et al (editors): *The Addison-Wesley Manual of Nursing Practice*. Addison-Wesley, 1983.

Spiro H: *Clinical Gastroenterology*. Macmillan, 1983.

Swearingen PL: *The Addison-Wesley Photo-Atlas of Nursing Procedures*. Addison-Wesley, 1984.

Thorpe CJ, Caprini JA: Gallbladder disease: Current trends and treatments. *AJN* 1980; 80:218.

Turnbull RB, Weakley FL: *Atlas of Intestinal Stomas*. Mosby, 1967.

Weinsier RL, Butterworth CE, Jr: *Handbook of Clinical Nutrition*. Mosby, 1981.

Whitney EN, Cataldo CB: *Understanding Normal and Clinical Nutrition*. West Publishing, 1983.

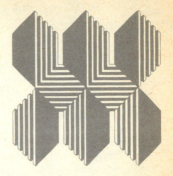

7

Hematologic Disorders

▶ Section One **Disorders of the Red Blood Cells**

The erythrocyte, or red blood cell (RBC), is the transport mechanism for hemoglobin, which carries oxygen from the heart and lungs to the tissues, exchanges it for carbon dioxide, and then returns to the heart and lungs. RBCs are very flexible and capable of bending, elongating, and squeezing through tiny capillaries. Normal RBCs can travel under high pressure and speed, are extremely active metabolically, and have an average life of 120 days. The bone marrow produces and replaces RBCs every day and can respond to the increased need for RBCs by increasing production. However, with increased production, immature RBCs (reticulocytes) are often released into the circulation; a high level of immature RBCs often aids in the diagnosis of RBC disorders.

Anemia is a common hematopoietic disorder defined as a reduced number of RBCs and/or a reduced amount of hemoglobin. The general effects of anemia result from a deficiency in the oxygen-carrying mechanism, although some effects are related to varied etiologies and pathogenesis. Three basic types of anemias are discussed in this section.

I. Pernicious Anemia

Vitamin B_{12} is supplied by diet and stored in the liver to be used for maturation of RBCs. Deficiency of this vitamin leads to the development of immature erythrocytes, a chronic condition known as pernicious anemia. Decreased dietary intake of animal products, increased need for this vitamin with pregnancy or a tumor, presence of parasites, or surgery involving the small intestine where the vitamin is absorbed are conditions that can lead to vitamin B_{12} deficiency. The most common condition is the decrease in production by the gastric mucosa of *intrinsic factor,* a microprotein, which when combined with vitamin B_{12} facilitates absorption and use of the vitamin by body cells, particularly in the bone marrow, GI tract, and nervous system.

A. Assessment

Chronic indicators: Brittle nails, smooth tongue, numbness and tingling of the extremities, fatigue, and dysphagia. However, because of slow progression, many patients remain asymptomatic. Anorexia, weight loss, jaundice from destruction of malformed erythrocytes, and gingivitis from absence of vitamin B_{12} also can occur.

Acute indicators: Dyspnea on exertion, irritability, palpitations, and dizziness in the presence of severe deficiency. In addition, because the nervous system is particularly sensitive to the lack of vitamin B_{12}, degenerative changes of the cerebral cortex and spinal cord can occur, seen mainly in the form of paresthesias.

Physical exam: Presence of oral lesions and gingivitis, tachycardia, unsteady gait, and clumsiness.

B. Diagnostic Tests

1. <u>Schilling's test:</u> Patient is given radioactive-tagged vitamin B_{12}, and urine concentration of tagged B_{12} is then measured. For normal individuals, B_{12} is absorbed and excreted in the urine. In the presence of pernicious anemia, B_{12} is not absorbed and urine levels will be low (<3%).

2. <u>Trial administration of vitamin B_{12}:</u> May be given to evaluate patient's response. In the presence of pernicious anemia, symptoms will be relieved.

3. <u>Serial hemoglobin and erythrocyte counts:</u> Initially will be decreased.

4. <u>Bone marrow aspiration:</u> Will reveal hyperplasia with increased numbers of large-sized megaloblasts.

5. <u>Gastric analysis:</u> Will reveal decreased volume of gastric secretions. Atrophic gastritis is characteristic of pernicious anemia.

6. <u>LDH:</u> May be increased.

C. Medical Management

1. **Vitamin B$_{12}$ replacement:** Dosage depends on the individual and the response to treatment. For example, 100 mg cyanocobalamin may be given IM qd × 7 days. If improvement occurs, it is given qod × 7 days and then q3–4 days × 2–3 weeks.

2. **Concurrent treatment of underlying disorder:** If present, eg, gastric mucosal problem.

3. **Serial measurements of reticulocytes:** To determine effectiveness of treatment.

D. Nursing Diagnoses and Interventions

Alteration in bowel elimination: Diarrhea or constipation related to gastrointestinal mucosal atrophy secondary to reduced hematocrit

Desired outcomes: Patient does not experience constipation or diarrhea. Patient can verbalize knowledge of therapeutic measures to promote normal bowel elimination.

1. If patient is constipated, implement the following:

   □ Assist patient with establishing a regular bowel pattern, for example, by increasing fluids (to at least 2–3 L/day) and dietary fiber and initiating a regular exercise program.

   □ For other interventions, see **Alteration in bowel elimination:** Constipation, p. 536, in "Caring for Patients on Prolonged Bed Rest," "Appendix One."

2. If diarrhea occurs, teach patient to avoid high-roughage foods, administer prescribed antidiarrheal medications, and encourage increased intake of fluids to prevent dehydration.

Potential for infection related to increased susceptibility secondary to decreased leukocyte production (associated with decrease in all blood elements)

Desired outcomes: Patient does not exhibit signs of infection. Patient and SOs can verbalize understanding of the indicators of and measures to prevent infection.

1. Maintain strict asepsis when performing invasive procedures. Wash hands well before caring for patient.

2. Teach patient and SOs the technique for handwashing.

3. Be alert to indicators of respiratory infection to report to MD: cough; changes in the amount, color, and consistency of sputum; increased respiratory rate; and presence of crackles (rales), rhonchi, and fever. Teach these indicators to patient and SOs.

4. To prevent stasis of secretions in the lung, which can lead to infection, teach patient how to perform effective coughing and deep breathing.

5. Teach patient and SOs the indications of wound infection and UTI.

Activity intolerance related to fatigue secondary to decreased oxygen-carrying capacity of the blood

Desired outcome: Patient increases activities to tolerance and exhibits physical findings within an acceptable range.

1. Provide frequent rest periods between care activities, allowing time for undisturbed rest.

2. As patient performs ADLs, be alert to indicators of decreased tissue oxygenation such as dyspnea on exertion, dizziness, palpitations, and headaches.

3. Reassure patient that usually, symptoms are relieved and tolerance for activity is increased with therapy.

4. As patient's condition improves, encourage increase in activities to tolerance.

Set specific goals with patient, for example, "Today I would like you to try to walk from your room to the nurses' station and back three (or appropriate number, depending on patient's tolerance) times."

Alteration in nutrition: Less than body requirements related to decreased intake secondary to fatigue, impairment of oral mucosa, and/or anorexia

Desired outcome: Patient does not exhibit signs of malnutrition or weight loss.

1. If patient is easily fatigued, encourage small, frequent meals.
2. If oral lesions/cracks are present, encourage soft and bland foods. For more information, see "Stomatitis," pp. 272–274, in Chapter 6, "Gastrointestinal Disorders."
3. For patient with decreased appetite, encourage SOs to bring in patient's favorite foods and stay with patient during meals to encourage eating.

Potential for injury related to risk of sensorimotor deficit secondary to inability to absorb and utilize vitamin B_{12}

Desired outcome: Patient does not exhibit signs of injury caused by neurologic deficit.

1. Assess for sensory deficit and protect patient from extremes of heat and cold if deficit is noted. As needed, orient patient to all activities and surroundings at frequent intervals.
2. Assess strength and motor ability before allowing patient to ambulate unassisted.
3. Teach patient and SOs the signs and symptoms of neurologic deficit and the importance of reporting them to staff or MD promptly. Reassure patient that neurologic deficit usually reverses with therapy.

E. Patient–Family Teaching and Discharge Planning

Provide patient and SOs with verbal and written information for the following:

1. Necessity of vitamin B_{12} replacement for life, even when symptoms resolve.
2. Technique for administering vitamin B_{12} or arrangement for monthly clinic visits for injection.
3. For injections that will be performed by patient or SOs, the need for a supply of vitamin B_{12}, 22-gauge needles, 3-cc syringes, and alcohol sponges.
4. Importance of regular medical follow-up, including serial monitoring of blood levels.

II. Hemolytic Anemia

Hemolytic anemia is characterized by abnormal or premature destruction of RBCs. Hemolysis can be intrinsic or result from conditions such as infection or radiation. *Sickle cell anemia* is a form of chronic hemolytic anemia characterized by abnormal, crescent-shaped, rigid, and elongated erythrocytes. These "sickle" RBCs interfere with circulation because they cannot get through the microcirculation and are destroyed in the process. Sickle cell anemia can affect almost every body system due to decreased oxygen delivery, decreased circulation caused by occlusion of the vessels by RBCs, and inflammatory process. This disorder occurs when the gene is inherited from both parents (homozygous); a carrier state exists when it is inherited from one parent (heterozygous). Medical treatment has improved the prognosis for this disorder, which is seen predominantly in blacks. *Thalassemia* is another type of chronic hemolytic anemia. In this disorder, hemoglobin A is manufactured in less-than-normal amounts, although the hemoglobin itself is of normal morphology. This is an inherited disorder passed on through an autosomal gene. Severity depends on whether the inheritance is heterozygous or homozygous. It occurs most often in individuals of Mediterranean descent, eg, Greeks and Italians. If the condition is severe *(thalassemia major)*, the patient seldom survives to adulthood. Individuals with intermediate and minor forms develop normally and usually can expect a normal life span. *Acquired hemolytic anemia* is usually the result of an abnormal immune response that causes premature destruction of RBCs. Hemolysis can occur as a result of a foreign antigen such as from a transfusion reaction, or an autoimmune reaction in which the hemolytic agent is intrinsic to the patient's body. Other possible causes include exposure to radiation and ingestion of drugs such as sulfisoxazole (eg, Gantrisin), phenacetin, and methyldopa (eg, Aldomet).

Hemolytic crisis: Patients with chronic hemolytic anemia can do relatively well for a period of time, but many factors can precipitate a hemolytic crisis or acute hemolysis. For example, an individual with mild hemolytic anemia can become severely anemic with an acute infectious process, or with any other physiologic or emotional stressor, including surgery, trauma, or emotional upset. Widespread hemolysis causes an acute decrease in oxygen-carrying capacity of the blood, resulting in decreased oxygen delivery to the tissues. Organ congestion from the hemolyzed blood cells occurs, and this affects organ function and precipitates a shock state.

A. Assessment

Chronic indicators: Pallor (eg, conjunctival), fatigue, dyspnea on exertion, and intermittent dizziness, all of which depend on the severity of the anemia

Acute indicators: Fever, visual blurring, temporary blindness, abdominal pain, lymphadenopathy, splenomegaly, and decreased urinary output (signs and symptoms of hemolytic crisis). Peripheral nerve damage can result in paralysis or paresthesias, vomiting, and chills.

B. Diagnostic Tests

1. Sickle cell test: To screen for sickle cell anemia.
2. Hemoglobin and hematocrit: Decreased.
3. Serum tests: LDH and bilirubin will be elevated.
4. Urine and fecal urobilinogen: Increased and are more sensative indicators of RBC destruction than serum bilirubin levels.
5. Bone marrow aspiration: Will reveal erythroid hyperplasia, especially with chronic hemolytic anemia.
6. Hemoglobin electrophoresis: Will diagnose hemoglobin AS, a sickle cell trait.

C. Medical Management

1. **Elimination or discontinuation of causative factor:** If possible, eg, chemical, drug, incompatible blood.
2. **Supportive therapy of shock state:** If it occurs.
3. **Transfusion:** If circulatory failure or severe anemic anoxia occurs.
4. **Corticosteroids:** Usually 50–100 mg prednisone, given with antacids.
5. **Folic acid:** To help prevent hemolytic crisis in patients with chronic hemolytic anemias.
6. **Splenectomy:** To provide relief, depending on the cause of the anemia. The spleen is the site of RBC destruction.

D. Nursing Diagnoses and Interventions

Potential impairment of skin integrity related to vulnerability secondary to occlusion of the vessels and impaired oxygen transport to the tissues and skin

Desired outcomes: Patient's skin does not exhibit signs of breakdown or trauma. Patient can verbalize knowledge of the importance of preventing tissue trauma.

1. Use a bed cradle to keep pressure of bed linen and blankets off patient's skin.

2. Caution patient about the importance of avoiding trauma or injury to the skin and tissues.

3. Apply dry, sterile dressings or dressing materials such as Op-Site and Tegaderm to areas of tissue breakdown. Use aseptic technique to help prevent infection.

Alteration in tissue perfusion: Renal, related to decreased circulation secondary to hemolytic obstruction

Desired outcome: Patient's I&O and other physical findings are within acceptable limits.

1. Monitor I&O. Report urine output <0.5 mL/kg/h in the presence of adequate intake.

2. In the absence of renal or cardiac failure, encourage fluid intake to maintain adequate glomerular blood flow. Assist patient with ROM exercises to help promote circulation.

3. Deliver IV fluid as prescribed to maintain fluid balance and renal perfusion.

Alteration in tissue perfusion: Peripheral and cardiopulmonary related to decreased circulation secondary to inflammatory process and occlusion of blood vessels with RBCs

Desired outcome: Patient's VS and physical findings are within acceptable limits.

1. Assess BP at frequent intervals and report significant drops (>10 mm Hg from baseline readings).

2. Assess amplitude of peripheral pulses as an indicator of peripheral perfusion.

3. Be alert to signs of cardiac depression, including decreased BP, increased heart rate, decreased pulse amplitude, dyspnea, and decreased urine output.

4. Assess for and report indicators of hypoxia and/or respiratory dysfunction, such as increased respiratory rate, dyspnea, SOB, and cyanosis.

5. Assist patient with ROM exercises to enhance tissue perfusion as well as increase joint mobility. **Caution:** Exercise should be avoided if any early signs of hemolytic crisis appear because exercise can aggravate hemolysis.

6. Report significant findings to MD.

Alteration in comfort: Pain related to hemolysis in joints

Desired outcome: Patient relates a reduction in discomfort and does not exhibit signs of uncontrolled pain.

1. Monitor for the presence of pain; administer pain medications as prescribed.

2. Reassure patient that pain will subside when acute hemolytic episode is over.

3. Elevate extremities to enhance comfort.

4. Apply moist heat packs to the joints to increase circulation and decrease pain.

5. Apply elastic stockings or wraps, if prescribed, to support joints and enhance circulation.

Potential for injury related to risk of sensorimotor deficit secondary to peripheral nerve hypoxia

Desired outcomes: Patient does not exhibit signs of injury from neurologic deficit. Visual disturbance, which can signal hemolytic crisis, is detected and reported to MD promptly, resulting in immediate treatment and absence of injury to patient.

1. Monitor motor strength and coordination, and report changes in peripheral sensation. Protect patient from extremes of heat and cold if impaired sensation is noted.

2. Accompany patient during ambulation; provide physical support as necessary.

3. Assess patient for visual disturbances, reporting immediately the presence of blurred vision or blindness, which are indicators of hemolytic crisis.

4. Teach patient and SOs the indicators of sensorimotor dysfunction, including gait unsteadiness, uncoordination, paresthesia, and paralysis.

Knowledge deficit: Factors that can precipitate hemolytic crisis and measures that can help prevent it

Desired outcome: Patient can verbalize knowledge of factors that precipitate hemolytic crisis as well as measures that can help prevent it.

1. Teach patient and SOs the indicators of hemolytic crisis, including jaundice, dyspnea, SOB, joint or abdominal pain, decreasing BP, or increased heart rate.

2. Explain to patient and SOs that stress and anxiety can precipitate hemolytic crisis. Stress the importance of maintaining a calm environment for the patient.

3. Teach patient stress reduction techniques such as meditation and relaxation exercises.

4. Discuss with SOs the importance of avoiding stressful and emotional topics with patient.

5. Caution patient to avoid physical stress, which also can precipitate a crisis.

See "Pernicious Anemia" for the following: **Potential for infection**, p. 341, and **Activity intolerance**, p. 341.

E. Patient–Teaching Planning and Discharge Planning

Provide patient and SOs with verbal and written information for the following:

1. Side effects of steroids, if prescribed, including weight gain, headache, and increased appetite.

2. Support groups available for sickle cell anemia and thalassemia.

3. Factors that precipitate hemolytic crisis, such as stress and trauma or chemicals and drugs, depending on etiology.

4. Importance of avoiding infectious processes such as URIs and getting prompt medical attention should infection occur.

5. Medications, including drug name, purpose, schedule, dosage, precautions, and potential side effects.

6. Importance of medical follow-up.

III. Hypoplastic (Aplastic) Anemia

This type of anemia results from inability of erythrocyte-producing organs, specifically the bone marrow, to produce erythrocytes. The causes of hypoplastic anemia are varied but can include use of antineoplastic or antimicrobial agents, infectious process, pregnancy, hepatitis, and radiation. Approximately half of the patients with hypoplastic anemia have had exposure to drugs or chemical agents, while the remaining half have had immunologic disorders. Hypoplastic anemia also can involve pancytopenia, the depression of production of all three bone marrow elements: erythrocytes, platelets, and granulocytes. Usually the onset of hypoplastic anemia is insidious, but it can evolve quickly in some cases. Prognosis is usually poor for these patients.

A. Assessment

Chronic indicators: Weakness, fatigue, pallor, dysphagia, and numbness and tingling of the extremities (indicators of anemia).

Table 7-1 Commonly Used Blood Products

Product	Approximate Volume	Indications	Precautions/Comments
Whole Blood (WB)	500–510 mL (450 WB; 50–60 antico-agulants)	Acute, severe blood loss; hypovolemic shock. Increases both red cell mass and plasma	Must be ABO and Rh com-patible. Do not mix with dextrose solutions; always prime tubing with normal saline. Observe for dys-pnea, orthopnea, cya-nosis, and anxiety as signs of circulatory overload; monitor VS. Hepatitis risk = 2*
Packed Red Blood Cells (RBCs)	250 mL	Increases RBC mass and oxygen-carrying capacity of the blood	Must be ABO and Rh com-patible. Less immunologic risk than with WB because some donor antibodies are removed. Less volume, reducing risk of fluid over-load. Hepatitis risk = 2*
Fresh Frozen Plasma (FFP)	250 mL	Treatment of choice for combined coagula-tion factor deficien-cies and factor V and XI deficiencies; alternate treatment for factor VII, VIII, IX, and X deficiencies when concentrates are not available	Must be ABO compatible. Supplies clotting factors. Usual dose is 10–15 mL/kg body weight. Hepatitis risk = 2**
Platelet Concen-trate	25–50 mL (volumes may vary; usual adult dose is 5–6 U)	Treatment of choice for thrombocytopenia. Also used for leuke-mia and hypoplastic anemia	Usual dose is 0.1 U/kg body weight to increase platelet count to 25,000. Admin-ister as rapidly as toler-ated. ABO compatibility is preferable, but is expen-sive and usually not prac-tical. Effectiveness is de-creased by fever, sepsis, and splenomegaly. Febrile reactions are common. Use special "platelet" tub-ing and filter. Hepatitis risk = 2**
Platelet Concen-trate by Platelet Pheresis	200 mL, but may vary	Treatment for thrombo-cytopenic patients who are refractory to random donor platelets	Involves removing donor's venous blood 200 mL at a time, removing the platelets by centrifuge, and returning the blood to patient. This is performed approximately six times to yield 200 mL platelets. Uses special donors, who usually are human leu-kocyte antigen (HLA)

Table 7-1 continued

Product	Approximate Volume	Indications	Precautions/Comments
			matched to the patient. Hepatitis risk = 2*
Cryoprecipitate (factor VIII)	10–25 mL	Routine treatment for hemophilia (factor VIII deficiency) & fibrinogen deficiency (factor XIII deficiency)	Made from FFP. Infuse immediately upon thawing. Hepatitis risk = 2*
AHG (factor VIII) Concentrates	20 mL	Alternative treatment for hemophilia A	Allergic and febrile reactions occur frequently. Administer by syringe or component drip set. Can store at refrigerator temperature, making it convenient for hemophiliacs during travel. Hepatitis risk = 3**
Factor II, VII, IX, X Concentrate	20 mL	Treatment of choice for hemophilia B & factor IX deficiencies	Can precipitate clotting. Allergic and febrile reactions occur occasionally. Contraindicated in liver disease. Hepatitis risk = 3**
Albumin	50 or 250 mL	Hypovolemic shock, hypoalbuminemia, plasma replacement for burn patients	Osmotically equal to 5X its volume of plasma. Used as a volume expander or in hypoalbuminemic states. Commercially available. Hepatitis risk = 0*
Plasma Protein Fraction (PPF)	250 mL (83% albumin with some alpha and beta globulins)	Volume expansion	Commercially available; expensive. Certain lots reported to have caused hypotension, possibly related to vasoactive amines used in preparation. Hepatitis risk = 0*
Granulocyte Transfusion (collected from a single pheresis donor)	200 mL, but may vary	Leukemia with granulocytopenia related to treatment	Not a common treatment. Febrile and allergic symptoms are frequent. Must be ABO compatible. Hepatitis risk = 3*

*Relative hepatitis risk: 0, no risk, 1 and 2, moderate to high risk, 3, maximum risk.
**Risk is greater because multiple donors are used.

Acute indicators: Fever and infection (because of decreased neutrophils); bleeding (because of thrombocytopenia); and dizziness, dyspnea on exertion, progressive weakness, and oral ulcerations.

History of: Exposure to chemical toxins or radiation, use of antibiotics such as chloramphenicol.

B. Diagnostic Tests

1. <u>CBC with differential:</u> Low levels of hemoglobin, WBCs, and RBCs; however, RBCs usually appear to be normal morphologically.

2. <u>Platelet count:</u> Low.

3. <u>Bleeding time:</u> Prolonged.

4. <u>Bone marrow aspiration:</u> Will reveal hypocellular or hypoplastic tissue with a fatty and fibrous appearance and depression of erythroid elements.

C. Medical Management

1. **Determine cause of anemia.**

2. **Transfuse packed RBCs or frozen plasma:** See Table 7-1, p. 346.

3. **Transfuse concentrated platelets:** To keep platelet count $>20,000/mm^3$. Hemorrhage occurs less frequently when platelet count is above this level (see Table 7-1, p. 346).

4. **Granulocyte transfusion:** For life-threatening sepsis (see Table 7-1, p. 347).

5. **Cultures:** If infection is suspected.

6. **Antibiotic therapy:** If infection is found.

7. **Reverse isolation:** If granulocytes count is $<200/mm^3$.

8. **Steroid therapy:** To stimulate granulocyte production, although results with adults are not always successful.

9. **Oxygen:** If anemia is severe.

10. **Bone marrow transplantation:** Performed in a few centers in the US. In this procedure, $500-700$ mL of bone marrow are aspirated from the pelvic bones of the donor and then filtered and infused into the patient. The donated marrow must be antigen-compatible and therefore the donor is usually a twin or sibling. The procedure involves significant risk and requires isolation, asepsis, specialized staff, and extensive supportive therapy such as platelet transfusions and RBC transfusions.

11. **Androgen therapy:** An attempt to stimulate bone marrow activity.

▶ **Note:** Because of the potential for antibody formation, all blood products and transfusions are avoided, if possible, if there is any possibility of later bone marrow transplantation.

D. Nursing Diagnoses and Interventions

Potential for infection related to increased susceptibility secondary to decreased leukocytes

Desired outcome: Patient does not exhibit signs of infection.

1. Perform meticulous handwashing before patient contact.

2. If appropriate, maintain protective/reverse isolation, using gloves, gown, and masks; make sure that visitors do the same. Discourage delivery of plants and flowers to the room.

3. Report any signs of systemic infection (eg, fever); obtain prescription for blood, wound, and urine cultures as indicated.

4. Monitor for and report any signs of local infection, such as sore throat or reddened or draining wounds. **Note:** With decreased or absent granulocytes, pus may not form. Therefore it is important to look for other signs of infection.

5. Provide oral care at frequent intervals to prevent oral lesions, which may result in bleeding and infection.

6. Provide and encourage adequate perianal hygiene to prevent rectal abscess. Avoid giving medications or taking temperature rectally.

7. Avoid invasive procedures, if possible.

8. Encourage ambulation, deep breathing, turning, and coughing to prevent problems of immobility, which can result in pneumonia and skin breakdown.

9. Arrange for patient to have a private room when possible.

10. Teach patient and SOs signs and symptoms of infection and the importance of notifying staff or MD promptly if they are noted.

Knowledge deficit: Potential for bleeding (caused by low platelet count) and measures that can help prevent it

Desired outcome: Patient can verbalize knowledge of the potential for bleeding, as well as measures that can prevent it.

1. Teach patient about the potential for bleeding and the importance of monitoring for hematuria, melena, frank bleeding from the mouth, epistaxis, or coughing up of blood and notifying staff promptly should they occur.

2. Teach patient to use an electric razor and soft-bristled toothbrush.

3. Explain the importance of maintaining regularity with bowel movements to prevent straining and potential bleeding.

4. Teach patient to avoid potentially traumatic procedures such as enemas and rectal temperatures.

Activity intolerance related to fatigue and weakness secondary to decreased oxygen-carrying capacity of the blood

Desired outcome: Patient increases activities to tolerance and exhibits physical findings within acceptable limits.

1. Plan frequent rest periods, providing time for periods of undisturbed rest.

2. Administer oxygen as prescribed to augment oxygen delivery to the tissues. Also encourage deep breathing, which may increase oxygenation by enhancing gas exchange.

3. Administer blood components (usually RBCs) as prescribed. Double-check typing with a colleague, and monitor for and report signs of transfusion reaction.

4. Encourage gradually increasing activities to tolerance as patient's condition improves. Set mutually-agreed upon goals with patient. For example, "Let's plan this morning's activity goals. Do you feel you could walk up and down the hall once or twice?" (or appropriate amount, depending on patient's tolerance).

Alteration in tissue perfusion: Peripheral and cerebral related to tissue hypoxia secondary to decreased production of erythrocytes

Desired outcome: Patient's neurologic checks and other physical findings are within acceptable limits.

1. Perform neurologic checks and assess patient's orientation as indicators of cerebral perfusion. If signs of decreasing cerebral perfusion occur, establish precautionary measures, eg, keeping siderails up and the bed in the lowest position to protect patient from injury. Request restraints, if indicated.

2. Assess sensorimotor status to help evaluate nervous system oxygenation.

3. Prevent injury from heat or cold applications for patients with decreased sensations.

4. Deliver oxygen as prescribed.

5. Teach patient deep-breathing exercises, which may increase oxygenation by enhancing gas exchange.

6. Promptly report indicators of a worsening condition to MD.

See "Pernicious Anemia" for the following: **Alteration in nutrition**, p. 342.

E. Patient–Family Teaching and Discharge Planning

Provide patient and SOs with verbal and written information for the following:

1. Medications, including drug name, purpose, dosage, schedule, precautions, and potential side effects.
2. Indicators of systemic infection, including fever, malaise, fatigue, as well as signs and symptoms of URI, UTI, and wound infection.
3. Importance of avoiding exposure to individuals known to have acute infections; preventing trauma, abrasions, and breakdown of the skin; and maintaining good nutritional intake to enhance resistance to infections.
4. Signs of bleeding/hemorrhage, which necessitate medical attention: melena, hematuria, epistaxis, ecchymosis, and bleeding of gums.
5. Measures to prevent hemorrhage, such as using electric razor and soft-bristled toothbrush and avoiding activities that can traumatize the tissues.
6. Importance of reporting general symptoms of anemia, including fatigue, weakness, paresthesia, blurred vision, palpitations, and dizziness.

IV. Polycythemia

Polycythemia is a chronic disorder characterized by excessive production of RBCs. As the number of RBCs increases, blood volume, blood viscosity, and hemoglobin concentration increase, causing excessive workload of the heart and congestion of organ systems such as the liver and kidney. *Secondary polycythemia* results from an abnormal increase in erythropoietin production, for example, secondary to hypoxia that occurs with chronic lung disease, or it can occur inappropriately, such as with renal tumors. *Polycythemia vera* is a primary disorder of unknown etiology, resulting in increased RBC mass, leukocytosis, and slight thrombocytosis. Because of the increased viscosity and decreased microcirculation, mortality rate is high if the condition is left untreated. In addition, there is a potential for this disorder to evolve into other hematopoietic disorders such as leukemia.

A. Assessment

Signs and symptoms: Headache, dizziness, visual disturbances, dyspnea, thrombophlebitis, joint pain, fatigue, chest pain, and a feeling of "fullness," especially in the head.

Physical exam: Hypertension, crackles (rales), cyanosis, ruddy complexion, hepatosplenomegaly.

B. Diagnostic Tests

1. <u>CBC:</u> Increased RBC mass (8–12 million/mm^3); increased hemoglobin; leukocytosis.
2. <u>Platelet count:</u> Increased.
3. <u>Bone marrow aspiration:</u> Will reveal RBC proliferation.
4. <u>Uric acid levels:</u> May be increased because of increased nucleoprotein, an end product of RBC breakdown.

C. Medical Management

1. **Phlebotomy:** Blood withdrawn from the vein to decrease blood volume (and decrease hematocrit to 45%).
2. **Myelosuppressive agents such as radiophosphorus:** To inhibit proliferation of RBCs.

3. **Alkylating (myelosuppressive) agents such as busulfan and chlorambucil:** To decrease bone marrow function.

D. Nursing Diagnoses and Interventions

Potential alteration in tissue perfusion: Peripheral and cerebral related to decreased circulation secondary to phlebotomy

Desired outcome: Patient's VS and physical findings are within acceptable limits.

1. During procedure, keep patient recumbent to prevent dizziness or hypotension.
2. Assess for tachycardia, hypotension, or dizziness during procedure; notify MD of significant findings.
3. After the procedure, assist patient with sitting position for 5–10 minutes before ambulation to prevent orthostatic hypotension.
4. Teach patient about the potential for orthostatic hypotension and the need to use caution when standing for at least 2–3 days after the phlebotomy.

Alteration in nutrition: Less than body requirements related to decreased intake secondary to feelings of "fullness" (associated with congestion of organ systems)

Desired outcome: Patient does not exhibit signs of malnutrition or weight loss.

1. Encourage patient to eat small, frequent meals.
2. Request that SOs bring in patient's favorite foods if they are unavailable in the hospital.
3. Advise patient to eat mild foods, which are better tolerated, and to avoid spicy foods, which can cause irritation.

Alteration in comfort: Headache, angina, and abdominal and joint pain related to decreased circulation secondary to hyperviscosity of the blood

Desired outcome: Patient verbalizes a reduction in discomfort and does not exhibit signs of uncontrolled pain.

1. Assess patient for the presence of headache, angina, abdominal pain, and joint pain.
2. In the presence of joint pain, elevate the extremity; apply moist heat to ease discomfort.
3. Administer analgesics as prescribed.
4. Encourage use of nonpharmacologic pain control, such as relaxation and distraction.
5. Be alert to indicators of peripheral thrombosis such as calf pain and tenderness.
6. Report significant findings to MD.

Alteration in tissue perfusion: Peripheral and renal related to decreased circulation secondary to hyperviscosity of the blood

Desired outcome: Patient's I&O and physical findings are within acceptable limits.

1. Monitor I&O; report urine output <0.5 mL/kg/h in the presence of adequate intake, which can signal congestion and decreased perfusion.
2. In the absence of signs of cardiac and renal failure, encourage fluid intake to decrease viscosity.
3. Encourage patient to exercise and ambulate to tolerance to enhance circulation.
4. Monitor patient for indicators of impending neurologic damage such as muscle weakness and decreases in sensation and LOC.
5. Report significant findings to MD.

E. Patient–Family Teaching and Discharge Planning

Provide patient and SOs with verbal and written information for the following:

1. Need for continued medical follow-up, including potential for phlebotomy q1–3 mo.
2. Medications, including drug name, purpose, dosage, schedule, precautions, and potential side effects.
3. Importance of augmenting fluid intake.
4. Signs and symptoms that necessitate medical attention: angina, muscle weakness, numbness and tingling of extremities, decreased tolerance to activity, and joint pain.
5. Nutrition: importance of maintaining a balanced diet to increase resistance to infection and limiting intake of iron to help minimize abnormal RBC proliferation.

► Section Two   **Disorders of Coagulation**

The formation of a visible fibrin clot is the conclusion of a complex series of reactions involving different clotting factors in the blood that are identified by Roman numerals I–XIII. All are plasma proteins except factor III (thromboplastin) and factor IV (calcium ion). When a vessel injury occurs, these factors interact to form the end product, a clot. The clots that are formed are eventually dissolved by the fibrinolytic system.

Platelets play a role in coagulation by releasing substances that activate the clotting factors. At the time of vascular injury, platelets migrate to the site and adhere to each other to form a temporary plug to stop the bleeding.

I. Thrombocytopenia

Thrombocytopenia is a common coagulation disorder, which results from a decreased number of platelets. It can be congenital or acquired, and it is classified according to cause. Common causes include deficient formation of thrombocytes, which occurs with bone marrow disease or destruction; accelerated platelet destruction, loss, or increased utilization such as in hemolytic anemia, diffuse intravascular coagulation, or damage by prosthetic heart valves; and abnormal platelet distribution such as in hypersplenism and hypothermia. Potential triggers include autoimmune disorder, severe vascular injury, and spleen malfunction. In addition, thrombocytopenia can occur as a side effect of certain chemotherapeutic agents and antibiotics. Regardless of the cause or trigger, the disorder affects coagulation and hemostasis. With chemical-induced thrombocytopenia, prognosis is good after withdrawal of the offending drug. Prognosis for other types of thrombocytopenia is dependent on the individual's response to treatment. The acute idiopathic form of thrombocytopenia occurs more frequently in children and is usually self-limiting. *Thrombocytopenic purpura*, also termed *idiopathic thrombocytopenic purpura* (ITP), occurs when blood extravasates into tissue and mucous membranes due to increased destruction or decreased formation of thrombocytes.

A. Assessment

Chronic indicators: Long history of mild bleeding or hemorrhagic episodes. Increased bruising, gum bleeding, and petechiae also may be noted.

Acute indicators: Fever, splenomegaly, acute and severe bleeding episodes, weakness, lethargy, malaise, hemorrhage into mucous membranes, gum bleeding, and GI bleeding. Prolonged bleeding can lead to a shock state with tachycardia, SOB, and decreased LOC.

History of: Recent infection; vaccination; use of chlorothiazide, digitalis, quinidine, rifampin, sulfisoxazole, chloramphenicol, phenytoin.

B. Diagnostic Tests

1. Platelet count: Can vary from only slightly decreased to nearly absent. Less than 100,000 is significantly decreased; <20,000 results in a serious risk of hemorrhage.
2. CBC: Low hemoglobin and hematocrit levels; WBC within normal range.
3. Template bleeding time: Increased.
4. Bone marrow aspiration: Will reveal increased number of megakaryocytes (platelet precursors) in the presence of ITP, but may be decreased with certain causes of thrombocytopenia.
5. Platelet antibody screen: May be positive. The test is not generally available.

C. Medical Management and Surgical Interventions

1. **Treatment of underlying cause or removal of precipitating agent.**
2. **Platelet transfusion:** Unless platelet destruction is the cause of the disorder (see Table 7-1, p. 346).
3. **Corticosteroids:** To enhance vascular integrity or diminish platelet destruction.
4. **Splenectomy:** Removal of an organ responsible for platelet destruction. This is considered viable treatment unless patient has acute bleeding, a severe deficiency of platelets, or a cardiac disorder that contraindicates surgery.

D. Nursing Diagnoses and Interventions

Potential for injury related to increased risk of bleeding secondary to decreased platelet count

Desired outcomes: Patient does not exhibit signs of bleeding. Patient can verbalize knowledge of measures that can help prevent bleeding.

1. Teach patient to use electric razor and soft-bristled toothbrush.
2. When appropriate, protect patient from injury by keeping siderails up and padding them.
3. When possible, avoid venipuncture. If performed, apply pressure on site for 5–10 minutes or until bleeding stops.
4. Avoid IM injections. If performed, use small-gauge needles when possible.
5. Monitor platelet count daily.
6. Advise patient to avoid straining at stool or coughing, which increases intracranial pressure and can result in intracranial hemorrhage. Obtain prescription for stool softeners, if indicated, to prevent constipation. Teach patient anticonstipation routine as described in **Alteration in bowel elimination: Constipation,** p. 536, in "Caring for Patients on Prolonged Bed Rest," "Appendix One."
7. Administer corticosteroids as prescribed.
8. Monitor patient for hematuria, melena, epistaxis, hematemesis, or severe ecchymosis. Teach patient to be alert to and report these indicators promptly.
9. Administer platelets as prescribed and be alert to transfusion reaction (see Table 7-1, p. 346).
10. Alert MD to significant findings

Alteration in comfort: Malaise and joint pain related to hemorrhagic episodes and/or blood extravasation into the tissues

Desired outcome: Patient relates a reduction in discomfort and does not exhibit signs of uncontrolled pain.

1. Monitor patient for signs of fatigue or malaise.
2. Maintain a calm, restful environment; provide periods of undisturbed rest.
3. Elevate legs to minimize joint discomfort in the lower extremities.
4. Administer analgesics as prescribed. **Caution:** Aspirin is contraindicated because of its antiplatelet action.

Potential fluid volume deficit related to loss secondary to postsplenectomy bleeding/ hemorrhage

Desired outcome: Patient does not exhibit signs of hypovolemia or excessive bleeding.

1. Monitor postoperative VS for changes that may indicate bleeding, eg, decreasing BP and increased heart rate. Be alert to restlessness as well.
2. Inspect abdomen for presence of distention, and question patient about abdominal pain or tenderness, which can signal internal bleeding.
3. Inspect operative site for the presence of frank bleeding.
4. Monitor postoperative platelet count. Approximately 60–70% of postsplenectomy patients have increased platelet counts.
5. Report significant findings to MD.

If surgery is performed, see nursing diagnoses and interventions for the care of preoperative and postoperative patients, pp. 528–532, "Appendix One."

E. Patient–Family Teaching and Discharge Planning

Provide patient and SOs with verbal and written information for the following:

1. Importance of preventing trauma, which can cause bleeding.
2. Seeking medical attention for *any* signs of bleeding or infection. Review the signs and symptoms of common infections, such as URI, UTI, and wound infection.
3. Importance of regular medical follow-up for platelet counts.
4. If discharged on corticosteriods, the potential side effects that necessitate medical attention: acne, moon face, buffalo hump, hypertension, gastric upset, weight gain, thinning of arms and legs, edema, and mood changes. Stress the importance of *not* discontinuing steroids unless directed by MD.
5. Other medications, including drug name, dosage, purpose, schedule, precautions, and potential side effects.

II. Hemophilia

Hemophilia is a type of hereditary bleeding disorder characterized by a deficiency of one or more clotting factors. Classic hemophilia is caused by deficiency of factors VIII (hemophilia A) and IX (hemophilia B). Both types of hemophilia are sex-linked inherited disorders. Individuals affected are usually males, whereas their mothers and sisters are asymptomatic carriers. This disorder also can occur in females if it is inherited from an affected male and a female carrier or if it is due to X chromosome inactivation during embryologic development. Intracranial hemorrhage is the most common cause of death.

A. Assessment

Chronic indicators: Bruising after minimal trauma, joint pain.

Acute indicators: Acute bleeding episodes after minimal trauma. Hemarthrosis is the most common and debilitating symptom, causing painful and swollen joints. Large ecchymoses can occur, as well as bleeding from the gums, tongue, GI tract, urinary tract, or from cuts in the skin. Shock can result from severe bleeding.

B. Diagnostic Tests

1. <u>Partial thromboplastin time (PTT):</u> Prolonged.
2. <u>Bleeding time:</u> Prolonged.
3. <u>Platelet count:</u> Usually normal.
4. <u>Activated clotting time:</u> Prolonged.
5. <u>Assays of factors VIII and IX:</u> Will reveal low activity.

C. Medical Management

1. **Factor transfusion:** For hemophilia B (see Table 7-1, p. 347).
2. **Transfusion of fresh frozen plasma:** See Table 7-1, p. 346.
3. **Cryoprecipitate:** For infusion of factor VIII with classic hemophilia A. (See Table 7-1, p. 347.) Synthetic plasma has less risk of reaction.
4. **Antilytic agents such as desmopressin (DDAVP) and aminocaproic acid:** To enhance intrinsic mechanisms and decrease the need for factor replacement.

D. Nursing Diagnoses and Interventions

Potential for injury related to increased risk of bleeding secondary to clotting factor deficiency

Desired outcome: Patient does not exhibit signs of bleeding.

1. Monitor VS for signs of bleeding, including hypotension and increased heart rate. Also be alert to patient restlessness.
2. Monitor patient for evidence of bleeding, including swollen joints, abdominal pain, hematuria, hematemesis, melena, and epistaxis.
3. If signs of bleeding occur, elevate the affected area if possible, and apply cold compresses and gentle pressure to the site.
4. When indicated, institute measures to minimize the risk of bleeding from trauma, such as keeping siderails up and padded, assisting with ambulation, and limiting invasive procedures if possible.
5. Teach patient to use electric razor and soft-bristled toothbrush.
6. Do not administer aspirin; caution patient about its anticoagulant action.
7. Administer clotting factors as precribed.
8. To enhance joint mobility, assist patient with ROM exercises; however, avoid them for the first 48 hours after a bleeding episode to minimize the risk of recurrence. Factor VIII prophylaxis may be required to control hemarthrosis from ROM exercises.

Alteration in comfort: Pain related to swollen joints (hemarthrosis)

Desired outcome: Patient verbalizes a reduction in discomfort and does not exhibit signs of uncontrolled pain.

1. Apply splints or other supportive devices to joints, immobilizing them in slight flexion.
2. Elevate and/or position pillows under affected joints for comfort.
3. Administer analgesics as prescribed; avoid aspirin because of its anticoagulant action.
4. Assist patient with ambulation as needed.
5. Ice may be used for its topical analgesia and vasoconstriction. **Caution:** Avoid use of warm thermotherapy for these patients, as it would increase swelling.

E. Patient-Family Teaching and Discharge Planning

Provide patient and SOs with verbal and written information for the following:

1. Importance of avoiding trauma and necessity of seeking medical attention for *any* bleeding.
2. Phone numbers to call in the event of emergency.
3. Procedure in the event of bleeding: application of cold compresses and gentle, direct pressure; elevation of affected part if possible; seek medical attention promptly.
4. Importance of notifying MD if dental procedures need to be done.
5. Importance of lifetime medical follow-up and regular factor transfusions.

In addition:

6. In patients for whom factor VIII prophylaxis is used, patient and SOs will require instruction in the IV administration of factor VIII.
7. Explain the importance of frequent assessment of joint function to allow rapid identification and treatment of hemophilic arthritis.

III. Disseminated Intravascular Coagulation

Disseminated intravascular coagulation (DIC) is an acute coagulation disorder characterized by paradoxical clotting and hemorrhage. The sequence usually progresses by massive clot formation, depletion of the clotting factors, and activation of diffuse fibrinolysis, followed by hemorrhage. DIC occurs secondary to widespread coagulation factors in the bloodstream caused by extensive surgery, burns, shock, neoplastic diseases, and abruptio placenta; extensive destruction of blood vessel walls caused by eclampsia, anoxia, and heat stroke; or damage to blood cells caused by hemolysis, sickle cell disease, and transfusion reactions. Prompt assessment of the disorder can result in a good prognosis. Usually, affected patients are transferred to ICU for careful monitoring and aggressive therapy.

A. Assessment

Clinical indicators: Bleeding of abrupt onset, oozing from venipuncures sites, bleeding from surgical sites. Symptoms of hypoperfusion can occur, including decreased urine output and abnormal behavior.

Risk factors: Infection, burns, trauma, hepatic disease, hypovolemic shock, severe hemolytic reaction, obstetric complications, and hypoxia.

B. Diagnostic Tests

1. <u>Serum fibrinogen:</u> Low because of abnormal consumption of clotting factors.
2. <u>Platelet count:</u> Will be <250,000 because of platelet's role in clot formation.
3. <u>Fibrin split products (FSP):</u> Increased, indicating widespread dissolution of clots.
4. <u>PT:</u> Increased because of depletion of clotting factors.
5. <u>PTT:</u> High because of depletion of clotting factors.
6. <u>Peripheral blood smear:</u> Will show fragmented RBCs.
7. <u>Bleeding time:</u> Prolonged because of decreased platelets.

C. Medical Management

1. **Identify and treat primary disorder.**
2. **Anticoagulant therapy:** With IV heparin, which interferes with the coagulation process and minimizes consumption of the coagulation factors as well as activation of the fibrinolytic system. Heparin dose is regulated and determined by PTT.
3. **Compartment replacement of platelets and clotting factors:** Instituted after heparin therapy has been initiated, because otherwise the transfused factors would enhance the clotting process.

4. **Thrombolytic agents such as streptokinase:** To increase circulation in throm-bosed vessels after the acute phase has resolved.

D. Nursing Diagnoses and Interventions

Potential alteration in tissue perfusion: Peripheral, cerebral, and renal, related to altered circulation secondary to coagulation/fibrinolysis processes

Desired outcome: Patient's VS and physical findings are within acceptable limits.

1. Monitor VS. Be alert to and report decreased BP, increased heart rate, or decreased amplitude of peripheral pulses, which signal that coagulation is occurring.

2. Monitor I&O; report output <0.5 mL/kg/h in the presence of adequate in-take, another indicator of the coagulation process.

3. Perform neurologic checks and assess LOC to evaluate cerebral perfusion. If signs of impaired cerebral perfusion occur, protect patient from injury by in-stituting measures such as keeping bed in the lowest position and siderails up.

4. Monitor for hemorrhage from surgical wounds, GI tract, and mucous mem-branes, which can occur after fibrinolysis.

5. Report significant findings to MD; prepare to transfer patient to ICU if con-dition worsens.

See "Pulmonary Embolism" in Chapter 1, "Respiratory Disorders," for the following: **Potential for injury** related to increased risk of bleeding secondary to anticoagulant therapy, p. 9.

E. Patient–Family Teaching and Discharge Planning

See primary diagnosis

▶ Section Three   **Neoplastic Disorders of the Hematopoietic System**

White blood cells (WBCs), also called leukocytes, are the blood cells responsible for both immunity and the body's response to infectious organisms. Different types of WBCs are classified according to structure, specialized function, and response to dye in the laboratory. The three main classifications of WBCs are granulocytes, lym-phocytes, and monocytes, all of which may undergo malignant transformations. The bone marrow has a reserve of approximately 10 times the number of circulat-ing WBCs, which are released into the circulation during an infectious process.

I. Hodgkin's Disease

Hodgkin's disease is a tumor of the lymph tissue. It is distinguished from other lym-phomas by the presence of large, variable cells called Reed-Sternberg cells, which proliferate and invade normal lymph tissue throughout the body. Lymph tissue is found in the spleen, liver, bone marrow, lymph nodes, and lymph channels, which connect virtually all tissues. Clinical presentation depends on the degree of malig-nant cell growth, extent of the invasion, and tissues that are affected. Hodgkin's dis-ease frequently affects young people, and it can be treated successfully, particularly with early diagnosis and intervention. The etiology of the disorder is unclear, al-though a hereditary component has been implicated. Although no infectious or-ganism has been identified, infection has been suggested as a potential cause. Long-term survival (20 years) is now possible. *Non-Hodgkin's lymphomas* also can occur, but they tend to affect individuals around the age of 50. This disorder involves an abnormal, malignant lymphocytic invasion of the lymph nodes; however, Reed-Sternberg cells are not involved in the malignancy.

A. Assessment

Chronic indicators: Nonspecific symptoms such as persistent fever, night sweats, malaise, weight loss, and pruritis.

Acute indicators: Worsening of the above symptoms, in addition to unexplained pain in the lymph nodes after drinking alcohol.

Physical exam: Enlarged (painless) lymph nodes in the cervical area; possible splenomegaly and hepatomegaly.

B. Diagnostic Tests

1. <u>CBC:</u> Decreased hemoglobin and hematocrit (confirming anemia); increased, decreased, or normal levels of WBCs.

2. <u>Platelet count:</u> May be low.

3. <u>Lymph node biopsy:</u> May reveal presence of characteristic Reed-Sternberg cells.

4. <u>Lymphangiogram:</u> To determine extent of involvement. Cannulas are inserted into the lymph vessels and contrast medium is injected. Before the procedure, assessment must be made regarding patient allergy to contrast medium.

5. <u>Biopsy of the bone marrow, lung, liver, pleura, or bone:</u> May be performed to determine involvement.

6. <u>Serum alkaline phosphatase:</u> If elevated, will indicate liver or bone involvement.

7. <u>Erythrocyte sedimentation rate (ESR):</u> Will be elevated.

8. <u>Staging laparotomy with splenectomy and liver biopsy:</u> To determine extent of the disease and plan of care.

9. <u>Chest x-ray and/or abdominal CT scan:</u> To help determine presence of nodal involvement.

C. Medical Management

1. **Staging:** To determine extent of the disease. A simplified description of staging follows (based on Ann Arbor Staging Classification):

   ☐ *Stage I:* Limited to a single lymph node region or a single extralymphatic organ.

   ☐ *Stage II:* Involves two or more lymph node regions on the same side of the diaphragm or localized involvement of an extralymphatic organ.

   ☐ *Stage III:* Involves lymph node regions on both sides of the diaphragm, accompanied by involvement of an extralymphatic region and/or the spleen.

   ☐ *Stage IV:* Diffuse involvement of one or more extralymphatic region or tissue.

2. **Radiation therapy to lymph node regions:** For stages I and II.

3. **Chemotherapy in combination with radiation:** For stages III and IV. One common combination of chemotherapeutic agents includes mechlorethamine hydrochloride (nitrogen mustard), vincristine, prednisone, and procarbazine. For non-Hodgkin's lymphoma, a variety of antineoplastic drugs are currently being used, including cytoxan, vincristine, prednisone, procarbazine, doxorubicin, and bleomycin.

D. Nursing Diagnoses and Interventions

See "Pernicious Anemia" for the following: **Activity intolerance**, p. 341, and **Alteration in nutrition:** Less than body requirements, p. 342. See "Hypoplastic Anemia" for the following: **Potential for infection**, p. 348. See nursing diagnoses and interventions for the care of patients with cancer and other life-disrupting illnesses, pp. 544–551, and the care of preoperative and postoperative patients, pp. 528–532, "Appendix One."

E. Patient–Family Teaching and Discharge Planning

Provide patient and SOs with verbal and written information for the following:

1. For patients in stage I or II, the resumption of normal lifestyle with minor adjustments, as prescribed.
2. Continuing radiation or chemotherapy, if prescribed, which is given on an outpatient basis; confirm date and time of next appointment.
3. Signs and symptoms that necessitate medical attention: persistent fever, weight loss, enlarged lymph nodes, malaise, and decreased exercise tolerance.
4. Importance of preventing infection and avoiding exposure to individuals with infection, which is essential because of alterations in WBC count and patient's decreased resistance to infection secondary to therapy. Teach patient the indicators of common infections such as UTI, URI, and wound infection.
5. Diet: importance of maintaining good nutritional habits to increase resistance to infection.
6. Referral to American Cancer Society and local support groups.
7. Avoiding trauma, which can cause bruising, especially in presence of thrombocytopenia.
8. If appropriate, measures to assist patient with ADLs.

II. Acute Leukemia

Acute leukemia is an abnormal, malignant proliferation of WBC precursors, also called "blasts." These abnormal cells accumulate in bone marrow, body tissues, and blood vessels and eventually cause malfunction by encroachment, hemorrhage, or infection. In addition, they function inappropriately in response to infection and prevent normal WBC maturation. The two most common types of acute leukemia are *myelogenous* (arising from the myeloblast, which matures into a neutrophil) and *lymphoblastic* (arising from the lymphoblast, which matures into a lymphocyte). Untreated, acute leukemia is invariably fatal, and even with treatment the prognosis varies. Acute lymphoblastic leukemia (ALL) most often affects children under 15 years old, and acute myelogenous leukemia usually affects individuals older than 20 years.

A. Assessment

Chronic indicators: Fever, pallor, chills, and weakness, which can be present for days, weeks, or months before acute crisis occurs.

Acute indicators: High fever, diffuse petechiae, ecchymosis, epistaxis, anorexia, headaches, visual disturbances, weakness, feeling of abdominal fullness, and lethargy.

Physical exam: Sternal and bone tenderness on palpation, splenomegaly, hepatomegaly, palpable lymph nodes, pallor, and diffuse bleeding of mucous membranes.

B. Diagnostic Tests

1. <u>CBC:</u> Hemoglobin will be decreased; WBC value may be low, normal, or elevated, and will include many immature cells.
2. <u>Bone marrow aspiration:</u> Will reveal increased numbers of myeloblasts or lymphoblasts.
3. <u>Platelet count:</u> Will be decreased.
4. <u>Uric acid:</u> Increased secondary to rapid cell destruction.

C. Medical Management

The goal is the complete remission or reduction in the number of malignant cells and increased number of normal leukocytes by normal hematopoiesis. Secondary management goals are to return the erythrocyte index and thrombocyte count to normal.

1. **Chemotherapy/pharmacotherapy:** Used in combination to produce remission (less than 5% blast cells and no identifiable leukemic cells in the bone marrow). Treatment may be continued for 1½–2 years after remission occurs. **Note:** For children with ALL, treatment may last up to 3 years.

   □ *For acute lymphoblastic leukemia:* Vincristine sulfate and prednisone, asparaginase, and doxorubicin and methotrexate for CNS prophylaxis.

   □ *For acute myelogenous leukemia:* Daunorubicin hydrochloride, cytarabine, and thioguanine.

2. **Transfusion of packed RBCs:** To restore erythrocytes. Leukocyte-poor packed RBCs is preferable to whole blood because febrile reactions to WBCs or platelet antibodies are prevented. Because of possible antibody formation and increased transfusion reactions over time, transfusions are given conservatively, especially in patients for whom long-term transfusions of platelets and granulocytes are anticipated Therefore, patients may need to tolerate a certain degree of anemia. (See Table 7-1, p. 346.)

3. **Platelet transfusion:** To restore platelet levels to >20,000 mm^3. (See Table 7-1, p. 346.)

4. **Bone marrow transplantation:** Available in specialized centers. (See discussion in "Hypoplastic Anemia," p. 348.)

D. Nursing Diagnoses and Interventions

Potential for infection related to increased susceptibility secondary to myelosuppression from disease process or therapy

Desired outcome: Patient does not exhibit signs of infection.

1. Perform meticulous handwashing before caring for patient.
2. Be aware that as the neutrophil count decreases, the risk of infection increases. When the patient becomes neutropenic, perform reverse (protective) isolation using a gown, mask, and gloves; provide a private room.
3. Avoid all invasive procedures (eg, catheterization) unless absolutely necessary. When such procedures are performed, use strict asepsis.
4. Assist patient with ambulation when possible. Institute turning, coughing, and deep breathing at frequent intervals to help prevent problems of immobility that can result in infection, such as skin breakdown and respiratory dysfunction.
5. Provide oral hygiene and perianal care at frequent intervals.
6. Monitor patient's temperature at frequent intervals. In the presence of any suspected infections, obtain prescription for a culture.
7. Administer antibiotic therapy if prescribed.
8. Deliver transfusion of granulocytes if prescribed.

Potential for injury related to increased risk of bleeding secondary to decreased platelet count

Desired outcomes: Patient does not exhibit signs of bleeding. Patient can verbalize knowledge of the signs and symptoms of bleeding and the importance of seeking medical attention promptly should they occur.

1. Monitor platelet counts. Counts <50,000 dramatically increase the risk of bleeding.
2. Request that patient alert staff to oozing from the gums.

3. Inspect patient's skin, mouth, nose, urine, feces, sputum, emesis, and IV sites for signs for bleeding. Test all excretions for the presence of occult blood.

4. Monitor VS at frequent intervals and be alert to signs of bleeding such as hypotension and increased heart rate.

5. Limit invasive procedures to those that are absolutely necessary.

6. Use small-gauge needles when possible. Maintain gentle pressure on injection site until bleeding stops.

7. If bleeding occurs, elevate the affected part, if possible, and apply cold compresses and gentle pressure.

8. Pad siderails to prevent trauma.

9. Administer platelet transfusions as prescribed.

10. Teach patient the signs and symptoms of bleeding and the importance of notifying staff promptly should they occur.

Activity intolerance related to fatigue and weakness secondary to decreased oxygen-carrying capacity of the blood

Desired outcome: Patient increases activities to tolerance and exhibits physical findings within acceptable range.

1. If prescribed, administer packed RBCs to restore normal erythrocyte level.

2. Assist patient with ADLs as necessary.

3. Provide periods of undisturbed rest.

4. Minimize restlessness, which increases oxygen utilization, by providing frequent comfort measures such as backrubs.

5. Administer oxygen, if prescribed. Encourage deep-breathing exercises, which may promote oxygenation by enhancing gas exchange.

6. As patient's condition improves, encourage activities to tolerance. Set mutually agreed-upon goals, for example, "Can you walk the length of the hall two or three times (or appropriate number, depending on tolerance) this morning?"

Alteration in tissue perfusion: Renal related to decreased circulation secondary to destruction of RBCs and their precipitation in kidney tubules

Desired outcome: Patient's I&O and physical findings are within acceptable limits.

1. Monitor for and report signs of renal insufficiency, including positive fluid balance, weight gain, and urinary output <0.5 mL/kg/h in the presence of adequate intake.

2. Maintain adequate hydration to enhance urinary flow and decrease precipitation.

3. Encourage ambulation or in-bed exercises to patient's tolerance to promote renal circulation.

4. Alert MD to significant findings.

See nursing diagnoses and interventions for the care of patients with cancer and other life-disrupting illnesses, pp. 544–551, "Appendix One."

E. Patient–Family Teaching and Discharge Planning

Provide patient and SOs with verbal and written information for the following:

1. Importance of avoiding infections and bleeding and measures to prevent same, including the following: Avoid exposure to individuals with infection, maintain good hygiene, avoid situations with high risk of trauma or injury, and report *any* signs of infection to MD (eg, fever, chills, and malaise).

2. Side effects of chemotherapy: constipation, alopecia, nausea and vomiting, anorexia, diarrhea, stomatitis, skin rash, nail changes, hyperpigmentation of the skin, weight gain from steroid use, ecchymosis, and cystitis.

3. Importance of good nutrition, eating small and frequent meals, consuming 2–3 L/day of fluids (unless contraindicated by cardiac or renal disorder), and using soft-bristled toothbrush and electric razor.

4. Referrals to American Cancer Society, Leukemia Society of America, local support groups, and home care or hospice groups, if appropriate.

III. Chronic Leukemia

Chronic leukemias are characterized by malignant proliferation of abnormal immature WBCs. These abnormal cells eventually infiltrate body tissues and organs and prevent maturation of normal WBCs, thus preventing usual and necessary WBC function. Chronic leukemic cells are a more mature form than is seen in acute leukemias and accumulate much more slowly. The two most common types of chronic leukemia are *chronic myelogenous* (involves the myelocyte, precursor of the neutrophil) and *chronic lymphatic* (involves the lymphocyte). Causes of chronic leukemia are unclear, although chromosomal abnormality is suspected in many cases of myelogenous leukemia. Also implicated are hereditary factors and immunologic defects.

A. Assessment

Chronic indicators: Fatigue, anorexia, weight loss, feeling of heaviness in the spleen area, malaise, unexplained low-grade fever, and lymph node enlargement.

Acute indicators: High fever, diffuse petechiae, ecchymosis, epistaxis, anorexia, headaches, visual disturbances, weakness, feeling of abdominal fullness, and lethargy.

B. Diagnostic Tests

1. CBC with differential: Elevated WBC; decreased hemoglobin and neutrophils.

2. Platelet count (thrombocytes): Low.

3. Bone marrow aspiration: Usually identifies abnormal distribution and/or increased number of cells.

C. Medical Management and Surgical Interventions

For chronic lymphocytic leukemia:

1. **Chlorambucil and prednisone:** To produce remission.

2. **Total body or local irradiation of spleen and lymph nodes.**

For chronic myelogenous leukemia:

1. **Chemotherapy**

   □ *Busulfan and hydroxyurea:* During the stable, chronic phase.

   □ *Daunorubicin, cytarabine, vincristine, prednisone, and thioguanine:* During the acute phase.

2. **Splenectomy:** May be necessary if the spleen is destroying platelets.

D. Nursing Diagnoses and Interventions

See "Acute Leukemia," p. 360.

▶ **Note:** Although patients survive longer and the severity of symptoms is less with chronic leukemias, the same principles and nursing interventions apply.

See nursing diagnoses and interventions for the care of patients with cancer and other life-disrupting illnesses, pp. 544–551, and the care of preoperative and post-operative patients (if splenectomy is performed), pp. 528–532, "Appendix One."

E. Patient–Family Teaching and Discharge Planning

See same section in "Acute Leukemia," p. 361.

▶ Selected References

Abramowicz M (editor): *The Med Let Drugs Ther* Feb 15, 1985; 27:13–20.

Aiso N, Floyd R: Drug-induced hemolytic anemia. *California Pharmacist* July 1982; XXX:18–23.

Bonadonna G, Santoro A: *Current Diagnosis and Treatment of Malignant Lymphomas.* Bristol-Myers, 1983.

Brandt B: A nursing protocol for the client with neutropenia. *Oncology Nursing Forum* 1984; 11:24–28.

Campbell JB, Preston R, Smith KY: The leukemias: Definition, treatment, and nursing care. *Nurs Clin North Am* Sept 1983; 18:523–542.

Carpenito LJ: *Handbook of Nursing Diagnosis.* Lippincott, 1983.

Darovic J: Disseminated intravascular coagulation. *Crit Care Nurse* Nov-Dec 1982; 2:36–46.

Dwyer JE, Held DM: Home management of the adult patient with leukemia. *Nurs Clin North Am* Dec 1982; 17:665–676.

Fischbach F: *A Manual of Laboratory Diagnostic Tests,* 2nd ed. Lippincott, 1984.

Hays K, Rafferty DC: Care of the patient with malignant lymphoma. *Nurs Clin North Am* Dec 1982; 17:677–696.

Houlihan N, Feeley A: The acute and chronic leukemias. *Cancer Nursing* Aug 1981; 4:323–338.

Hutchinson MM: Aplastic anemia: Care of the bone marrow failure patient. *Nurs Clin North Am* Sept 1983; 18:543–552.

Jones DA, Dunbar CF, Jirovec MM: *Medical Surgical Nursing: A Conceptual Approach.* McGraw-Hill, 1982.

Kinney MR et al (editors): *AACN's Clinical Reference for Critical Care Nursing.* McGraw-Hill, 1981.

McLeod BC: Immunologic factors in reactions to blood transfusions. *Heart Lung* July-August 1980; 9:675–681.

Pack B (editor): Symposium on sickle cell disease. *Nurs Clin North Am* March 1983; 18:129–230.

Vogelpohl RA: Disseminated intravascular coagulation. *Crit Care Nurse* May-June 1981; I:38–43.

Walter J: Care of the patient receiving antineoplastic drugs. *Nurs Clin North Am* Dec 1982; 17:607–630.

Wessler R: Care of the hospitalized adult patient with leukemia. *Nurs Clin North Am* Dec 1982; 17:649–664.

Wintrobe MM et al: *Clinical Hematology,* 8th ed. Lea & Febiger, 1981.

Woods ME, Kowalski JD: Symposium on oncologic nursing practice. *Nurs Clin North Am* Dec 1982; 17:535–784

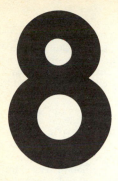

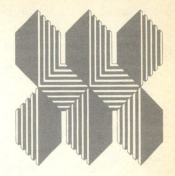

8

Musculoskeletal Disorders

▶ Section One **Inflammatory Disorders**

Arthritis is inflammation of a joint. There are many forms, including osteoarthritis, gouty arthritis, rheumatoid arthritis, Reiter's syndrome, ankylosing spondylitis, systemic lupus erythematosus, and psoriatic arthritis. Osteoarthritis, gouty arthritis, and rheumatoid arthritis are frequently seen in hospitalized patients and therefore are discussed in this section.

I. Osteoarthritis

Osteoarthritis, also known as degenerative joint disease (DJD), is an extremely prevalent disorder. It is a chronic, progressive disease characterized by increasing pain, deformity, and loss of function. It can be found in any age group, usually following trauma or as a complication of congenital malformation. True joint inflammation is seldom present (except in the distal interphalangeal joints). Hereditary and mechanical factors are suspected to be the primary causes of this process.

Primary osteoarthritis is idiopathic and occurs in the distal interphalangeal joints (DIP), proximal interphalangeal joints (PIP), the carpometacarpal joints (CMC), hip, knee, first metatarsophalangeal joint (MTP), and the cervical and lumbosacral spine. *Secondary arthritis* can occur in any joint and usually follows some form of intra-articular injury or extra-articular cause that affects joint dynamics. Examples include joint fractures and chronic insults such as poor posture, obesity, occupational abuse, or a metabolic disease that affects the joint (ochronosis, osteitis deformans, or hyperparathyroidism).

A. Assessment

Involvement can range from incidental findings on x-ray to pervasive disease that affects the patient's independence in the performance of ADLs.

Signs and symptoms: Onset is insidious, beginning with joint stiffness. It evolves into joint pain, which worsens with activity and is relieved with resting the joint. Signs of local inflammation are usually absent, except occasionally in the DIP, PIP, and CMC joints. Usually, there are no specific systemic signs or symptoms.

Physical exam: Characteristic findings include Heberden's nodes (enlargement of the DIP joint), Bouchard's nodes (enlargement of the PIP joint), varus or valgus deformity of the knee, bony enlargement of the joint, and flexion contracture of the knee. Frequently, crepitation is found.

B. Diagnostic Tests

There are no characteristic laboratory studies associated with this disorder.

X-ray studies: May reveal narrowing of the joint space, osteophytosis (bony projections) of the joint margins, bone cysts, bony erosions, and dense subchondral bone.

C. Medical Management and Surgical Interventions

1. **Rest:** The principal therapy for preventing progression. The patient is advised to avoid activities that will further stress the joint. Use of ambulatory assistive devices, splints, or orthotics may be prescribed to allow rest or decreased stress on affected joints, and the patient is instructed in methods that prevent postural strain. Regular rest periods of 30–60 minutes are often advised for patients prone to overworking.

2. **Weight reduction:** For patients for whom excessive weight contributes to the pathology.

3. **Local moist heat:** To decrease stiffness and provide some subjective pain relief. Hydrotherapy with warm water is especially useful in aiding range of motion (ROM) exercises. Patients who cannot afford to purchase a device to

supply moist heat may be required to use a traditional heating pad. Some patients find greater subjective relief from cold packs than from moist heat.

4. **ROM and muscle-strengthening exercises:** May be useful in selected cases to increase joint function and supplement joint strength. Exercises may include passive ROM, active ROM, active-assisted ROM, and isometric and isotonic exercises. The maxim that is followed for the appropriate amount of exercise is that pain that lasts until the next exercise period (or several hours) indicates the exercise was too strenuous.

5. **Intra-articular steroids:** Used by some MDs to provide transient relief of symptoms. However, they do not halt the progression of the disease and run the risk of introducing refractory infections.

6. **Pharmacotherapy:** Includes the use of analgesics and anti-inflammatory agents. Analgesics may be necessary to combat the pain associated with DJD. Aspirin, acetaminophen, and the nonsteroidal anti-inflammatory agents (see Table 8-1, p. 370) are usually satisfactory, but occasionally, narcotic analgesics are required for short periods following physical therapy or surgical interventions.

7. **Surgical interventions:** Various orthopedic surgeries may be utilized to correct underlying congenital anomalies or defects created by trauma. Arthroplastic surgery allows damaged joint surfaces to be augmented, repaired, or replaced, while periarticular tissues may be repaired to improve joint strength. Joint replacement has been used to replace most joints, but the greatest success has been found with the hip (see p. 412) and knee (see p. 415) implant arthroplasties. In joints that are chronically infected or not amenable to standard or implant arthroplasties, an arthrodesis (joint fusion) may provide joint stability and permit some function.

8. **Splints and orthotic devices:** May be used to supplement joint strength or protect the joint from excessive strain.

9. **Assistive devices:** A great variety have been developed to help patients perform ADLs independently, even in cases of significant joint function loss. Examples include stocking helpers, built-up eating utensils, pickup sticks, and raised toilet seats.

D. Nursing Diagnoses and Interventions

Alteration in comfort: Pain related to inflammatory process or corrective therapy

Desired outcome: Patient verbalizes a reduction in discomfort and does not exhibit signs of uncontrolled pain.

1. Administer analgesics and anti-inflammatory agents as prescribed and document their effectiveness.

2. Instruct the patient in the use of nonpharmacologic methods of pain control, including guided imagery; graduated breathing (as in Lamaze); enhanced relaxation; massage; biofeedback; cutaneous stimulation (via a counterirritant such as oil of wintergreen); transcutaneous electrical nerve stimulation (TENS) device; warm or cool thermotherapy; and tactile, auditory, visual, or verbal distraction.

3. Use traditional nursing interventions to counteract the pain, including backrubs, repositioning, and encouraging the patient to verbalize feelings.

4. Incorporate rest, local warmth, and elevation of the affected joints, when possible, to help control arthritic pain.

5. Advise patient to coordinate the time of peak effectiveness of the anti-inflammatory agent with periods of exercise or mandatory use of arthritic joints.

6. Instruct patient in the use of moist heat and hydrotherapy, which will help reduce long-term discomfort.

Knowledge deficit: Proper use of a heating device

Desired outcome: Patient can verbalize and demonstrate proper use of the heating device.

1. Provide patient with instructions for the proper use of moist or dry heat. Because older individuals may have decreased neuronal function and skin that is more easily traumatized, instruct them in the use of a thermometer (with adequate-size numbers for reading) or a controlled warming device.

2. Caution the patient about the potential for increasing his or her tolerance to heat. This can occur when the heat has been used for long periods of time, and may cause the patient to feel the need for a higher degree of heat than that which is safe.

Impaired physical mobility related to adjustment to a new walking gait with an assistive device

Desired outcomes: Patient can demonstrate adequate upper body strength for use of an assistive device. Patient demonstrates appropriate use of the assistive device on flat and uneven surfaces.

1. Before ambulation, ensure the necessary strength of the patient's upper extremities for using the assistive device by incorporating the interventions listed in **Potential impairment of physical mobility**, p. 535 in "Appendix One." Triceps strength is especially important for ambulation with crutches or a walker. Having patients push down on the bed as they extend their arms to lift their buttocks off the bed will strengthen the triceps muscles.

2. Provide a thorough discussion with a demonstration to teach the patient how the assistive device is used.

3. Once the assistive device is in position, repeat the the instructions and then supervise the ambulation. Ambulation should begin in small increments on level ground and eventually progress to all surfaces the patient is expected to encounter after hospital discharge.

4. Ensure that before discharge, the patient is able to demonstrate independence in ambulation with the assistive device on level surfaces and stairs and with getting in and out of a car.

See "Appendix One" for nursing diagnoses and interventions for the care of patients on prolonged bed rest, pp. 533–537.

E. Patient–Family Teaching and Discharge Planning

Provide patient and SOs with verbal and written information for the following:

1. Medications, including drug name, dosage, purpose, schedule, precautions, and potential side effects.

2. Importance of systemic rest as well as rest of the affected joints.

3. Weight reduction, if it is appropriate for the patient.

4. Proper use of moist heat.

5. Necessity of ROM and muscle-strengthening exercises.

6. Use of splints or orthotics, including care and cleansing and where to get replacements.

7. Use, care, and replacement of assistive devices.

8. If surgery was performed, the precautions related to the procedure, wound care, and the indicators of wound infection or complications of surgery.

9. Importance of follow-up care and the date of the next appointment and a phone number to call should any questions arise.

II. Gouty Arthritis

Gout is a crystal-induced synovitis that results from an abnormal amount of urates. *Primary gout*, an inherited metabolic disorder, is caused by either excess production or underexcretion of urates. *Secondary gout* results from other conditions in which uric acid is retained or excessively produced, such as lead poisoning, use of thiazide diuretics, chronic renal disease, myeloproliferative disease, hemoglobinopathies, cancer chemotherapy, and multiple myeloma. The pathophysiology involves the formation of tophus (nodular deposition of monosodium urate monohydrate crystals), which causes a pronounced inflammatory response. Tophi may be found in synovial tissues, cartilage, periarticular tissues, tendon, bone, and the kidneys. Although the relationship between high serum levels of uric acid (hyperuricemia) and gouty arthritis is unclear, there appears to be some relationship between rapid fluctuations in the level of serum uric acid and an acute gouty attack. Uric acid renal calculi, nephrosclerosis, and gouty nephritis can accompany this process.

A. Assessment

Chronic indicators: Joint changes similar to those of osteoarthritis (see p. 366). Uncontrolled or untreated gout results in a progressive, chronic disorder that causes severe joint deformity and loss of function. Hypertension, renal calculi, and renal failure also may be seen.

Acute indicators: Sudden onset, acute inflammation, and an excruciatingly painful joint that presents with erythema, joint effusion, restricted motion, warmth, and tenderness. Systemic indicators include tachycardia, anorexia, fever, headache, and malaise. Although it is usually monoarticular, polyarticular attacks have been noted with this disorder.

Physical exam: Tophi may be noted as subcutaneous nodules on the hands, feet, olecrannon bursa, prepatellar bursa, and ears. The most commonly affected joint is the metatarsophalangeal joint of the great toe, but the feet, ankles, and knees are also commonly affected.

History of: Recent surgery, oral intake high in purines, alcoholic excess, infection, and use of diuretics.

B. Diagnostic Tests

1. <u>Serum tests:</u> Uric acid is frequently elevated above the normal 7.5 mg/dL during an acute attack unless the patient is taking medications that depress the serum levels of uric acid (large doses of A.S.A., methyldopa, phenothiazines, sulfinpyrazone, or clofibrate). There also will be leukocytosis and an elevated sedimentation rate.

2. <u>Joint fluid aspiration:</u> Allows compensated polariscopic examination of wet smears to reveal presence of sodium urate crystals.

3. <u>Tophus aspiration:</u> Provides identification of typical sodium urate crystals.

4. <u>X-ray:</u> Will demonstrate no change early in the disease, but with chronic disease there will be radiolucent urate tophi (which look like punched-out areas on the x-ray) adjacent to soft tissue tophi.

C. Medical Management and Surgical Interventions

1. Pharmacotherapy

□ *Colchicine:* Drug of choice during the acute phase. It is believed that it mediates the inflammatory response caused by the urate crystals. Usual dosage is 0.5 mg qh or 1 mg q2h until either the pain is controlled or side effects appear. Side effects include nausea, vomiting, abdominal cramping, and diarrhea. To reduce the incidence of side effects, the initial dose may be given IV. Colchicine is contraindicated in patients with inflammatory bowel disorders, significant hepatic disease, or renal disease.

Table 8-1 Nonsteroidal Anti-Inflammatory Agents

Generic Name	Common Trade Names	Usual Daily Dosage (mg)
acetylsalicylic acid	Aspirin	650–1300 q4h
choline salicylate	Arthropan	650 q4–6h
choline magnesium trisalicylate	Trilisate	1000–1250 bid
fenoprofen calcium	Nalfon	300–600 qid
ibuprofen	Motrin, Advil, Nuprin	200–400 qid
indomethacin	Indocin	20–50 tid
magnesium salicylate	Mobidin	600–1200 tid or qid
meclofenamate sodium	Meclomen	50 tid or qid
mefenámic acid	Ponstel	250 qid
naproxen	Naprosyn	250–375 qid
naproxen sodium	Anaprox	275 q6–8h
oxyphenbutazone	Tandearil	100 tid
piroxicam	Feldene	20 qd
sulindac	Clinoril	150–200 bid
tolmetin sodium	Tolectin	200–400 mg tid

☐ *Corticosteroids:* May control acute attacks but must be combined with colchicine because discontinuation of the steroid often results in a relapse.

☐ *Nonsteroidal anti-inflammatory agents:* May be used for chronic or acute forms of the disease (see Table 8-1).

☐ *Analgesics such as acetaminophen with codeine or oxycodone preparations:* To control the pain of gout, which is usually excruciating.

2. **Joint rest:** Mandatory in acute phases and should include complete bed rest with elevation of the inflamed joint. Sometimes, topical cooling (ice applications to the joint) is prescribed to aid in reducing inflammation.

3. **Management between attacks:** May be accomplished with the following:

☐ *Colchicine:* Prophylactic or interim use.

☐ *Uricosuric agents such as probenecid or sulfinpyrazone:* The dosage is determined by the patient's serum uric acid levels. Nonrestricted patients should maintain a fluid intake of at least 2–3 L/day or use an alkalinizing agent such as sodium bicarbonate, which maintains urinary pH above 6.0 to prevent uric acid calculi. Salicylate drugs are avoided because they antagonize the effects of uricosuric agents.

☐ *Allopurinol, a xanthine oxidase inhibitor:* Lowers serum uric acid, decreases the concentration of uric acid in the urine, and mobilizes the uric acid crystals in tophi. Dosage varies, depending on serum uric acid levels. Because hepatotoxicity and renal calculi can occur, the drug is used cautiously in patients with renal and/or hepatic disease.

4. **Diet therapy:** Complete restriction of purines (metabolic precursors to uric acid) is seldom prescribed because purines are found in most protein foods, and rigid dietary restriction would be unhealthy. However, alcoholic beverage intake is frequently curtailed because of its connection with the precipitation of acute attacks.

5. **Surgical intervention:** Gouty tophi are excised when they erode through the skin or cause mechanical impairment. Chronic joint involvement may require the surgical interventions discussed in "Osteoarthritis," p. 367.

D. Nursing Diagnoses and Interventions

Knowledge deficit: Disease process, medication regimen, and potential drug side effects

Desired outcome: Patient can verbalize knowledge of the disease process, medication regimen, and potential drug side effects.

1. Assess patient's knowledge of the disease process, medication regimen, and potential side effects of the drugs. As appropriate, teach the pathophysiology of the disease. In addition, when secondary gout is suspected, inform patient about the primary disease causing the gout.

2. Provide thorough instructions for the medication therapy, including rationale, dosage, schedule, precautions, and potential side effects.

3. When initiating colchicine treatment for an acute attack, assess patient carefully for pre-existing bowel, liver, or renal disease. Instruct patient to notify the staff promptly when pain has abated or nausea, vomiting, abdominal cramping, or diarrhea occur. Colchicine dosages are usually decreased or terminated at the onset of any of these indicators.

4. For patients taking uricosuric agents, stress the potential for the development of uric acid renal calculi and the need for at least 2–3 L/day of fluid in non-restricted patients and/or the use of an alkaline ash diet or an alkalinizing agent such as sodium bicarbonate to ensure that the urine pH remains >6. Instruct these patients in the use of pH test tape to check urine pH.

5. Caution patients taking allopurinol of the potential for renal and hepatic complications.

6. Caution patients taking narcotic analgesics of the potential for altered sensorium, and advise them to avoid using machinery, driving, or performing other activities requiring alertness.

Knowledge deficit: Proper care of inflamed joints

Desired outcomes: Patient can verbalize knowledge of the importance of resting the joint during periods of inflammation and can demonstrate elevation of the joint, assisted ROM, and use of thermotherapy.

1. Elevate the inflamed joint with pillows, above the level of the heart. Explain the rationale to the patient.

2. Perform passive ROM of the joints bid (or have the patient perform assisted ROM). Explain the rationale to the patient.

3. Instruct patient to increase joint ROM as the inflammation subsides, following the process described under the nursing diagnosis **Potential impairment of physical mobility**, p. 535, in "Appendix One."

4. Advise patient to use thermotherapy as prescribed, using care to ensure adequate protection of the involved skin.

Knowledge deficit: Signs and symptoms of, and preventive measures for, uric acid renal calculi

Desired outcome: Patient can verbalize knowledge of the signs and symptoms of, and preventive measures for, uric acid renal calculi.

1. Teach the patient the indicators of renal calculi, eg, severe renal colic, costovertebral angle tenderness, chronic UTI, urinary retention, nausea, vomiting, and pain located in the flank, side, lower back, suprapubic area, groin, labia, or scrotum. Instruct patient to alert MD if any of these signs and symptoms occur after hospital discharge.

2. Ensure that patient is knowledgeable about preventive measures, including a fluid intake of at least 2–3 L/day in nonrestricted patients, alkalinating measures to ensure urinary pH >6, and use of pH test tape to monitor urinary pH.

Alteration in nutrition: More than body requirements related to excessive intake of purines and/or alcohol

Desired outcome: Patient can demonstrate knowledge of the prescribed dietary regimen by planning three meals a day for three successive days.

1. In severe disease forms, it may be necessary to restrict the patient's intake of purine-containing foods. High-purine-content foods include bouillon, broth, consomme, gravy, organ meats, mackerel, yeast, poultry, meats, fish, shellfish, scallops, asparagus, beans, lentils, mushrooms, peas, and spinach. Ensure that the patient receives consultation, with verbal instruction in the dietary regimen as well as written instructions to take home.

2. Inform patient that excessive use of alcohol has been known to precipitate gout attacks.

See "Osteoarthritis" for the following: **Alteration in comfort,** p. 367. See "Appendix One" for nursing diagnoses and interventions for the care of preoperative and postoperative patients, pp. 528–532, and for the care of patients on prolonged bed rest, pp. 533–537.

E. Patient–Family Teaching and Discharge Planning

Provide patient and SOs with verbal and written information for the following:

1. Pathophysiology of the patient's form of gout.
2. Medications, including drug name, purpose, dosage, schedule, precautions, and potential side effects.
3. Indicators of renal calculi.
4. Diet therapy if appropriate, and the importance of avoiding excessive alcohol consumption.
5. Use of therapeutic local and systemic rest

III. Rheumatoid Arthritis

Rheumatoid arthritis (RA) is a systemic disease characterized by remissions and exacerbations of inflammation of the connective tissue throughout the body. Although many connective tissues have potential for involvement (heart, blood vessels, lungs, spleen, and kidney) and generalized systemic effects may be noted, this discussion centers on the arthritic aspects of this process. RA most commonly affects the synovial joints, but the effects of this disease are highly variable. The etiology is unknown, but theories include autoimmune process, food allergies, hereditary deficit, and slow viral infections. The disease onset and progression can be rapid and fulminating or slow and chronic.

The inflammatory process results in chronic synovitis with the formation of pannus, an inflammatory exudate that accumulates over the surface of the synovial membrane, eventually eroding cartilage, bone, ligaments, and tendons. Involvement of connective periarticular tissues results in loss of support structures and leads to characteristic joint changes, which further contribute to the pathology.

A. Assessment

Acute indicators: Morning stiffness lasting >30 minutes, symmetrical joint involvement, joint effusion, periarticular edema, pain, local warmth, and erythema. Joint stiffness is usually worsened by stress placed on the joint, and it can follow periods of inactivity as well. Prodromal signs and symptoms may incude malaise, weight loss, vague periarticular pain, low-grade fever, and vasomotor disturbances resulting in paresthesia and Raynaud's phenomenon. Sometimes, an acute exacerbation is related to stress such as infection, surgery, trauma, or emotional strain.

Chronic indicators: Progressive thickening of the periarticular tissues, subluxation, fibrous ankylosis, atrophy of skin and muscle, severe limitation of ROM with progressive loss of function, joint and muscle contractures, dryness of the eyes and mucous membranes, and subcutaneous nodules. Some patients develop splenomegaly and enlarged lymph nodes.

B. Diagnostic Tests

1. <u>Serologic and other blood studies:</u> Many are performed to detect certain macroglobulins, which make up the rheumatoid factor.

   □ *Latex fixation test:* Positive in 75% of the individuals with RA. Higher titers are associated with more severe clinical disease. Because false positives are common, a definite diagnosis cannot be made on this test alone.

   □ *ESR:* If elevated, is an indicator of inflammation.

   □ *Immunoglobulins, especially IgM and IgG:* If elevated, strongly suggest an autoimmune process as the cause of RA.

   □ *Normocytic hypochromic anemia:* Usually present secondary to long-standing inflammation.

   □ *WBC count:* Usually normal or slightly elevated, but leukopenia can be present, especially in the presence of splenomegaly.

2. <u>Fluid aspiration from the involved joint:</u> May reveal synovial fluid greater in volume than normal, opaque and cloudy yellow in appearance, glucose level lower than serum level, and elevated WBCs and leukocytes in the presence of RA.

3. <u>X-ray studies of the involved joints:</u> In the early phases will illustrate soft tissue swelling, erosion of joint surfaces normally covered by articular cartilage, and osteoporosis of adjacent bone. In long-standing disease, the joint will show periarticular weakness, subluxation, joint space narrowing, bone cyst formation, and concurrent osteoarthritic joint changes. Special attention is paid to upper cervical vertebrae, where subluxation of C1 or C2 can result in life-threatening neurologic complications.

4. <u>Radionuclide joint scanning:</u> To identify inflamed synovium in patients with appropriate symptoms.

C. Medical Management and Surgical Interventions

1. **Systemic rest:** Mandatory throughout all phases of this disease. In exacerbations, bed rest may be required until significant clinical joint findings have decreased for 2 weeks. During this period, proper joint positioning is essential to prevent contractures. Concurrent physical therapy is prescribed to put joints through passive ROM at least once a day. During remissions, the patient should receive 8 hours of sleep each night and 1–2 hours rest at midday. Any increase in symptomatology necessitates increasing the amount of rest.

2. **Emotional support:** To lessen stress and help patients deal with fear, disability, and the many losses they will incur.

3. **Rest of inflamed joints:** Imperative. Unstable joints should be splinted or braced to provide support and put through passive ROM at least daily while inflamed.

4. **Joint exercise:** Essential to maintain joint function and muscle strength, with the amount increasing as inflammation decreases. A graded exercise program should include the following: passive ROM, active-assisted ROM, active ROM, and resistive ROM with gradually increasing levels of resistance. Isometric exercise is used to maintain muscle strength during active joint inflammation. Any signs of increasing joint inflammation are cause for regression to a less stressful exercise until joint inflammation has again decreased. Inflamed weight-bearing joints should be protected from stress by orthotics and ambulatory adjuncts (cane, crutches, and walker, or a wheel chair if imperative).

5. **Thermotherapy:** To relax muscles and reduce pain. Cold therapy is used during inflammatory stages to reduce pain. Moist heat (especially warm tub baths) is useful to exercise stiffened joints, using the heat and buoyancy to aid motion. When submersion is not possible, use of moist warm cloths before exercise will decrease the patient's discomfort.

6. **Assistive devices:** For example, stocking helpers, raised toilet seats, pickup sticks.

7. **Anti-inflammatory agents:** See Table 8-1, p. 370. **More potent anti-inflammatory agents**, also used in the treatment of RA, include the following:

    □ *Antimalarials (chloroquine phosphate, 250 mg/day; or hydroxychloroquine sulfate, 200 mg/day):* Result in long-term control of symptoms for some patients. Side effects include keratitis and retinitis, necessitating periodic ophthalmic examinations for early assessment of complications.

    □ *Chrysotherapy (use of medicinal gold salts):* Benefits up to 60% of patients with RA through an unknown mechanism of action. Contraindications include severe drug allergies, previous gold toxicity, hepatotoxicity, or hematologic pathology. It is administered by weekly injections of increasing dosage (up to 50 mg/week) until clinical results are noted or toxic reactions are encountered. A significant anti-inflammatory effect often takes several months of therapy. Potential toxic reactions include exfoliative dermatitis, bone marrow depression, stomatitis, and nephritis. Before each injection, the patient should have a urinalysis (for proteinuria and microscopic hematuria) and CBC with differential for hemoglobin, platelet levels, and WBC count. The patient also should be assessed for skin or mucous membrane lesions. Periodic hepatic function tests should be done, and the patient should be advised to avoid direct sunlight.

    □ *Corticosteroids:* Control the symptoms of RA, but they do not substantially alter the progression of the disease. Removal of the steroid frequently results in exacerbation of symptoms, so steroids are usually used only to carry the patient through a severe flareup or to control concurrent connective tissue disease (eg, eye lesions, pericarditis). They are used cautiously at the lowest dose possible to control signs of inflammation. Intra-articular steroids may be used on occasion (no more than 4× year) for especially troublesome joints.

    □ *Penicillamine:* Used *only after* all other methods have been ineffective in controlling symptoms. Fifty percent of patients taking this drug will develop side effects, including thrombocytopenia, leukopenia, aplastic anemia, nephrotic syndrome, and immune complex disease (myasthenia gravis). This medication is taken between meals to aid absorption.

8. **Surgical interventions**

    □ *Synovectomy:* To remove the inflamed synovium and prevent pannus formation. This may be performed either by surgical excision or instillation of a radioactive solution to "burn" the synovium.

    □ *Arthroplasty:* To correct periarticular weakness, which in turn will correct subluxation and external stressors on the diseased joint.

    □ *Osteotomy:* To correct disruptive force vectors placed on the joint surfaces or to correct bony malalignments.

    □ *Carpal tunnel release, tarsal tunnel release, ganglionectomy, tendon repair, and removal of Baker's cyst:* Examples of surgeries performed to correct concurrent connective tissue defects associated with RA.

    □ *Implant arthroplasty:* Significantly increases functional capabilities for selected RA patients. They are used for many joints, but the greatest success has been seen with the hip and knee. The rate of success is dependent on the joint, patient's general condition, stage of disease, and rate of compliance with therapy.

□ *Arthroscopy:* May be used for diagnosis and/or treatment. Bodies may be excised, plica (redundant tissue) incised, and cartilage abraided (or "shaved") through an arthroscope.

9. **Experimental therapies under trial in the United States:** Include additional nonsteroidal anti-inflammatory agents, an anthelmintic agent (Levamisole), cyclophosphamide, azathioprine, chlorambucil, plasmapheresis, leukapheresis, and irradiation of the lymph nodes. Experimental surgeries include various new implant designs and joint transplantation.

D. Nursing Diagnoses and Interventions

See "Osteoarthritis" for the following: **Alteration in comfort**, p. 367, **Knowledge deficit:** Proper use of a heating device, p. 368, and **Impaired physical mobility** related to adjustment to a new walking gait, p. 368. See "Gouty Arthritis" for the following: **Knowledge deficit:** Disease process, medication regimen, and potential drug side effects, p. 370, and **Knowledge deficit:** Proper care of inflamed joints, p. 371. See "Ligamentous Injuries" for the following: **Knowledge deficit:** Need for elevation of the involved extremity, use of thermotherapy, and exercise, p. 376, **Knowledge deficit:** Care and assessment of the casted extremity, p. 377, and **Knowledge deficit:** Potential for joint weakness, and the techniques for applying elastic wraps and assessing neurovascular status, p. 378. See "Torn Anterior Cruciate Ligament" for the following: **Potential fluid volume deficit** related to abnormal loss secondary to postsurgical hemorrhage or hematoma, p. 383. See "Fractures" for the following: **Self-care deficit**, p. 393, and **Knowledge deficit:** Potential for disuse osteoporosis, p. 394. See "Amputation" for the following: **Knowledge deficit:** Postsurgical exercise regimen, p. 406. See "Total Hip Arthroplasty" for the following: **Knowledge deficit:** Potential for infection (foreign body reaction), p. 413. See "Herniated Nucleus Pulposus" in Chapter 4 for the following: **Knowledge deficit:** Pain control measures, p. 168. See "Appendix One" for nursing diagnoses and interventions for the care of preoperative and postoperative patients, pp. 528–532, and the care of patients on prolonged bed rest, pp. 533–537.

E. Patient—Family Teaching and Discharge Planning

Provide patient and SOs with verbal and written information for the following:

1. Treatment regimen, including physical therapy, systemic rest, rest of inflamed joints, exercise, and thermotherapy.

2. Medications, including drug name, dosage, schedule, precautions, and potential side effects.

3. Potential complications of the disease and therapy and the need to recognize and seek medical attention promptly should they occur.

4. Potential concurrent pathology (pericarditis, ocular lesions) and need to report them promptly to health care professional.

5. Use and care of splints and orthotics, including return demonstration.

6. Use of adjunctive aids as appropriate, such as pickup sticks, long-handled shoe horn, crutches, walker, and cane, including return demonstration.

7. As necessary, referral to visiting or public health nurses for ongoing care after discharge.

8. Phone numbers to call should questions or concerns arise about therapy or disease after discharge.

9. Treatment and facilities available for these patients, which can be obtained by writing to Arthritis Foundation, 1314 Spring Street NW, Atlanta, Georgia 30309.

▶ Section Two **Muscular and Connective Tissue Disorders**

Most hospitalized patients with muscular or connective tissue disorders have had some form of injury or have been hospitalized for the care of the sequellae of the disease, for example, the need for tendon transfers or joint fusions. This section relates exclusively to traumatic muscular and connective tissue disorders.

I. Ligamentous Injuries

Ligaments are collections of fascial tissues that connect bone to bone, thereby supplementing joint stength. Ligament tears usually result from direct trauma or transmission of a force to the joint. The degree of trauma incurred will vary with the strength of the involved ligament. For example, strong ligaments will require more force before tearing than will a ligament weakened by previous injury or disease. Tears can be longitudinal, transverse, tangential, complete, or partial, or they can involve avulsion fractures of their origin or insertion.

A. Assessment

Signs and symptoms: Localized ecchymosis, edema, tenderness, weakness, pain, joint effusion, limited ROM, or joint instability. A diagnosis is based primarily on consideration of the patient's complaints, the mechanism of the injury, and the physical assessment.

B. Diagnostic Tests

1. <u>X-ray studies:</u> Stressing the weakened joint during x-ray exam may reveal an enlarged joint space.
2. <u>Arthrogram (instillation of a radiopaque dye or radiolucent gas into the joint):</u> May identify torn or weakened ligaments.
3. <u>Arthroscopy:</u> To rule out concurrent intra-articular pathology or trauma.

C. Medical Management and Surgical Interventions

1. **Treatment for uncomplicated ligamentous injuries:** Rest of the joint, elevation, immobilization, local applications of cold followed by heat, and control of pain. Immobilization is usually accomplished with an elastic wrap, splint, or cast.
2. **Surgical repair:** For injuries resulting in grossly unstable joints. The surgery involves removal of the nonviable ligament and suture repair or reefing of the stretched ligament, using strong, absorbable suture material. An avulsion injury without fracture may be reinserted onto its bony insertion site by using bone staples or passing a suture through holes drilled into the bony insertion site.
3. **ROM and muscle-strengthening exercises:** Begun after an appropriate period of immobilization of the injured area (a minimum of 3 weeks).

D. Nursing Diagnoses and Interventions

Knowledge deficit: Need for elevation of the involved extremity, use of thermotherapy, and exercise regimen

Desired outcome: Patient can verbalize understanding of the rationale for treatment, including the exercise regimen and the use of elevation, medications for pain, and thermotherapy.

1. Teach patient the pathophysiology of the injury and the concomitant inflammatory response.
2. Instruct patient to keep the injured extremity elevated until edema is no longer a problem (usually 3–7 days). Explain that the involved extremity

should be kept above the level of the heart, with each successively distal joint elevated above the level of the preceding joint.

3. Explain that thermotherapy involves the application of ice and warmth. Ice is usually applied for the first 48 hours to prevent excessive edema. Warmth is then applied until the patient is comfortable without it (usually 3–5 days after the injury). Both are contraindicated for patients with peripheral vascular disease, decreased local sensation, coagulation disorders, or similar pathology that increases the potential for thermal injury. Advise the patient to apply thermotherapy with at least 2 thicknesses of terry cloth to protect the skin from injury. Explain that habituation to heat can cause the patient to apply increasingly warmer applications and that doing so is a potential source of injury.

4. Explain each prescribed exercise in detail, including the rationale. The optimal method is to teach it to the patient, demonstrate it, and then have the patient return the demonstration. Provide written instructions that review the exercise and list the frequency and number of repetitions for each. Include a phone number, should the patient have questions after hospital discharge.

Knowledge deficit: Care and assessment of the casted extremity

Desired outcomes: Patient can verbalize understanding of the care of the casted extremity and demonstrate knowledge of self-assessment of neurovascular status, use of ambulatory aids, exercise, and general cast care.

1. Explain the function the patient's cast is performing.

2. Instruct patient in the rationale and procedure for neurovascular checks of the casted extremity. Explain that they should be performed q2–4h for the first 2 days, and then qid until the cast is removed. Advise patient to be alert to and promptly report paleness, cyanosis, coolness, decreased pulse and/or capillary refill, increasing pain, decreasing sensation, and/or paralysis of the distal portion of the casted limb.

3. Ensure that the patient demonstrates independence in ADLs and ambulation before discharge. If ambulatory aids (crutches, walker, cane) are used, make sure their independent use is demonstrated on all surfaces the patient is likely to encounter and that the precautions are understood and verbalized by the patient.

4. Instruct patient to exercise the parts of the extremity that are not immobilized by the cast, for example, by wiggling the toes or fingers and putting the most proximal joints through complete ROM unless doing so is contraindicated by the MD. Isometric exercises for muscles beneath the cast will be prescribed for some patients. When prescribed, provide patient with the rationale and instructions for these exercises, including written instructions that review the information and explain the frequency and number of repetitions.

5. Provide patient with a phone number of the appropriate person to call if problems or questions arise after discharge.

6. Instruct patient in the basic components of cast care:

With plaster of Paris cast:

□ Use plastic bags while showering or in the rain to avoid getting cast wet. Damp cloths can be used on soiled cast surfaces but saturation must be avoided.

□ Use white shoe polish *sparingly* to cover stains.

□ Petal the cast edges with tape if edges are rough or cast crumbs are falling into the cast. If the edges continue to irritate the skin, they can be padded with moleskin, sheepskin, or foam rubber. However, continued irritation should be brought to the attention of the MD.

☐ Avoid putting anything inside the cast, because skin under the cast is more susceptible to injury.

☐ Report any changes in sensation, drainage on the cast, or foul odor because they can indicate the presence of pressure necrosis.

With synthetic cast material:

☐ Immersion in water may be permitted by MD, depending on the materials used, the type of injury, and whether or not surgery was performed. If immersion is permitted, it is necessary to dry the cast thoroughly (using a hair dryer on a cool setting) to prevent skin maceration.

☐ If permitted, dirt or sand can be rinsed from the cast.

☐ Avoid over-exercising the casted extremity; perform the exercises within the prescribed range.

☐ Avoid putting anything inside the cast, because skin under the cast is more susceptible to injury.

☐ Report any changes in sensation, drainage on the cast, or foul odor because they can indicate the presence of pressure necrosis.

Knowledge deficit: Potential for joint weakness, and the techniques for applying elastic wraps and assessing neurovascular status

Desired outcomes: Patient can verbalize understanding of the potential for joint weakness and can demonstrate knowledge of applying elastic wraps and self-checking neurovascular status.

1. Advise patient about the potential for joint weakness and the need for limiting or omitting activities that aggravate the condition.

2. If the MD has prescribed elastic wraps, elastic supports, or orthotic devices to supplement joint strength until exercise has compensated for the joint laxity, explain and demonstrate their use and application. Show the patient how to apply elastic wraps diagonally from the distal to proximal areas with an overlap of two-thirds to one-half of the width of the wrap for each successive layer.

3. Teach patient how to self-check neurovascular status 15 minutes after application and to rewrap the joint if a deficit is found.

4. Ensure that the patient receives two wraps, supports, or orthotic devices to allow for cleaning. Typically, these devices are washed with mild soap and water and allowed to to air dry without stretching (or see manufacturer's recommendations).

If surgery was performed, see "Torn Anterior Cruciate Ligament " for the following: **Potential fluid volume deficit** related to abnormal loss secondary to postsurgical hemorrhage or hematoma, p. 383. See "Appendix One" for nursing diagnoses and interventions for the care of preoperative and postoperative patients, pp. 528–532.

E. Patient–Family Teaching and Discharge Planning

Provide patient and SOs with verbal and written information for the following:

1. Prescribed therapies, such as elevation, thermotherapy, cast care, exercise, and elastic wraps.

2. Potential complications, including subluxation/dislocation, wound infection, and neurovascular deficit, all of which necessitate immediate medical attention.

3. **ADLs and ambulation:** Ensure that patient demonstrates independence before hospital discharge.

4. **Medications,** including drug name, rationale, dosage, schedule, precautions, and side effects.

II. Dislocation/Subluxation

A dislocation occurs when the joint surfaces are completely out of contact. A subluxation is an incomplete dislocation in that some of the joint surfaces remain in contact. Most dislocations and subluxations are the result of trauma and can involve significant periarticular damage, including fractures. Some subluxations are associated with pronounced connective tissue disease such as ulnar deviation of the phalanges and metacarpals, which is seen with severe rheumatoid·arthritis.

A. Assessment

Signs and symptoms: Vary with the joint involved. Although any joint can dislocate, some joints are more prone than others. One finding common to most forms of dislocation is limb shortening. Usually there is significant pain, ecchymosis, loss of normal bony contour, edema, and loss or limitation of joint ROM. Complications include recurrent dislocation, joint contracture, neurovascular injury, or eventual traumatic arthritis.

B. Diagnostic Tests

1. <u>X-rays:</u> Both anterior/posterior and lateral views are commonly used. Occasionally, an oblique view or other special approach (such as mortise or femoral notch views) is required. Because muscle spasms frequently force the dislocated bones back into normal alignment, it is sometimes necessary to stress the joint to permit visualization of the injury (called a "stress film").

2. <u>Arthrogram:</u> Use of radiopaque dye or radiolucent gas to outline the joint cavity to visualize injured ligaments, capsule, or intra-articular structures such as the menisci.

C. Medical Management and Surgical Interventions

Interventions vary with the degree of subluxation or dislocation and the joint involved. Many patients are discharged from the hospital with instructions for the use of thermotherapy, elevation, and pain medication.

1. **Dislocation of the sternoclavicular joint:** Usually reduced manually with local anesthesia. After reduction, the joint is immobilized with a clavicular strap (figure-8 bandage) for 2–6 weeks. Occasionally, an open reduction with internal fixation (ORIF) using screws, pins, or wire is necessary to maintain reduction.

2. **Uncomplicated subluxation or dislocation of the acromioclavicular (AC) joint:** May be immobilized with a clavicular strap or might require ORIF. After satisfactory joint stability has been achieved, the patient is started on a regimen of progressively more rigorous exercise to regain muscle strength and ROM.

3. **Dislocation of the shoulder:** Reduced with anesthesia or significant sedation and then immoblized in a Velpeau bandage, sling and swathe binder, or spica cast of the shoulder, all of which support the arm while immobilizing the shoulder. Immobilization is usually continued for 3–6 weeks, followed by progressive exercises to regain muscle strength and ROM. Surgical procedures usually include reefing (taking up redundant ligament with sutures) of the articular capsule and transferring or shortening the subcapsular muscle to tighten the periarticular tissues (also see p. 410).

4. **Dislocation of the elbow:** Frequently associated with fractures of the humerus, ulna, and/or radius. The elbow and fractures are carefully reduced, usually with general anesthesia, and the area is immobilized in a posterior

splint for 3–8 weeks. ORIF may be required. Because of the area of the injury, these patients are at risk for Volkmann's ischemic contracture (ischemic myositis), and therefore the extremity must be monitored carefully for evidence of neurovascular deficit. (See "Ischemic Myositis," p. 385.) Progressive exercises are used to regain muscle strength and ROM.

5. **Dislocation of the radioulnar or radiocarpal joints:** Usually reduced with regional anesthesia and then immobilized in a posterior splint or long arm cast for 2–4 weeks. However, an ORIF may be performed. Progressive exercise is used to regain muscle strength and ROM.

6. **Dislocations of the finger:** Usually reduced with regional or digital block anesthesia. The finger may be splinted with a metal splint or taped to an adjacent finger, followed by progressive mobilization. Surgery might be performed to reef the stretched periarticular tissues, followed by transfixion of the joint during the healing period, usually 10–14 days.

7. **Dislocation of the hip:** Usually requires general anesthesia with significant muscle relaxation for reduction. Immobilization is typically accomplished via balanced suspension traction for 3–6 weeks, followed by progressive ambulation, mobilization of the joint, and muscle-strengthening exercises. Open reduction with surgical repair of the torn capsule and ligaments might be required for severe or recurrent dislocations. A fractured acetabulum may require replacement via total hip arthroplasty.

8. **Dislocation of the patella:** Often self-limiting, in that the patella usually reduces itself. Immobilization may be accomplished with a knee immobilizer, posterior splint, cylinder cast, or long leg cast for 10–21 days, followed by progressive mobilization and quadriceps setting exercises. Surgery may be required to reef the periarticular tissues or reinsert the insertion of the patellar tendon to overcorrect distorted joint vectors that cause recurrent dislocation.

9. **Dislocation of the ankle:** Usually reduced under regional or general anesthesia and the joint is immobilized in a long leg plaster cast for 6–12 weeks. Surgery may be necessary to reef stretched periarticular tissues. Progressive mobilization and exercises are used to regain motion and strength.

10. **Dislocation of the toe:** Usually reduced with regional anesthesia. Often, the toe is immobilized for 3–5 days using an adjacent toe as a splint (taping the toes together).

D. Nursing Diagnoses and Interventions

See "Osteoarthritis" for the following: **Alteration in comfort**, p. 367, and **Impaired physical mobility** related to adjustment to a new walking gait, p. 368. See "Ligamentous Injuries" for the following: **Knowledge deficit:** Need for elevation of the involved extremity, use of thermotherapy, and exercise, p. 376, and **Knowledge deficit:** Care and assessment of the casted extremity, p. 377. If surgery was performed, see "Torn Anterior Cruciate Ligament" for the following: **Potential fluid volume deficit** related to abnormal loss secondary to postsurgical hemorrhage or hematoma, p. 383. See "Bunionectomy" for the following: **Potential alteration in tissue perfusion:** Peripheral, related to impaired circulation secondary to compression from circumferential casts or dressings, p. 404. See "Appendix One" for nursing diagnoses and interventions for the care of preoperative and postoperative patients, pp. 528–532, and for the care of patients on prolonged bed rest, pp. 533–537.

E. Patient–Family Teaching and Discharge Planning

Provide patient and SOs with verbal and written information for the following:

1. Therapy that will be used at home, including thermotherapy, elevation, use of immobilization devices, exercises, cast care (p. 377), and medications.

2. Potential complications that should be observed for at home, such as recurrent dislocations, neurovascular deficit, or wound infection.

3. Precautions that should be taken at home, including activity limitations (as directed by MD), monitoring for changes in neurovascular status qid, assessing wounds for indicators of infection, and following the guidelines described for cast, splint, or orthotic care.

4. Medications, including the drug name, rationale, dosage, schedule, precautions, and potential side effects.

III. Meniscal Injuries

Meniscal injuries involve the intra-articular fibrocartilages on the medial or lateral side of the knee's tibial plateau. These halfmoon-shaped cartilages facilitate joint motion while also absorbing some of the stress placed on the joint. There are a variety of cartilage injuries that can occur, and all involve a tear to varying degrees. Most commonly, a meniscal injury is the result of trauma to the knee or, less frequently, degeneration of the joint secondary to arthritis. Medial meniscus injuries are the most common and usually follow a knee movement involving internal rotation. Injuries to the lateral meniscus are more commonly associated with external rotation that occurs while the knee is partially flexed.

A. Assessment

Chronic indicators: Same as those seen with arthritis because arthritis will follow untreated or severe meniscal injuries. There may be weakness and atrophy of the quadriceps muscle group from disuse caused by joint pain.

Acute indicators: Occur after knee trauma that causes joint effusion and limited ROM. If the tear is large enough, it may result in locking, which is the inability to fully extend the joint. Joint pain or pain along the joint margins will occur. It may be possible to delineate point tenderness along the joint margin in the area of the tear.

B. Diagnostic Tests

1. McMurray's test for a torn medial meniscus: With the patient's leg fully flexed, the foot externally rotated, and the leg abducted, the examiner's index finger and thumb are positioned along the joint margins of the knee. The knee is then gradually extended. Clicks or pops accompanied by patient complaints of pain as the leg is extended are indicative of a medial meniscal tear. A lateral meniscus tear is tested for by placing the thumb and index finger along the joint margin of the knee with the patient's leg flexed and adducted and the foot internally rotated. Clicks or pops with patient complaints of pain as the leg is extended are indicative of lateral meniscus injury.

2. Apply grinding test: Performed with the patient prone and the knee flexed at 90°. With one hand, the examiner forces the foot and lower leg down on the femur while rotating the foot internally and externally. The examiner's other hand is positioned to palpate the joint margins as described in McMurray's test. Grinding or crepitus is usually indicative of a meniscal injury.

3. Arthrogram: Involves injection of radiopaque dye and radiolucent gas (usually air) into the joint to outline the area of injury and provide diagnosis of a meniscal tear as evidenced by absence of normal contour.

4. Arthroscopy: To diagnose and treat meniscal injuries. Under sterile conditions, the arthroscope is introduced into the joint to allow direct visualization of the meniscus. The patient is given local, regional, or general anesthesia for this procedure.

C. Surgical Interventions

Because the fibrocartilages tend to heal poorly, the usual treatment involves a menisectomy via arthroscope.

Arthroscopic surgery: Preferred for partial meniscectomy (over the outdated knee arthrotomy) because it is the least traumatic, allows retention of some of the anatomical meniscus for normal joint function, and allows a more rapid return to normal level of health. The patient is usually discharged same evening as surgery and placed on weightbearing as tolerated for 5–21 days using some form of external support for the knee, either an elastic wrap or knee immobilizer. Knee exercises (quadriceps setting and leg lifts) are prescribed for regaining muscle strength.

D. Nursing Diagnoses and Interventions

See "Osteoarthritis" for the following: **Alteration in comfort**, p. 367, and **Impaired physical mobility** related to adjustment to a new walking gait, p. 368. See "Ligamentous Injuries" for the following: **Knowledge deficit:** Need for elevation of the involved extremity, use of thermotherapy, and exercise regimen, p. 376. See "Torn Anterior Cruciate Ligament" for the following: **Potential fluid volume deficit** related to abnormal loss secondary to postsurgical hemorrhage or hematoma, p. 383. See "Bunionectomy" for the following: **Potential alteration in tissue perfusion:** Peripheral, related to impaired circulation secondary to compression from circumferential cast or dressing, p. 404.

E. Patient–Family Teaching and Discharge Planning

Provide patient and SOs with verbal and written information for the following:

1. Use of elevation and thermotherapy as prescribed.

2. Use of external support devices (elastic wraps or knee immobilizer), including care of the device, care of the skin beneath the device, and monitoring for areas of irritation and neurovascular deficit.

3. Cast care (see p. 377).

4. Prescribed exercise regimen, including rationale, demonstration, number of repetitions, and frequency.

5. Prescribed medications, including drug name, rationale, dosage, schedule, precautions, and potential side effects.

6. Indicators of wound infection, which necessitate medical attention: erythema, edema, joint effusion, purulent discharge, local warmth, pain, and fever.

7. Ambulation and use of assistive device.

IV. Torn Anterior Cruciate Ligament

A torn anterior cruciate ligament (ACL) is a common knee injury. The ACL prevents excessive forward motion and internal rotation of the tibia. Injury to this ligament can result in strain with microtears, partial tears, complete tears, or avulsion of the tibial or femoral attachments. Stresses that can result in tears include forceful contraction of the quadriceps muscles combined with restricted extension, "clipping" injuries incurred in football, forced pivoting on the knee, or excessive forward motion of the tibia, which can occur when stopping quickly while running.

A. Assessment

Chronic indicators: Untreated tears of the ACL result in gross instability, which eventually can cause osteoarthritis (see osteoarthritis assessment, p. 366).

Acute indicators: Sensation of the knee "giving way," joint effusion, restricted ROM, and joint instability and pain.

B. Diagnostic Tests

1. <u>Lachman test:</u> Positive if the ACL is torn. The patient's knee is partially flexed at 10–15° and the foot is planted flat on the examining table. The examiner then pulls the tibia forward while holding the femur stable. Excessive

forward movement of the tibia is evidenced by a convex curve of the patellar tendon, which is indicative of an ACL tear.

2. Drawer test: Performed with the knee flexed at 60° and the foot planted flat on the table. The tibia is pulled forward as the femur is stabilized. Excessive forward movement indicates a tear. The test is then repeated with the foot externally rotated 15° to assess concurrent injury of medial joint structures (meniscus or periarticular ligaments). Finally, the test is repeated with the foot internally rotated 30° to assess concurrent lateral joint injury.

3. Arthrography: Outlines tears via injection of radiopaque dye and radiolucent gas.

4. Radiography of the knee (including anterior/posterior, lateral, tunnel, and skyline views, with and without stress on the joint): Evaluates for the presence of abnormal joint contours.

5. Arthroscopy: Allows direct visualization of the ACL injury to determine degree of injury and assess need for surgery.

C. Medical Management and Surgical Interventions

The type of therapy is determined by the type of injury, length of time since the original injury, concurrent joint pathology, and the patient's age and functional goals.

1. **Bracing:** To provide primary support for an incompletely torn ACL or to supplement adjunctive joint support structures (posterior oblique ligament, collateral ligaments, lateral capsular ligament, and the menisci). Any of several commercial braces can be used to provide anteriorposterior, lateral, and rotational stability of the joint. They also may be used during joint rehabilitation following surgical intervention. Concurrent physiotherapy is provided to strengthen periarticular structures and muscles.

2. **Primary ACL repair:** Involves direct suturing of the torn ligament via an arthrotomy. The suture is heavy and nonabsorbable and is used in repairing tears that are less than six weeks old.

3. **ACL reconstruction:** Involves the use of either anatomic grafts or prosthetics. Regardless of the surgical procedure used, an arthrotomy requires prolonged knee immobilization (6–12 weeks in flexion in a long leg cast and/or a splint), followed by extensive physiotherapy and bracing. Physiotherapy is continued until the knee is functionally normal. In addition, many patients return from surgery with a closed wound drainage system consisting of a wound drain, tubing, and a reservoir. Most MDs bring the drainage tubing out through the area using a separate stab wound.

D. Nursing Diagnoses and Interventions

Potential fluid volume deficit related to abnormal loss secondary to postsurgical hemorrhage or hematoma formation

Desired outcomes: Patient does not exhibit signs of hypovolemia or excessive bleeding. If hematoma occurs, it is detected and reported promptly.

▶ **Note:** A hematoma is a collection of extravasated blood within the tissues following surgery (or trauma). During most orthopedic surgeries, a tourniquet is used to restrict blood flow from the operative field. Sometimes the tourniquet is left inflated until after the dressing or cast has been applied, and therefore major bleeding might not be noted during surgery. Even when the tourniquet is deflated, it is possible that a significant bleeding vessel may be overlooked or that bleeding will begin later during the patient's recovery.

1. Monitor drainage from the drainage system as well as that on the dressings or cast. Report output from the drainage system that exceeds 50 mL/h.

2. Because outlining the amount of drainage on the cast does not always provide an accurate assessment of drainage beneath the cast, carefully evaluate the patient's VS, subjective complaints, and neurovascular status.

3. Be alert to and report patient complaints of sensations of warmth beneath the cast or dressing, things "crawling" under the cast, aching, increasing pressure or pain, or coolness distal to the area of surgery, which can occur with hemorrhage or hematoma formation.

4. Monitor for and report VS indicative of shock or hemorrhage, including hypotension and increasing pulse rate.

5. Monitor for pallor, decreased posterior tibial or dorsalis pedis pulses, slowed capillary refill, or coolness of the distal extremity, which can occur with hemorrhage or hematoma formation.

6. If hemorrhage or hematoma formation is suspected, notify MD promptly. If the limb is casted, elevate it above the level of the patient's heart to slow the bleeding. If the limb is not casted, apply an elastic wrap for direct pressure on the site of bleeding.

7. If hemorrhage or hematoma formation is suspected and the patient's VS are indicative of shock but an MD is unavailable, the surgical area should be exposed by windowing the cast or loosening the dressing to allow direct inspection of the area. Direct pressure usually will control hemorrhage; if not, apply a thigh blood pressure cuff over sheet wadding to serve as a tourniquet until the MD arrives for definitive therapy.

See "Osteoarthritis" for the following: **Alteration in comfort**, p. 367, and **Impaired physical mobility** related to adjustment to a new walking gait, p. 368. See "Ligamentous Injuries" for the following: **Knowledge deficit:** Need for elevation of the involved extremity, use of thermotherapy, and exercise regimen, p. 376. See "Bunionectomy" for the following: **Potential alteration in tissue perfusion:** Peripheral, related to impaired circulation secondary to compression from circumferential casts or dressings, p. 404. See "Appendix One" for nursing diagnoses and interventions for the care of preoperative and postoperative patients, pp. 528–532.

E. Patient–Family Teaching and Discharge Planning

Provide patient and SOs with verbal and written information for the following:

1. Telephone number of appropriate person for patient's questions after hospital discharge.

2. Use of external support devices (elastic wraps or knee immobilizer), including care of the device, care of the skin beneath the device, and monitoring for areas of irritation and neurovascular deficit.

3. Cast care, as described in the nursing diagnosis **Knowledge deficit:** Care and assessment of the casted extremity, in "Ligamentous Injuries," p. 377.

4. Prescribed exercise regimen, including the rationale, how it is performed, the number of repetitions, and the frequency.

5. Prescribed medications, including drug name, rationale, dosage, schedule, precautions, and potential side effects.

6. Indicators of wound infection, which necessitate medical attention: erythema, edema, joint effusion, purulent discharge, local warmth, pain, and fever.

7. Ambulation with assistive device, including patient's demonstration of independence on level and uneven ground and stairs.

V. Ischemic Myositis (Compartment Syndrome)

Ischemic myositis is a progressive degeneration of muscle that occurs because of a severe interruption in blood flow to an area. Volkmann's ischemic contracture of the forearm and anterior tibial compartment syndrome (ATCS) are associated with this process. Edema within an anatomic compartment (either of the forearm or the anterior tibial compartment) can eventually occlude arterial blood supply and cause ischemic myositis. Similarly, impaired venous return from a compartment can lead to edema, which can impinge on arterial blood supply.

An iatrogenic compartment syndrome can result from any circumferential cast or dressing that adversely affects the circulation of tissues encompassed within. This syndrome is most commonly seen in trauma or surgery involving the elbow, wrist, knee, or ankle. Because muscle tissue requires large amounts of blood to meet the muscle's demands, necrosis will occur within 6–8 hours if the blood supply is inadequate. If not corrected quickly, ischemic myositis can result in a severely contracted, functionally useless, and disfiguring limb distal to the area of injury.

A. Assessment

Signs and symptoms: The five P's: pain, paresthesia, paralysis, pallor, and pulselessness. The pain is especially diagnostic because it increases in severity, exceeds that expected for the incurred trauma, and might not be controlled by narcotics. Passive movement of the involved distal extremity will result in severe pain. Paresthesias may include sensations of numbness, decreased sensation, or burning. Paralysis can involve pseudoparalysis because of the patient's avoidance of movements that stress the involved compartment, or frank paralysis of muscle that is ennervated by injured nerves in the involved compartment. Pallor and pulselessness are associated with lost circulation through the compartment; slowed capillary refill and impaired venous return can be prodromal signs.

B. Diagnostic Tests

1. <u>Compartment pressure:</u> Can be measured via a large-bore catheter that is introduced into the compartment and attached to a saline-primed manometer. Tissue pressures that exceed 30–40 mm Hg are indicative of compartment syndrome. Continuous monitoring devices may be used to monitor the pressure within the compartments of high-risk patients to warn of impending ischemic myositis.

2. <u>Arteriogram:</u> To rule out vasospasm or arterial trauma, which can result in ischemic myositis, especially in patients with supracondylar fractures of the humerus.

C. Medical Management and Surgical Interventions

1. **Conservative measures:** Used initially when ischemic myositis is suspected. The constriction limiting the swelling (eg, cast, splint, or circumferential dressing) is loosened down to skin level. However, if a fracture is involved, adequate immobilization should not be compromised. The limb is elevated to enhance venous return, and ice is applied to cause vasoconstriction in the area of the injury and inhibit further edema formation. Often, larger-than-normal levels of narcotics with potentiation, such as aspirin, acetaminophen, promethazine, or hydroxyzine, are required.

2. **Fasciotomy:** Necessary if conservative measures fail to control the progressive symptoms. This involves the complete removal of the anatomic restrictions in the involved compartment. After several days the fasciotomy is closed primarily or the area is grafted with skin.

3. **Surgical repair of a lacerated artery:** Performed if the cause is arterial injury. If vasospasm is the suspected cause, some surgeons will expose the involved artery and apply topical papaverine to control the problem; if un-

successful, resection of the involved artery with reanastomosis is frequently necessary.

D. Nursing Diagnoses and Interventions

See "Osteoarthritis" for the following: **Alteration in comfort**, p. 367. See "Ligamentous Injuries" for the following: **Knowledge deficit:** Need for elevation of the involved extremity, use of thermotherapy, and exercise, p. 376. See "Bunionectomy" for the following: **Potential alteration in tissue perfusion:** Peripheral, related to impaired circulation secondary to compression from circumferential casts or dressings, p. 404. If surgery was performed, see "Appendix One" for nursing diagnoses and interventions for the care of preoperative and postoperative patients, pp. 528–532.

E. Patient–Family Teaching and Discharge Planning

Provide patient and SOs with verbal and written information for the following:

1. Phone number of appropriate person to call for questions after hospital discharge.

2. Instructions regarding the process of ischemic myositis and the use of elevation, ice, and loosening of restrictive dressings.

3. Discharge instructions for patients with fractures (see "Fractures," p. 396).

4. Importance of seeking medical attention if signs and symptoms of wound infection occur.

► Section Three   **Skeletal Disorders**

I. Osteomyelitis

Osteomyelitis is an acute or chronic infection involving a bone. *Primary osteomyelitis* is a direct implantation of micro-organisms into bone via compound fractures or penetrating wounds, or from surgery. *Secondary or acute hematogenic osteomyelitis* is an infection of bone that occurs through its own blood supply or from infection from contiguous soft tissues or joints involved with septic arthritis. Although osteomyelitis often remains localized, it can spread through the marrow, cortex, and periosteum. Conditions favoring the development of osteomyelitis include recent bone trauma or bone with low oxygen tension such as found in sickle cell anemia. Acute hematogenic osteomyelitis is most frequently caused by *Staphylococcus aureus* (90–95%), but it also can result from *Escherichia coli*, *Pseudomonas* species, *Klebsiella*, *Enterobacter*, *Proteus*, *Streptococcus* (group A), and *Hemophilus influenzae*. Chronic osteomyelitis is comparatively rare and is characterized by persistent, multiple draining sinus tracts.

A. Assessment

Acute osteomyelitis: Abrupt onset of pain in the involved area, fever, malaise, and limited motion. Pseudoparalysis is especially indicative of osteomyelitis in children who refuse to move an adjacent joint because of pain.

Chronic osteomyelitis: Bone infection that persists intermittently for years, usually flaring up after minor trauma to the area or lowered systemic resistance. Edema and erythema over the involved bone, weakness, irritability, and generalized signs of sepsis can occur. Sometimes the only symptom is persistent purulent drainage from an old pocket or sinus tract.

History of: Total joint replacement, compound fracture, use of external fixator, vascular insufficiency (eg, with diabetes mellitus), recurrent UTIs.

B. Diagnostic Tests

1. <u>CBC:</u> Will reveal leukocytosis and anemia in the presence of osteomyelitis.

2. <u>ESR:</u> Elevated in the presence of osteomyelitis.

3. <u>Blood or sequestrum cultures:</u> To identify the causative organism. Sequestrum is a piece of necrotic bone that is separated from surrounding bone as a result of osteomyelitis.

4. <u>X-rays:</u> May reveal subtle areas of radiolucency (osteonecrosis) and new bone formation. No x-ray changes will be evident until the disease has been active at least 5 days in infants, 8–10 days in children, and 2–3 weeks in adults.

5. <u>Radioisotope scanning:</u> May reveal areas of increased vascularity (called "hot spots"), which are indicative of osteomyelitis.

C. Medical Management and Surgical Interventions

1. **IV anti-microbial therapy:** Continued for at least 6 weeks.

2. **Bed rest.**

3. **Immobilization of affected extremity:** With splint, cast, or traction to relieve pain and decrease the potential for pathologic fracture.

4. **Blood transfusions:** To correct any accompanying anemia.

5. **Removal of internal fixation device or endoprosthesis, if present:** To help control the infection.

6. **Surgical decompression of infected bone:** May be followed by primary closure, myocutaneous flaps to cover the denuded bone, or leaving the area open to drain and heal by secondary intention or with secondary closure.

7. **Drains:** May be inserted into the affected bone to drain the site or act as ingress-egress tubes to funnel topical antibiotics directly into the area of infection.

8. **Topical antibiotics:** May be used via continuous or intermittent infusion and are continued until three successive drain cultures have been negative.

9. **Long-term IV antibiotic therapy:** May be continued for 3–6 months.

10. **Hyperbaric oxygen:** May be used in selected patients with accessible areas of involvement to improve local oxygen supply.

11. **Amputation:** Although rarely performed, it may be required for extremities in which persistent infection severely limits function.

D. Nursing Diagnoses and Interventions

Potential for infection (for others) related to risk of cross-contamination; (for patient) related to susceptibility secondary to disease chronicity

Desired outcomes: Patient, other patients, and staff do not exhibit signs of infection. Patient can verbalize knowledge of the potential chronicity of the disease and the importance of strict adherence to the prescribed antibiotic therapy.

1. When appropriate for the infecting organism, isolate the patient from other patients, especially those with orthopedic disorders.

2. Ensure that the patient's drainage system is properly handled and that careful handwashing is observed between patients to prevent cross-contamination.

3. Teach patient about the disease and potential for chronic infection. Stress the importance of adherence to the prescribed antibiotic therapy.

4. As a general rule, use meticulous sterile technique when performing irrigations, dressing changes, or handling contaminated dressings. Wash hands well between patients.

Knowledge deficit: Adverse side effects from prolonged use of potent antibiotics

Desired outcome: Patient can verbalize knowledge of potential side effects of antibiotic therapy and precautions that must be taken.

Aminoglycoside antibacterials: Gentamicin sulfate, kanamycin sulfate, neomycin, streptomycin, and tobramycin are used to combat gram-negative organisms. Potential toxic reactions include ototoxicity (exhibited by dizziness, vertigo, tinnitus, and decreased auditory acuity); nephrotoxicity (evidenced by rising BUN and serum creatinine levels from progressive renal tubular necrosis, which can progress to renal failure if untreated); and superimposed infections, which occur because of loss of normal body flora protection against bacterial overgrowth.

1. Teach patient about the potential complications and the need to report symptoms as early as possible.

2. Advise patient that with long-term therapy, a baseline audiogram with weekly audiograms should be performed to identify potential hearing deficit; serum creatinine and BUN should be drawn weekly while patient is on aminoglycosides; and weights should be checked daily to help assess for fluid retention. Monitor I&O during patient's hospitalization to help assess renal function.

3. Advise patient to observe for superimposed infections, especially fungal infections, by assessing for fever, black or furry tongue, nausea, diarrhea, oral monilial growth, or vaginal monilial growth. If a Hickman catheter or similar device is used for antibiotic administration, the infusion site should be closely monitored for the presence of irritation that does not respond to usual treatments with topical antibiotics. During hospitalization, consult with MD about culturing suspicious areas of inflammation.

Penicillins: Ampicillin, carbenicillin, cyclacillin, methacillin, and oxacillin are used to combat organisms that demonstrate sensitivity to them. Potential toxic reactions include anemia, hypersensitivity reactions, and overgrowth of nonsusceptible organisms.

1. Teach patient about the potential complications and the need to report symptoms promptly.

2. Use penicillin cautiously in patients with allergies or allergic pathologies such as asthma, hayfever, or dermatitis. Erythematous, maculopapular rash; urticaria; and anaphylaxis can occur. Caution patient about these potential reactions.

3. Instruct patient to seek medical attention if rash, fever, chills, or signs of infection/inflammation develop.

Cephalosporins: Cefazolin, cephalothin, cephapirin, cephradine, cefoxitin, and cefamandole are used in the treatment of susceptible organisms. Potential toxic reactions include overgrowth of nonsusceptible organisms, photosensitivity, increased BUN, and hepatotoxicity.

1. Advise patient about the potential complications, which necessitate prompt medical attention.

2. Explain that patients with suspected renal or hepatic disease should have baseline and serial (weekly) serum liver enzymes (LDH, SGOT, SGPT), BUN, and serum creatinine evaluations. I&O should be monitored along with daily weight to determine hydration status. Scleral and skin icterus, as well as darkening of the urine (from increased urobilinogen), should be noted.

3. Advise patient to avoid direct sunlight or ultraviolet light sources. Suggest the use of sunscreening agents to help prevent photosensitivity reactions.

4. When oral medications are used, instruct patient to avoid intake with dairy or iron products because they can inhibit absorption from the gut.

Sulfonamides: Sulfadiazine, sulfamethoxazole, sulfapridine, and sulfisoxazole can cause toxic reactions, including disruption of intestinal flora, which results in decreased production of metabolically active vitamin K and hemorrhagic tendencies; agranulocytosis; nephrotoxicity; and crystaluria.

1. Teach patient about the potential complications and the importance of seeking prompt medical attention if they occur.

2. Advise patients on long-term therapy to have baseline BUN and serum creatinine level determinations along with weekly levels to rule out nephrotoxicity. Baseline and serial (weekly) granulocyte determinations also should be performed. Agranulocytosis can manifest as lesions of the throat, mucous membranes, GI tract, and skin. Daily weight and I&O evaluation should be watched to help assess hydration status.

3. Teach patient how to monitor for bleeding, especially epistaxis, bleeding gums, hemoptysis, hematemesis, melena, hematuria, prolonged bleeding from wounds, and ecchymosis. During patient's hospitalization, guaiac suspicious secretions, or send them to the lab if prescribed, to determine if blood is present.

4. Advise patient to consume at least 2–3 L/day of fluids (unless contraindicated by cardiac or renal disease) to prevent crystaluria. Teach the indicators of urinary calculi and the importance of getting medical attention should they occur: hematuria, pyuria, retention, frequency, urgency, and pain in the flank, lower back, perineum, thighs, groin, labia, or scrotum.

Knowledge deficit: Potential for infection and air embolus related to use of Hickman catheter or similar device for long-term intermittent antibiotic therapy

Desired outcomes: Patient can demonstrate care of the catheter and verbalize knowledge of the indicators of infection and/or air embolus.

1. Teach patient how to care for the catheter and monitor the entry site for indicators of infection/inflammation if therapy is to be continued at home. Use sterile technique for dressing changes, following hospital protocol for the procedure, which usually includes defatting the skin with acetone/alcohol, applying povidone-iodine, and covering the site with an air-occlusive dressing. Have patient or SO return the demonstration before hospital discharge. If appropriate, arrange a visit by a home health care nurse.

2. Caution patient about the importance of keeping the tubing clamped unless he or she is aspirating or injecting solutions into the catheter. Teach patient and SOs to be alert to indicators of air embolism: labored breathing, cyanosis, cough, chest pain, and syncope. Explain that if air embolism is suspected, the patient should be rolled immediately to the left side and placed in Trendelenburg's position while reclamping the catheter.

3. Teach patient the importance of preventing inadvertent puncture or breakage of the tubing and checking for kinks or cracks daily. Explain the necessity of taping all tubing junctures to prevent accidental separation and positioning the clamp over tape tabs to minimize stress on the tubing.

See "Osteoarthritis" for the following: **Alteration in comfort**, p. 367. See "Appendix One" for nursing diagnoses and interventions for care of preoperative and postoperative patients, pp. 528–532, the care of patients on prolonged bed rest, pp. 533–537, and the care of patients with life-disrupting illnesses, pp. 544–546.

E. Patient–Family Teaching and Discharge Planning

Provide patient and SOs with verbal and written information for the following:

1. Necessary patient care after hospital discharge, for example, dressing changes, warm soaks, ROM exercises. Involve SOs in patient care during hospitalized period to familiarize them with care that will be required after discharge.

2. When parenteral antibiotic therapy is to be done at home (usually via a Hickman catheter or similar long-term IV device), the method of administering medications and care of the device used.

3. Medications, including drug name, route, dosage, purpose, schedule, precautions, and potential side effects.

4. Involving a public health nurse, visiting nurse, or similar home health care service professional to ensure adequate follow-up at home.

5. Indicators of potential complications, such as recurring infection, pathologic fracture, joint contracture, pressure necrosis, and medication reactions or toxic effects

II. Fractures

A fracture is a break in the continuity of a bone. It occurs when stress is placed on the bone that exceeds the bone's biologic loading capacity. Most commonly, the stress is the result of trauma. *Pathologic fractures* are the result of decreased biologic loading capacity, so that even normal stress can result in a break.

A. Assessment

Chronic indicators: These are rare. Osteoporotic fractures of the vertebral column may be found incidental to an x-ray in an asymptomatic patient or in a patient who complains of back discomfort. Delayed union is a failure of the bone to unite within the normally accepted timeframe for that bone's healing, and a chronic fracture may result. Nonunion is demonstrated by nonalignment and lost function secondary to lost bony rigidity.

Acute indicators: Patient complains of sudden pain, which is usually associated with trauma or physical stress such as jogging or strenuous exercise. In pathologic fractures, the patient may describe signs and symptoms associated with the underlying pathology (see "Benign Neoplasms," p. 397, and "Malignant Neoplasms," p. 398)

Physical examination: Loss of normal bony or limb contours, edema, ecchymosis, limb shortening, decreased ROM of adjacent joints, false motion (movement that occurs outside of a joint), and crepitus, which should not be elicited purposely because of the risk of injury to surrounding soft tissues. Complicated and complex fractures can present with signs and symptoms of perforated viscus, neurovascular deficit, joint effusion, or excessive joint laxity.

▶ **Note:** Any patient with a suspected fracture should be treated as though a fracture is present until it is ruled out. Interventions should include immobilization and elevation of the involved area, application of ice, and careful monitoring of the neurovascular status distal to the injury.

B. Diagnostic Tests

Most fractures are identified easily with standard AP and lateral x-rays. Occasionally, it is necessary to involve special techniques such as the mortise view to demonstrate bimalleolar ankle fractures or x-rays through the open mouth to identify fractures of the odontoid process. Bone scans, tomograms, CT scans, stereoscopic films, and arthrograms also can be used.

C. Medical Management and Surgical Interventions

The choice of treatment varies with the complexity of the fracture, the patient's age and concurrent health problems, and functional goals. The goal of treatment is to provide immobilization of the bone until healing occurs. The length of time for immobilization varies with the type of fracture. The following is a brief overview of common examples of treatment interventions that may be utilized.

1. **Bed rest:** May be all that is required to maintain reduction for simple, uncomplicated fractures.

2. **Traction**

   □ *Cervical fractures:* Skeletal traction via Turner, Cone, Vinke, or Crutchfield tongs, which are inserted into the outer plate of the cranial vault. An alternative is the halo vest, which allows the insertion of four pins into the outer plate of the cranium. The pins are attached to a halo device that is connected to four metal posts encompassed within a body jacket, cast, or orthosis. This "four posted" jacket allows exposure of the head and neck, yet maintains immobilization of the fracture. Cervical collars can be used to provide skin traction for simple fractures.

   □ *Humeral fractures:* Dunlop's side arm or overhead 90/90 traction.

   □ *Pelvic fractures:* Pelvic sling or pelvic belt may be used for nondisplaced fractures, while skeletal traction with pins in the ilium and/or femur may be required for displaced fractures.

   □ *Femoral fractures:* Skin traction (Buck's extension, Russell's traction, or balanced suspension traction) may be applied until skeletal traction can be used or the fracture is internally fixated. Skeletal traction may involve a Steinmann pin or Kirshner wire positioned through the distal femur or proximal tibia. When skeletal traction is used, it is provided in combination with balanced suspension or Russell's traction and is used for 1–4 months.

   □ *Tibial fractures:* Temporary traction can be accomplished with Buck's extension or, for longer periods of time, with a pin placed through the distal tibia or calcaneus, augmented with balanced suspension or Russell's traction.

3. **Immobilization devices**

   □ *Uncomplicated, simple fractures of the cervical vertebrae:* Soft or hard cervical collars or a minerva jacket cast for less stable fractures.

   □ *Dorsal and lumbar vertebral fractures:* Plaster of Paris body cast.

   □ *Clavicular fractures:* Figure-8 dressing, modified Velpeau dressing (a wrap that holds the arm against the thorax with the elbow flexed at 90° or 45°), sling and swathe shoulder immobilizer, clavicular straps.

   □ *Humeral fractures:* Velpeau cast, shoulder spica cast (which abducts or extends the upper arm), or Caldwell's hanging plaster cast, which is a long arm cast with additional layers of plaster of Paris that provide weight to distract fracture fragments and aid in alignment. Patients in Caldwell's casts need to be instructed to allow the cast to be dependent, which will help ensure adequate fracture distraction.

   □ *Ulnar or radial fractures:* Long arm casts for proximal fractures or short arm casts for distal fractures. In the presence of significant edema, a sugar tong splint may be used. This is applied over heavy padding and consists of one long plaster splint that extends from the back of the wrist, bends around the elbow, covers the underside of the forearm to the wrist, and is held in place with an elastic wrap.

   □ *Hand fractures:* Short arm posterior splints until edema subsides, and then a short arm cast can be applied.

   □ *Femoral fractures:* Spica cast that extends from the thorax and completely encompasses the affected leg and opposite leg to the midthigh, or a long leg cast may be applied instead. After sufficient callous has formed, it may be possible to use a cast brace to allow motion of the knee and weight-bearing stress, which can facilitate bony union in certain fractures.

   □ *Patellar fractures:* Cylinder cast for nondisplaced fractures. Following any knee surgery, the leg is immobilized in a Jones dressing, which includes AP and lateral splints over bulky padding and is held in place with an elastic wrap. Once swelling subsides, a cylinder or long leg cast is applied.

☐ *Tibial fractures:* Cylinder or long leg cast; short leg cast for easily stabilized fractures.

☐ *Fibular shaft fractures:* While some fibular fractures may not require casting, a short leg walking cast is often applied if adequate support is not provided by the tibia.

☐ *Malleolar fractures:* Short leg cast that is converted to a walking cast after callous has formed; long leg cast for nondisplaced bimalleolar fractures.

☐ *Avulsion fractures of the insertion of the Achilles tendon from the calcaneous:* Often require a long leg cast with the knee flexed at 30° and the ankle slightly plantarflexed to reduce stress on the Achilles tendon.

☐ *Tarsal and metatarsal fractures:* Short leg cast that can be converted to a walking cast; a stiff-soled shoe or slipper cast may also be used.

☐ *Phalangeal fractures:* Splints made of plaster, metal, or plastic; or the toe can be immobilized by taping it to an adjacent toe.

4. **Closed reduction:** Allows for manipulation of displaced fragments to their normal anatomic alignment. It can be done under general, regional, local, or hematoma-block anesthesia.

5. **Open reduction with internal fixation (ORIF):** Indicated for fractures that are grossly unstable or for patients who cannot tolerate prolonged bed rest or traction. Internal fixation may be accomplished with screws, pins, wires, plates, bone grafts, methylmethacrylate, or rods.

6. **External fixation:** Consists of skeletal pins that penetrate the fracture fragments and are attached to universal joints, which in turn are attached to rods to provide stabilization. These rods form a frame around the fractured limb for immobilization. The external fixator is left in place until sufficient soft tissue repair or bony callus formation allows either application of a cast or complete removal of any form of immobilization. Sometimes the skeletal pins are left in place (after removing the external fixation rods) and incorporated into a cast that immobilizes the limb until the fracture has healed. The external fixator can be used to treat massive open comminuted fractures with extensive soft tissue injury and/or neurovascular injury in which there is increased risk of infection. It is also the treatment of choice for infected nonunion, segmental bone loss, limb-lengthening procedures, arthrodesis (joint fusion), and multiple trauma with injuries involving other body systems.

7. **Coaptation splint:** Provides immobilization for patients with significant nerve damage or edema while compensating for the edema to prevent iatrogenic compartment syndrome (see "Ischemic Myositis," p. 385). These splints involve the application of sheet wadding (padding), cotton pads (ABDs), and anterior and posterior plaster splints, which are held in place with an elastic wrap. Examples are the sugar tong splint used on the forearm or the Jones dressing that is applied to the knee.

8. **Progressive ROM and muscle-strengthening exercises:** Begun after the designated period of immoblization to help the patient regain joint function.

9. **Continuous passive motion (CPM):** A motor-driven device developed to place a joint through repeated extension and flexion. It is used as an adjunctive treatment for such injuries as femoral condyle and tibial plateau fractures.

D. Nursing Diagnoses and Interventions

See "Osteoarthritis" for the following: **Alteration in comfort**, p. 367, and **Impaired physical mobility** related to adjustment to a new walking gait, p. 368 (useful for any patient with spinal or lower-extremity injuries). See "Ligamentous Injuries" for the the following: **Knowledge deficit:** Need for elevation of the involved extremity, use of thermotherapy, and exercise, p. 376 (useful for patients discharged after a recent fracture or surgery), and **Knowledge deficit:** Care and assessment of the casted extremity, p. 377 (applies to any patient in a cast). See "Torn Anterior Cruciate Ligament" for the following: **Potential fluic volume deficit** related to abnormal loss secondary to postsurgical hemorrhage oɪ hematoma, p. 383 (for patients with open reduction and internal fixation). See "Bunionectomy" for the following: **Potential alteration in tissue perfusion:** Peripheral, related to impaired circulation secondary to compression from circumferential casts or dressings, p. 404 (relates to iatrogenic compartment syndrome and builds on information provided under "Ischemic Myositis," p. 385). See "Amputation" for the following: **Knowledge deficit:** Postsurgical exercise regimen, p. 406 (applies to any patient begun on exercise therapy). See "Repair of Recurrent Shoulder Dislocation" for the following: **Potential impairment of skin integrity** related to maceration of the axillary skin, p. 411 (useful for any patient with moist areas trapped by a therapeutic device that is necessary to treat a fracture). See "Total Hip Arthroplasty" for the following: **Knowledge deficit:** Potential for and mechanism of THA dislocation, p. 413 (for patients undergoing hemiarthroplasty for replacement of the femoral head), **Knowledge deficit:** Potential for infection caused by foreign body reaction to endoprosthesis, p. 413 (useful for any patient with an internal fixation device, especially large devices), and **Potential alteration in tissue perfusion**, p. 414 (can be adapted for any patient in traction). See "Herniated Nucleus Pulposus" in Chapter 4 for the following: **Knowledge deficit:** Pain control measures, p. 168. See "Appendix One" for nursing diagnoses and interventions for the care of preoperative and postoperative patients, pp. 528–532, and for the care of patients on prolonged bed rest, pp. 533–537.

Specific nursing diagnoses for patients with casts, traction, open reduction and internal fixation, and external fixators:

Self-care deficit: Inability to perform ADLs related to physical limitations secondary to cast and/or surgical procedure (applies to patients with casts, open reduction with internal fixation, and external fixators)

Desired outcome: Patient demonstrates independence with performing ADLs.

1. For patients with insufficient strength to manipulate casted extremities to allow independence in self-care, incorporate a structured exercise regimen that will increase strength and endurance. Direct the regimen toward development of those muscle groups necessary for the patient's activity deficit. See the guidelines described in **Potential impairment of physical mobility** related to inactivity secondary to prolonged bed rest, p. 535, in "Appendix One" and **Knowledge deficit:** Postsurgical exercise regimen, p. 406, in "Amputation."

2. Use assistive devices liberally. These include stocking helpers, Velcro fasteners, builtup handles on eating utensils, pickup sticks, raised toilet seats, and similar self-help devices.

3. As appropriate, ask social services department of hospital for assistance with funding for purchasing assistive equipment.

4. Because pain control is an essential element in enhancing self-care activities, ensure that the patient is as comfortable as possible (see **Alteration in comfort:** Pain related to inflammatory process or corrective therapy, p. 367, in "Osteoarthritis").

5. When needed, teach SOs how to assist patient with self-care.

6. If economic assistance is needed for home help, consult with social services for intervention.

7. As appropriate, utilize adaptive clothing (eg, garments with Velcro fasteners for easy removal and application) that is designed to accommodate the cast.

Potential impairment of skin integrity related to irritation secondary to the presence of a cast (applies to patients with casts and ORIF)

Desired outcomes: Patient denies the presence of discomfort under the cast and does not exhibit evidence of skin irritation or breakdown once the cast is removed. Patient can verbalize knowledge of the indicators of pressure necrosis.

1. When assisting with cast application, ensure that adequate padding is put on the affected extremity before the cast is applied.

2. While the cast is curing, handle it only with the palms of the hands to avoid pressure points caused by finger indentations. Ensure that the cast surface is exposed to air as much as possible to facilitate drying.

3. Petal the edges of plaster casts with tape or moleskin to prevent cast crumbs from falling beneath the cast and causing pressure necrosis.

4. Instruct patient never to insert anything between the cast and skin. In the presence of severe itching, advise patient to notify MD, who may prescribe a medication to relieve itching.

5. Ensure that the patient can verbalize understanding of the indicators of pressure necrosis beneath the cast: pain, burning sensation, foul odor from cast opening, or drainage on the cast.

Knowledge deficit: Potential for disuse osteoporosis (appropriate for patient with cast or traction)

Desired outcome: Patient can verbalize knowledge of the process of and measures to prevent disuse osteoporosis.

1. Ensure that the patient can verbalize understanding of the process of disuse osteoporosis, gearing the explanation to the patient's level of understanding: The immobilized limb has insufficient stress to stimulate osteoblastic (bone building) activity.

2. Instruct patient to report any indictors of pain in the immobilized limb or findings of spontaneous fracture such as bony deformity, pain, lost function, edema, and ecchymosis.

3. Consult with patient's MD about appropriate alternative methods of bone stress, and teach them to the patient. These can include use of a tilt table, sandbags applied intermittently against the bone, or having patient push against a footboard or perform isometric exericise of the immobilized limb.

Potential alteration in tissue perfusion: Peripheral, cerebral, or cardiopulmonary, related to impaired circulation secondary to fat embolization (applies to patients with multiple trauma, multiple fractures, or surgical repair of fractures)

Desired outcome: Patient's VS and physical findings are within acceptable limits.

1. Ensure strict maintenance of fracture immobilization to help prevent embolization.

2. Carefully monitor patient for the initial 72 hours following injury or surgery for indicators of fat embolism: tachycardia, tachypnea, cyanosis, fever, petechial rash (involving the conjunctiva, trunk, neck, and axilla), progressive mental dysfunction (confusion, disorientation), and the presence of fat globules in the retina of the eye. The hematocrit may drop, serum lipase will rise, and fat may be noted on urinalysis. The chest x-ray will show diffuse pulmonary infiltrate.

3. Because fat embolism is a life-threatening emergency, notify MD immediately should any of the above occur. Inform patient and SOs of these potential indicators so that they can notify the staff if they occur.

4. If a fat embolism occurs, perform prescribed respiratory support measures (eg, delivery of oxygen and rigorous pulmonary hygiene). Intubation with ventilation using positive end-expiratory pressure (PEEP) may be necessary.

5. Administer IV steroids, diuretics, and dextran as prescribed.

Knowledge deficit: Potential for infection related to orthopedic procedure and/or presence of internal or external device (appropriate for patients with ORIF, external fixators)

Desired outcomes: Patient can verbalize knowledge of the potential for infection, list the indicators that may occur, and relate the importance of reporting them immediately.

1. Advise patient about the potential for infection, which can occur as a result of the surgical procedure.

2. Be sure patient can verbalize understanding of the following indicators of infection and knows to report them immediately: persistent redness, swelling, increasing pain, wound drainage, local warmth, foul odor from beneath the cast, sensation of burning beneath the cast, drainage from the cast, and fever.

3. For patients with internal fixation devices, alert them to the potential for infection for as long as the implant is present. Instruct them to report any of the above indicators promptly.

Knowledge deficit: Potential for refracture due to vulnerability from presence of internal fixator (applies to patients with ORIF)

Desired outcomes: Patient can verbalize knowledge of the potential for refracture and demonstrates adherence to the prescribed regimen for prevention.

1. Advise patient that while the internal fixation device supplements strength of the bone at the fracture site in the early stages of healing, the implant will compromise the bone's strength later. Larger internal fixation devices alter the vectors of stress placed on the bone, reducing the normal physiologic balance between osteoblasts and osteoclasts, which results in a bone that is made weaker in the long run by the implant.

2. Be sure the patient verbalizes understanding of this process and demonstrates adherence to the prescribed regimen of limb usage and/or ambulation.

3. Ensure patient is aware that intramedullary nails or rods and large plates probably will be removed within a year.

Knowledge deficit: Function of external fixation, pin care, and signs and symptoms of pin site infection

Desired outcomes: Patient can verbalize knowledge of the rationale for the external fixator and can demonstrate ways to adapt his or her lifestyle around the fixator. Patient can demonstrate knowledge of pin care and verbalize knowledge of the indicators of infection.

1. Teach patient the rationale for use of the fixator with his or her type of fracture, emphasizing benefits for the patient.

2. Discuss ways in which the patient can adapt his or her lifestyle to accommodate the fixator, eg, by wearing adaptive clothing that fits the device.

3. Instruct patient and SOs in pin care as prescribed by MD. Some MDs prescribe daily pin site care with hydrogen peroxide or skin prep solutions such as pHisoHex, alcohol, or povidone-iodine. Some MDs prescribe that buildup of crusts from serous drainage be removed when cleansing pin sites, while others request that the crust be left intact to minimize the risk of infection. If prescribed, teach the patient how to apply antibacterial ointments and small dressings to the pin site. **Note:** Literature supplied with some external fixators cautions against the use of iodine-based mixtures, which may cause corrosion of the device.

4. Teach patient how to monitor the pin sites for indicators of infection, including persistent redness, swelling, drainage, pain, and local warmth, and to be alert to pin migration or "tenting" of the skin on the pin, which can signal

movement of the pin or infection. Instruct patient to report significant findings promptly to MD.

5. Advise patient of the need for follow-up care to ensure that the device is functioning properly and maintaining adequate immobilization of the fracture(s).

E. Patient—Family Teaching and Discharge Planning

Provide patient and SOs with verbal and written information for the following:

1. Medications, including the name, dosage, purpose, schedule, precautions, and potential side effects.

2. Importance of rest, elevation, and use of thermotherapy.

3. Rationale for the individual's therapy after discharge and how that therapy will be accomplished, for example, casting, external fixation, internal fixation.

4. Precautions of therapy

   □ *Casts:* Caring for the cast, monitoring neurovascular status of the distal extremity, watching for evidence of pressure necrosis beneath the cast, performing prescribed exercises, preventing skin maceration, and preventing disuse osteoporosis (see p. 377).

   □ *Internal fixation devices:* Caring for the wound, noting signs of wound infection, preventing refracture of the limb, performing prescribed exercises, and monitoring for delayed infection from the implant.

   □ *External fixator:* Demonstrating understanding of pin care, knowing when to notify MD of problems with the fixator, performing prescribed exercises, monitoring neurovascular status of the limb, and monitoring pin site for indicators of infection.

5. Ways in which patient can control discomfort.

6. Use of assistive devices and/or ambulatory aids. Ensure that the patient can perform a return demonstration.

7. Materials that are necessary for care at home and agencies that can supply materials.

In addition:

8. For patients who require home help, a collaborative effort between hospital nurses and community care agencies should be made to ensure continuity of care. Appropriate agency should see patient before hospital discharge.

III. Benign Neoplasms

The three most common benign bone tumors are osteochondromas, enchondromas, and giant cell tumors. *Osteochondromas* are the most common, representing 45% of all benign tumors. Usually they are found in the metaphysis (wider portion of the shaft) of the long bones, typically the distal femur or proximal humerus, although they also can occur in a rib or vertebra. Individuals under the age of 20 are most commonly affected. Some osteochondromas are the result of an inheritable autosomal dominant trait that causes concurrent growth retardation and bowing of the long bones. *Enchondromas* (chondromas) are most commonly found in the hand (metacarpals or phalanges) or the proximal humerus. They represent approximately 10% of all diagnosed benign tumors. Although they occur most commonly in the thirties, they may be seen at any time. *Giant cell tumors* are found most often around the proximal humerus, distal radius, or the knee in the area of the fused epiphyseal growth plate. Ten percent of these tumors degenerate into malignancy with a potential for metastasis. Tumors recur 40% of the time.

A. Assessment

Osteochondromas: Indicators arise from mechanical irritation of surrounding musculotendinous structures, and include pain upon specific movements of the involved areas or from irritation.

Enchondromas: Local pain. Unless the growth is in an area with little soft tissue, the growth is usually not palpable.

Giant cell tumors: Pain occurs before the mass becomes palpable.

B. Diagnostic Tests

AP and lateral x-rays are most commonly used for preliminary diagnosis. CT scans, tomograms, contrast radiography, and angiograms can be used to clarify the extent of the tumor.

C. Medical Management and Surgical Interventions

All three types of tumors are best treated with surgical removal. Resection can require allografting, prosthetic replacement, or use of methylmethacrylate to replace resected bone. When removal is impossible, curettage (scraping) of the lesion is usually done. In some giant cell tumors, radiation therapy is used to inhibit recurrence.

D. Nursing Diagnoses and Interventions

Knowledge deficit: Disease process and potential for recurrence (if appropriate)

Desired outcomes: Patient can verbalize understanding of the disease process. Patients with giant cell tumors can verbalize understanding of the potential for recurrence and slight chance of malignancy.

1. Provide patient with a clearly understood description of the disease process. Drawings, models, books, and other references should be used to enhance patient's learning.
2. Validate that the patient clearly understands the disease process and does not confuse it with a malignant tumor.
3. Be sure that patients with giant cell tumors are aware of the potential for recurrence and slight potential for degeneration to malignancy, as well as the importance of reporting renewed indicators of tumor to MD.

See "Osteoarthritis" for the following: **Alteration in comfort**, p. 367. See "Appendix One" for nursing diagnoses and interventions for the care of preoperative and postoperative patients, pp. 528–532.

E. Patient–Family Teaching and Discharge Planning

Provide patient and SOs with verbal and written information for the following:

1. Description of the disease process.
2. For surgical patients, the indicators of wound infection (swelling, persistent redness, wound drainage, pain, local warmth, and fever) and the necessity of reporting these indicators promptly to MD.
3. For patients with casts and orthotics, the care of the extremity and immobilization device (see p. 377).
4. Medications, including the name, dosage, purpose, schedule, precautions, and potential side effects.
5. Post-hospitalization therapy and the importance of follow-up.

IV. Malignant Neoplasms

The most common malignant tumors affecting bones are osteogenic sarcoma, primary chondrosarcoma, and myeloma. *Osteogenic sarcoma* is the most common of the three, occurring most frequently in adolescents. It is found (in order of prevalance) in the distal femoral metaphysis, proximal tibial metaphysis, proximal humeral metaphysis, pelvis, and proximal femur. This tumor is associated with early metastasis to the lung, lymph involvement, and rapid death unless rigorous treatment is begun early in the disease process. The current survival rate following resection and adjunctive chemotherapy is 60%. *Chondrosarcomas* occur half as frequently as osteogenic sarcomas and are usually seen between ages 50 and 60. Most of these tumors originate in the pelvic girdle, ribs, or shoulder girth. Resection of all of the tumor results in an excellent 5-year cure rate; however, inadequate resection frequently results in recurrence and late metastasis to the lung. *Myelomas* arise from bone marrow and thus are not truly bone tumors; however, they are the most common malignant tumor that affects the bones. The peak time of onset is the sixth and seventh decades. Myelomas can occur in any bone, although they are seen less frequently in smaller bones. Average survival after diagnosis is 1–2 years.

A. Assessment

Osteogenic sarcomas: Pain, tenderness, limited ROM, and swelling near a joint. Night pain is usually more severe.

Chondrosarcomas: Localized pain, rarely with a demonstrable mass.

Myelomas: Symptoms of anemia, as well as weight loss, significant pain, tenderness, backache, or pathologic and spontaneous fracture.

B. Diagnostic Tests

1. <u>Standard x-rays, CT scans, tomograms, and radioisotope (Gallium) uptake tests:</u> To delineate extent of the disease.

For myelomas:

2. <u>Standard blood and electrolyte tests:</u> May reveal moderate normocytic anemia and a markedly elevated sedimentation rate. Serum calcium levels, PTT, and PT are usually elevated.

3. <u>Bence Jones protein:</u> Urine will be positive in 40% of patients with myeloma.

4. <u>Bone marrow aspiration:</u> May reveal plasma cells with large nuclei and nucleoli.

5. <u>Immunoelectrophoresis:</u> Will show an abnormal amount of either IgG or IgA produced by the tumor cells.

C. Medical Management and Surgical Interventions

1. **Osteogenic sarcoma:** Treated with resection of the tumor, most commonly by amputation. Recent attempts to perform less radical resections, including therapy with chemotherapeutic agents and occasionally radiotherapy, have met with some success.

2. **Chondrosarcoma:** Usually treated with resection, with the degree of resection dependent on the stage of tumor development. Radiotherapy and chemotherapy have not proven to be effective in treating this disease.

3. **Multiple myeloma:** Requires extensive therapy with radiation and chemotherapy. Radiation is used to control localized bone pain and treat areas with pathologic fractures. Chemotherapy with melphalan, prednisone, and vincristine has been shown to be helpful. Occasionally, hypercalcemia requires additional therapy with increased volumes of IV fluids, furosemide, prednisone, or mithramycin. Laminectomy may be required for spinal cord compression caused by vertebral lesions. Blood transfusions and potent analgesics are usually required.

D. Nursing Diagnoses and Interventions

See "Osteoarthritis" for the following: **Alteration in comfort**, p. 367, and **Impaired physical mobility** related to adjustment to a new walking gait, p. 368. See

"Torn Anterior Cruciate Ligament" for the following: **Potential fluid volume deficit** related to abnormal loss secondary to postsurgical hemorrhage or hematoma, p. 383. See "Appendix One" for nursing diagnoses and interventions for the care of preoperative and postoperative patients, pp. 528–532, and care of patients with cancer and other life-disrupting illnesses, pp. 544–551. **Note:** When postoperative casts, use of orthotics, exercises, or similar therapies are prescribed, refer to appropriate nursing diagnoses throughout this chapter. If the patient undergoes amputation, refer to "Amputation," p. 405.

E. Patient–Family Teaching and Discharge Planning

Provide patient and SOs with verbal and written information for the following:

1. Medications, including the name, rationale, dosage, schedule, precautions, and potential side effects.

2. For surgical patients, the following indicators of wound infection and the importance of notifying MD should they occur: persistent redness, swelling, local warmth, fever, discharge from the wound, or pain.

3. For patients with casts, orthotics, prosthetics, ambulatory aids, assistive devices, or similar therapies: instructions for their use, including a return demonstration by patient and a phone number to call should any questions arise after hospital discharge.

4. Referral to hospice or agency that provides home help. This should occur before discharge planning begins to ensure continuity of care between the hospital and home or hospice.

V. Osteoporosis

Osteoporosis is a condition in which the amount of bony mass decreases while the size of the bone remains constant. It is a major health problem in the United States, potentially affecting as many as 15–20 million Americans and causing over a million fractures a year in people over the age of 45. The risk of osteoporosis increases with age and is higher in females than in males. Factors in the development of osteoporosis include menopause, reduced activity, and decreased dietary intake of calcium.

A. Assessment

Signs and symptoms: Documented loss of bone density, most commonly found in conjunction with pathologic fractures secondary to osteoporosis. Most fractures occur in the dorsal (thoracic) and lumbar vertebral bodies (usually D8 through L2), the neck and intertrochanteric regions of the femur, and the distal radius. Vertebral compression fractures can develop gradually, resulting in loss of height, kyphosis, back discomfort, and constipation. Fractures of the hip result in significant morbidity and mortality.

B. Diagnostic Tests

1. <u>Standard AP and lateral x-rays of the spine:</u> Provide a diagnosis for osteoporotic fractures. Bone density loss is not easily demonstrated by standard radiographs because 20–30% of bone density must be lost before it can be noted on x-ray.

2. <u>Radiogrammetry, photodensitometry, single- and dual-photon absorptiometry, neutron activation, and single- and dual-energy computed tomography:</u> These are examples of some of the sophisticated noninvasive tests that can be used to determine bone density. However, the availability and cost of these tests make their routine use prohibitive.

C. Medical Management and Surgical Interventions

1. **Oral estrogen:** Doses as low as 0.625 mg have been shown to be effective in preventing osteoporosis in postmenopausal women. Use of cyclic estrogen/progesterone also may reduce the risk of endometrial cancer.

2. **Calcium intake:** Should exceed 1000–1500 mg/day for women approaching menopause. Each 8-oz glass of milk provides 275–300 mg of calcium, indicating that an intake of 4–6 glasses/day is ideal. Vegetable calcium sources (eg, dark green, leafy vegetables; sesame seeds) are also good. For lactose-intolerant patients or those unable to consume dietary calcium, calcium supplementation is prescribed. Some antacids (eg, Tums) contain calcium and may serve as a calcium supplement. **Note:** Because smoking and a high-sugar, high-meat diet affect the phosphorus-calcium ratio, and therefore calcium utilization, individuals who do not smoke or eat red meat or sugar have a lower calcium requirement (Walker, 1972).

3. **Vitamin D:** Necessary to allow adequate intestinal absorption and usage of calcium. The recommended daily intake of this vitamin is 600–800 U twice daily. Because excessive vitamin D is associated with significant toxicity, higher intake is discouraged without clear documentation of need.

4. **Moderate weightbearing exercise:** To stress bones and activate osteoblastic bone formation, because inactivity has been shown to result in disuse osteoporosis. Williams' back exercises, pectoral stretching, isometric abdominal exercises, and walking are often recommended.

5. **A variety of treatment modalities under investigation for use in combating osteoporosis:** Include sodium fluoride, calcitrol, calcitonin, weekly androgenic anabolic steroids, thiazides, and bisphosphonates. However, their efficacy has not been proven yet.

D. Nursing Diagnoses and Interventions

Knowledge deficit: Disease process and the importance of compliance with the prescribed therapy

Desired outcome: Patient can verbalize knowledge of the disease process and demonstrates compliance with the therapy.

1. Ensure that patient is aware of the silent nature of this disorder and realizes that by the time symptoms arise, it is too late for effective treatment.

2. Teach patient that even in the absence of symptoms, it is essential to comply with therapy.

Alteration in nutrition: Less than body requirements related to increased need for calcium and vitamin D

Desired outcome: Patient demonstrates intake of adequate amounts of calcium and vitamin D and plans a 3-day menu that provides sufficient intake of both.

1. Ensure that the patient can verbalize understanding of the foods that are high in calcium, including cheese, milk, dark green leafy vegetables, eggs, peanuts, sesame seeds, and oysters. Provide patient with a list of these foods, including the relative amounts of calcium for each.

2. Teach patient how to plan menus that provide sufficient daily intake of calcium and vitamin D-fortified foods such as eggs, halibut, herring, fortified dairy products, liver, mackerel, oysters, salmon, and sardines.

3. Provide patient with sample menus that include adequate daily amounts of calcium and vitamin D. Have patient plan a 3-day menu that incorporates these foods.

4. Provide patient with a phone number to call should questions arise after hospital discharge.

See "Amputation" for the following: **Knowledge deficit:** Postsurgical exercise regimen, p. 406.

E. Patient—Family Teaching and Discharge Planning

Provide patient and SOs with verbal and written information for the following:

1. Medications, including the name, dosage, purpose, schedule, precautions, and potential side effects.
2. Instructions for the prescribed dietary regimen, including the rationale for the diet and foods to include and foods to avoid, if appropriate.
3. Prescribed exercise regimen, including how to perform the exercise, number of repetitions of each, and frequency of exercise periods.

VI. Paget's Disease (Osteitis Deformans)

Paget's disease is an idiopathic process suspected of being caused by a slow viral infection. Three to four percent of the population over age 40 have some Pagetic findings, and 20% over age 80 have some Pagetic bone. This disorder results from an aberrant function of osteoclasts (bone-resorbing cells) and osteoblasts (bone-building cells), resulting in bone that is high in mineral content, weaker, of poor quality, grossly deformed, and thickened. Active lesions have increased vascularity, and have been attributed to high-output cardiac failure in extensive disease.

A. Assessment

Signs and symptoms: Most patients are asymptomatic except for pain at the involved site(s), which can be difficult to differentiate from osteoarthritis or myalgia. Some patients develop pathologic fractures through the Pagetic lesions, or the process can be an incidental finding on x-rays taken to rule out other processes. Cranial enlargement or radiculoneuropathy can result in the following: oculomotor deficits, visual deficits, deafness, dysphagia, dysphasia, hemifacial paresthesia, or paralysis. Vertebral involvement is evidenced by kyphoscoliosis or stenotic lesions of the spinal cord or nerves, resulting in radiculoneuropathy of these structures.

B. Diagnostic Tests

1. <u>Standard x-rays:</u> May reveal typical mosaic-appearing lesions, osteoporosis circumscripta (an area of radiolucency surrounded by normal bone), protrusio acetabuli (protrusion of the acetabulum into the pelvis), pseudofractures, microfractures, incomplete transverse fractures, sclerotic bony lesions, invaginated foramen magnum, and pathologic fractures.
2. <u>Serum tests:</u> Will reveal an elevated serum alkaline phosphatase, indicating new bone formation.
3. <u>Urine assay:</u> Will reveal elevated hydroxyproline, indicating bony lysis.
4. <u>Bone biopsy:</u> Can be used to confirm the diagnosis in questionable cases.

C. Medical Management and Surgical Interventions

Treatment is restricted to patients who have pervasive disease and/or significant symptoms of involvement in critical areas because the treatments carry significant risk. Suppressive therapy is restricted to patients with radiculoneuropathy, imminent complications, highly resorptive lesions, and who are immobilized or require surgery on involved areas.

1. **Nonsteroidal anti-inflammatory agents:** May be used to control pain (see Table 8-1, p. 370).
2. **Suppressive therapy:** May include the following

   □ *Synthetic salmon calcitonin:* 50–100 MRC (Medical Research Council) units SC, 3 times a week. This hormone inhibits bone resorption while combating parathyroid gland action. Side effects include nausea, a feeling of warmth following injection, and flushing.

□ *Etidronate disodium (EHDP):* Daily dosages of 5 mg/kg of body weight. It is theorized that EHDP coats bone surfaces to prevent bony resorption and formation. Side effects include cramps, diarrhea, and nausea. EHDP should be given on an empty stomach for optimal absorption. This medication is contraindicated in patients with new fractures or who are immobilized, and it can increase the risk of pathologic fracture in patients with extensive disease.

□ *Mithramycin:* A cytotoxic agent given in short courses (10 doses) of 25 μg/kg IV. It is theorized that this medication suppresses the action of osteoclasts in bone resorption. Side effects include anorexia, nausea, vomiting; elevated SGOT, BUN, and creatinine; and depressed platelets and leukocytes.

3. **Surgical interventions:** Restricted to repair of pathologic fractures. Surgery on involved bones requires adequate preparation via typing and crossmatching of several units of blood, meticulous hemostasis during surgery, and careful monitoring for hemorrhage after surgery.

D. Nursing Diagnoses and Interventions

Knowledge deficit: Potential complications of Paget's disease

Desired outcome: Patient can verbalize knowledge of the disease pathology and awareness of the importance of promptly reporting untoward indicators to MD.

1. Teach patient the disease pathology, including the signs and symptoms of potential complications such as renal calculi, significant cranial or spinal radiculoneuropathy (decreased hearing, headache, paresthesia, weakness, paralysis, visual defects, dysphasia, dysphagia, oculomotor weakness); hydrocephalus (headache, pupillary inequality, altered LOC); and alterations in gait.

2. Advise patient of the importance of promptly reporting untoward indicators to MD.

See "Gouty Arthritis" for the following: **Knowledge deficit:** Signs and symptoms and preventive measures for uric acid renal calculi, p. 371. See "Torn Anterior Cruciate Ligament" for the following: **Potential fluid volume deficit** related to loss secondary to postsurgical hemorrhage or hematoma, p. 383.

E. Patient–Family Teaching and Discharge Planning

Provide patient and SOs with verbal and written information for the following:

1. Medications, including drug name, purpose, dosage, schedule, potential side effects, and precautions.

2. Signs to monitor for and report while on suppressive therapy, especially ecchymosis, melena, hematoma, and hematuria, as well as indicators of prolonged bleeding, hemorrhage, and superimposed infections.

3. Indicators to monitor for and report related to complications of the disease (see **Knowledge deficit**, above).

▶ Section Four   **Musculoskeletal Surgical Procedures**

I. Bunionectomy

Bunionectomy is surgery to correct hallux valgus. Hallux refers to the great toe and valgus means that it is bent outward, away from the midline. The bunion is actually a prominence of the first metatarsal head, resulting from altered joint dynamics as the hallux subluxates laterally. Although a bunion can occur because of hereditary intrinsic joint weakness, the most frequent cause is improperly fitting footwear.

A. Assessment

Signs and symptoms: Can range from mild varus deformity to severe varus deformity with altered gait. In acute conditions, the patient has inflammation of the adventitial bursa, resulting in erythema, local warmth, and tenderness. The patient has great difficulty fitting shoes. X-rays are often used to define bony involvement and displacement of the lateral sesamoid bone.

B. Medical Management and Surgical Interventions

1. **Conservative treatment:** Begins with appropriately fitted footwear to accommodate the deformity.

2. **Bunionectomy:** Performed when the patient has significant pain and alterations in ambulation affecting ADLs. Many forms of surgery can be used, but the main elements include removal of the projecting metatarsal head, excision of the displaced sesamoid bone, release of the adductor hallucis tendon, and tightening of the medial periarticular tissues to prevent recurrence. Ambulation with appropriate immobilization of the involved foot is begun within 2–5 days of surgery. A short leg cast, slipper cast, or bunion boot is used for immobilization.

C. Nursing Diagnoses and Interventions

Knowledge deficit: Disease process and therapeutic regimen

Desired outcome: Patient can verbalize knowledge of bunion formation, preventive measures, prescribed postoperative immobilization, and potential complications.

1. Assess patient's level of understanding about the disease process and treatment modalities involved.

2. Provide instructions about causes and progression of bunion formation, role of improperly fitting shoes in bunion formation, role of surgery in bunion correction, rationale for the postoperative regimen of care, need for immobilization of the surgical area to promote healing and maintain realignment, technique for caring for the casted extremity, and indicators of wound infection.

3. As appropriate, provide written material for cast care, indicators of wound infection and neurovascular deficit, wound care, and use of appropriate pain medication. For further information on cast care, see the nursing diagnosis **Knowledge deficit:** Care and assessment of the casted extremity, p. 377 in "Ligamentous Injuries."

4. Allow time for patient's questions and expressions of anxiety. Be supportive and reassuring.

Impairment of physical mobility related to immobilization device and/or non-weightbearing secondary to bunionectomy

Desired outcomes: Patient demonstrates compliance with elevation of the operant extremity above the level of the heart during the early postoperative period. Patient demonstrates use of safety measures while ambulating with the immobilization device.

1. Following surgery, the patient will be permitted bathroom privileges with a walker or crutches, with weightbearing as tolerated. Otherwise, ensure that the operant extremity is kept elevated higher than the level of the heart to facilitate reduction of postoperative edema. **Note:** Patients with plaster of Paris casts are restricted to nonweightbearing ambulation until 48 hours after the cast has been applied.

2. The patient will begin ambulation wearing a cast or bunion boot that is worn for 3–6 weeks following surgery. Caution patient to ambulate with care in the device until it becomes an integral part of ambulation. Special care should be exercised on stairs, hills, and uneven surfaces.

Potential alteration in tissue perfusion: Peripheral, related to impaired circulation secondary to compression from circumferential casts or dressings

Desired outcomes: Patient does not exhibit signs of impaired neurovascular status. Patient can verbalize knowledge of the signs of impaired neurovascular status and awareness of the importance of getting prompt treatment should they occur.

1. Assess the operant extremity for the integrity of neurovascular status each time VS are taken (or at least q4h). Impaired neurovascular status requires nursing interventions such as elevation, loosening restrictive dressings, or promptly notifying the MD if these measures are ineffective.

2. Ensure that the patient can verbalize the signs and symptoms of impaired neurovascular status and knows how to call the MD should they occur after hospital discharge. These include persistent changes in color (pallor, cyanosis, redness), coolness, delayed capillary refill, paresthesia (numbness, tingling), or inability to move distal areas (the great or second toe).

See "Osteoarthritis" for the following: **Alteration in comfort**, p. 367.

D. Patient–Family Teaching and Discharge Planning

Provide patient and SOs with verbal and written information for the following:

1. Technique for ambulation with the casted extremity or bunion boot. Be sure the patient demonstrates independence in ADLs before hospital discharge.

2. Medications, including name, rationale, dosage, schedule, precautions, and potential side effects.

3. Indicators of wound infection and impaired neurovascular status and the importance of notifying MD promptly should they occur.

4. Phone number to call should patient have questions after hospital discharge.

II. Amputation

Today, amputation is less frequently required as an orthopedic surgical intervention than it was before the advent of antibiotics and microsurgery techniques. However, amputation is still required for certain disorders, such as atherosclerotic arterial occlusive disease, osteomyelitis, severe trauma, malignant tumors, or congenital anomalies. In the United States, most amputations are performed for advanced atherosclerotic arterial occlusive disease, especially in patients with diabetes mellitus or over age 60. When it is possible to increase an individual's function with a prosthesis, amputation is sometimes offered as an optional treatment. The majority of amputations are of the lower extremity.

A. Assessment

Signs and symptoms: Patients with advanced atherosclerotic arterial occlusive disease often have gangrene, a chronic stasis ulcer, or an infected wound that fails to heal. The patient usually complains of pain and there can be rubor (a dark red color) when the limb is dependent, as well as atrophy of the skin and subcutaneous tissues.

See "Osteomyelitis," p. 386, and "Malignant Neoplasms," p. 397, in this chapter and "Atherosclerotic Arterial Occlusive Disease," p. 77, in Chapter 2, as appropriate.

B. Diagnostic Tests

1. <u>Angiography:</u> Confirms inadequacy of circulation.
2. <u>CT scan:</u> Determines the degree of neoplastic or osteomyelitic involvement.
3. <u>Biopsy:</u> May be used to confirm presence of osteomyelitis or neoplasm.
4. <u>Extensive evaluations by OT for fine motor function and by PT for gross motor function:</u> To document functional loss and potential for rehabilitation.

C. Medical Management and Surgical Interventions

1. **Amputation:** The actual procedure used for amputation depends on the area of the limb involved. Generally, the surgical goals are to remove the least amount of tissue possible, provide adequate tissue for a viable myocutaneous flap to create a stump, and ensure adequate provision for a prosthetic device. Large blood vessels are individually identified and suture-ligated. Nerves are stretched and then suture-ligated to allow them to retract back into the residual limb (stump) to prevent trauma when the stump is used. Usually, bone ends are beveled to prevent trauma from sharp edges. Infected limbs are closed loosely to allow adequate drainage until infected tissues have been adequately treated.

2. **Postoperative period:** Immediately after surgery, a prosthesis may be used to promote wound healing, minimize stump edema, decrease the length of rehabilitation, and prevent complications of immobility after surgery. A cast is applied over the postoperative dressing, which incorporates a device that allows subsequent attachment of a pylon prosthesis to allow ambulation while the first prosthesis is being made. Early ambulation prevents flexion contractures; allows earlier gait training; improves psychologic state; prevents loss of muscle strength; and increases local circulation to improve wound healing, which subsequently decreases edema and pain.

D. Nursing Diagnoses and Interventions

Potential impairment of physical mobility related to contracture secondary to disuse of the extremity

Desired outcome: Patient does not exhibit signs of joint contracture.

1. Control patient's pain to ensure appropriate movement.
2. After providing elevation for the first 2 days postoperatively, intersperse elevation with periods of ROM to the remaining joints of the involved extremity. **Note:** Both elevation and ROM are performed with MD prescription.
3. Prevent flexion contractures of the knee and hip by assisting the patient with lying prone for an hour 3 times a day.
4. Another method for preventing flexion contractures is to have the patient perform exercises that increase the strength of the muscle extensors. Consult with MD regarding prescriptions for the following exercises:

   □ *Above-the-knee amputation:* Have patient attempt to straighten the hip from a flexed position against resistance and/or perform gluteal-setting exercises.

   □ *Below-the-knee amputation:* Have patient attempt to straighten the knee against resistance and/or perform hamstring-setting exercises. These patients also should perform the exercises described with above-the-knee amputations.

5. For other interventions, see **Potential impairment of physical mobility** related to inactivity secondary to prolonged bed rest, p. 535, in "Appendix One."

Impairment of physical mobility related to altered stance secondary to amputation of the lower limb

Desired outcome: Patient demonstrates use of muscle-tightening technique to enhance mobilization.

1. Inform patients with lower-extremity amputation that difficulty in adjusting to the altered stance may occur as a result of the amputation. Suggest that to prevent an altered stance, patient should tighten the gluteal and abdominal muscles while standing.

2. For other interventions, see **Impaired physical mobility** related to adjustment to a new walking gait with an assistive device, p. 368, in "Osteoarthritis."

Knowledge deficit: Postsurgical exercise regimen

Desired outcome: Patient can verbalize knowledge of the exercise regimen and return the demonstration independently.

1. To increase compliance with the prescribed exercise regimen, provide patient with an explanation of the rationale for the exercises, method of performing the exercises, and suggestions for adapting these exercises to home use. Most therapeutic programs include ROM and muscle-strengthening exercises.

2. Demonstrate each exercise until the patient is able to return the demonstration independently. Provide patient with written instructions that review each exercise and describe the number of repetitions and number of times a day it should be performed, and a phone number to call should any questions arise after patient is discharged.

3. If additional equipment is required, provide patient with information regarding where it can be purchased and, if necessary, seek financial assistance from social services.

Knowledge deficit: Care of the stump and prosthesis; signs and symptoms of skin irritation or pressure necrosis

Desired outcomes: Patient can verbalize knowledge of the care of the stump and prosthesis and independently return the demonstration of wrapping the stump. Patient can verbalize knowledge of the indicators of pressure necrosis and irritation from the wrapping device or prosthesis.

▶ **Note:** A stump that is inappropriately treated will become edematous and more easily prone to injury, which will delay proper fitting of the permanent prosthesis.

1. If molding of the stump for eventual prosthetic fitting is prescribed, instruct the patient in the technique for application of an elastic sleeve or wrap: Application of the elastic wrap is begun with a recurrent turn over the distal end of the stump and then diagonal circumferential turns are made, overlapping half to two-thirds of the width of the wrap. Traction applied to the wrap should ensure more pressure on the distal portion of the stump. The elastic device should be snug but not excessively so, since a tight wrap can impede circulation and healing. Rewrapping should be done q4h, combined with careful inspection of the stump. Areas prone to pressure, such as bony prominences or prominent tendons, should be assessed for evidence of excess pressure. Ensure that all tissue is contained by the elastic device. If any tissue is allowed to bulge, proper fitting of the prosthesis will be difficult.

2. Teach patient to monitor the stump for indicators of skin irritation or pressure necrosis caused by the elastic device or prosthesis, including blebs, abrasions, and erythemic or tender areas. Explain that if massage fails to alleviate the problem, the patient should seek the help of the public health nurse or visiting nurse or notify the MD.

3. For areas that are prone to pressure, provide extra padding with sheet wadding, moleskin, or lambswool to prevent irritation.

4. The day after the sutures have been removed (and assuming the incision is dry and intact) instruct the patient to cleanse the stump daily with mild soap and water. Caution against the use of emollients, which can create skin maceration beneath the prosthesis.

5. Advise patient that when molding is no longer necessary (after 1–6 months), he or she will be fitted with a stump sock, which allows air to circulate around the stump.

6. Ensure that patient receives complete instructions in the care of the prosthesis by the prosthetist or knowledgeable nurse.

Potential fluid volume deficit related to abnormal loss secondary to postsurgical hemorrhage

Desired outcomes: Patient does not exhibit signs of hypovolemia or excessive bleeding. Patient is aware of the importance of promptly reporting bleeding to the staff.

1. Inspect the postoperative dressing (or cast) for increasing drainage. If the stump is elevated, inspect dependent areas for evidence of bleeding. Inform patient of the need to report increasing bleeding to staff.

2. If a drain or drainage device is used, document the amount of drainage. Report drainage that exceeds 50 mL/h.

Alteration in comfort: Pain related to phantom limb sensations

Desired outcome: Patient relates a reduction in phantom limb sensations and does not exhibit signs of uncontrolled pain.

1. Explain to the patient that continued sensations often arise from the amputated part. Although they can be painful, irritating, or simply disconcerting, these sensations usually resolve with time.

2. Manage these painful sensations with the interventions discussed in **Alteration in comfort:** Pain, p. 367, in "Osteoarthritis." For this type of pain, counterirritation is especially useful. Other phantom limb sensations may respond to similar tactics, such as distraction, relaxation, or use of cutaneous stimulation via oil of wintergreen, heat, or massage.

3. Some MDs advocate vigorous stimulation of the end of the stump to alter the feedback loop of the resected nerve. Advise patient that this can be done by hitting the end of a *well-healed* stump with a rolled towel.

4. Chronic phantom limb sensation may require exploration of the stump to resect a neuroma at the site of the nerve resection. Inform patient that this may be a possibility if phantom limb sensations continue for more than 6 months.

Disturbance in self-concept related to alterations in body image and role performance secondary to amputation

Desired outcome: Patient begins to show adaptation toward loss of the limb and demonstrates role-related responsibilities.

1. Be aware that use of a prosthesis immediately after surgery allows patients to continue to perceive of themselves as ambulatory (and thus "whole") individuals.

2. Gently encourage patient to look at and touch the stump and verbalize feelings about the amputation. It is essential that the nurse and other caregivers show an accepting attitude as well as encourage SOs to accept the patient as he or she now appears.

3. Assist patient with adapting to the loss of the limb while maintaining a sense of what is perceived as the "normal" self. This may be accomplished by introducing patient to others who have successfully adapted to an amputation similar to that of the patient. In addition, teaching aids such as audiovisuals, books, pamphlets, and videotapes can be employed to demonstrate how others have adapted to the amputation.

4. For patients who continue to have difficulty adapting to the amputation, provide a referral to an appropriate resource person, such as a psychologist or psychiatric nurse.

> See "Osteoarthritis" for the following: **Alteration in comfort**, p. 367. See "Fractures" for the following: **Knowledge deficit:** Potential for infection, p. 395. See "Appendix One" for nursing diagnoses and interventions for the care of preoperative and postoperative patients, pp. 528–532, and for the care of patients with cancer and other life-disrupting illnesses, pp. 544–551.

E. Patient–Family Teaching and Discharge Planning

Provide patient and SOs with verbal and written information for the following:

1. How and where to purchase necessary supplies and equipment for self care.

2. Care of the stump and prosthesis.

3. Indicators of wound infection, which necessitate medical attention: swelling, persistent redness, discharge, local warmth, systemic fever, and pain.

4. Medications, including name, rationale, dosage, schedule, precautions, and potential side effects.

5. Phone number of a resource person, should questions arise after hospital discharge.

6. Prescribed exercises. Patient should be able to perform them independently before discharge.

7. Referral to appropriate resource person, should maladaptive behaviors associated with grieving or body image disturbance continue.

8. Ambulation with assistive device and prosthesis on level and uneven surfaces and on stairs. Patient should demonstrate independence before hospital discharge. For patients with an upper-extremity amputation, independence with ADLs should be demonstrated before discharge

III. Tendon Transfer

A tendon transfer involves the transference of the insertion site of a functioning muscle-tendon unit to a new position to change the action of that unit. This allows compensation of a deficit created by paralyzed or severed muscle. Because there is considerable overlap in function, in that multiple muscles often serve one purpose, tendon transfer may allow the patient to regain function without any concomitant loss of function.

A. Diagnostic Test

Electromyography: Can be used to ensure adequate muscle function of the units proposed for transfer.

B. Medical Management and Surgical Interventions

1. **Surgical procedure:** Involves transection of the tendon at an appropriate level, transfer to the new position, and fixation to the appropriate insertion site with permanent sutures, staples, screws, or wire. It is also possible to attach "new" tendon to the resected tendon above the insertion site using tendon repair suture techniques. Examples of disorders in which tendon transfer procedures are performed include radial paralysis, congenital talipes equinovarus (a form of clubfoot), and extensive injury to the extensor pollicis longus, which limits thumb extension.

2. **Postsurgical immobilization:** The operant area is immobilized until there has been sufficient healing of the tendon repair (2–6 weeks) or stabilization of the bony insertion site (4–12 weeks).

3. **Physical therapy regimen:** After immobilization, the patient is begun on an intense, progressive physical therapy regimen to regain strength in the transferred tendon, retrain new muscle function, and compensate for decreased strength at the site of the transfer. Various orthotics and special exercise rigs can be constructed to aid the patient in regaining function.

C. Nursing Diagnoses and Interventions

See "Osteoarthritis" for the following: **Alteration in comfort**, p. 367, and **Impaired physical mobility** related to adjustment to a new walking gait, p. 368. See "Ligamentous Injuries" for the following: **Knowledge deficit:** Care and assessment of the casted extremity, p. 377. See "Torn Anterior Cruciate Ligament" for the following: **Potential fluid volume deficit** related to loss secondary to postsurgical hemorrhage or hematoma, p. 383. See "Bunionectomy" for the following: **Potential alteration in tissue perfusion:** Peripheral, related to impaired circulation secondary to compression from circumferential casts or dressings, p. 404. See "Appendix One" for nursing diagnoses and interventions for the care of preoperative and postoperative patients, pp. 528–532.

D. Patient–Family Teaching and Discharge Plannning

Provide patient and SOs with verbal and written information for the following:

1. Use of therapies such as thermotherapy and elevation.
2. Use of external support devices such as elastic wraps, splints, or similar items. This should include care of the device, care of the skin beneath the device, monitoring the area for presence of irritation, and monitoring for neurovascular deficit.
3. Cast care instructions, if patient is discharged with a cast (see p. 377).
4. Prescribed exercise regimen, including rationale for the therapy, how it is accomplished, number of repetitions, and frequency of the exercise.
5. Medications, including name, rationale, dosage, schedule, precautions, and potential side effects.
6. Indicators of wound infection, which necessitate medical attention: persistent redness, swelling, wound discharge, local warmth, and increase in pain.
7. Use of ambulatory aid, if patient is discharged with one. This should include return demonstration of independence in ambulation on level and uneven surfaces and stairs before discharge.
8. Phone number of resource person, should questions arise after patient has been discharged.

IV. Bone Grafting

A bone graft procedure refers to the transfer of cancellous and/or cortical bone from one site to another. The bone can be from the patient (autogenic), another human (homogenic), or another species (heterogenic). Currently, the most successful results are achieved with autogenic grafts, but homogenic grafting is showing increasing promise as a therapeutic resource. Bone grafts can be required to create bony fusion of a joint (arthrodesis), compensate for lost or inadequately developed bone, or correct bony non-union of fractures.

Current microsurgical techniques permit myocutaneous-bone or muscle-bone grafts that involve bone, overlying muscle, and/or skin. These complex grafting techniques provide much greater potential for success for procedures that are used to rebuild large areas from which tissue has been lost due to trauma or necessary surgical resection. The following discussion is limited to traditional, simple autogenic bone grafting procedures.

A. Diagnostic Tests

The need for bone grafts can be documented by the following: AP x-rays, gallium scans (to rule out osteomyelitis), and angiograms to evaluate blood supply when myocutaneous–bone or muscle–bone grafts are to be done.

B. Medical Management and Surgical Interventions

1. **Bone graft procedure:** Most commonly, bone grafts are taken from the anterior or posterior iliac crest. However, bone grafts also can be harvested from the fibula, tibia, or ribs. The graft usually involves resection of a piece of cortical bone that is fashioned to replace the deficit or enhance bony fusion or fixation. Usually, cancellous bone is taken from the same site and packed in and around the cortical graft to facilitate new bone formation. The donor site frequently oozes blood, so a postoperative drain is often placed.

2. **Postoperative regimen:** Usually, the recipient site requires immobilization (most often with a cast) to prevent dislodging of the graft. Some bone grafts require internal fixation to hold them in place.

C. Nursing Diagnoses and Interventions

See "Osteoarthritis" for the following: **Alteration in comfort**, p. 367, and **Impaired physical mobility** related to adjustment to a new walking gait, p. 368. See "Ligamentous Injuries" for the following: **Knowledge deficit:** Care and assessment of the casted extremity, p. 377. See "Torn Anterior Cruciate Ligament" for the following: **Potential fluid volume deficit** related to loss secondary to postsurgical hemorrhage or hematoma, p. 383. See "Bunionectomy" for the following: **Potential alteration in tissue perfusion:** Peripheral, related to impaired circulation secondary to compression from circumferential casts or dressings, p. 404. See "Appendix One" for nursing diagnoses and interventions for the care of preoperative and postoperative patients, pp. 528–532.

D. Patient–Family Teaching and Discharge Planning

See "Tendon Transfer," p. 409.

V. Repair of Recurrent Shoulder Dislocation

The shoulder is a complex set of joints, including the glenohumeral, sternoclavicular, acromioclavicular, and thoracoscapular joints, all of which act in combination to allow function. Of these joints, the glenohumeral joint is most commonly affected by dislocation. Most glenohumeral dislocations originate with trauma. Once periarticular weakness and laxity are established, the shoulder can dislocate with minimal stress while abducting. A shoulder repair is necessary when the patient has significant pain and compromised function.

▶ **Note:** See "Dislocation/Subluxation," p. 379, for a discussion of assessment, diagnostic tests, and medical management.

A. Medical Management and Surgical Interventions

1. **Bristow procedure:** Transfers the short ends of the biceps and coracobrachialis muscular origin sites from the coracoid process to the scapular neck. The new positions allow these muscles to hold the head of the humerus in its anatomic position within the glenoid cavity.

2. **Bankart procedure:** Involves reattaching the anterior joint capsule to the

front rim of the glenoid cavity to reduce laxity and prevent anterior dislocation.

3. **Putti-Platt procedure:** Involves reefing (shortening) of the subscapularis tendon to prevent excessive lateral rotation, which can contribute to dislocation.

4. **Postoperative care:** After surgery, the patient is usually placed in a shoulder immobilizer for 7–14 days. If the patient has large shoulder muscles, a postoperative drain may be required. After immobilization, a regimen of progressive ROM exercises is begun, first to regain ROM and then to increase muscle strength.

B. Nursing Diagnoses and Interventions

Potential impairment of skin integrity related to maceration of the axillary skin secondary to shoulder immobilization

Desired outcomes: Patient does not exhibit signs of skin impairment. Patient can verbalize knowledge of the established plan of prevention and the signs and symptoms of maceration.

1. Assess patient's axillary skin before surgery to evaluate the potential for maceration, including open wounds, areas of irritation, and excessive perspiration.

2. Teach patient the rationale and interventions used for preventing maceration and the need to report indicators of maceration such as pain, burning, irritation, and foul odor.

3. Cleanse the axilla well before surgery.

4. Before the shoulder immobilizer is positioned, the operating room nurse will place a cotton (ABD) pad in the axilla. After 2–3 days, remove the pad. Then cleanse, thoroughly dry, and inspect the axilla (as well as possible) without abducting the shoulder. Usually, this can be done by holding a washcloth in the hand and sliding the hand into the axilla. Although talc can be used, its use should be judicious because it can build up and act as a reservoir for moisture. Replace the cotton pad with a new one and document the condition of the skin. If the patient is not allergic, a deodorant pad may be used instead.

Potential alteration in tissue perfusion: Peripheral, related to impaired circulation and compression of the musculocutaneous nerve secondary to pressure from the immobilization device

Desired outcomes: Patient does not exhibit signs of impaired nerve function. Patient can verbalize knowledge of the signs and symptoms of impaired sensorimotor function and the importance of notifying the staff promptly should they occur.

1. Unless it is contraindicated, encourage flexion and extension of the fingers and wrist to enhance perfusion to the muscles and nerves.

2. Monitor the wrist and upper arm for evidence of pressure and/or irritation from the immobilizer. However, be aware that the device must be sufficiently tight to ensure adequate immobilization.

3. With every VS assessment, evaluate upper extremity nerve function. Be especially alert to the patient's inability to contract the biceps muscle and to absent or abnormal sensations along the radial portion of the forearm. Notify MD of significant findings.

4. Instruct the patient to notify the staff promptly should any alterations in sensory or motor function occur.

See "Osteoarthritis" for the following: **Alteration in comfort**, p. 367. See "Amputation" for the following: **Knowledge deficit:** Postsurgical exercise regimen, p. 406. See "Appendix One" for nursing diagnoses and interventions for the care of preoperative and postoperative patients, pp. 528–532.

C. Patient–Family Teaching and Discharge Planning

Provide patient and SOs with verbal and written information for the following:

1. Prescribed exercise regimen, including rationale for each exercise, method of performing the exercise, number of repetitions for each, and frequency of the exercise periods. Be sure the patient can return the demonstration independently before discharge.

2. Indicators of wound infection, which necessitate medical attention: swelling, persistent redness, local warmth, fever, and pain.

3. For patients discharged with braces or immobilizers, the use and care of the device and care of the axilla on the operant side.

4. Medications, including name, rationale, dosage, schedule, precautions, and potential side effects.

5. Phone number of a resource person, should questions arise after hospital discharge.

VI. Total Hip Arthroplasty

Total hip arthroplasty (THA) is surgery involving resection of the hip joint and its replacement with an endoprosthesis. Conditions resulting in the need for a THA include osteoarthritis, rheumatoid arthritis, ankylosing spondylosis (Marie-Strumpell disease), Legg-Calve-Perthes disease, and severe hip trauma. Usually, THA is restricted to older patients because the duration of the implant life is unknown. However, younger patients with severe disease also undergo this procedure.

THA is performed when the joint has been severely affected by disease, resulting in significant pain and a femoroacetabular articulation without useful function. Because it is an irreversible procedure involving the removal of significant amounts of bone, several conditions should be met before the patient is considered a serious candidate. In addition to severe pain and loss of function, conservative therapies need to have been exhausted and the patient should demonstrate compliance to past therapeutic regimens and be free of any concurrent infectious process.

A. Diagnostic Tests

1. <u>Gallium scan and ESR:</u> May be indicated to rule out concurrent infection.

2. <u>Scintigraphy:</u> Can be used to document leg length discrepancy, which can be surgically compensated for by using alternative neck lengths on the femoral prosthesis.

B. Medical Management and Surgical Interventions

1. **Surgical procedure:** Although the actual surgical procedure for THA can be accomplished via a variety of approaches, it is most commonly done through a posterior lateral approach. Methylmethacrylate may be used as a grouting agent to hold the endoprosthesis in place, or special prosthetics coated with porous materials may be used to allow bony ingrowth to internally fix the devices. Once the prosthetic acetabulum is positioned, the femoral canal is reamed to accept the femoral prosthesis. A drain is then inserted into the deeper layers of the wound.

2. **Antibiotics:** Because the potential for infection is increased with the presence of the massive endoprosthesis, the patient is placed on prophylactic antibiotics before, during, and for at least 5 days after surgery. Infection of the THA may require its temporary or permanent removal.

3. **Postsurgical immobilization:** The patient is immobilized in a balanced suspension or similar device (A-frame, abduction pillow, or wedge abduction pillow) to prevent internal rotation, adduction, and flexion past 90°, which can cause dislocation of the endoprosthesis. If methylmethacrylate is used, the patient will be more readily mobile (usually within 5 days) because of the im-

mediate fixation of the device. If a porous-coated device is used, it is not immediately fixed in place and the patient may require longer immobilization (several days to several weeks). If the greater trochanter was removed to allow visualization or correct muscle weakness, it will require wiring and further immobilization for at least 3 weeks in balanced suspension or limited weight-bearing for several weeks.

4. **Progressive physical therapy:** To regain muscular strength and to ensure the patient has adequate upper extremity strength to allow ambulation with crutches or a walker. During postoperative immobilization, the patient begins muscle-strengthening exercises using balanced suspension (or a similar device). The patient must be reminded to avoid internal rotation, adduction, and flexion of the hip past 90°.

C. Nursing Diagnoses and Interventions

Knowledge deficit: Potential for and mechanism of THA dislocation, preventive measures, positional restrictions, prescribed ambulation regimen, and use of assistive devices

Desired outcomes: Patient can verbalize knowledge of the potential for, preventive measures for, and mechanism of THA dislocation and can demonstrate the prescribed regimen for ambulation and performance of ADLs without experiencing dislocation.

▶ **Note:** There is a high risk of dislocation until the periarticular tissues scar down around the endoprosthesis. If it occurs once, there is increased potential for recurrence because the periarticular tissues will have been stretched. Dislocation is treated with reduction under anesthesia and immobilization in balanced suspension for 3–6 weeks. Recurrent dislocation may require surgical intervention to tighten periarticular tissues or revise the THA. After 6 weeks, the properly placed THA has significantly decreased potential for dislocation. The following discussion relates to the posteriolateral approach for THA surgery. Other approaches require different positional restrictions.

1. Advise patient about the potential for dislocation and its implications in the preoperative period.
2. Show patient what the endoprosthesis looks like (using a model or similar implant) and how easily it can be dislocated when positional restrictions are not followed.
3. During the preoperative period, instruct patient in the use of ambulatory aids and ADL-assistive devices that allow independence without violation of positional restrictions. Explain the use of devices used to maintain positional restrictions.
4. After surgery, reinforce positional restrictions and restriction of activities that involve these positions, including pivoting on the affected leg, sitting on a regular-height toilet seat, bending over to tie shoelaces, or crossing the legs.
5. Advise patient about the need for long-handled shoe horn, pickup sticks, stocking helpers, and a raised toilet seat for use after discharge. Provide addresses for stores that retail these items.
6. Be sure the patient verbalizes and demonstrates understanding of the positional restrictions and is able to accomplish ambulation and performance of ADLs independently, using the assistive device.

Knowledge deficit: Potential for infection caused by foreign body reaction to the endoprosthesis

Desired outcome: Patient can verbalize knowledge of the ongoing potential for infection, its indicators, and the importance of seeking prompt medical care should they occur.

1. Advise patient that infection potential will be a permanent situation. Because of foreign body reaction and increased blood supply resulting from associated inflammatory response, these patients are at increased risk for hematogenic (blood borne) infection. Introduce this as a potential complication as part of the informed consent process and review it as part of preoperative teaching.

2. Before hospital discharge, ensure that the patient verbalizes understanding of the indicators of wound, urinary tract, upper respiratory, and dental infections. Include this information on a written handout that reviews the information and lists a phone number to call should questions arise after hospital discharge.

3. Advise patient to wear a Medic-Alert bracelet and always to request prophylactic antibiotics for procedures that can result in bacterial seeding of the bloodstream, such as minor or major surgery or dental extractions.

4. Advise patient to call MD promptly should indicators of infection of the THA occur. These can include drainage, pain, fever, local warmth, swelling, restricted ROM of the joint, and feelings of pressure in the hip.

Potential alteration in tissue perfusion: Peripheral, related to impaired circulation secondary to compression from traction or abduction device

Desired outcomes: Patient does not exhibit signs of impaired neurovascular status. Patient can verbalize knowledge of potential neurovascular complications and the importance of reporting indicators of impairment.

1. Because the traction sling or abduction device can press on neurovascular structures, it is imperative that neurovascular status of the leg in traction, especially peroneal nerve function, be assessed along with the VS. The peroneal nerve runs superficially by the neck of the fibula and can be assessed by gently pricking the dermatome of the first web space between the great and second toes and having patient dorsiflex the foot. Loss of sensation and/or movement signals impaired peroneal nerve function.

2. Be sure patient is aware of the potential for neurovascular impairment and the importance of reporting alterations in sensations and movements.

3. Encourage patient to reposition the leg within the restrictions of the sling and positional limitations.

4. Encourage patient to perform prescribed exercises as a means of stimulating circulation in the area.

See "Osteoarthritis" for the following: **Alteration in comfort**, p. 367, and **Impaired physical mobility** related to adjustment to a new walking gait, p. 368. See "Torn Anterior Cruciate Ligament" for the following: **Potential fluid volume deficit** related to loss secondary to postsurgical hemorrhage or hematoma, p. 383. See "Amputation" for the following: **Knowledge deficit:** Postsurgical exercise regimen, p. 406. See "Appendix One" for nursing diagnoses and interventions for the care of preoperative and postoperative patients, pp. 528–532, and care of patients on prolonged bed rest, pp. 533–537.

D. Patient–Family Teaching and Discharge Planning

Provide patient and SOs with verbal and written information for the following:

1. Prescribed exercise regimen, including rationale for each exercise, number of repetitions for each, and frequency of the exercise periods. Be sure patient verbalizes understanding of the exercises and gives a return demonstration before hospital discharge.

2. Indicators of the types of infections, including the following: *wound* (persistent redness, swelling, discharge, local warmth, restricted hip ROM, feel-

ings of hip pressure, fever, and pain); *urinary tract* (dysuria, pyuria, foul odor to the urine, cloudy urine, urgency, frequency, and pain in the suprapubic, flank, groin, scrotal, or labial area); *upper respiratory tract* (change in color or amount of sputum, cough, sore throat, malaise, fever); and *dental* (pain, swelling of the jaw, difficulty with mastication, fever). Advise patient to notify MD promptly if any of these indicators occur and to seek prophylactic antibiotics for minor surgical procedures.

3. Assistive devices (eg, pickup sticks, stocking helpers, long-handled shoe horns, and raised toilet seat). Ensure that patient demonstrates independence in their use before hospital discharge.

4. Ambulation with crutches on level and uneven surfaces.

5. Getting in a car safely without risking dislocation. The patient should be able to demonstrate this procedure before hospital discharge.

6. Medications, including name, rationale, dosage, schedule, precautions, and potential side effects.

7. Phone number of a resource person should questions arise after hospital discharge

VII. Total Knee Arthroplasty

Total knee arthroplasty (TKA) is surgery that involves resection of the knee joint and its replacement with an endoprosthesis. Several pathologic conditions can result in the need for TKA, including osteoarthritis, rheumatoid arthritis, gouty arthritis, hemophilic arthritis, and severe knee trauma. Generally, TKA is restricted to older patients because the life span of the implant is unknown. However, younger patients also undergo this procedure, depending on the severity of the disease, amount of pain, and degree of functional deficit in the femorotibial and/or femoropatellar articulations. Because this procedure is irreversible and involves the removal of significant amounts of bone from the femur, tibia, and patella, several conditions must be met before the patient is considered a potential candidate. Conservative methods of therapy must have been exhausted and there has to be significant loss of function and pain that severely limit ambulation and ADL. In addition, the patient must have demonstrated compliance with past medical regimens and be free of any concurrent infectious process.

A. Diagnostic Tests

See discussion with "Total Hip Arthroplasty," p. 412. In addition, arthroscopy may be useful in confirming the extent of the pathology to identify the appropriate prosthesis.

B. Medical Management and Surgical Interventions

1. **Surgical procedure:** The approach varies with the type of prosthetic device used. During the procedure a skin flap is created. If the blood supply is compromised during surgery or from postoperative hematoma formation, the flap can necrose and jeopardize the success of the operation; therefore it requires careful monitoring. The implant is internally fixed with methylmethacrylate or bony ingrowth. The wound is sutured closed in layers and a drain is left in place.

2. **Postoperative immobilization:** Usually accomplished with a Jones dressing, which is composed of a bulky padding with anterior, posterior, and lateral plaster splints that are held in place with an elastic wrap. The Jones dressing ensures immobilization while allowing for edema formation to minimize the risk of iatrogenic compartment syndrome. If the implant is to be held in place with bony ingrowth, the leg may be immobilized within a cast after postoperative edema has subsided.

3. **Ambulation:** If methylmethacrylate was used to internally fix the implant, the patient may be permitted to ambulate without weightbearing within 3–5

days, slowly advancing to weightbearing as tolerated within 10–14 days. ROM of the knee is often done within 5 days under supervision of a physical therapist. For implants held in place with bony ingrowth, ambulation is not begun until after 10–14 days, and weightbearing may be contraindicated for as long as 6–12 weeks. If there is a cast, ROM is not begun until the cast has been removed.

4. **Continuous passive motion (CPM):** Usually advocated for patients who undergo a TKA. The CPM device is applied to the patient's bed and the operant extremity is positioned in a sling in the device. The device then moves the leg through preset limits of ROM in preset timed cycles. Use of CPM allows greater ROM with less pain. (The minimal flexion for a successful TKA is 90–110°).

C. Nursing Diagnoses and Interventions

See all nursing diagnoses (except **Knowledge deficit:** Potential for and mechanism of THA dislocation) in "Total Hip Arthroplasty," pp. 413–414.

D. Patient–Family Teaching and Discharge Planning

See "Total Hip Arthroplasty," p. 414.

► Selected References

Adams JC: *Outline of Orthopaedics*. Churchill-Livingstone, 1976.

Althoff DG: External fixation of the lower extremity: Care considerations. In: *Assessment and Fracture Management of the Lower Extremities*. Hilt N (editor). National Association of Orthopaedic Nurses, 1984.

Berger MR: Bunions: An overview. *Orthopaedic Nursing* Sept/Oct 1984; 3:17.

Dalinka MK, Aronchick JM, Haddad JG: Paget's disease. *Orthop Clin North Am* Jan 1983; 14:3.

Day LJ et al: Orthopedics. In: *Current Surgical Diagnosis and Treatment*, 6th ed. Way LW (editor). Lange, 1983.

DeHaven KE: Arthroscopy in the diagnosis and management of the anterior cruciate ligament deficient knee. *Clin Orthop* Jan/Feb 1983; 172:52–56.

Engleman EP, Shearn MA: Arthritis and allied rheumatic disorders. In: *Current Medical Diagnosis and Treatment 1983*. Krupp MA, Chatton MJ (editors). Lange, 1983.

Farrell J: Helping the new amputee. *Orthopaedic Nursing* May-June, 1982; 2:18.

Farrell J: *Illustrated Guide to Orthopedic Nursing*, 2nd ed. Lippincott, 1982.

Holden CEA: Simple bone grafts. In: *The Severely Injured Limb*. Ackroyd CE, O'Connor BT, de Bruyn PF (editors). Churchill-Livingstone, 1983.

Jergensen FH: Osteomyelitis. In: *Current Surgical Diagnosis and Treatment*. Way LW (editor). Lange, 1983.

Johnson RJ: The anterior cruciate ligament problem. *Clin Orthop* Jan/Feb 1983; 172:14–18.

Kennedy JC: Application of prosthetics to anterior cruciate ligament reconstruction and repair. *Clin Orthop* Jan/Feb 1983; 172:125–129.

Koerner ME, Dickinson GR: Arthritis: A look at some of its forms. *AJN* 1983; 83: 254.

Lane PL, Lee MM: New synthetic casts: What nurses need to know. *Orthopaedic Nursing* Nov-Dec 1982; 1:13.

Miller MC: Nursing care of the patient with external fixation therapy. *Orthopaedic Nursing* Jan-Feb 1983; 2:11–15.

Moye C: Nursing care of the amputee: An overview. *Orthopaedic Nursing* May/June 1982; 2:33.

Ross DG: Anatomy and assessment of the knee. In: *Lower Extremity Assessment and Fracture Management* (monograph). National Association of Orthopaedic Nurses (editors). 1984:14–21.

Ross DG: Diagnostic overview: Paget's disease. *Orthopaedic Nursing* May-June 1984; 3:41.

Ross DG: Musculoskeletal nursing. In: *Current Medical Surgical Nursing*. Sitzmann J (editor). Lange, 1986.

Rutan F: Preprosthetic program for the amputee. *Orthopaedic Nursing* May-June 1982; 2:14.

Spickler LL: Knee injuries of the athlete. *Orthopaedic Nursing* Sept/Oct 1983; 2:11.

Steadman JR: Rehabilitation of acute injuries of the anterior cruciate ligament. *Clin Orthop* 1983; 172:129–132.

Tanagho EA, Smith DR: Urology. In: *Current Surgical Diagnosis and Treatment*, 6th ed. Way, LW (editor). Lange, 1983.

Walker ARP: Human requirements of calcium: Should low intakes be supplemented? *Am J Clin Nutrition* 1972; 25:518.

Wallerstein RO: Blood. In: *Current Medical Diagnosis and Treatment*, 1983. Krupp MA, Chatton MJ (editors). Lange, 1983.

Zangara RJ: Arthritis and related disorders. In: *Manual of Medical Therapeutics*, 24th ed. Campbell JW, Frisse M (editors). Little, Brown, 1983.

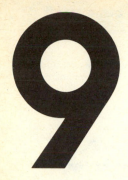

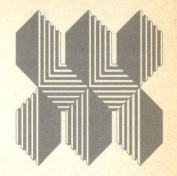

9

Reproductive Disorders

> ► Section One **Surgeries and Disorders of the Breast**

I. Breast Augmentation

Breast augmentation is the implantation of suitable material into the breast to increase breast size. The decision for surgery is made by the patient, who then seeks a qualified practitioner, usually a plastic surgeon, to perform the surgery.

A. Assessment

Clinical indicators: Because the procedure is elective, there are no specific indicators. Frequently, the patient has had a decrease in breast size following weight loss, or she may never have been satisfied with the size of her breasts. The patient should not have unrealistic expectations for the surgery such as saving a marriage or offsetting a problem such as obesity.

Physical examination: The breasts may be small, or there may be some muscle looseness that causes them to sag. There should be no signs of breast disease such as nipple discharge and puckering of the skin. (See "Malignant Disorders of the Breast," p. 426, for other signs.)

B. Diagnostic Tests

There are no tests specific for breast augmentation. However, routine laboratory tests may be performed to confirm the patient's physical readiness for surgery.

C. Surgical Intervention

An inframammary incision is made into the breast, positioned so that the scar will not be evident. An implant, usually a silastic envelope containing silicone gel, is inserted into the submuscular pocket subpectorally or subcutaneously.

D. Nursing Diagnoses and Interventions

Disturbance in self-concept related to body image secondary to small breast size

Desired outcome: Patient expresses positive and realistic reasons for having breast augmentation and is supported in her decision to have this surgery.

   1. Review the patient's expectations for the outcome of surgery. The patient should not have unrealistic expectations as evidenced by statements such as "Surgery will change my life or marriage."
   2. Provide support for the patient's decision to have this surgery by spending time with her and allowing her to verbalize fears and concerns.
   3. If appropriate, allow the patient to express feelings such as being "self-centered." Be nonjudgmental about her feelings.

Alteration in comfort: Pain related to surgical procedure

Desired outcome: Patient relates a reduction in discomfort and does not exhibit signs of uncontrolled pain.

   1. Assess and document location, quality, and duration of the pain.
   2. Medicate the patient with analgesics as prescribed; evaluate and document the response.
   3. Provide ice packs to decrease swelling in the early postoperative period.
   4. Ensure that the patient has a comfortable bra that adequately supports her breasts.
   5. Teach the patient relaxation techniques such as slow, diaphragmatic breathing and guided imagery.
   6. Provide distractions such as television or soothing music.
   7. Encourage activity as tolerated.

Knowledge deficit: Incisional site care and the potential for postoperative capsular contracture

Desired outcome: Patient can verbalize knowledge of incisional site care and the potential for capsular contracture.

1. Instruct patient to cleanse the incisional site after the sutures have been removed, using basic hygiene such as soap and water. Explain that heavy lotions, medications, or creams should not be used unless specified by MD.
2. In preparation for hospital discharge, instruct patient in self-examination techniques for signs of fibrotic capsular formation, which can be evidenced by displacement of the implant and hardening of the breast.
3. If prescribed, teach the procedure for breast massage to help prevent capsular contraction: Using a gentle rotary motion, squeeze and then flatten the breast. Typically, this is performed twice daily, either immediately after the surgery or after the wound heals. Have the patient demonstrate the procedure before discharge from the hospital if it has been prescribed for the immediate postoperative period.

See "Appendix One" for nursing diagnoses and interventions for the care of preoperative and postoperative patients, pp. 528–532.

E. Patient–Family Teaching and Discharge Planning

Provide patient and SOs with verbal and written information for the following:

1. Medications, including the drug name, purpose, dosage, schedule, precautions, and potential side effects.
2. Indicators of wound infection, which must be reported to the MD: persistent redness, pain, swelling, and drainage at the incisional area.
3. Care of the incision site, including cleansing and dressing, if indicated.
4. Importance of monthly breast self-examination (BSE). Teach the technique to patients who do not know it.
5. Activity restrictions, which may include limited use of the arm for 2 weeks postoperatively with resumption of full activity after 3 weeks.
6. Breast massage, if prescribed as a prophylaxis for capsular contraction.

II. Breast Reconstruction

After a mastectomy, a woman may elect to have breast reconstruction in an attempt to create a breast "mound" in place of the lost breast. Although there is no medical indication for breast reconstruction, psychologic benefits may result. Breast reconstruction can usually be performed at the time of mastectomy. However, when positive axillary nodes are discovered, reconstruction is delayed at least 3 months to avoid poorer cosmetic results secondary to radiation or chemotherapy. This surgery has become more popular in recent years because the technique continues to improve and patients are becoming more aware of the procedure and its benefits.

A. Assessment

Clinical indicators: Absence of the breast, patient's desire for surgery, sufficient tissue present, and absence of progressive disease.

Physical exam: There should be no evidence of infection, and healing of the mastectomy scar should be complete if a surgical delay was indicated.

B. Diagnostic Tests

There are no diagnostic tests specific to reconstruction; however, routine laboratory tests may be performed to confirm the patient's physical readiness for surgery.

C. Medical Managment and Surgical Interventions

1. **Analgesics and possibly narcotics:** To control postsurgical discomfort.

2. **IV therapy:** To treat dehydration secondary to surgery.

3. **Balanced diet:** As tolerated to enhance tissue restoration.

4. **Surgical procedure:** Varying procedures may be involved, depending on the amount of tissue left at the reconstruction site. When there is sufficient tissue, an implant is placed under the pectoralis and serratus muscles. If a radical mastectomy has been performed, there is usually inadequate soft tissue, muscle, and skin on which to place the implant. It then becomes necessary to graft tissue from other locations, such as the latissimus dorsi flap or rectus abdominis musculocutaneous flap. Latissimus dorsi flap reconstruction involves the transfer of the muscle, skin, and subcutaneous tissue from the back to the mastectomy site. The rectus abdominis musculocutaneous flap involves the transfer of one of the rectus abdominis muscles, as well as overlying skin, subcutaneous fat (lipectomy), and artery to the mastectomy site. With this procedure an implant also may be needed, depending on the amount of tissue available. If a nipple is desired on the reconstructed breast, it can be created from skin of the inner thigh, buttock, labia, or the other nipple.

5. **Suction apparatus:** Placed in the wound to minimize the chance of hematoma formation.

D. Nursing Diagnoses and Interventions

Knowledge deficit: The surgical procedure, preoperative care, and postoperative regimen

Desired outcome: Patient can verbalize knowledge of the surgical procedure and expected results as well as preoperative care and the postoperative regimen.

1. Explain that after surgery a suction apparatus will be present, which removes blood to minimize the potential for hematoma formation. This is usually removed when drainage is less than 10–20 mL over 24 hours.

2. Consult with the MD to arrange a visit by a woman who has had breast reconstruction surgery to share feelings and demonstrate the cosmetic results.

3. Explain that movement and activity may be restricted following surgery, depending on the procedure used. When an implant is placed under ample tissue, recovery is rapid and hospitalization is usually 1–3 days; flap reconstruction is more involved and movement and activity may be more restricted. Patients with a latissimus flap reconstruction are usually discharged after 2–5 days, when the drains are removed. A rectus abdominis procedure is more extensive, and because of the lipectomy the patient is usually on bed rest for several days and discharged after a week.

4. For other interventions, see the same nursing diagnosis in "Caring for Preoperative and Postoperative Patients," "Appendix One," p. 528.

Knowledge deficit: Potential for postoperative fibrotic capsular contraction and the technique for breast massage

Desired outcome: Patient can verbalize knowledge of the potential for fibrotic capsular contraction and demonstrate the technique for breast massage.

1. Explain to the patient that fibrotic capsular contraction is a potential complication of breast reconstruction surgery.

2. To minimize the risk of fibrotic capsular contracture, teach breast massage by the second or third postoperative day. This involves using a gentle rotary motion to squeeze and flatten the breast. Usually it is performed at least three times a day.

Potential fluid volume deficit related to abnormal loss secondary to postsurgical hemorrhage or hematoma formation

Desired outcomes: Patient does not exhibit signs of excessive bleeding/drainage. If a hematoma is present, it is detected and reported promptly.

1. Assess for the appearance of a hematoma as evidenced by swelling, pain, and possibly a bluish discoloration of the skin. Report significant findings to the MD.

2. Assess the suction apparatus for patency, and document the amount and character of the drainage. Report drainage that exceeds 50 mL/hr for 2 hours. Re-establish suction as necessary. Usually the suction apparatus is removed when the total drainage is less than 10–20 mL in 24 hours. Report significant findings to the MD.

Disturbance in self-concept related to altered body image secondary to breast reconstruction surgery

Desired outcomes: Patient relates realistic expectations before surgery and demonstrates movement toward acceptance of body changes after surgery.

1. Review with patient her expectations for the outcome of surgery.

2. Discuss the emotional responses that women often have following breast reconstruction, such as elation during the early postoperative period followed by depression and confusion.

3. Explain that some of the depression and confusion may be a result of the memory of the mastectomy and fear of cancer. Reassure patient that these feelings are normal and usually disappear after a short time.

4. Provide emotional support by being with the patient when the dressing is first removed. Explain that the reconstructed breast will not look like the other breast at first because of the molding process that takes place during the recovery period.

See "Appendix One" for nursing diagnoses and interventions for the care of preoperative and postoperative patients, pp. 528–532, and patients with cancer and other life-disrupting illnesses, pp. 544–551.

E. Patient–Family Teaching and Discharge Planning

Provide patient and SOs with verbal and written information for the following:

1. Care of the incision, including applying a gauze dressing until the sutures are removed on about the 7th day. After the sutures are removed, micropore tape strips are usually placed over the incision until healing has taken place, and they should be replaced when they become loose. Instruct patient to notify MD if signs of infection, including persistent redness, pain, swelling, or drainage, appear at the incision site.

2. Taking showers, which is usually permitted after the suction catheter is removed. If present, the dressing should be removed from the operative site and replaced after bathing.

3. Activity restriction for the first 4–6 weeks or as directed, including strenuous exercise, contact sports, excessive stretching, and heavy lifting (>5 lb).

4. Avoiding putting pressure on the chest wall for 4–6 weeks. For example, patient should use superior position during coitus.

5. Importance of breast massage (at least 3 times a day) for the first year after surgery. Explain that it takes 3–6 months for the reconstructed breast to appear natural in contour.

6. Importance of not wearing a bra for 3 months to allow for unrestricted movement of the implant.

7. The importance of applying prescribed lotion to the nipple daily if a nipple transplant was performed.

8. Importance of monthly breast self-examination (BSE) of both breasts. If patient does not know the examination technique, teach her the procedure.

9. Medications, including drug name, purpose, dosage, schedule, precautions, and potential side effects.

III. Benign Breast Disease

The most common breast masses are those caused by fibrocystic disease, fibroadenomas, and intraductal papilloma; all are evaluated for potential malignancy.

Fibrocystic disease: Can be either a simple cyst(s) caused by normal changes in the lining of the duct and the secretion of fluid or a premalignant condition caused by hyperplasia of the cells. Fibrocystic disease is the most common breast lesion in women. It usually develops at about age 20–25 and often regresses with menopause.

Fibroadenomas: Solid masses that may occur at age 15–60, with peak occurrence at 21–25 years.

Intraductal papilloma: A benign condition of the ductal system of the breast. It occurs infrequently and is found most often in women 35–45 years of age.

A. Assessment

Signs and symptoms: With fibrocystic disease there often are bilateral, multiple masses that are painful and tender. They change in size relative to the menstrual cycle and are most evident just before menstruation. The masses are firm, mobile, and smooth or regular in shape. Fibroadenomas are painless masses and are usually unilateral. The mass itself is mobile, solid, firm, well circumscribed, and usually spherical, but it can be lobulated or dumbbell-shaped. The most frequent symptom of intraductal papilloma is serosanguineous or serous nipple discharge. A mass is usually not present.

Physical exam: With fibrocystic disease, masses usually can be palpated in the upper outer quadrants of the breasts. Fibroadenomas are often discovered by the patient and are usually 2–2.5 cm in diameter. An intraductal papilloma often involves a 1 cm area that circumvents the nipple; discharge also may be found on physical exam.

History of: Benign breast masses. There is potential for recurrence of both fibrocystic disease and fibroadenomas.

B. Diagnostic Tests

1. Mammography: A roentgenographic test used to identify cancerous masses, which appear as small densities with stippled calcifications. There is a slight risk of false-positive and false-negative results.

2. Xeroradiography: A noninvasive test that uses a lesser radiation dose than mammography; however, there is a higher risk of false-positive or false-negative results.

3. Thermography: Presents a picture of normal and abnormal temperatures in the breast. Malignant masses are warmer because of increased vascularity in the area. Again, there is the risk of false-positive and false-negative results. Thermography is not as accurate as mammography and cannot be substituted for it.

4. Ultrasound mammography: Uses sound waves to delineate the internal pattern of the breast. It is used when cysts and enlarged ducts are suspected. It is 98% accurate in diagnosing cysts and enlarged ducts.

5. Magnetic resonance (MR): Experimental technique that uses the interaction between magnetism and radio waves (without ionizing radiation) to show the structure of the breasts. It can image breast cancers that are large and palpable.

6. Aspiration biopsy: Involves aspirating the contents of the mass via a large-bore needle. The aspirate is then placed on a slide for Papanicolaou evaluation.

7. Incisional biopsy: Involves the surgical removal of part of the mass for histologic evaluation.

8. Excisional biopsy: Involves the removal of the entire mass as well as marginal breast tissue. This procedure results in the most accurate diagnosis.

C. Medical Management and Surgical Interventions

1. **Diet:** For fibrocystic disease, the promotion of nutritious foods and the elimination of methylxanthine substances such as coffee, tea, and chocolate to decrease the pain and size of the cysts. Vitamin E therapy may be helpful in reducing the incidence of recurrent cysts. It is theorized that a diet low in fat and high in fiber helps prevent breast cancer.

2. **Excisional biopsy:** Not only useful in diagnosis, it removes the breast mass as well.

3. **Wedge resection of the breast:** Resection of the lobe that is involved in the intraductal papilloma.

D. Nursing Diagnoses and Interventions

Fear related to the possibility of cancer, change in body image, surgical or diagnostic procedure, and pain

Desired outcome: Patient is able to discuss fears and demonstrates increasing psychologic comfort.

1. Reassure patient that >90% of breast masses are benign.

2. Explain the diagnostic, preoperative, and postoperative procedures as necessary.

3. If appropriate, inform patient that a local anesthetic might be used during the biopsy and that sensations of pulling and probing may be felt.

4. Provide support by allowing time for the verbalization of feelings, and answer questions.

5. If patient is at high risk of malignancy, see **Fear** in "Malignant Disorders of the Breast," p. 428.

Alteration in comfort: Pain related to biopsy

Desired outcome: Patient relates a reduction in discomfort and does not exhibit signs of uncontrolled pain.

1. Assess and document the location, quality, and duration of the pain.

2. Medicate with the prescribed analgesics; evaluate and document the patient's response.

3. To help decrease swelling, apply a wrapped ice pack to the involved breast.

4. Ensure that the patient has a comfortable bra that supports the breast adequately.

See "Appendix One" for nursing diagnoses and interventions for the care of preoperative and postoperative patients, pp. 528–532.

E. Patient–Family Teaching and Discharge Planning

Provide patient and SOs with verbal and written information for the following:

1. Medications, including the drug name, purpose, dosage, schedule, precautions, and potential side effects.

2. Indicators of wound infection, which necessitate MD notification. These include persistent redness, pain, swelling, and discharge at the operative site.

3. Care of the incision site, including cleansing. After sutures are removed, soap and water should be used for gentle cleansing

4. Resumption of daily activities to patient's tolerance.

5. Diet as tolerated; importance of eliminating methylxanthine products if fibrocystic disease is diagnosed.

6. Scheduled date for the completed pathology report, or an explanation of the diagnosis, if already available.

7. Importance of BSE. Teach the procedure to patients who do not know it.

IV. Malignant Disorders of the Breast

Breast cancer is one of the three most common types of breast disease, second only to fibrocystic disease in occurrence. In the United States, it is the most frequently occurring type of reproductive cancer in females. Breast cancer is usually diagnosed between 40 and 70 years, with 54 the median age. However, in the last few years there has been an increase in newly diagnosed cases in women in their 20s and 30s.

The histopathology of breast tumors involves the progression of the tumor from a local preinvasive disease state to invasive malignancy. The changes that occur in the breast are due primarily to hyperplasia of the epithelium. Although carcinoma in situ is usually noninvasive, it too can develop into invasive carcinoma. The differentiation between noninvasive and invasive cancer requires extensive examination of tissue cells obtained during excisional biopsy.

A. Assessment

Signs and symptoms: The earliest indicator is the presence of a palpable mass. Signs of advanced disease include nipple retraction, change in breast contour, nipple discharge, redness or heat of the breast, palpable lymph glands, dimpling of the skin of the breast, and *peau d'orange* or orange peel appearance of the breast. Ulceration also may be a sign of advanced disease.

Physical exam: Palpable mass, which is usually located in the upper outer quadrant of the breast. The mass is usually not painful, and it is unilateral, irregular in shape, poorly delineated, and usually nonmobile. There may be signs of edema, venous engorgement, and abnormal contours.

Risk factors: Previous breast cancer in the contralateral breast; family history of cancer and breast cancer, especially a mother or sister, particularly if the family member was affected at an early age or had bilateral disease; being over age 50; postmenopausal weight gain; early age at menarche (11 or younger); late age of menopause (after 52 years); nulliparity or late age at first full-term delivery (over 30). In addition, it is theorized that exposure to carcinogens, use of estrogens, and a high-fat diet are other factors in the development of breast cancer.

B. Diagnostic Tests

The most specific test for detection of breast disease is the excisional breast biopsy. (See "Benign Breast Disease," p. 425.) Mammography can be used as a screening method in women who are at high risk, and it may detect breast masses in patients who do not have a palpable mass. However, there is the risk of false-negative and false-positive results. The American Cancer Society recommends a baseline mammogram for women age 35–40, and a mammogram q1–2 years for women 40–49 and annually for women over age 50.

C. Medical Management and Surgical Interventions

1. **Staging of the tumor:** Provides a means for formulating the prognosis and treatment plan. The size of the tumor, the appearance of the cancer in the

Table 9-1 Cancer Staging*

Stage A
Absence of skin edema, ulceration, or solid fixation of the tumor to chest wall; axillary nodes negative.

Stage B
Same as A, except involvement of axillary nodes occurs, with <2.5 cm transverse diameter; nodes are not fixed to overlying skin or to deeper axillary structures.

Stage C
Presence of any one of the following five signs of advanced cancer:
1. Edema of less than a third of the breast skin.
2. Ulceration of the breast skin.
3. Tumor solidly fixed to the chest wall.
4. Axillary node involvement (2.5 cm or more in transverse diameter).
5. Axillary nodes fixed to overlying skin or deeper structures.

Stage D
More advanced cancer than stage C:
1. Any two or more of the signs described under stage C.
2. Edema of more than a third of the breast skin.
3. Satellite skin nodules.
4. Inflammatory carcinoma.
5. Supraclavicular lymph node involvement.
6. Parasternal tumor.
7. Edema of the involved arm.
8. Metastases to other sites.

*Based on Columbia Clinical Classification and Staging System.

axillary nodes, the histopathologic examination, and the presence of distant metastases determine the degree of staging (see Table 9-1).

2. **Radiation therapy:** Can be used either in metastatic disease or in the treatment of early breast cancer. In early breast cancer, the tumor is excised along with some of the adjacent tissue, followed by external radiation and/or radioactive implants.

3. **Radical mastectomy or Halstead procedure:** The most extensive surgical procedure. It involves the removal of the breast, nipple and areola, axillary lymph nodes, and the pectoralis minor and major muscles.

4. **Modified radical mastectomy:** Removal of the breast tissue, nipple and areola, the tumor and surrounding skin, the axillary lymph nodes, and possibly the pectoralis minor muscle.

5. **Total mastectomy or simple mastectomy:** Involves the removal of the breast, but the lymph nodes are left intact.

6. **Partial mastectomy (lumpectomy, tylectomy, or segmental resection):** Refers to the excision of the tumor and a small amount of tissue surrounding it. Axillary nodal dissection is usually done.

7. **Quadrectomy:** Removal of the entire quadrant of the breast where the tumor is located. Axillary nodal dissection is usually done.

8. **Chemotherapy:** Includes the use of either a single agent or a combination of agents. This management pattern is used either as an adjunct to surgery or in advanced disease when metastases have occurred or positive lymph nodes have been identified. The use of cytotoxic drugs has been found to be more effective when used in combination. These combinations include the following:

☐ *Cyclophosphamide, methotrexate, and fluorouracil:* Used in metastatic or recurrent disease.

    □ *Cyclophosphamide, doxorubicin, and fluorouracil:* Used in metastatic disease.

9. **Hormonal therapy:** The hormone used depends on whether the tumor is estrogen-receptor-positive or estrogen-receptor-poor, and it is also used in advanced disease as adjuvant therapy for stage II breast disease. Some of the hormonal agents used include:

    □ *Tamoxifen citrate:* An anti-estrogen used in estrogen-receptor-positive tumors.

    □ *Diethylstilbestrol:* Used in women at least 5 years postmenopausal when the tumor is estrogen-receptor-poor.

    □ *Fluoxymesterone:* Used in women at least 5 years postmenopausal with estrogen-receptor-poor tumors who also have bone metastasis and estrogen failure.

D. Nursing Diagnoses and Interventions

Fear related to the possibility of cancer and its treatment

Desired outcome: Patient freely expresses fears and anxieties and relates increasing psychologic comfort.

1. Assess the patient's understanding of the potential diagnosis and treatment plan; clarify and explain as appropriate.

2. Provide time for patient to express feelings and fears.

3. Evaluate the patient's emotional status, and explore with the patient what her breasts mean to her. The breast may represent nurturance, sexuality, femininity, and desirability.

4. Assess your own feelings about the diagnosis of cancer and the psychologic meaning of the breast. Your attitudes may be reflected in the patient's care, and therefore a positive attitude is essential for optimal patient support.

5. Provide a nonthreatening, relaxed atmosphere for the patient and SOs by using therapeutic communication techniques such as open-ended questions and reflection.

Ineffective individual coping related to depression secondary to diagnosis of breast cancer

Desired outcomes: Patient demonstrates comfort with expressing her feelings, identifies positive coping patterns, and accepts the support of others.

1. Assist patient with developing a support system.

2. If an extensive mastectomy was performed, recognize the signs of grief, such as denial, anger, withdrawal, or inappropriate affect. Provide emotional support, and describe the stages of grief to the patient and SOs. Provide explanations to SOs, who may misunderstand the meaning of the patient's behavior or actions

3. Consult with the surgeon regarding a visit by a woman who has had a diagnosis similar to that of the patient. "Reach to Recovery" volunteers from the American Cancer Society are trained to share their experiences with breast cancer patients.

Potential impairment of physical mobility related to risk of alterations in the upper extremity secondary to postmastectomy complications

Desired outcomes: Patient complies with the therapeutic regimen to prevent joint contractures, lymphedema, and infection, and does not experience impaired mobility in the involved upper extremity.

1. Consult with the surgeon before the mastectomy to determine the type of surgery anticipated. Together, you can develop an individualized exercise program specific to the patient's needs that can be implemented as soon as the patient returns from the recovery room.

2. Passive ROM can be initiated in the recovery room, and you can teach the patient assisted ROM on the involved shoulder as soon as she returns to her room. Encourage finger, wrist, and elbow movement to aid circulation and help minimize edema.

3. Encourage progressive exercise by having the patient use the affected arm for personal hygiene and ADLs the morning after surgery. Other exercises (clasping the hands behind the head and "walking" the fingers up the wall) should be added as soon as patient is ready. Once the sutures have been removed (usually around the 2nd postoperative week), patient should begin exercises that will enhance external rotation and abduction of the shoulder. Before hospital discharge, the patient should be able to achieve maximum shoulder flexion by touching her fingertips together behind her back. With the surgeon's consent, a "Reach for Recovery" volunteer can visit and provide patient with verbal instructions and written handouts for these exercises.

4. Assist patient with ambulation until her gait is normal. Encourage correct posture, with the back straight and shoulders back.

5. To minimize the risk of lymphedema and/or infection, avoid giving injections, measuring BP, or taking blood samples from the affected arm. Remind the patient about her lowered resistance to infection and the importance of promptly treating any breaks in the skin. To help prevent infection after hospital discharge, advise patient to treat minor injuries with soap and water and to notify the MD if signs of infection occur.

6. Advise patient to wear a Medic-Alert bracelet that cautions against injections and tests in the involved arm.

7. To protect the hand and arm from injury, advise the patient to wear a protective glove when gardening or doing chores that require exposure to harsh chemicals such as cleaning fluids. Explain that cutting cuticles should be avoided and that lotion should be used to keep the skin soft.

Disturbance in self-concept related to altered body image secondary to loss of a breast

Desired outcome: Patient demonstrates movement toward acceptance of the loss of a breast.

1. Recognize that loss of a breast is perceived in different ways by different women. It is frequently more traumatic for the young adult.

2. Provide emotional support by being with the patient when the surgical dressing is removed.

3. As appropriate, explain that sexual dysfunction often occurs after mastectomy and that it can be minimized with resumption of sexual relations as soon as the pain has decreased. Assure patient that relations that were positive before surgery usually remain positive. However, be aware that sexual relationships that were weak before the surgery may not tolerate the added stress.

4. Recognize the need for a supportive person, such as a "Reach for Recovery" volunteer, who has experienced the same procedure. Consult with the MD regarding a visit by this individual, if indicated. Support systems also should be made available to SOs.

5. If indicated, provide the patient with a breast prosthesis after surgery to help her feel "normal." A temporary prosthesis, made of nylon and filled with dacron fluff, can be worn until the incision heals. Provide the patient with information on where to get a breast prosthesis. The American Cancer Society has lists of distributors and types of prostheses available.

6. Be aware that use of touch often enhances the patient's self-concept.

7. Provide information and answer questions about breast reconstruction.

Alteration in comfort: Pain related to the surgical procedure

Desired outcome: Patient expresses a reduction in discomfort and does not exhibit signs of uncontrolled pain.

1. Assess and document the location, quality, and duration of the pain.
2. Medicate patient with the prescribed analgesics before the pain becomes too severe. Evaluate and document the response.
3. Reassure patient that phantom breast sensations are normal.
4. Provide a comfortable in-bed position, and support the affected arm with pillows.
5. Encourage movement of the fingers on the affected arm to increase circulation. Inform the patient that although progressive exercise will cause some discomfort, it will aid in the mobility of the affected arm and enhance recovery.
6. Reassure the patient that exercise movements will be adapted to her level of tolerance.
7. If appropriate, instruct the patient in relaxation techniques and use of guided imagery.
8. Provide distraction, such as television, radio, or books.
9. Use touch to help relieve tension, for example, by giving a gentle massage.

See "Appendix One" for nursing diagnoses and interventions for the care of preoperative and postoperative patients, pp. 528–532, and patients with cancer and other life-disrupting illnesses, pp. 544–551.

E. Patient–Family Teaching and Discharge Planning

Provide patient and SOs with verbal and written information for the following:

1. Medications, including drug name, purpose, dosage, schedule, precautions, and potential side effects.
2. Type and dates of follow-up treatment.
3. Resumption of sexual activity, which usually can occur as soon as pain is diminished.
4. Care of the incision site, including cleansing. Explain the components of good hygiene.
5. Progressive exercise regimen, which should be continued at home. Advise patient to stop the exercise movement if a pulling sensation or pain is felt.
6. Informing health care professionals to avoid measuring BP or giving injections in the affected arm.
7. Indicators of infection and the importance of reporting them to MD.
8. Permanent breast prosthesis, including distributors and types available.
9. Name and telephone number of a support person who can be called during the first postoperative year. An ideal individual is a "Reach for Recovery" volunteer.
10. Performing monthly BSE.

▶ Section Two   **Neoplasms of the Female Pelvis**

Cancers of the cervix and ovaries are frequently occurring reproductive cancers in women. 1984 statistics of the American Cancer Society show 55,000 new cases of uterine cancer (16,000 of cervical cancer, 39,000 of endometrial cancer) and 18,000 new cases of ovarian cancer. Women of all ages can develop cancer of these structures, although it is most often found in individuals between the ages of 40 and 60.

I. Cancer of the Cervix

Cervical cancer is one of the most frequently occurring cancers in women. Although the cause is unknown, the following risk factors have been associated with this disease: early age of first coitus, early age of first pregnancy, multiple pregnancies, intercourse with males who practice poor hygiene, multiple sexual partners, herpesvirus type II, and family history. The two types of cervical cancer are squamous cell, which is the most common, and adenocarcinoma. *Preinvasive* describes cancerous cells that are limited to the cervix; *invasive* refers to cancer that is present in the cervix, in other pelvic structures, and possibly in the lymphatic system as well. Preinvasive cancer of the cervix typically is found in women age 30–40; invasive cancer usually appears between the ages of 40 and 50. Treatment of preinvasive cancer has a greater success rate.

A. Assessment

Preinvasive: Patient asymptomatic; Pap smear abnormal.

Invasive: Abnormal vaginal bleeding; persistent, watery vaginal discharge; postcoital pain and bleeding; abnormal Pap smear.

B. Diagnostic Tests

1. Pap smear: Cells are collected from the endocervix, cervix, and upper vagina with an applicator, placed on a slide, and sent to the lab for analysis. Pap smear results are reported as follows:

    ☐ *Stage I:* Normal; negative for malignant cells.

    ☐ *Stage II:* Negative for malignant cells but containing atypical elements (infection).

    ☐ *Stage III:* Markedly atypical cells suggestive of malignancy.

    ☐ *Stage IV:* Malignant cells probably present.

    ☐ *Stage V:* Malignancy present.

2. Colposcopy: Procedure providing a three-dimensional view of the cervix and allowing for cervical staining with an iodine solution (Schiller's test). Cells that do not absorb the stain are considered abnormal and are sent to the lab for further examination. This procedure takes approximately 20 minutes.

3. Conization biopsy: Surgical procedure performed under general anesthesia in which a cone-shaped area of the cervix is biopsied for lab analysis to determine the extent of the malignancy.

4. Lymphography: Radiologic exam, which grades the stages of cervical cancer. Contrast dye is injected into the dorsal aspect of the foot so that lymphatic vessels and nodes can be visualized. The procedure can take up to 4 hours, during which time the patient must remain very still. X-ray films are taken at the time of the injection of the dye and 24 hours later to evaluate the lymph nodes. If the nodes are positive for cancer cells, the size of the lymph nodes will change, as will their architecture (foamy appearance with "bites" taken out of them). Because the contrast dye remains in the lymph nodes for up to 15 months, evaluation of changes can be done over a period of time without repeating the dye injection.

5. Chest x-ray: May reveal presence of metastasis to the lungs.

6. Staging of the disease: The following parameters are used (based on clinical classification of the International Federation of Gynecology and Obstetrics):

☐ *Stage O:* Carcinoma in situ; preinvasive.

☐ *Stage I:* Cancer cells in the cervix only.

Stage IA: Cervical cancer with <3 mm spread.

Stage IB: Cervical cancer with definite invasive areas.

☐ *Stage II:* Cancer involving cervix and vagina but not the pelvic wall.

Stage IIA: No involvement of uterine tissue.

Stage IIB: Involvement of uterine tissue.

☐ *Stage III:* Involvement of the pelvic wall or lower third of the vagina.

Stage IIIA: No extension onto the pelvic wall.

Stage IIIB: Extension onto pelvic wall and/or kidney secondary to hydronephrosis (obstructed flow of urine to kidney producing kidney atrophy).

☐ *Stage IV:* Cancer in bladder, rectum, and other organs of the pelvis.

Stage IVA: Metastasis to rectum, bladder.

Stage IVB: Metastasis to distant organs.

▶ **Note:** Metastasis to lymph nodes occurs in 15% of stage I and up to 60% of stage IV cases.

C. Medical Management and Surgical Interventions

1. **External radiation therapy:** The best treatment for invasive cancer of the cervix; all stages of cancer are treated with this therapy, which is performed on an outpatient basis in the nuclear medicine department. Dosage and length of treatment are determined by MD specializing in nuclear medicine.

2. **Radium implants:** Used to destroy cervical cancer that is graded stage II–IV. While the patient is anesthetized, an applicator is positioned into the vagina through the cervix and its position is confirmed by x-ray. After the patient returns to her room the radiologist inserts a radioactive isotope and leaves it in place for 1–3 days. During this time the patient is in a private room and remains in isolation.

   A combination of external radiation and implants gives the best therapeutic results. While the implant is in place, the patient is kept on strict bed rest, has an indwelling catheter, is on a low-residue diet, and is given analgesia (usually non-narcotic) and diphenoxylate hydrochloride with atropine sulfate (Lomotil) or paregoric to control diarrhea, which often occurs. After the implant has been removed, the patient is allowed to ambulate.

3. **Hysterectomy:** Often the treatment of choice. The uterus and cervix are removed surgically via an abdominal or vaginal approach. Patient usually returns to the room with an indwelling catheter.

D. Nursing Diagnoses and Interventions

Alteration in comfort: Pain related to surgery or radiation implant

Desired outcome: Patient expresses relief from discomfort and does not exhibit signs of uncontrolled pain.

1. Provide back rubs, which are especially helpful for patients who were in the lithotomy position during surgery. Massage the shoulders and upper back for patients with radium implants, who are not allowed position changes.

2. For other interventions, see similar nursing diagnosis in "Caring for Preoperative and Postoperative Patients" "Appendix One," p. 528.

Potential fluid volume deficit related to abnormal loss secondary to postoperative or postimplant bleeding

Desired outcomes: Patient does not exhibit signs of excessive bleeding or shock. Patient and SOs can verbalize knowledge of the signs of excessive bleeding and are aware of the need to alert staff promptly if they are noted.

1. Monitor VS q2–4h during the first 24 hours. Be alert to indicators of hemorrhage and impending shock: hypotension, increased pulse and respirations, pallor, and diaphoresis.

2. Assess postoperative bleeding q2–4h by noting amount and quality of drainage on dressings if abdominal approach was used, or on perineal pads if vaginal approach was used. If an implant is in place, check for vaginal bleeding, a sign that erosion is occurring.

3. Inspect the abdomen for distention and assess patient for presence of severe abdominal pain; both are indicators of internal bleeding.

4. Review CBC values for evidence of bleeding: decreases in hemoglobin and hematocrit. Notify MD of significant findings.

5. Inform patient and SOs about the signs of excessive bleeding and the need to alert staff immediately should they occur.

Potential alteration in pattern of urinary elimination related to inadequate intake or obstruction of indwelling catheter

Desired outcomes: Patient has a patent indwelling catheter and demonstrates an adequate I&O.

1. Monitor I&O and document q shift. Notify MD if urinary output falls below 30 mL/h over 2 hours in the presence of an adequate intake. Along with low back pain, this can be indicative of ureteral ligation during surgery.

2. Ensure patency of the indwelling catheter. See "Appendix One," **Potential for infection**, p. 532, for interventions related to the care of patients with indwelling catheters.

3. Administer oral and/or parenteral fluids as prescribed. Ensure totals of 2–3 L/day in nonrestricted patients.

4. Assess for bladder distention by inspecting the suprapubic area and percussing or palpating the bladder. **Caution:** For patients with radiation implants, bladder distention can result in radiation burns to the bladder.

Disturbance in self-concept related to altered body image and role performance expectations secondary to diagnosis of cancer

Desired outcomes: Patient can verbalize her perceptions of past, present, and future role expections. Patient exhibits adaptation to her situation and begins to assume self-care as her condition allows.

1. Anticipate patient's concern about loss of uterus, presence of cancer and the potential for recurrence, and "loss of womanhood." Provide emotional support and an unhurried atmosphere for patient and SOs to ask questions and express concerns, frustrations, and fears.

2. Recognize the covert signs of grief that can accompany self-concept disturbances: anger, withdrawal, demanding behavior, or inappropriate affect. Give support to SOs who might misinterpret patient's coping mechanisms.

3. To enhance patient's sense of control over her situation, encourage her to perform ADLs and begin self-care as soon as her condition warrants.

4. Provide materials from organizations such as the American Cancer Society and arrange for a contact person (role model) from such an organization, if appropriate.

See "Appendix One" for nursing diagnoses and interventions for the care of preoperative and postoperative patients, pp. 528–532, and patients with cancer and other life-disrupting illnesses, pp. 544–551.

E. Patient–Family Teaching and Discharge Planning

For patients with radium implants: Provide verbal and written information for the following:

1. Necessity of notifying MD if the following problems occur: vaginal bleeding, rectal bleeding, foul-smelling vaginal discharge, abdominal pain and/or distention, hematuria.

2. Resumption of sexual intercourse, typically 6 weeks after surgery or as directed by MD.

3. Medications, including drug name, dosage, purpose, schedule, precautions, and potential side effects.

4. Need for follow-up care; confirm date and time of next medical appointment if known.

5. Patient is *not* radioactive once the implant has been removed.

For patients who have had a hysterectomy:

1. Necessity of notifying MD if the following indicators of infection occur: incisional swelling, redness, purulent drainage or vaginal bleeding, abdominal pain.

2. Care of the incision.

3. Restriction of activities as directed, such as heavy lifting (>5 lb) and sexual intercourse. Advise patient to get maximum amounts of rest and avoid fatigue.

4. Medications, including drug name, dosage, purpose, schedule, precautions, and potential side effects.

5. Need for follow-up care; confirm date and time of next MD appointment if known.

II. Ovarian Tumors

The etiology of ovarian tumors is unknown, but there is a strong relationship between their development and familial incidence. They can occur in females of all ages, but are most common between the ages of 20 and 45. If left untreated, the disease can spread through the lymphatic system and into the bloodstream, or it can proliferate by peritoneal seeding, in which malignant cells spread to peritoneal lymph nodes. *Benign ovarian tumors* seen most frequently include fibromas, which are found most often in postmenopausal women, and cystadenomas, which are the most common ovarian tumor, occurring in 70% of cases.

Malignant solid ovarian tumors are rarely diagnosed early because the patient tends to be asymptomatic. Survival rate is low because the tumor is usually not detected until an advanced stage. These tumors are the most lethal type of gynecologic cancer.

A. Assessment

Benign ovarian tumors: Abdominal enlargement and complaints of abdominal fullness.

Solid ovarian tumors: Abdominal enlargement and pressure; pelvic pressure and discomfort.

Signs and symptoms for both classifications: Amenorrhea, postmenopausal vaginal bleeding, and other menstrual irregularities; urinary frequency and urgency; constipation.

Physical exam: Abdominal distention; an enlarged ovary, which is highly suspicious in postmenopausal women.

B. Diagnostic Tests

1. <u>Abdominal x-ray:</u> Will reveal presence of an ovarian tumor.

2. <u>Ultrasound of the abdomen:</u> Will reveal an ovarian mass.

3. <u>Culdoscopy:</u> A surgical procedure done under general anesthesia. A culdoscope, an instrument with a light source, is passed through the vagina to visualize pelvic organs. There is no surgical incision and the procedure can be done on an outpatient basis.

4. <u>Laparoscopy:</u> Uses a laparoscope, an instrument with a telescope and light source, to visualize the pelvic organs through an incision made near the umbilicus. This procedure is done under general anesthesia, usually on an outpatient basis.

5. <u>Cytologic examination of the pelvic washings/ascites:</u> May show presence of malignant cancerous cells.

6. <u>Staging of ovarian tumors (dependent on surgical exploration):</u> The following parameters are used (based on clinical classification of the International Federation of Gynecology and Obstetrics):

   □ *Stage I:* Tumors limited to the ovaries.

   Stage IA: Growth limited to one ovary; no ascites.

   Stage IB: Tumors limited to both ovaries; no ascites.

   □ *Stage II:* Tumors involving one or both ovaries with presence of malignant cells in pelvic organs.

   Stage IIA: Involvement of uterus and/or fallopian tubes with presence of malignant cells.

   Stage IIB: Presence of malignant cells in other pelvic tissues.

   □ *Stage III:* Tumors involving one or both ovaries with metastasis outside the pelvis and/or positive retroperitoneal nodes. Tumor limited to retroperitoneal lymph nodes. Malignant cells found in small bowel omentum.

   □ *Stage IV:* Tumors involving one or both ovaries with metastasis to distant organs.

C. Medical Management and Surgical Interventions

1. **Wedge resection:** Surgical procedure in which a benign tumor is removed, leaving normal ovarian tissue. It is done under general anesthesia using an abdominal or vaginal approach.

2. **Salpingo-oophorectomy:** Removal of the ovary and fallopian tube on the affected side. It is performed under general anesthesia using an abdominal approach. Solid tumors of the ovary are treated with this procedure.

3. **Total hysterectomy and bilateral salpingo-oophorectomy:** Performed if both ovaries are affected. If the disease has invaded other abdominal organs, **radiation therapy** also is used. Postoperative care includes adequate hydration and pain management; prophylactic antibiotics, depending on the extent of the surgical procedure and the risk of infection; and ambulation, usually the first evening after surgery.

4. **Chemotherapy:** Used when the disease has spread to distant organs. Chemotherapeutic medications include doxorubicin, platinol, and cyclophosphamide. Chemotherapy is a palliative rather than curative measure.

D. Nursing Diagnoses and Interventions

See "Cancer of the Cervix" for the following: **Alteration in comfort**, p. 432, **Potential fluid volume deficit** (blood loss), p. 433, **Potential alteration in pattern of urinary elimination**, p. 433, and **Disturbance in self-concept**, p. 433. See "Appendix One" for nursing diagnoses and interventions for the care of preoperative and postoperative patients, pp. 528–532, and patients with cancer and other life-disrupting illnesses, pp. 544–551.

E. Patient–Teaching Teaching and Discharge Planning

Provide patient and SOs with verbal and written information for the following:

1. Medications, including drug name, dosage, schedule, purpose, precautions, and potential side effects.
2. Importance of reporting indicators of infection (depending on the surgery) to the MD: fever; vaginal bleeding and discharge; abdominal pain and distention; and incisional redness, purulent drainage, local warmth, and swelling.
3. Activity restrictions related to heavy lifting (>5 lb), exercise, sexual intercourse, or housework, as directed by MD.
4. Necessity of follow-up appointments; confirm date and time of next MD appointment if known.

III. Endometrial Cancer

Endometrial (uterine) cancer typically occurs in postmenopausal women between the ages of 50 and 70. It is a slow-growing cancer that can take up to 10 years to metastasize. Risk factors for developing uterine cancer include obesity, hypertension, diabetes mellitus, history of uterine polyps, sterility, menopausal estrogen therapy, and nulliparity; it is more common in Caucasian women. *Adenocarcinoma* is the most common endometrial cancer, and its growth is estrogen-dependent in the early stages. The tumor can be found in any location within the uterus and it is considered cancer in situ. The invasive stages of uterine cancer are not estrogen-dependent and can spread to the vagina, pelvic lymph nodes, ovaries, lungs, brain, and bones. Recurrence most frequently is seen in the vagina. When an early diagnosis is made the prognosis is good, with successful treatment occurring in 80–90% of the cases.

A. Assessment

Signs and symptoms: Abnormal bleeding, including spotting; watery, unpleasant serosanguineous discharge.

Physical exam: Presence of a palpable uterine mass, uterine polyps; obvious increase in uterine size in advanced disease.

B. Diagnostic Tests

1. Dilation and curettage (D&C): Surgical procedure in which the cervical opening is widened by a dilating instrument and the uterine lining is scraped with a curette to obtain a specimen for examination.
2. Endometrial biopsy: Procedure in which a specimen is obtained from the endometrial surface for biopsy. In premenopausal women, it is obtained 12 hours after the onset of the menses because the cervix is easier to enter at that time.
3. Hysteroscopy: Examination via an endoscope, which enters the uterus through the vagina, allowing visualization, biopsy, and photography with a camera. The patient is anesthetized with a pericervical block.
4. Chest x-ray: To detect metastasis to the lungs.

5. <u>Proctosigmoidoscopy:</u> Visualizes the distal sigmoid colon, rectum, and anal canal with an endoscope, allowing biopsy of tissue for detecting metastasis to pelvic structures.

6. <u>Cystoscopy:</u> Visualizes the bladder via the insertion of a cystoscope through the urethra. A biopsy is done to detect cancerous cells in the bladder.

7. <u>IVP:</u> To rule out spread of disease to other organs.

8. <u>Staging of the disease.</u> The following parameters are used (based on clinical classification of the International Federation of Gynecology and Obstetrics):

□ *Stage O:* Carcinoma in situ. Histologic findings suggestive of malignancy.

□ *Stage I:* Carcinoma confined to the corpus of the uterus.

□ *Stage IA:* Cancer measuring 8 cm in length from the external os to the upper point of the uterus.

□ *Stage IB:* Cancer measuring >8 cm in length from the external os to the upper point of the uterus.

□ *Stage II:* Cancer involving the corpus and cervix but not extending beyond the uterus.

□ *Stage III:* Cancer extending beyond the uterus but confined to the true pelvis.

□ *Stage IV:* Cancer extending outside the true pelvis or obviously involving the mucosa of the bladder or rectum.

C. Medical Management and Surgical Interventions

1. **Total hysterectomy with bilateral salpingo-oophorectomy:** Performed in patients who have a well-defined stage I tumor without cervical involvement. The uterus, cervix, fallopian tubes, ovaries, and a part of the vaginal cuff are removed.

2. **Radical hysterectomy with bilateral pelvic lymph node dissection:** Performed for patients with stage II uterine cancer.

3. **Radiation therapy:** Used if the cancer stage is difficult to determine. If an implant is used, the applicator is positioned in the uterus through the vagina while the patient is anesthetized. After the patient returns to her room, the radioisotope is placed in the applicator by a radiologist. External radiation of the uterus and pelvic nodes is performed on an outpatient basis for a period of time that is determined by the radiologist. When surgery and radiation therapy are used in combination, radiation therapy is done preoperatively (usually about 6 weeks before) to destroy cancer cells in the pericervical lymphatics and inhibit recurrence. This treatment is used for stage II and stage III cancers.

4. **Chemotherapy:** Used for advanced and recurrent disease. Chemotherapeutic drugs include doxorubicin, vincristine sulfate, cyclophosphamide, and d-actinomycin. Combinations of drugs and the dosage and length of treatment are determined by the patient's response to treatment and the severity of recurrence.

5. **Progestin therapy:** Used for in situ endometrial cancers (stages I and II) that are estrogen dependent, and it produces a remission in 35% of the cases. It is used as palliative treatment for stage IV cancers. Medroxyprogesterone (Depo-Provera) is the hormone that is usually used.

D. Nursing Diagnoses and Interventions

See "Cancer of the Cervix," p. 432.

E. Patient–Family Teaching and Discharge Planning

See "Cancer of the Cervix," p. 434.

▶ Section Three   **Disorders of the Female Pelvis**

Endometriosis is often seen in younger women; cystocele, rectocele, and uterine prolapse are associated with women who are postmenopausal. These conditions occur when there is misplacement of structures or tissue within the female pelvis.

I. Endometriosis

Endometriosis is a condition in which endometrial tissue is present outside of the uterus. Typically it is found on the ovaries or in the peritoneal cul-de-sac. It might also be found in the vagina, vulva, uterosacral ligaments, or bowel. In extreme cases it is found in the lungs, bones, and other organs of the body. Endometriosis is considered a benign disease; it most often occurs in nulliparous women 30–40 years of age and in those who have had their first child at a later age. Its cause is unknown but it is theorized that the tissue travels up the fallopian tubes and into the perineum during the menstrual cycle, or that during surgical procedures such as a cesarean section the tissue becomes implanted and grows at the surgical site.

A. Assessment

Signs and symptoms: Dysmenorrhea 5–7 days before and 2–3 days after menses, hypermenorrhea (prolonged, excessive, and/or frequent menses), infertility, painful defecation during menses, sacral backache, and dyspareunia. Patient may be asymptomatic.

Physical exam: Palpation of the peritoneal cul-de-sac and ovaries may reveal presence of nodules or masses with extensive disease. Nodularity and tenderness of the uterosacral ligaments are common. The pelvic exam is performed several days before the menstrual cycle.

B. Diagnostic Tests

1. Laparoscopy: Confirms presence of endometriosis at pelvic organs by passing a lighted instrument through an incision made near the umbilicus.
2. Culdoscopy: Also confirms the presence of endometriosis by passing a lighted instrument through the vagina to visualize the pelvic organs.

C. Medical Management and Surgical Interventions

1. **Encourage pregnancy in women wishing to have children:** Pregnancy softens and atrophies the diseased areas as a result of hormone production. Pregnancy (or pseudopregnancy) stops the spread of endometriosis, and in most cases remission occurs following delivery.
2. **Pharmacotherapy:** Estrogens are not used because of their side effects. *Danazol* (400 mg bid) is an androgen given to suppress ovulation and, hence, endometriosis. It is the current treatment of choice.
3. **Surgical procedures:** Determined by the patient's age and desire to have children, and by extent of the disease. They are performed if medical treatment is unsuccessful.

   □ *For women without extensive disease who wish to have children, one of the following is performed:* Cauterization of endometrial implants, uterine suspension, lysis of adhesions, or removal of endometrial implants. These procedures are usually performed via an abdominal approach, although uterine suspension also can be performed by a vaginal approach.

   □ *For women who are not menopausal but do not wish to have children:* A hysterectomy is performed, leaving the ovaries intact so that normal hormonal balance is maintained.

   □ *When there is extensive disease:* A total hysterectomy with bilateral salpingo-oophorectomy is performed. The ovaries are removed because they are the hormone-carrying organs, which influence the development and progression of the disease.

D. Nursing Diagnoses and Interventions

See "Cancer of the Cervix" for the following: **Alteration in comfort**, p. 432, **Potential fluid volume deficit** (blood loss), p. 433 and **Potential alteration in pattern of urinary elimination**, p. 433. See "Appendix One" for nursing diagnoses and interventions for the care of preoperative and postoperative patients, pp. 528–532.

E. Patient–Family Teaching and Discharge Planning

See "Ovarian Tumors," p. 436.

II. Cystocele

A cystocele is the bulging of the posterior bladder wall into the vagina. It is caused by the stretching and tearing of the pelvic connective tissue during childbirth. Most often it occurs as a result of the delivery of a very large baby or after several deliveries. Symptoms usually do not appear until middle age. A rectocele also might be present (see "Rectocele," p. 440).

A. Assessment

Signs and symptoms: Sensation of vaginal fullness, inability to empty bladder after voiding, urinary frequency, dysuria, stress incontinence, incontinence resulting from urgency, and recurrent cystitis.

Physical exam: Manual pelvic exam will reveal prolapsed cervix and a soft mass that bulges into the anterior vagina. The mass increases in size with straining.

B. Diagnostic Tests

1. Cystogram: May show the presence of bladder herniation.
2. Measurement of residual urine via intermittent urinary catheterization: May reveal >60 mL.
3. Urine culture and sensitivity: May reveal presence of bladder infection caused by retention.

C. Medical Management and Surgical Interventions

1. **Urinary catheterization:** To empty a distended bladder. This is an emergency measure rather than a permanent correction.
2. **Antibiotics:** Given if urinary retention results in an infection.
3. **Estrogen therapy:** Conjugated estrogen (Premarin) is sometimes given in small doses daily for 3 weeks each month in postmenopausal women to maintain hormonal levels. A lack of hormones results in weakness of the anterior vaginal wall, which allows the development of a cystocele.
4. **Kegel isometric exercises:** To help with bladder control. See discussion, p. 137.
5. **Weight control:** Overweight women are encouraged to lose weight.
6. **Anterior colporrhaphy:** Surgical procedure via vaginal approach to suspend the bladder. It involves separating the anterior vaginal wall from the bladder and urethra, suturing the bladder wall to reduce herniation, and excising the thinned vaginal wall. If a cystocele and rectocele (see "Rectocele," p. 440) are both present, an anterior and posterior colporrhaphy (A&P repair) is performed.
7. **Pessary:** Used as an internal support for some patients (see discussion in "Uterine Prolapse," p. 442).

D. Nursing Diagnoses and Interventions

See "Cancer of the Cervix" for the following: **Potential fluid volume deficit** (blood loss), p. 433. See "Urinary Incontinence" in Chapter 3, "Renal–Urinary Disorders", for nursing diagnoses and interventions pertaining to incontinence, p. 136. See "Appendix One" for nursing diagnoses and interventions for the care of preoperative and postoperative patients, pp. 528–532.

E. Patient–Family Teaching and Discharge Planning:

Provide patient and SOs with verbal and written information for the following:

1. Medications, including drug name, purpose, dosage, schedule, precautions, and potential side effects.

2. Activity limitations during the first 6 weeks or as directed, including no heavy lifting (>5 lb) or strenuous exercises.

3. Abstinence from sexual intercourse for 6 weeks or as prescribed if vaginal surgery was performed.

4. Notifying MD of the following indicators of infection: persistent pain; purulent, foul-smelling drainage.

5. Importance of follow-up appointments; confirm date and time of next appointment if known.

III. Rectocele

A rectocele is a rectovaginal hernia that develops when the connective tissue between the rectum and vagina is ruptured during the delivery of a large baby, a rapid or forceps delivery, or a breech presentation. If there is straining with defecation or the patient is obese, the condition is aggravated and progresses. The symptoms of this condition often do not become apparent until the woman is 35–40 years old.

A. Assessment

Signs and symptoms: Continuous urge to have a bowel movement, sensation of rectal and vaginal fullness, constipation, incontinence of flatus and/or feces, and the presence of hemorrhoids and/or fecal impaction.

Physical exam: A nontender fullness can be felt by depressing the perineum as the patient strains; manual rectal examination will reveal the presence of a rectocele.

B. Diagnostic Test

Barium enema: Will reveal the presence of a rectocele.

C. Medical Management and Surgical Interventions

1. **Promote bowel elimination:** With laxatives, stool softeners, and a high-fiber diet.

2. **Posterior colporrhaphy:** This surgical procedure separates the posterior vaginal wall from the rectum and reduces the rectal herniation. If both a cystocele and rectocele are present, an anterior and posterior colporrhaphy (A&P repair) is performed. (See "Cystocele," p. 439.)

D. Nursing Diagnoses and Interventions

Alteration in bowel elimination: Constipation related to restriction against straining, low-residue diet, and/or pain with defecation secondary to surgical procedure

Desired outcomes: After the early postoperative period, patient relates the presence of bowel movements within her normal pattern, with minimal discomfort. Patient can verbalize knowledge of the rationale for alerting staff before and after bowel movements, and for not straining during defecation.

1. Assess patient for the presence of constipation; administer stool softeners or mild laxatives as prescribed.

2. The patient will be on a low-residue diet during the early postoperative period to minimize the potential for disruption of the surgical site. As indicated after the early postoperative period, consult with the MD regarding the introduction of high-residue foods to promote bowel movements.

3. Instruct patient not to strain when having a bowel movement, as this can disrupt the surgical repair.

4. Advise patient that defecation may be painful and to alert staff as soon as the urge to defecate is felt so that she can be medicated prior to the bowel movement.

5. As prescribed, use a heat lamp to help reduce perineal swelling, promote healing, and reduce discomfort.

6. Avoid the use of enemas and/or rectal tubes, which can disrupt the surgical repair.

7. Provide sitz baths as a comfort measure.

8. Request that the patient notify staff after each bowel movement; document accordingly.

See "Cancer of the Cervix" for the following: **Potential fluid volume deficit** (blood loss), p. 433. See "Appendix One" for nursing diagnoses and interventions for the care of preoperative and postoperative patients, pp. 528–532.

E. Patient–Family Teaching and Discharge Planning

Provide patient and SOs with verbal and written information for the following:

1. Medications, including drug name, purpose, dosage, schedule, precautions, and potential side effects.

2. Limitation of activities during the first 6 weeks as directed by MD, including heavy lifting (>5 lb) and exercising. Abstinence from sexual intercourse is usually recommended for 6 weeks. Advise patients that initially coitus may be painful.

3. Indicators of infection: abdominal or rectal pain, foul-smelling vaginal discharge, and/or fever.

4. Importance of follow-up care; confirm date and time of next medical appointment if known.

IV. Uterine Prolapse

A uterine prolapse is a bulging of the uterus through the pelvic floor into the vagina. It results from an injury to the cervical and uterosacral ligaments, which can occur with childbirth, surgical trauma, or atrophy of the supportive tissue during menopause. A prolapse also can develop as a result of uterine tumors, diabetic neuropathy, neurologic injury to the sacral nerves, obesity, or ascites. A prolapse will progress unless surgically repaired.

A prolapse is graded in the following way:

□ *Grade I:* Cervix remains within the vagina; the uterus partially descends into the vagina. This is a slight prolapse.

□ *Grade II:* Cervix protrudes through the entrance to the vagina. This is a moderate prolapse.

□ *Grade III:* Entire uterus protrudes through the entrance of the vagina with vaginal inversion. This a severe prolapse, occurring most frequently in postmenopausal, multiparous women and often along with a rectocele, cystocele, and enterocele (a hernia containing a loop of small intestine or the sigmoid colon that bulges into the upper posterior vagina).

A. Assessment

Signs and symptoms: Patient complaints of heaviness in the pelvis, low bachache, "dragging" sensation in the inguinal region, and involuntary loss of urine with coughing/sneezing.

Physical exam: Pelvic examination is performed with the patient either standing or supine. As patient bears down, a firm mass can be palpated in the lower vagina. This exam also can confirm diagnosis of a rectocele and cystocele, if present.

B. Medical Managment and Surgical Interventions

1. **Vaginal pessary:** A rubber device that is inserted into the vagina to support the pelvic structures. It is used if there is a slight or moderate prolapse and/or if surgery is contraindicated or unwanted by patient.

2. **Weight loss:** If patient is obese.

3. **Estrogen suppositories:** To maintain tone of the pelvic floor.

4. **Antibiotics:** If patient has a urinary tract infection.

5. **High-fiber diet:** To aid in bowel elimination.

6. **Vaginal hysterectomy:** To correct uterine prolapse. For severe prolapse with rectocele and cystocele, a hysterectomy with an anterior/posterior colporrhaphy is performed.

C. Nursing Diagnoses and Interventions

Disturbance in self-concept related to changes in body image and role performance expectations secondary to hysterectomy

Desired outcomes: Patient can verbalize her perceptions of past, present, and future role expectations. Patient relates beginning adaptation to her hysterectomy and begins to assume self-care as her condition allows.

1. Assess the patient's concern with body image and role performance expectations as a result of the hysterectomy. Be alert to verbal and nonverbal responses. Provide emotional support and an unhurried milieu for the patient and SOs to express feelings.

2. Anticipate questions and provide information in a caring manner. Be sensitive to the patient's concerns.

3. Recognize the covert signs of grief that can accompany self-concept disturbances: anger, withdrawal, demanding behavior, or inappropriate affect. Give support to SOs who may misinterpret the patient's coping mechanisms.

4. Enhance patient's sense of control over her situation by encouraging her to perform ADLs and begin self-care as her condition warrants.

5. If appropriate, refer the patient to a psychosocial health care professional.

See "Rectocele" for the following: **Alteration in bowel elimination:** Constipation, p. 440. See "Cancer of the Cervix" for the following: **Potential fluid volume deficit** (blood loss), p. 433. See "Appendix One" for nursing diagnoses and interventions for the care of preoperative and postoperative patients, pp. 528–532.

D. Patient–Family Teaching and Discharge Planning

See "Rectocele," p. 441.

▶ Section Four   **Interruption of Pregnancy**

The following conditions or surgical procedures involve women of childbearing age and can result in continued problems with childbearing and/or sterilization.

I. Spontaneous Abortion

A spontaneous abortion, or miscarriage, occurs in approximately 15% of pregnancies. It is the expulsion of the products of conception before the 24th week of gestation and it is classified in the following ways:

Threatened abortion: Vaginal bleeding and cramping during the first trimester and part of the second. Either the symptoms disappear or an abortion occurs.

Inevitable abortion: Vaginal bleeding, cramping, and dilation and effacement of the cervix; cannot be halted.

Incomplete abortion: Expulsion of products of conception, with continued vaginal bleeding, indicating that part or all of the placenta remains attached to the uterus.

Complete abortion: Expulsion of all products of conception, with minimal vaginal bleeding.

Missed abortion: Presence of a dead fetus in the uterus, without expulsion.

Habitual abortion: Three or more pregnancies that are spontaneously aborted by the same woman.

There are three primary causes of spontaneous abortion: *fetal*, which includes defective development and faulty implantation of the fertilized ovum; *maternal*, including infection, malnutrition, and endocrine abnormalities and incompetent cervix; and *placental*, which includes abruptio placenta (premature separation of placenta) and incorrect placental implantation.

A. Assessment

Signs and symptoms: Vaginal bleeding, cramping, low back pain, no increase in size of uterus, anorexia.

Physical exam: A pelvic examination will reveal the size of the uterus and show either that products of conception are intact or have been expelled.

B. Diagnostic Tests

1. <u>CBC:</u> Will reveal a decrease in hemoglobin and hematocrit. There is a potential for elevation in leukocyte count, which would signal an infection.

2. <u>Lab examination of products of conception:</u> To confirm results of pelvic examination.

3. <u>Ultrasound:</u> Will confirm the presence of a dead fetus in a missed abortion as evidenced by absence of fetal movement.

4. <u>Endocrine studies:</u> Human chorionic gonadotropin (HCG), estrogen, and progesterone titers will be minimal or absent.

C. Medical Management and Surgical Interventions

1. **Blood and/or blood products:** Administered for excessive blood loss.

2. **Parenteral fluid administration:** For excessive fluid loss.

3. **Analgesics:** For pain management.

4. **Antibiotics:** When indicated, to prevent or treat infection.

5. **Dilation and currettage (D&C):** Procedure done in the first trimester to remove products of conception. Under general or local anesthesia, the canal of the cervix is dilated to allow a curette to pass through the cervix into the

uterus and scrape out any products of conception that remain. A **suction evacuation**, which utilizes a suction apparatus rather than a curette, may be performed instead.

6. **IV oxytocin:** To induce labor after 12 weeks' gestation. Oxytocin contracts the uterus by stimulating the smooth muscles.

7. **Shirodkar procedure:** Performed early in the second trimester to manage an incompetent cervix when patient has a history of repeated second trimester abortions. With this technique, the cervix is reinforced with a purse-string suture. The suture is released at term (or immediately if labor begins) to allow a vaginal delivery. This procedure is not performed in the presence of membrane rupture, cramping, vaginal bleeding, or a cervical dilation greater than 3 cm.

8. **RhoGAM:** an Rh_o (D) immune globulin given to prevent Rh sensitization in Rh-negative women whose partners are Rh-positive.

D. Nursing Diagnoses and Interventions

Potential fluid volume deficit related to abnormal loss secondary to postsurgical or post-abortion bleeding

Desired outcome: Patient does not exhibit signs of excessive blood loss or shock.

1. Assess and document BP, pulse, and respirations at frequent intervals (typically q15min × 4; q30min × 2; q1–2h until stable; and then q4h). Notify MD of significant changes. Be alert to hypotension, changes in LOC, and increasing pulse and respiration rates.

2. Monitor I&O at least q4h. Be alert to decreasing urinary output, which can signal the onset of shock.

3. Administer parenteral fluids, blood, and blood products as prescribed.

4. Inspect perineal pads and note and document the amount and quality of bleeding. If vaginal bleeding increases or there is expulsion of the products of conception, notify MD at once. Save any tissue or clots that are expelled. **Note:** Bleeding is considered excessive if more than two perineal pads are saturated in 1 hour.

5. If prescribed, administer oxytocin to assist with the contraction of the uterus and expulsion of the fetus.

6. After expulsion of the contents of conception has occurred, palpate the uterine fundus to assess its tone. If it feels soft and boggy, provide light massage by rubbing in a circular motion. **Caution:** Avoid massaging a uterus that is well contracted, because this can result in muscle fatigue and uterine relaxation.

Alteration in comfort: Acute pain related to uterine contractions

Desired outcome: Patient verbalizes reduction in discomfort and does not exhibit signs of uncontrolled pain.

1. Monitor and document number and length of contractions. Assess and document the patient's level of pain and response to pain management.

2. Administer analgesics as prescribed. Provide backrubs, which are especially relaxing.

3. Instruct patient in alternative methods of pain relief, including deep breathing, relaxation techniques, and guided imagery.

4. Assist patient with ADLs as appropriate.

Potential for infection related to increased susceptibility secondary to retention of some or all of the products of conception

Desired outcomes: Patient does not exhibit signs of infection. If an infection is present, it is detected and reported promptly.

1. Assess temperature q4h; notify MD if an elevation occurs.

2. Be alert to the presence of foul-smelling vaginal discharge, an indicator of infection.

3. Administer antibiotics as prescribed.

4. Ensure that perineal care is performed after every voiding and bowel movement.

Disturbance in self-concept related to altered expectations for role performance secondary to loss of fetus

Desired outcomes: Patient verbalizes realistic acceptance of change in her role or verbalizes plans for adaptation. Patient demonstrates communication with SOs.

1. Provide emotional support for patient and SOs. Provide time and a supportive atmosphere for patient to feel comfortable with expressing feelings and concerns.

2. Assist patient with identifying concerns, if present, with role performance as a wife and/or childbearer. Assist patient with developing plans for adaptation.

3. Involve social services if needed.

Grieving related to anticipated or actual fetal loss

Desired outcomes: Patient is able to express feelings about the (potential) loss, is able to share her grief with SOs, and does not demonstrate evidence of ineffective coping.

1. Assess the stage of grieving patient is experiencing. Be aware that feelings may be complicated by emotions that preceded the (impending) fetal loss. For example, if the woman experienced joy regarding her pregnancy, her grief may be more than anticipated. Conversely, if the pregnancy was viewed as a negative experience, she may experience feelings of guilt and/or self-blame.

2. Assist patient and SOs with acknowledging the loss by taking the time to sit and talk with them.

3. Offer emotional support and encourage the patient and SOs to discuss the loss among themselves, as well.

4. Ensure privacy for the patient and SOs.

5. Refer the patient to community-based parent support group.

6. Provide for pastoral or other supportive care if indicated.

E. Patient–Family Teaching and Discharge Planning

Provide patient and SOs with verbal and written information for the following:

1. Medications, including drug name, purpose, dosage, schedule, precautions, and potential side effects.

2. Vaginal bleeding, which should taper gradually during the first 10 days. Advise patient that increasing bleeding is abnormal and necessitates medical attention.

3. Indicators of infection, which necessitate medical attention: temperature 100F or greater and foul-smelling vaginal discharge.

4. Activity limitations as directed by MD, including strenous exercise and sexual intercourse.

5. Importance of follow-up care; confirm date and time of next medical appointment if known.

6. Name and address of community resources.

II. Tubal (Ectopic) Pregnancy

A tubal pregnancy is an implanted fertile ovum in the fallopian tube or, more rarely, in the peritoneum, ovary, or cervix. In the fallopian tube, the implanted ovum causes a weakening of the tubal wall, resulting in a rupture that can cause bleeding into the peritoneum, a medical emergency. Factors that predispose toward ectopic pregnancy include pelvic inflammatory disease (PID); a tumor in the fallopian tube, resulting in tubal distortion; surgical scarring of the fallopian tube; tubal endometriosis; and gonorrhea. These pathologies may interfere with the structure and function of the fallopian tube and cause a delay in the passage of the ovum into the uterus, which can result in a tubal pregnancy.

Tubal pregnancies occur in 1 out of every 200 pregnancies.

A. Assessment

Signs and symptoms: Indications of pregnancy, including amenorrhea, nausea, breast enlargement, urinary frequency. The following acute symptoms occur during the 6th week of gestation: mild to moderate vaginal bleeding with unilateral lower abdominal cramping that becomes increasingly sharp and constant, referred shoulder pain caused by irritation of the diaphragm from the pooling of blood in the peritoneum, and fever. **Caution:** Immediate intervention is necessary to prevent loss of blood, which can lead to shock and death.

Physical exam: Abdominal palpation may reveal a unilateral lower quadrant tenderness; auscultation may reveal decreased bowel sounds. **Note:** Pelvic examination is deferred until the patient is anesthetized or has received pain medication because of the severe pain that can be elicited.

B. Diagnostic Tests

1. <u>CBC:</u> May reveal a decreased hemoglobin and hematocrit and an increased leukocyte count.
2. <u>Serum pregnancy test:</u> Usually positive.
3. <u>Ultrasound:</u> May identify the presence of a gestational sac.
4. <u>Culdocentesis:</u> May reveal the presence of blood in the peritoneum. In this test, fluid is aspirated from the vaginal cul-de-sac.
5. <u>Laparoscopy:</u> Will confirm the presence of ectopic pregnancy and allow immediate treatment.

C. Medical Management and Surgical Interventions

1. **Whole blood or packed cells:** To replace loss if necessary.
2. **Broad spectrum IV antibiotics:** May be administered prophylactically.
3. **Analgesics/narcotics:** For pain management.
4. **Laparotomy with salpingectomy:** Performed to remove the affected tube and its contents if the ectopic pregnancy has not ruptured.
5. **Unilateral salpingectomy (removal of the fallopian tube) or salpingo-oophorectomy (removal of the fallopian tube and ovary):** Performed if the ectopic pregnancy ruptures. A ruptured ectopic pregnancy is considered a surgical emergency because of the inevitable loss of blood into the peritoneum. The type of surgical procedure used is dependent on the extent of structural involvement.
6. **RhoGAM:** If indicated, is given to Rh-negative mothers after ectopic pregnancy.

D. Nursing Diagnoses and Interventions

Potential fluid volume deficit related to abnormal loss secondary to bleeding/hemorrhage with ectopic rupture

Desired outcome: Patient does not exhibit signs of excessive bleeding or shock.

1. Assess VS at frequent intervals, noting changes in BP, pulse, and respiratory rate. Be alert to hypotension and increases in pulse and respiratory rates as indicators of impending shock.

2. Assess the amount and quality of vaginal bleeding. Bright red, frank bleeding, along with abnormal VS, should be reported to the MD at once.

3. Review results of CBC, noting values of hemoglobin and hematocrit, which are decreased with blood loss

4. Infuse parenteral and/or blood products as prescribed.

Potential for infection related to increased susceptibility secondary to ectopic rupture

Desired outcome: Patient does not exhibit signs of infection; or, if they appear, they are detected and reported promptly.

1. Monitor leukocyte count, which will be elevated with infection.

2. Monitor the patient's temperature q4h; note and report significant elevations to MD.

3. Administer antibiotics as prescribed.

See "Spontaneous Abortion" for the following: **Disturbance in self-concept**, p. 445, and **Grieving**, p. 445. See "Appendix One" for nursing diagnoses and interventions for the care of preoperative and postoperative patients, pp. 528–532.

E. Patient–Family Teaching and Discharge Planning

Provide patient and SOs with verbal and written information for the following:

1. Medications, including drug name, purpose, dosage, schedule, precautions, and potential side effects.

2. Importance of monitoring vaginal drainage, including the amount, color, consistency, and odor; and reporting significant changes to MD.

3. Activity limitations as directed by MD, including strenuous exercise, housework, and sexual intercourse.

4. Indicators of incisional infection including persistent redness, swelling, warmth, fever, purulent discharge, and incisional/abdominal pain.

5. Importance of follow-up care; confirm time and date of next medical visit if known.

▶ Section Five   **Disorders and Surgeries of the Male Pelvis**

I. Benign Prostatic Hypertrophy

The prostate is an encapsulated gland that surrounds the male urethra below the bladder neck and produces a thin, milky fluid during ejaculation. As a man ages, the prostate gland grows larger. Although the exact cause of the enlargement is unknown, one theory is that hormonal changes affect the estrogren–androgen balance. This noncancerous enlargement is common in men over age 50, and as many as 75% of men over the age of 70 are believed to have symptoms of prostatic enlargement.

A. Assessment

Chronic indicators: Urinary frequency, hesitancy, and dribbling; decreased force of stream; nocturia; hematuria.

Acute indicators: Anuria, nausea, vomiting, abdominal tenderness, pain that is sharp and intense.

Physical exam: Bladder distention, "kettle-drum" sound with percussion over the distended bladder. Rectal exam will reveal a smooth, firm, and elastic enlargement of the prostate.

B. Diagnostic Tests

1. <u>Urinalysis</u> tests the integrity of urinary function and <u>urine culture and sensitivity</u> verifies presence of infection; the results will specify the type of organism and determine the most effective antibiotic.

2. <u>Phenolsulfonphthalein (PSP):</u> Tests adequacy of renal blood flow and tubular function. PSP is injected into a vein and urine is collected via indwelling catheterization at least three times post-injection. **Note:** Because high fluid intake is necessary for patients undergoing this test, closely monitor patients who have cardiac or renal insufficiencies.

3. <u>CBC, other blood tests:</u> Results might indicate mild anemia from local bleeding, elevated creatinine if renal function has been affected, and elevated blood urea nitrogen (BUN) if renal function is compromised.

4. <u>Cystoscopy:</u> To visualize the prostate gland, estimate its size, and ascertain the presence of any damage to the bladder wall secondary to an enlarged prostate. **Note:** Because patients undergoing cystoscopy are susceptible to septic shock, it is contraindicated in patients with acute UTI because of the danger of introducing gram negative bacteria into the bladder.

5. <u>Intravenous pyelography (IVP)/excretory urogram:</u> Evaluates the structure and function of the kidneys, ureters, and bladder, and reveals calculi if they are present. **Note:** Two complications of IVP are allergic reaction to dye and acute renal failure induced by the contrast medium. Exposure to contrast medium might worsen existing renal insufficiency, especially in elderly, dehydrated, or diabetic patients. Before the study, patients should be queried about allergies to shellfish or reactions to previous dye studies. After IVP, patients should be monitored for indicators of renal failure.

▶ **Note:** All urine specimens should be sent to the laboratory immediately after they are obtained, or refrigerated if this is not possible. Urine left at room temperature has a greater potential for bacterial growth, turbidity, and alkaline pH, any of which can distort the test results.

C. Medical Management and Surgical Interventions

1. **Catheterization:** To relieve urinary retention.

2. **Antibiotics and antimicrobial agents:** To treat infection, if one is present.

3. **Antiandrogen (estrogen) therapy:** May be initiated to lower the levels of testosterone if this is the cause of the prostate's enlargement. Occasionally, an orchiectomy is performed for the same purpose. **Note:** The patient will become impotent while on estrogen therapy; however, an orchiectomy will *not* affect the patient's ability to have intercourse.

4. **Reducing prostatic congestion via rectal massage of the prostate gland:** This is performed only if there is substantial congestion. Hot sitz baths are also prescribed to relieve congestion.

5. **Restricting rapid intake of fluids:** Particularly alcohol, which can result in episodes of acute urinary retention from loss of bladder tone secondary to rapid distention.

6. **Prostatectomy:** Removal of enlarged prostatic tissue.
   □ *Transurethral resection of the prostate (TURP):* Prostatic tissue is scraped away

via cystoscopy. This is the most common approach, especially in patients who are poor surgical risks. It is done under spinal anesthesia.

◻ *Suprapubic transvesical prostatectomy:* Prostatic tissue is removed via incision high in the bladder (abdominal approach). This is indicated for a large prostate that cannot be removed transurethrally.

◻ *Retropubic extravesical prostatectomy:* Prostatic tissue is removed via low abdominal incision without entry into the bladder.

7. **Prostatic cryosurgery:** Prostatic tissue is frozen and destroyed by the instillation of liquid nitrogen through an indwelling catheter. The tissue begins to slough off after 2–3 days and will continue to do so even after the catheter is removed. This procedure may be chosen for patients who are very poor surgical risks. It is done under local anesthesia.

D. Nursing Diagnoses and Interventions

Knowledge deficit: Potential for infection/shock after cystoscopy or TURP

Desired outcome: Patient and/or SOs can verbalize knowledge of the indicators of shock/infection and are aware of the need to alert staff immediately should they occur.

1. Patients who have had a cystoscopy and/or TURP are at increased risk for septic shock because of the surgical instrumentation. Teach the following indicators to the patient and/or SOs and explain the importance of alerting the staff immediately should they occur: low-grade temperature (100–101F), warm extremities, rapid pulse and respiration rates, restlessness, unusual anxiety, irritability, and disorientation.

2. Teach the following indicators of UTI: chills, fever, flank pain, diaphoresis, and cloudy and/or foul-smelling urine.

3. Explain to patient and SOs that with the first stages of septic shock the skin will remain warm, dry, and pink, but will become cool and clammy with reduced cardiac output. In addition, as shock progresses, urinary output decreases.

Potential fluid volume deficit related to abnormal loss secondary to bleeding/hemorrhage due to surgical procedure and/or pressure on the prostatic capsule

Desired outcomes: Patient does not exhibit signs of excessive bleeding. Patient can verbalize knowledge of actions that might result in hemorrhage of the prostatic capsule.

1. Upon patient's return from the recovery room, monitor VS q15min for first hour; if stable, check q30min for an hour and then q4h for 24 hours. Be alert to increasing pulse, decreasing BP, diaphoresis, pallor, and increasing respirations, which can occur with hemorrhage and impending shock.

2. Monitor catheter drainage closely for the first 24 hours. Watch for dark red drainage that does not lighten to reddish-pink or drainage that remains thick in consistency after irrigation, which can signal venous bleeding within the operative site.

3. Be alert to bright red, thick drainage at any time, which can occur with arterial bleeding within the operative site.

4. Do not measure temperature rectally or insert rectal tubes or enemas into the rectum. Instruct patient not to strain with bowel movements or sit for long periods of time. Any of these actions can result in pressure on the prostatic capsule and potentially lead to hemorrhage. Obtain prescription for and provide stool softeners or cathartics as necessary.

5. The surgeon may establish traction on the indwelling urethral catheter in the operating room to help prevent bleeding. Maintain the traction for 4–8 hours after surgery, or as directed.

Potential fluid volume excess: Edema related to retention secondary to administration of high volumes of irrigating fluid

Desired outcomes: Patient does not exhibit signs of fluid overload or electrolyte imbalance, or, if they occur, they are detected and reported promptly. Patient and SOs can verbalize the indicators of fluid overload and are aware of the need to alert the staff immediately should they occur.

1. Monitor and record I&O. To determine the true amount of urinary output, subtract the amount of irrigant from the total output. Report discrepancies that indicate fluid retention.
2. Monitor the patient's mental and motor status. Assess for the presence of muscle twitching, convulsions, and changes in mentation. These are signs of water intoxification and/or electrolyte imbalance, which can occur within 24 hours of surgery because of the high volumes of fluid that are used in irrigation. Alert patient and SOs to the potential for these indicators.
3. Promptly report indications of fluid overload and/or electrolyte imbalance to the MD.

Potential impairment of skin integrity related to irritation secondary to wound drainage

Desired outcome: Patient does not exhibit evidence of skin impairment at the wound site.

1. Monitor incisional dressings frequently during the first 24 hours and change or reinforce as needed. If the incision has been made into the bladder, excoriation can result from prolonged contact of urine with the skin.
2. Use Montgomery straps rather than tape to secure the dressing.
3. If the drainage is copious after drain removal, apply a wound drainage or ostomy pouch with a skin barrier over the incision. Use a pouch with an anti-reflux valve to prevent contamination from reflux.

Alteration in comfort: Pain related to bladder spasms

Desired outcome: Patient relates a reduction in discomfort and does not exhibit evidence of uncontrolled pain.

1. Assess and document the quality, location, and duration of pain.
2. Medicate the patient with prescribed analgesics, narcotics, and antispasmodics as appropriate; evaluate and document the patient's response.
3. Provide warm blankets, heating pad to affected area, or warm baths to increase regional circulation and relax tense muscles.
4. Teach technique for slow, diaphragmatic breathing to relax patient and help ease pain.
5. Provide backrubs and encourage use of other nonpharmacologic methods of pain relief such as guided imagery, distraction, relaxation tapes, and soothing music.
6. Monitor for leakage around the catheter, which can signal the presence of bladder spasms.
7. If the patient has spasms, assure him they are normal and can occur because of irritation of the bladder mucosa by the catheter balloon or from a clot that results in backup of urine into the bladder with concomitant irritatation of the mucosa. Encourage fluid intake, as this will help prevent spasms. If the MD has prescribed catheter irrigation for the removal of clots, follow instructions carefully to prevent discomfort and injury to patient.

Potential for sexual dysfunction related to fear of impotence secondary to lack of knowledge of postsurgical sexual function

Desired outcome: Patient can verbalize knowledge of accurate information regarding sexual function.

1. Assess patient's level of readiness to discuss sexual function; provide opportunities for patient to discuss fears and anxieties.

2. Assure patient who has had a simple prostatectomy that his ability to attain and sustain an erection is unaltered. Retrograde ejaculation or "dry" ejaculation occurs in most patients, but this ends after a few months. It does not, however, affect the ability to achieve orgasm.

3. Encourage communication between patient and his SO.

4. Be aware of your own feelings regarding sexuality. If you are uncomfortable discussing sexuality, request that another staff member take responsibility for discussing feelings and concerns with the patient.

See "Cancer of the Bladder" in Chapter 3, "Renal–Urinary Disorders," for the following: **Potential alteration in pattern of urinary elimination** related to obstruction of suprapubic catheter, p. 130. See "Appendix One" for nursing diagnoses and interventions for the care of preoperative and postoperative patients, pp. 528–532.

E. Patient–Family Teaching and Discharge Planning

Provide patient and SOs with verbal and written information for the following:

1. Medications, including drug name, purpose, dosage, schedule, precautions, and potential side effects.

2. Indicators that necessitate medical attention: cloudy or foul-smelling urine, fever, pain, dysuria.

3. Care of incision, if appropriate, including cleansing, dressing changes, and bathing. Advise patient to be aware of indicators of infection: persistent redness, increased warmth along incision, or purulent drainage.

4. Care of catheters or drains if patient is discharged with them.

5. Daily fluid requirement of at least 2–3 L/day in nonrestricted patients.

6. Consuming foods or juices that produce an acid ash in the urine to help minimize the potential for UTI. These include cranberries, plums, and prunes.

7. Importance of increasing dietary fiber or taking stool softeners to minimize the risk of damage to the prostatic capsule by preventing straining with bowel movements.

8. Avoiding the following activities for the period of time prescribed by MD: sitting for long periods of time, heavy lifting (>5 lb), and sexual intercourse.

9. Perineal exercises to help regain urinary sphincter control.

II. Prostatitis

Prostatitis is inflammation of the prostate gland. Acute bacterial prostatitis is the form most frequently seen in the hospital setting. It is caused by the introduction of bacteria into the prostate via the bloodstream, urethra, or the kidneys. The urethra is the most common avenue for introduction of bacteria, and patients undergoing urethral instrumentation such as cystoscopy or catheterization are at increased risk. Statistics show an increased risk of prostatitis with advancing age and increased prostate size.

A. Assessment

Signs and symptoms: Chills, fever (moderate to high), urinary urgency and frequency, dysuria, perineal and low back pain, and purulent urethral discharge. Mental confusion might be seen in older patients because of decreased oxygenation in the brain due to infection.

Physical exam: Presence of tender, enlarged, boggy prostate gland palpated on rectal exam.

B. Diagnostic Tests

1. <u>WBC count:</u> To reveal presence of infection.
2. <u>Urinalysis and urine culture:</u> To detect the presence of urinary tract infection (UTI) and identify the offending bacteria.
3. <u>BUN and creatinine:</u> Show evidence of renal involvement when the test results are elevated.
4. <u>Culture and sensitivity of the prostatic and urethral exudate:</u> Identifies the causative bacteria and determines the most appropriate antibiotic.

▶ **Note:** All urine specimens should be sent to the laboratory immediately after they are obtained, or refrigerated if this is not possible. Urine left at room temperature has a greater potential for bacterial growth, turbidity, and alkalinity, any of which can distort the test results.

C. Medical Management and Surgical Interventions

1. **Pharmacotherapy** may include the following:

   □ *Antispasmodics:* Such as propantheline bromide or oxybutynin chloride.

   □ *Stool softeners:* To prevent pressure on the prostatic capsule from straining.

   □ *Antipyretics:* For fever associated with infections.

   □ *Urinary analgesics:* Such as phenazopyridine hydrochloride to alleviate burning with urination.

   □ *Antibiotics:* Often given in combination (eg, trimethoprim-sulfamethoxazole) to control gram-negative bacteria. The erythromycins usually are given for gram-positive bacteria, and gentamicin or tobramycin sulfate is used for more severe infections. If sepsis is suspected, ampicillin or amoxicillin is given.

2. **Bed rest:** Either strict or with bathroom privileges during the first 24–48 hours to relieve perineal and suprapubic pain.
3. **Intravenous fluids:** For hydration.
4. **Serial urine cultures, urinalysis, and WBC:** To monitor the infection and determine bacterial level.
5. **Sitz baths:** To relax perineal muscles and reduce risk of urinary retention.
6. **Suprapubic drainage system:** For relief of continued urinary retention.
7. **Restriction of sexual intercourse:** During the acute phase.

▶ **Note:** During the acute phase of bacterial infection, urethral instrumentation is contraindicated.

D. Nursing Diagnoses and Interventions

Alteration in comfort: Pain related to infectious process

Desired outcome: Patient verbalizes relief of discomfort and does not exhibit signs of uncontrolled pain.

1. Assess and document the quality, location, and duration of pain.

2. Medicate patient as prescribed with analgesics for urinary burning and anti-spasmodics for spasms.

3. Provide sitz baths or apply warm blankets or heating pad to patient's perineum to improve circulation and relax tense muscles.

4. Teach patient the technique for slow, diaphragmatic breathing for pain control.

Potential alteration in pattern of urinary elimination related to dysuria or anuria secondary to obstruction associated with prostatitis

Desired outcome: Indications of acute urinary retention, should they occur, are detected and reported promptly.

1. Patient may have frequency or urgency with urination; record time and amount of each voiding. Assess the character of the urinary output, which should be straw colored with a characteristic urine odor.

2. Assess the patient's abdomen and note any indicators of distention, tenderness, or discomfort. Percuss abdomen for evidence of "kettle-drum" sound, which occurs with distention. Because retention can occur secondary to edematous prostatic tissue, notify MD if patient exhibits signs of retention or has not voided in >6 hours.

3. If retention persists, it may be necessary to prepare patient for percutaneous insertion of suprapubic catheter or trocar cystotomy. These procedures are performed by the MD at the bedside after an injection of a local anesthetic into the suprapubic area. Administer narcotic or analgesic as prescribed to relax the patient before the procedure

Sensory-perceptual alterations related to confusion secondary to infectious process

Desired outcome: Patient can verbalize orientation to time, place, and person.

1. Because confusion is a side effect of infection, especially in individuals over age 65, assess the patient's mentation by asking questions that require more than "yes" or "no" answers. Orient patient to reality as necessary.

2. If the patient is confused, keep urinal and other necessary items such as the call light within reach. Keep the siderails up.

3. If mentation is severely affected and the patient is unable to follow simple commands or is confused, arrange to have an SO stay with patient. If this is not possible, obtain a prescription for restraints if appropriate.

4. Do not administer heavy sedatives because the patient may forget where he is and become incontinent or attempt to get up.

See "Cancer of the Bladder" in Chapter 3, "Renal–Urinary Disorders," for the following: **Potential alteration in pattern of urinary elimination** related to obstruction of suprapubic catheter, p. 130.

E. Patient–Family Teaching and Discharge Planning

Provide patient and SOs with verbal and written information for the following:

1. Medications, including drug name, purpose, dosage, schedule, precautions, and potential side effects.

2. Indicators of infection, which necessitate medical attention: cloudy or foul-smelling urine, fever, pain.

3. Care of catheters if patient is discharged with them.

4. Intake of fruits such as cranberries, plums, and prunes to produce an acid ash in the urine to lower urinary pH and help minimize the risk of UTI.

5. Avoidance of methylxanthine-containing foods or fluids, such as alcohol, coffee, caffeinated colas, tea, chocolate, and spices, which can cause diuresis or increase prostatic secretions.

6. Activity restrictions as directed by MD (eg, no prolonged sitting).

III. Prostatic Neoplasm

Cancer of the prostate is the second most common cancer in men over age 50. Because most prostatic neoplasms develop in the posterior portion of the gland, they can be detected in the early stages of development; therefore, rectal examinations should be a part of every man's regular health checks after the age of 40. When it is treated before metastasis occurs, the survival rate is good (70%), but when it is detected after metastasis, the survival rate drops to 35%. Unfortunately, symptoms occur only after prostatic cancer is well advanced, and medical treatment is often not sought until the tumor has affected urinary status or produced back or hip pain, recurring cystitis, or urinary obstruction.

A. Assessment

Signs and symptoms (in the later stages of development): Dysuria, dribbling, anuria, hematuria, nocturia, burning with urination, urgency, chills, fever, and cloudy and foul-smelling urine.

Physical exam: Bladder distention; "kettle-drum" sound with percussion over distended bladder. Rectal exam may reveal a large, hard, fixed prostate with irregular nodules.

B. Diagnostic Tests

1. Urinalysis and urine culture: Verify presence of infection.

2. Phenolsulfonphthalein (PSP): Tests adequacy of renal blood flow and tubular function. PSP is injected into a vein and urine is collected via indwelling catheterization at least three times after injection. **Note:** Because high fluid intake is necessary for patients undergoing this test, closely monitor patients who have cardiac or renal insufficiencies.

3. CBC: Results may reveal presence of marked anemia if bone marrow is being replaced by tumor growth.

4. Creatinine and BUN: Will be elevated if renal function is compromised.

5. Serum acid phosphatase: Will be elevated if metastasis has occurred. Because prostate tissue is rich in this enzyme, the spread of the disease results in an increase in the amount of acid phosphatase in the blood.

6. Serum alkaline phosphatase: Will be elevated if metastasis has spread to the bones.

7. IVP/excretory urogram: Evaluates the structure and function of the kidneys, ureters, and bladder. Other findings may include ureteral obstruction caused by metastasis to the pelvic lymph nodes or direct invasion by the tumor. (See discussion of the complications of IVP on p. 457.)

8. Needle biopsy of prostate: Performed under general anesthesia to remove a portion of the diseased gland for lab analysis. The area to be biopsied is identified digitally via the rectum and the biopsy needle is inserted through the perineal skin directly into the area that has been identified. No dressing is applied, but an indwelling catheter might be inserted if bleeding is expected.

9. CT scan: May show presence of metastasis to the bones. Patient might experience a flushed or burning sensation if contrast medium is administered.

▶ **Note:** All urine specimens should be sent to the laboratory immediately after they are obtained, or refrigerated if this is not possible. Urine left at room temperature has a greater potential for bacterial growth, turbidity, and alkalinity, any of which can distort the test results.

C. Medical Management and Surgical Interventions

1. **Staging of the disease** [based on International Union Against Cancer: Tumor, Nodes, and Metastasis (TNM) System]:

   □ *Stage I:* Cancer is diagnosed by biopsy; no clinical signs or symptoms.

   □ *Stage II:* Cancer is confined to prostatic capsule; can be felt on rectal exam as a hard, stony mass; tumor confined to one lobe of prostate.

   □ *Stage III:* Cancer passes into tissues surrounding the prostate; might reach the lymph nodes or be confined within prostatic capsule; high serum phosphatase levels indicating increased tumor activity; patient might be symptomatic, with dribbling and difficulty starting stream, and/or have recurrent cystitis and urinary retention.

   □ *Stage IV:* Cancer has spread to the bone or into lymph nodes and beyond; presence of high serum phosphatase levels. Patient exhibits signs of advanced disease: uremia, anemia, anorexia, urinary retention, and possibly severe bone pain if bone metastasis has occurred .

2. **External radiation therapy:** Performed both for curative and palliative therapy, depending on the stage of the neoplasm. Treatment occurs over a 6-week period, and patients can expect to remain sexually potent after treatment. This therapy also is used to shrink a tumor, thereby relieving obstruction in the urinary tract.

3. **Interstitial irradiation of the prostate:** Uses gold, chromium, or iodine implantation to destroy the prostate tumor at its origin. It will not, however, affect other areas if metastasis has occurred.

4. **Estrogen therapy:** Might be initiated to reduce plasma testosterone levels, since it is believed that testosterone is involved in the development of prostate cancer. Typically, diethylstilbestrol (DES) is given daily. Estrogen therapy causes 100% impotence during treatment. **Note:** Because DES can cause fluid retention, it must be given cautiously to patients with a history of cardiac disease or renal problems. Estramustine phosphate, a combination of estradiol and nitrogen mustard, might be used if estrogen therapy is ineffective. This drug does not cause impotence and its side effects are few, although patients tend to experience anorexia and nausea.

5. **Chemotherapy:** Might be used either as a curative or palliative measure.

6. **Surgical procedures** might include the following:

   □ *Radical prostatectomy with or without pelvic node dissection:* Using either the perineal or retropubic approach, the entire prostate gland is removed along with the seminal vesicles and a portion of the bladder neck. This procedure is done for stage II and stage III tumors. Occurrence of impotence is 80–100%.

   □ *Bilateral orchiectomy:* Although rarely done, it may be implemented along with estrogen therapy to depress testosterone production.

D. Nursing Diagnoses and Interventions

Knowledge deficit: Side effects of estrogen therapy and/or bilateral orchiectomy

Desired outcome: Patient can verbalize knowledge of the extent and duration of body changes.

1. Inform patient of side effects of estrogen therapy and orchiectomy, for example, breast enlargement, breast tenderness, loss of sexual desire, and/or impotence.

2. For patients on estrogen therapy, provide reassurence that side effects will disappear after therapy has been discontinued.

3. If appropriate, explain to patient that before initiating estrogen therapy, MD may prescribe radiation therapy to the areolae of the breasts to minimize painful gynecomastia. However, this will not decrease other side effects.

4. Assure the patient undergoing orchiectomy that the procedure will not affect his ability to have an erection but that he will not ejaculate.

Grieving related to sexual dysfunction secondary to radical prostatectomy

Desired outcome: Patient can verbalize feelings regarding his impotence.

1. Assess the patient's level of readiness to discuss sexual function; provide opportunities for the patient to discuss feelings and anxieties.

2. Monitor for signs of grief such as hostility, depression, and/or demanding behavior. Conversely, be alert to a patient who is taking the diagnosis too well, which may signal avoidance or denial.

3. Describe the stages of grief to the patient and SO: anger, denial, bargaining, depression, and acceptance; and explain that everyone involved may experience a different stage of grief at a given time.

4. Encourage communication between patient and SO.

5. Be aware of your own feelings regarding sexuality. If you are uncomfortable discussing sexual matters, request that a capable staff member take responsibility for discussing feelings and concerns with the patient.

6. When appropriate, and after discussing the situation with MD, arrange for professional counselling.

See "Benign Prostatic Hypertrophy" for the following: **Potential fluid volume deficit** (blood loss), p. 449, and **Potential impairment of skin integrity**, p. 450. See "Prostatitis" for the following: **Alteration in comfort**, p. 452. See "Appendix One" for nursing diagnoses and interventions for the care of preoperative and postoperative patients, pp. 528–532, and patients with cancer and other life-disrupting illnesses, pp. 544–551.

E. Patient–Family Teaching and Discharge Planning

See "Benign Prostatic Hypertrophy," p. 451.

IV. Testicular Neoplasm

Cancer of the testes is most often found in men in their 20s and 30s. Usually it is discovered by accident, often after a traumatic injury to the groin for which professional examination was warranted. Self-examination is the best method of early detection of this disorder. It is believed that men with an undescended testicle are at higher risk than the general male population. Individuals who have had surgery at an early age to correct this condition have a higher than normal chance of developing the cancer; however, they are also better able to check for lumps and thickenings in the testis after it has been surgically descended.

The most common testicular tumors are seminomas, which spread slowly through the lymphatic system to the iliac and periaortic nodes. Embryonal tumors, on the other hand, metastasize quickly. Other tumor types include teratocarcinoma, adult teratoma, choriocarcinoma, and Leydig cell. Most testicular cancers are combinations of two forms of cancer, which can make treatment difficult.

A. Assessment

Signs and symptoms: Initially, the abnormal lump or thickening in the testis is usually painless, but aching or a heavy sensation is often described. Later, patient may experience abdominal pain from bowel or ureteral obstruction, coughing caused by metastasis to the lungs, weight loss, and anorexia. In addition, growth of breast tissue may occur because of the reduction of testosterone.

Physical exam: Palpation of symmetrical, firm scrotal mass; presence of supra-clavicular or abdominal mass caused by enlargement of lymph nodes in those areas.

B. Diagnostic Tests

1. <u>Hematocrit and hemoglobin:</u> Drawn preoperatively to assess for the presence of anemia, which can occur because of metastasis.

2. <u>24-hour urine collection for 17-ketosteroids (17-KS):</u> Measures level of testosterone, which is elevated with testicular cancer. **Note:** Instruct patient and staff to save all urine for 24 hours in a special receptacle that contains preservatives. Refrigerate urine during the test period and send it to the lab as soon as the 24-hour period has lapsed.

3. <u>Serum alpha-fetoprotein (AFP) and human chorionic gonadotropin (HCG) levels:</u> If elevated, confirm the diagnosis.

4. <u>Chest x-ray:</u> May show presence of metastasis to the lungs.

5. <u>IVP/excretory urogram:</u> May show displacement of the kidney or ureters by masses of carcinomatous lumbar nodes, which cause ureteral stenosis.

6. <u>Lymphangiograms:</u> May reveal enlarged iliac and periaortic lymph nodes if disease has spread. In this procedure, contrast medium is injected into the dorsal aspects of the feet to outline the lymphatic vessels. The contrast medium will discolor the patient's urine and stool for 24–48 hours after the procedure. The injection of this substance might be uncomfortable, and the injection site will be tender for a few days.

▶ **Note:** Two complications of IVP and lymphangiogram are allergic reactions to the dye and contrast-medium-induced acute renal failure. Exposure to contrast medium may worsen existing renal or cardiac insufficiency, especially in the elderly, dehydrated, or diabetic patient. Before the study, query the patient about allergies to shellfish and reactions to previous dye studies. After the test, monitor patient for signs of renal failure.

C. Medical Management and Surgical Interventions

1. **Radiation therapy:** To irradiate lymph nodes if there is little evidence of metastasis. It is used with or without surgery to treat seminomas, which are the most radiosensitive, and can be used after surgery for other types of testicular cancers.

2. **Chemotherapy:** Used if cancer has spread outside of the testicle. It is used for radioresistant tumors (choriocarcinoma) with or without surgery. Most types of testicular carcinomas appear to be sensitive to chemotherapy, particularly to cisplatin, dactinomycin, methotrexate, and vinblastine sulfate.

3. **Serial AFP and HCG levels:** Drawn routinely over a 2-year period. Levels drop toward normal if the neoplasm has been eradicated, and rise if it has not.

4. **Staging of the disease:** Necessary for guiding treatment and evaluating the prognosis. The following parameters are used (based on Walter Reed General Hospital Staging System):

   □ *Stage I:* Tumor confined to testis, with no clinical or radiologic evidence that it has spread.

   □ *Stage II:* Clinical or radiologic evidence that tumor has spread to lymph nodes distal to the diaphragm.

   □ *Stage III:* Clinical or radiologic evidence that tumor has spread to lymph nodes superior to the diaphragm (mediastinal and supraclavicular nodes).

   □ *Stage IV:* Clinical or radiologic evidence that tumor has metastasized beyond lymphatic system into viscera.

5. **Biopsy:** To confirm the presence of malignancy. In the absence of malignancy, the abnormal benign lump is removed but the testicle is left. If the lump proves to be malignant, an **orchiectomy** is performed to remove the diseased testicle. A small incision is made at the inguinal area on the affected side rather than in the scrotum itself. This permits high ligation of the cord at the inguinal ring to allow for removal of the whole testis, which other approaches do not allow. The patient may return from surgery with an indwelling catheter and incisional drain for removal of excess exudate.

6. **Retroperitoneal lymph node dissection or lymphadenectomy:** Performed if there is evidence of metastasis to the lymph nodes that has not responded to other forms of treatment such as radiation therapy or chemotherapy. It is performed a few days after the orchiectomy to remove nodes from the kidney to the inguinal area on the affected side. Because of the possible manipulation of bowel and the length of time under general anesthesia, the patient may experience postoperative ileus. An NG tube is used to help prevent this and it is left in place until peristalsis returns.

D. Nursing Diagnoses and Interventions

Disturbance in self-concept related to actual and perceived changes in sexual function secondary to impending orchiectomy

Desired outcomes: Patient verbalizes feelings and frustrations regarding the orchiectomy. Patient can verbalize knowledge of realistic rather than perceived changes that will occur.

1. Provide a calm, unhurried atmosphere for patient and SOs. Use facilitative communication techniques, such as open-ended questions, reflective statements, and rephrasing of patient's statements for clarification.

2. Encourage communication between patient and SOs.

3. Encourage patient to verbalize feelings, fears, and frustrations regarding sexual attractiveness, feared impotence, and infertility. Explain that the *surgery* will not impair fertility or potency; however, his fertility may be compromised during radiation or chemotherapy, which can last for 2 years. If he also will have a lymphadenectomy, explain that ejaculatory failure may occur, depending on the amount of lymph gland that will be removed.

4. If appropriate, explain that a silicone prosthesis may be placed in the scrotum to achieve a normal appearance. Consult with MD regarding the potential for this procedure.

5. For patient undergoing radiation or chemotherapy, explain that he can store sperm in a sperm bank. However, the rate of pregnancy is only 50% by this method because some sperm do not survive the freezing process.

Alteration in comfort: Pain related to scrotal swelling secondary to orchiectomy and/or lymphadenectomy

Desired outcome: Patient verbalizes a reduction in discomfort from swelling in the scrotal area and does not exhibit signs of uncontrolled pain.

1. Assess and document the quality, duration, and location of the pain.

2. Administer prescribed analgesics as indicated. Note and document the patient's response.

3. Adjust the scrotal support as needed to enhance the patient's comfort. The scrotal support elevates and supports the scrotum to minimize the amount of edema.

4. Apply wrapped ice gloves or packs to the scrotum to reduce swelling.

Potential fluid volume deficit related to abnormal loss secondary to postsurgical bleeding

Desired outcomes: Patient does not exhibit signs of hypovolemia or excessive blood loss; if excessive bleeding occurs, it is detected and reported promptly.

1. Monitor the patient's VS q15min for 1 hour upon return from the recovery room. Once stable, check q30min for 1 hour and then q4h for 24 hours (or according to hospital protocol).

2. Be alert to increasing pulse, decreasing BP, diaphoresis, pallor, and increasing respiratory rate, which signal hemorrhage and/or impending shock.

3. Monitor I&O. In nonrestricted patients, ensure a fluid intake of at least 2–3 L/day. Immediately after surgery, fluids are intravenous and then advanced to oral. Measure and document urine, NG, and drainage apparatus output; record output amounts separately.

4. Check the dressing at frequent intervals after surgery, and change it when it become damp. Document color and amount of drainage. Notify MD if drainage is heavy (saturates dressings within 1 hour after changing), becomes bright red, or forms clots on the dressings, any of which can occur with arterial or venous bleeding.

See "Appendix One" for nursing diagnoses and interventions for the care of preoperative and postoperative patients, pp. 528–532, and patients with cancer and other life-disrupting illnesses, pp. 544–551.

E. Patient–Family Teaching and Discharge Planning

Provide patient and SOs with verbal and written information for the following:

1. Medications, including drug name, purpose, dosage, schedule, precautions, and potential side effects.

2. Care of incision, including cleansing and dressing changes. Advise patient to be alert to signals of infection, such as persistent redness, swelling, pain, warmth or puffiness along incision, and purulent drainage.

3. Care of drains or catheters if patient is discharged with them.

4. Review of postoperative activity restrictions as directed by MD, such as no heavy lifting (>5 lb), driving, or sexual intercourse for 4–6 weeks.

5. Necessity of continued care, such as radiation therapy, chemotherapy, serial lab work; confirm date and time of next appointment if known.

6. Importance of self-examination of remaining testicle, since it is possible to get unrelated cancer in remaining testis.

V. Penile Implants

Impotence is the inability of the male to attain or sustain an erection for satisfactory intercourse. Its causes are either psychologic or physiologic. Physiologic factors include vascular, endocrine, or neuromuscular disorders such as diabetes mellitus, radical pelvic surgery, hypogonadism, spinal cord trauma, or multiple sclerosis. Drug or alcohol use also can affect potency.

Before surgery the patient must meet the following criteria:

□ *Have desire for sexual intercourse, including penetration.*

□ *Have penile sensation and the ability to achieve some kind of orgasm:* The presence of these factors increases the potential for gratification after an implant.

□ *Lack any prostatic or urinary tract problems:* After implantation, endoscopic or transurethral procedures are difficult to perform.

A. Implantation Procedures

1. **Insertion of rigid or semirigid penile implants:** Silicone rods are placed into the corpora cavernosa through an incision at the base of the dorsal surface of

the penis. With this procedure the penis stays semirigid but will not be notice-able under clothing or interfere with ADLs.

2. **Insertion of inflatable penile implant:** Two silicone tubes are placed into the corpora cavernosa via a suprapubic incision. A reservoir containing a radi-opaque fluid is sutured into the abdominal fascia and a bulb is inserted into one scrotal sac. To initiate an erection the man must squeeze the scrotal bulb, which fills the rods with radiopaque fluid from the reservoir. Compression of the release bulb, which is located in the lower part of the scrotal sac, allows the erection to subside.

B. Nursing Diagnoses and Interventions

Alteration in comfort: Pain related to the surgical procedure

Desired outcome: Patient verbalizes a reduction in discomfort and does not exhibit signs of uncontrolled pain.

1. Assess and document quality, location, and duration of pain. Immediately after surgery, the pain can be severe and can last for as long as a week. Mild pain might be present for several weeks after that. Medicate the patient with analgesics or narcotics as prescribed.

2. Apply ice packs or gloves to the area to reduce swelling; but closely monitor patient's reaction as the weight of the ice might increase discomfort.

3. Assist patient with slow, diaphragmatic breathing and other nonpharmaco-logic pain control methods such as guided imagery, distraction, relaxation tapes, and/or backrubs.

4. Medicate the patient about one-half hour before major moves such as am-bulation and when MD first inflates the implant, which is done a few days after surgery and repeated several times a day for about a week.

5. Use a bedcradle or hoop to prevent discomfort caused by weight of bed linens.

Disturbance in self-concept related to altered body image secondary to the pres-ence of the penile implant

Desired outcomes: Patient expresses his feelings regarding the presence of the im-plant and exhibits a reduction in self-consciousness by participating in care activities that involve the implant. Patient with semirigid implant can verbalize measures for disguising its appearance.

1. Encourage the patient to discuss his feelings, fears, and frustrations regard-ing the implant.

2. Recognize that impotence threatens a man's self-concept, regardless of the reason for the impotence.

3. Provide a calm and accepting environment by discussing the procedure with patient openly and objectively. Reassure him that this surgery is not unusual or bizarre.

4. Promote acceptance of the implant by encouraging the patient to look at it and assist with dressing changes or other appropriate measures.

5. For patients with semirigid implants, explain that wearing jockey briefs rather than boxer or bikini briefs will better disguise the appearance of the penis.

6. If the patient feels self-conscious with his appearance in street clothes, en-courage him to wear loose fitting trousers until he finds clothing that better suits him.

7. Assure patient that he will be able to participate in any sport he chooses and that work will not be affected by the prosthesis.

See "Appendix One" for nursing diagnoses and interventions for the care of preoperative and postoperative patients, pp. 528–532.

C. Patient–Family Teaching and Discharge Planning

Provide patient and SO verbal and written information for the following:

1. Medications, including drug name, purpose, dosage, schedule, precautions, and potential side effects.

2. Indicators that necessitate medical attention, such as cloudy or foul-smelling urine, fever, increased pain and/or swelling in scrotum or penis.

3. Care of incision, including cleansing and dressings. Advise patient to be alert to signals of infection: persistent redness, pain, increased warmth along incision line, and puffiness.

4. Activity restrictions established by MD, such as sitting for long periods of time, heavy lifting (>5 lb), and strenuous exercise. Sexual activity can be resumed when all pain and edema have subsided, usually after 4–8 weeks.

5. Technique for operating inflatable device.

► Selected References

Aitken DR, Minton JP: Complications associated with mastectomy. *Surg Clin North Am* 1983; 63:1331.

Bernhard L: Endometriosis. *JOGN* 1982; 11:300–304.

Bonadonna G (editor): *Cancer Investigation and Management*, vol 1. *Breast Cancer: Diagnosis and Management*. Wiley, 1984.

Byrne C, et al: *Laboratory Tests: Implications for Nursing Care*, 2nd ed. Addison-Wesley, 1986.

Carpenito L: *Nursing Diagnosis: Application to Clinical Practice*. Lippincott, 1983.

Dinner MI, Dowden RV: Breast reconstruction: State of the art. *Cancer* 1984; 53:809.

Dunphy J, Way L: *Gynecology in Current Surgical Diagnosis and Treatment*, 5th ed. Lange, 1981.

Fogel CI, Woods NF: *Health Care of Women: A Nursing Perspective*. Mosby, 1981.

Gault PL: The prostate. *Nursing 77* 1977; 7:34–38.

Gault PL: Taking your part in the fight against testicular cancer. *Nursing 81* 1981; 11:47–50.

Gault-Catarrinho PL: Testicular cancer. *Crit Care Update* March 1983; 10:32–35.

Haggensen CD, Bodian C, Haggensen DE: *Breast Carcinoma: Risk and Detection*. Saunders, 1981.

Harris JR, Hillman S, Silen W: *Conservative Management of Breast Cancer: New Surgical and Radiotherapeutic Techniques*. Lippincott, 1983.

Harrison JH: *Campbell's Urology*, 4th ed. Saunders, 1978.

Hassey KM, Bloom LS, Burgess SL: Radiation alternative to mastectomy. *AJN* 1983; 83:1567.

Hawkins J, Higgins L: *Maternity and Gynecological Nursing: Women's Health Care*. Lippincott, 1981.

Hoeft RT, Jones AG: Treating metastasis with estramustine phosphate. *AJN* 1982; 82:828.

Holden L: Helping your patient through her hysterectomy. *RN* 1983; 46(9):42–46.

Howe J, et al: *The Handbook of Nursing*. Wiley, 1984.

Jewell HJ: Prostatic cancer: A personal view of the problem. *J Urol* 1984; 131: 845–849.

Jones J, et al: *Women's Health Management: Guidelines for Nurse Practitioners*. Reston, 1984.

Jones AG, Hoeft RT: Cancer of the prostate. *AJN* 1982; 82:826.

Leopold GR: *Clinics in Diagnostic Ultrasound*, vol 12: *Ultrasound in Breast and Endocrine Disease*. Churchill Livingstone, 1984.

Luckmann J, Sorensen K: *Medical-Surgical Nursing: A Psychophysiologic Approach*, 2nd ed. Saunders, 1980.

Mast M: Primary care of the mastectomy patient. *Nurse Pract* 1984; 2:27.

National Institutes of Health: *The Breast Cancer Digest*, 2nd ed. Department of Health and Human Services, Public Health Services. April, 1984. NIH Publication #84–1691.

Nurses' Clinical Library: Nursing 84 Books: *Renal and Urologic Procedures*. Springhouse, 1984.

Olds SB, London ML, Ladewig PA: *Maternal-Newborn Nursing*, 2nd ed. Addison-Wesley, 1984.

Patterson J: Colposcopy. *JOGN* 1983; 12:11–15.

Pfeiffer CH, Mulliken JB: *Caring for the Patient with Breast Cancer: An Interdisciplinary/ Multidisciplinary Approach*. Reston, 1984.

Reichel W (editor): *Clinical Aspects of Aging*, 2nd ed. Williams and Wilkins, 1982.

Rosenberg SJ, Culp DA, and Fallon B: Experience with Jonas penile prosthesis. *J Urol* 1984; 6:1087–1088.

Rutledge DN: Nurses' knowledge of breast reconstruction: A catalyst for earlier treatment of breast cancer? *Cancer Nurs* 1982; 5:469.

Senie RT, Rosen PP, Kinne DW: Epidemiologic factors associated with breast cancer. *Cancer Nurs* 1983; 6:367.

Sheahan SL: Management of breast lumps. *Nurse Pract* 1984; 2:19.

Small EC: Psychosocial issues in breast disease. *Clin Obstet Gynecol* 1982; 25:447.

Stanfil P: The psychosocial implications of hysterectomy. *JOGN* 1982; 11:318–320.

Swearingen PL: *The Addison-Wesley Photo-Atlas of Nursing Procedures*. Addison-Wesley, 1984.

Taber B: *Manual of Gynecologic and Obstetric Emergencies*. Saunders, 1979.

Tobiason SJ: Benign prostatic hypertrophy. *AJN* 1979; 79:286–290.

Tucker S, et al: *Patient Care Standards*, 3rd ed. Mosby, 1984.

Weatherley-White RC: *Plastic Surgery of the Breast*. Harper & Row, 1980.

Wood RY, Rose K: Penile implants for impotence. *AJN* 1978; 78:234–238.

Wynder E, Rose DP: Diet and breast cancer. *Hosp Prac* April 1984; 73.

10

Sensory Disorders

▶ Section One **Disorders and Surgeries of the Eye and Ear**

I. Cataract

A cataract is the clouding or opacity of the crystalline lens and/or its capsule. Cataracts are often bilateral and usually associated with aging. However, they are also seen in younger individuals and in these cases are associated with congenital, systemic, or traumatic factors. Cataracts can be categorized as follows:

Senile cataract: The most common type. This is a slow, progressive disorder characterized by a gradual opacity of the lens and decrease in visual acuity.

Congenital cataract: Probably genetically caused and can occur with systemic disease such as maternal rubella. These cataracts are usually bilateral. Surgery can be performed on individuals as young as 2–3 months to prevent amblyopia or delayed until young adulthood.

Traumatic cataract: Most commonly caused by a foreign body or blunt injury to the eye. Although it usually manifests itself immediately, the cataract can occur years after the original injury.

Systemic disease cataract: Can occur with galactosemia, hypoparathyroidism, diabetes mellitus, atopic dermatitis, and Werner's and Down's syndromes.

Toxic cataract: Uncommon cataract that may be caused by the use of dinitrophenol (an appetite suppressant), long-term corticosteroid use, or echothiophate iodide (used to treat glaucoma).

A. Assessment

Signs and symptoms: Blurred, decreased, or absent vision; inability to see in bright light; progressive loss of visual acuity.

Physical exam: On ophthalmoscopic evaluation, lens is gray/white and opaque in appearance and the retina may not be visible. A light directed laterally on the pupil of a normal eye will reveal an orange-red color (the red reflex), whereas the patient with a cataract may have partial or complete absence of red reflex because of lens opacity. The Snellen test chart will identify decreased clarity/acuity of distance vision.

B. Medical Management and Surgical Interventions

No known medical treatment is effective. Surgery is usually performed under local anesthetic. With bilateral cataracts the more affected eye is usually corrected first; if no complications ensue, the second surgery takes place 1–2 months later.

1. **Pharmacologic management:** Includes use of mydriatic eyedrops, systemic and local antibiotics, analgesics, and corticosteroids.

2. **Surgical procedures**

   ☐ *Phacoemulsification:* Usually done before extracapsular surgery. An ultrasonic needle emulsifies the lens nucleus prior to irrigation and removal of lens fragments.

   ☐ *Extracapsular:* Conservative and simple to perform, usually for traumatic or congenital cataracts. The lens capsule is incised and the lens is removed, leaving the posterior capsule in place.

   ☐ *Intracapsular:* The lens and entire capsule are removed either with a forcep or pencil-like probe that is cooled to −35C.

   ▶ **Note:** If medically indicated, a replacement (intraocular) lens is implanted after removal of the original.

3. **Eye patch and protective metal shield:** Usually prescribed for sleep up to 1 month after surgery. **Dark glasses** are recommended for temporary use once the eye dressings are removed. Temporary prescription lenses may be prescribed for the first 6−8 weeks after surgery, with permanent lenses or contacts 2−3 months later. For those patients who are not candidates for contact or intraocular lenses, permanent **cataract glasses** are prescribed. Cataract glasses tend to distort images, decrease and distort peripheral vision, and cause objects to appear a third larger than they actually are.

C. Nursing Diagnoses and Interventions

Knowledge deficit: Diagnosis, treatment plan, and surgical procedure

Desired outcomes: Patient can verbalize (and demonstrate, as appropriate) knowledge of the diagnosis, treatment plan, surgical procedure, and postoperative routine, and does not exhibit signs of harmful anxiety.

1. Assess patient's knowledge of the diagnosis, treatment plan, and surgical procedure and clarify or provide explanations as necessary. Provide time for patient to ask questions and express fears and anxieties.

2. Demonstrate deep-breathing exercises before surgery and explain their role in preventing postoperative respiratory complications. Explain that passive ROM and limb movements will be employed during the postoperative period to improve and increase circulation during period of bed rest. Have patient return demonstration of appropriate exercises. Coughing exercises are contraindicated, however, because they can increase intraocular pressure.

3. Explain that upon return from surgery, a semi-Fowler's position of up to 30° (confirm with MD) will be maintained to prevent increased introcular pressure and strain on suture line. If prescribed, patient can lie on unoperative side, as well.

4. Instruct patient not to touch, rub, or tightly shut eye or bend over after surgery to prevent infection and disruption of operative site.

5. Explain that an eye patch and shield are worn 1−5 days after surgery to prevent accidental injury to the eye.

Sensory-Perceptual alterations related to visual deficit secondary to disease process and/or presence of cataract glasses, eye shield, eye patch, or other measure that distorts or diminishes vision

Desired outcomes: Patient can verbalize orientation to time, place, and person and relates the attainment of adequate amounts of sensory stimulation.

1. Orient patient to surroundings before and after surgery.

2. Request that all individuals entering room identify themselves, state their purpose for being there, and inform patient when they are leaving.

3. Avoid touching patient without first announcing your intent.

4. Visit patient often; encourage SOs to spend as much time as possible with patient. Request that SOs bring in a radio to provide sensory stimulation and minimize patient's boredom.

5. Place all necessary articles within patient's reach. Encourage patient to utilize sense of touch to familiarize self with new objects and their placement.

6. Encourage patient to check temperature of food with fingers before eating. If possible, keep food groups in same position on plate during each meal, and explain food locations to patient (eg, meat is at 12:00). Provide individual packets of sugar and seasonings so that patient can better gauge amounts to use.

7. Teach patient to position fingers just inside rim of glass while filling to avoid overfilling.

8. Do not move furniture without alerting patient.

9. Keep doors either completely closed or completely open.

10. Ensure that side rails are kept up at all times.

11. Instruct patient to notify staff for assistance with ambulation once he or she is no longer on bed rest.

▶ **Note:** For patient with cataract glasses, explain that glasses can magnify objects >30% of actual size and will make them appear closer. Advise patient to compensate, for example, by pouring liquids in front of rather than over glass. Suggest use of nonbreakable dishes until accommodation occurs. Also explain that there are "blind spots" at approximately 11–20 feet at which objects will appear to pop in and out (jack-in-the-box phenomenon). Reassure patient that he or she will accommodate to this over time or that the lenses will be changed.

If patient has an intraocular lens implant, explain that it will help correct distance vision but that glasses will be needed for reading.

Potential for infection related to increased susceptibility secondary to invasive and therapeutic procedures

Desired outcome: Patient does not exhibit signs of infection.

1. Reinforce loose dressings with tape and reapply eye shield. Usually, the MD changes the dressing in the early postoperative period. After MD has removed the initial bandage, inspect the eye for signs of infection, including redness, swelling, or purulent discharge. Teach patient to alert staff to the presence of persistent pain.

2. Wash your hands well and use strict aseptic technique for eye care and instillation of ointment or drops.

3. Assist patient with maintaining a dry operative site; perform hygiene activities for patient as allowed by MD.

4. Remind patient not to touch or rub operative eye.

5. For uncooperative patients, request arm restraints to prevent handling of eye dressing and rubbing of operative eye.

▶ **Note:** If contact lenses are prescribed, use aseptic technique for lens insertion. Instruct patient in technique.

Knowledge deficit: Importance of avoiding increased intraocular pressure and activities that can cause it

Desired outcome: Patient can verbalize knowledge of the importance of avoiding increased intraocular pressure and activities that can cause it.

1. Explain that increased intraocular pressure can cause disruption of the operative site, and caution patient about the following:

   ☐ Avoid straining with bowel movements; request laxative/stool softeners as needed.

   ☐ Notify staff when nauseated so that antiemetics can be given.

   ☐ Avoid coughing and sneezing if possible; if unavoidable, do so with mouth and eyes open.

   ☐ Avoid heavy lifting, bending, or vigorous activity until approved by MD.

2. Teach patient the importance of maintaining prescribed position.

3. Instruct patient to notify staff immediately if persistent or sudden severe pain occurs in the operative eye, as this can signal increased ocular pressure.

Potential for injury related to increased risk of bleeding secondary to high vascularity of the ocular tissue

Desired outcomes: Patient does not exhibit signs of bleeding, or if it occurs, it is detected and reported promptly, resulting in immediate treatment and absence of injury to patient.

1. Inspect outer dressing for presence of bleeding. Instruct patient to alert staff to the presence of increased or sudden severe pain in the operative eye, which can signal hemorrhage.
2. When dressing is removed, be alert to and report presence of hyphema (bleeding in the anterior chamber of the eye).
3. Remind patient not to touch, rub, or tightly shut eye.
4. If bleeding does occur, position patient in semi-Fowler's position, alert MD, and keep patient calm.

Self-care deficit: Inability to perform ADLs related to imposed activity restrictions and visual deficit

Desired outcomes: Patient avoids ADLs that require use of ocular muscles and/or can cause increased intraocular pressure and assumes independence with ADLs as soon as these activities are permitted.

1. Instruct patient to avoid shaving, face washing, and hair combing early in the postoperative period as these activities require use of the ocular muscles. If allowed by MD, perform these activities for patient. When patient is able to perform these activities, place toilet articles on the nonoperative side.
2. Continue to perform activities for patient that require stooping and bending, such as putting on shoes and socks and washing feet.

See nursing diagnoses and interventions for the care of preoperative and postoperative patients, pp. 528–532 in "Appendix One."

D. Patient–Family Teaching and Discharge Planning

Provide patient and SOs with verbal and written information for the following:

1. Medications, including name of drug, rationale, procedure for eyedrop and ointment instillation, dosage, schedule, precautions, and potential side effects.
2. Indicators of infection that necessitate medical attention, including drainage, persistent redness, swelling, and continuous pain in the operative eye.
3. The function of eye glasses or intraocular lenses; importance of wearing dark glasses to minimize photophobia when mydriatics are used.
4. Importance of avoiding the following: heavy lifting (>5 lb); strenuous activities for 4–6 weeks, or as directed; rubbing, touching, or bumping the operative eye; and using OTC ophthalmic medications without MD approval.
5. Importance of follow-up appointments with MD; confirm date and time of next appointment if known.

When contact lenses are prescribed:

6. Importance of aseptic technique and proper insertion.
7. Need for Medic-Alert bracelet or ID card to identify patient as a contact lens wearer.

II. Intraocular Lens Implant Following Cataract Surgery

An intraocular lens implant is an elective procedure performed at the surgeon's and patient's discretion at the time of the surgery for removal of a cataract. It is an alternative for patients who do poorly with glasses or contact lenses. Complications include uveitis, glaucoma, retinal detachment, hemorrhage, and dislocation of the lens; and they occur more frequently with this procedure than with the standard cataract surgery. Advantages include permanent lens placement and decreased visual magnification and distortion.

A. Surgical Interventions

There are two methods of implantation. With the *anterior lens procedure*, the anterior chamber lens is inserted in front of the iris. With the *posterior lens procedure*, the posterior chamber lens is positioned in the posterior chamber lens capsule behind the iris. This is the more frequently performed surgery.

B. Nursing Diagnoses and Interventions

See "Cataract," pp. 465–467.

C. Patient–Family Teaching and Discharge Planning

1. Explain that there is usually no loss in depth perception with the implant. Remind patient that glasses will still be required for reading and close vision.

2. For other information, see teaching and discharge interventions in "Cataract," p. 467.

III. Corneal Ulceration

Corneal ulceration is a serious ocular disease caused by a breakdown in the epithelium of the cornea. As a result, transparency of the cornea is compromised, resulting in distortion of images to the retina. Potential causes include bacteria, trauma, virus, fungus, vitamin deficiency, and drug hypersensitivity. Because it causes paralysis of the lower lid, facial (cranial VII) nerve palsy also can cause corneal ulceration. Initially, the cornea becomes inflamed (keratitis). Progressive inflammation leads to ulceration with eventual corneal scarring, perforation, or intraocular infection. Approximately 10% of all known cases of blindness in the United States are caused by this condition.

A. Assessment

Signs and symptoms: Blurred, decreased, or absent vision; progressive loss of visual acuity; photophobia; increased lacrimation; bloodshot eye; and mild to severe pain with blinking. Purulent discharge occurs in the presence of severe infection.

Physical exam: Slit-lamp observation with staining reveals a bright green hue in the compromised area. Ophthalmoscopic evaluation identifies corneal changes, infection, or traumatic abrasion, and will reveal bloodshot eye, white or grey patches, and/or shadows on the cornea. Occasionally, visual inspection will reveal changes in light reflection or an area of opacity. The Snellen eye test identifies decreased clarity/acuity of vision.

B. Diagnostic Test

Corneal scrapings: To identify presence of bacterial or fungal source of ulceration.

C. Medical Management and Surgical Interventions

1. **Removal of foreign body:** If one is present.

2. **Pharmacotherapy**

   ☐ *Topical and systematic antibiotics:* To treat identified infection, usually after results of corneal scraping.

   ☐ *IV vitamin A:* If ulceration is caused by vitamin A deficiency, usually 10,000–15,000 U/day.

   ☐ *Topical steroids:* To treat hypersensitivity reactions, if indicated.

3. **Pain management:** Warm compresses. Atropine sulfate and scopolamine also may be used to decrease pain by dilating the pupil and thereby restricting movements of the iris and ciliary body.

4. **Other treatments:** May include taping or suturing eyelids shut to prevent blinking and minimize eye movements, or constructing a conjunctival flap to promote blood supply to the decompensated cornea. In the presence of infection, dressings are not used because they can promote bacterial growth. Dry dressings are used for clean abrasions or erosions, however.

5. **Surgery:** Considered only after medical management has failed and scarring or perforation has occurred. See "Corneal Transplant," p. 470.

D. Nursing Diagnoses and Interventions

Knowledge deficit: Diagnosis and treatment plan

Desired outcome: Patient can verbalize understanding of the diagnosis and treatment plan and does not exhibit signs of harmful anxiety.

1. Assess patient's knowledge of the diagnosis and treatment plan, and explain or clarify information as appropriate.

2. Encourage questions and provide time for expression of fears and anxieties.

3. Explain that the eyes may be patched, taped, or sutured shut to minimize eye movements.

4. Instruct patient not to rub, touch, or squeeze affected eye, which can spread infection and cause further trauma.

Alteration in comfort: Pain related to corneal ulceration/surgical procedure

Desired outcomes: Patient expresses relief from discomfort and does not exhibit signs of uncontrolled pain.

1. Monitor patient for presence of pain and medicate with prescribed medications as indicated.

2. Explain that decreasing eye movements will help minimize pain.

3. If prescribed, apply warm compresses to the eyes.

4. Discourage reading, which can increase pain; encourage use of alternatives such as talking books or radio to divert attention away from pain.

5. Provide other comfort measures such as backrubs.

6. Instruct patient to inform staff of increased or sudden, severe eye pain, which can signal that perforation has occurred. **Note:** In the presence of acute perforation, place a dry sterile dressing lightly over affected eye, place patient in dorsal recumbent position, and notify MD immediately.

Potential for noncompliance related to frustration secondary to frequency of antibiotic administration and lack of knowledge of its importance

Desired outcomes: Patient can verbalize knowledge of the importance of frequent antibiotic administration and exhibits compliance with the treatment plan. If indicated, patient and SOs can return demonstration of aseptic technique for administration of the medication.

1. Stress the importance and rationale for the medication, which is usually administered hourly.

2. Teach patient and/or SOs the technique for instillation of eye drops or ointment if the medication is to be continued after hospital discharge.

3. Teach and stress the importance of aseptic technique.

4. If indicated, teach SOs to assess patient's eyes for signs of continuing infection: persistent redness, swelling, and purulent drainage.

See "Cataract" for the following: **Sensory-Perceptual alterations**, p. 465, and **Self-care deficit**, p. 467. As appropriate, see nursing diagnoses and interventions for the care of preoperative and postoperative patients, pp. 528–532 in "Appendix One."

E. Patient–Family Teaching and Discharge Planning

Provide patient and SOs with verbal and written information for the following:

1. Medications, including drug name, purpose, dosage, schedule, route, precautions, potential side effects, and instructions for aseptic administration, if indicated.

2. Keeping a spare bottle or tube of medication on hand in case original is lost or depleted.

3. Importance of avoiding the following: use of OTC eye drugs without MD approval; rubbing, touching, or bumping the involved eye; and use of eye makeup without MD approval.

4. Reporting the following indicators of eye infection to MD: persistent redness, swelling, purulent drainage, and/or persistent pain.

5. Importance of follow-up care; confirm date and time of next appointment if known.

6. Using dark glasses with mydriatics to minimize photophobia and prevent eye trauma.

IV. Corneal Transplant

A corneal transplant (keratoplasty) is a surgical procedure that replaces a diseased cornea with corneal tissue from a human fetus or cadaver. Surgical goals include decreasing corneal opacity, increasing corneal transparency, and improving visual acuity. Surgical success and improved vision depend on the extent of damage, degree of corneal vascularization, age of the donor (the younger the better), and presence of any concurrent or recurrent infection. Approximately 30–40% of transplant patients have some form of graft reaction or rejection.

A. Assessment

See "Corneal Ulceration," p. 468.

B. Medical Management and Surgical Interventions

1. **Preoperatively:** Miotic agents may be prescribed to minimize lenticular trauma during surgery. An osmotic agent also may be used to soften the globe. The eyelashes are trimmed and an antibacterial face scrub is performed.

2. **Surgical procedure:** Performed either under general or local anesthesia. A button-sized piece of tissue is removed from the donor cornea and sutured into the recipient cornea with nonabsorbable sutures that are usually left in place for 6–12 months. Grafts are either full thickness (penetrating keratoplasty) or partial thickness (lamellar keratoplasty). The cornea is either partially or totally replaced. Visual acuity should improve immediately, but complete recovery can take up to 1 year.

C. Nursing Diagnoses and Interventions

Knowledge deficit: Diagnosis, surgery, precautionary measures, and treatment plan

Desired outcomes: Patient can verbalize (and demonstrate, as appropriate) knowledge of the diagnosis, surgical procedure, precautionary measures, and treatment plan, and does not exhibit signs of harmful anxiety.

1. Assess patient's knowledge of the diagnosis, surgery, and treatment plan. Clarify or provide explanations as appropriate. Encourage patient to ask questions; provide time for expression of fears and anxieties.

2. Explain that one or both eyes will be patched after surgery.

3. For patients with full-thickness keratoplasty, explain that activities will be restricted for at least 48 hours and a flat position is usually required.

4. To minimize the potential for injury or infection, instruct patient not to touch, rub, or tightly squeeze operative eye after surgery.

5. Explain that an eye patch and shield may be worn nightly for 1–2 weeks after surgery to protect the eye. They also may be worn daily for a few days.

6. Explain that to prevent increased intraocular pressure during the first 4–6 postsurgical weeks (or as directed by MD), patient should avoid lifting heavy objects (>5 lbs), bending, or any vigorous activity. Patient also should avoid coughing or sneezing with closed mouth and eyes, straining with bowel movements, and vomiting. Stress the importance of alerting staff to constipation or nausea so that appropriate medications can be given.

7. Instruct patient and/or SOs in aseptic technique for administration of eyedrops or ointment. Stress that good handwashing is necessary to minimize the potential for infection

8. Inform patient that watching TV is usually allowed, but reading should be avoided because it requires more frequent ocular movement.

9. Explain that patient probably will be allowed out of bed 1–2 days after surgery.

Alterations in comfort: Pain related to surgical procedure

Desired outcome: Patient expresses relief from discomfort and does not exhibit signs of uncontrolled pain.

1. Assess patient for pain and medicate with prescribed analgesics as necessary.

2. Explain that mild discomfort is normal after surgery. Instruct patient to notify staff of increased pain or sudden severe pain, which can signal complications such as hemorrhage, slipped graft, or compromise from tight dressings.

3. Provide comfort measures such as backrubs.

See "Cataract" for the following: **Self-care deficit**, p. 467, **Potential for infection**, p. 466, **Knowledge deficit:** Importance of avoiding increased intraocular pressure, p. 466, and **Sensory-Perceptual alterations**, p. 465. See nursing diagnoses and interventions for the care of preoperative and postoperative patients, pp. 528–532 in "Appendix One."

D. Patient–Family Teaching and Discharge Planning

Provide patient and SOs with verbal and written information for the following:

1. Medications, including route, purpose, dosage, schedule, precautions, and potential side effects.

2. Importance of avoiding the following: use of OTC ophthalmic medications without MD approval; heavy lifting (>5 lb) or strenuous activities for 4–6 weeks; rubbing, touching, or bumping the eye(s).

3. Reporting signs of infection to MD, including purulent drainage, pain, persistent redness, and swelling.

4. Need for follow-up care with MD; confirm date and time for removal of sutures if known.

V. Vitreous Disorders and Vitrectomy

The vitreous plays an important role in maintaining the form and transparency of the eye. With age, disease, or trauma it can degenerate and liquify, forming small fluid-filled cavities. As these cavities merge, the vitreous is pushed forward, causing traction on the retina. Ultimately this can lead to a collapsed or detached vitreous, retinal tears, or vitreous hemorrhage. Vitreous degeneration affects 65% of persons over age 60; and individuals with myopia, diabetes, or hypertension are especially susceptible. Indications for a vitrectomy include eye contusion, vitreous loss, hemorrhage, abscess, inflammation, retinal detachment with severe vitreous traction, and global rupture or penetration.

A. Assessment

Signs and symptoms: Complaints of floaters (spots, webs, or streaks) caused by vitreous particles, decreased vision, or flashing lights, which result from abnormal vitreous traction that stimulates the photoreceptors.

Physical exam: Floaters can be seen with ophthalmoscopy. Slit-lamp observation may reveal retraction, condensation, diabetic shrinkage, or injury.

B. Diagnostic Test

B-scan ultrasonography: Diagnoses posterior-segment disorders associated with gross vitreous opacification, intraocular foreign bodies, and vitreoretinal relationships.

C. Medical Management and Surgical Interventions

1. **Bed rest.**
2. **Bilateral eye patches.**
3. **Vitrectomy:** Surgical treatment of choice. A small slit is made in the sclera, and a significant amount of damaged vitreous is removed and replaced with fortified Ringer's solution. Abnormal fibrous traction bands and preretinal membranes can be cut to relieve retinal traction.

D. Nursing Diagnoses and Interventions

Knowledge deficit: Diagnosis, surgery, and treatment plan

Desired outcome: Patient can verbalize (and demonstrate, as appropriate) understanding of the diagnosis, surgery, precautions, and treatment plan, and does not exhibit signs of harmful anxiety.

1. Assess patient's knowledge of the diagnosis, surgical procedure, and treatment plan. Clarify and provide explanation as appropriate. Allow time for questions and expression of fears and anxieties.
2. Explain that the operative eye will be patched for several days after surgery.
3. Explain that patient will be restricted to a specified position for several days after surgery. Confirm position with MD.
4. Caution patient that rubbing, touching, or tightly squeezing the eye must be avoided to prevent dehiscence and spread of infection.
5. Caution patient that lifting, stooping, straining at stool, coughing and sneezing with closed mouth and eyes, and bending must be avoided to prevent increased intraocular pressure.
6. Teach patient deep-breathing exercises to help prevent postsurgical respiratory problems. Teach use of ROM and other exercises, including calf pumping, ankle circling, and isometrics of the gastrocnemius and quadriceps muscles to prevent lower-extremity venostasis. Have patient return the demonstration. Coughing exercises are contraindicated, however, because they increase intraocular pressure.

See "Cataract" for the following: **Sensory-Perceptual alterations**, p. 465, **Potential for infection**, p. 466, **Knowledge deficit:** Importance of avoiding increased intraocular pressure, p. 466, **Potential for injury** related to increased risk of bleeding, p. 467, and **Self-care deficit**, p. 467. See nursing diagnoses and interventions for the care of preoperative and postoperative patients, pp. 528–532 in "Appendix One."

E. Patient–Family Teaching and Discharge Planning

Provide patient and SOs with verbal and written information for the following:

1. Medications, including route, drug name, purpose, dosage, schedule, precautions, and potential side effects. Stress the importance of keeping a spare bottle or tube of eyedrops or ointment on hand.

2. Importance of reporting indicators of infection (purulent drainage, pain, persistent redness, swelling) to MD.

3. Necessity of avoiding the following: heavy lifting (>5 lb) and strenuous activities for 4–6 weeks, or as directed; rubbing, touching, or bumping the eye; and use of OTC ophthalmic medications without MD approval.

4. Need for follow-up medical care; confirm date and time of next appointment if known.

5. Wearing dark glasses to minimize photophobia.

VI. Glaucoma

Glaucoma is a condition in which the intraocular pressure of the aqueous humor is higher than normal (>25 mm Hg), causing atrophy of the optic disc, death of the nerve fibers, and irreversible loss of vision. This increase in pressure within the eye can be caused by excessive aqueous humor production or obstruction in the outflow pathway, preventing aqueous drainage. Glaucoma is usually genetically associated, and it is estimated that 1–2% of individuals over age 40 have some signs of this disease. Although glaucoma is usually bilateral, it can affect just one eye.

▶ **Note:** Glaucoma leads to blindness when it is left untreated.

Primary glaucoma: Usually caused by obstruction of the trabecular meshwork. There are two types: *chronic simple glaucoma* (open-angle) and *acute or chronic congestive glaucoma* (closed narrow-angle). Approximately 95% of individuals with glaucoma have the open-angle type.

Secondary glaucoma: Usually associated with trauma, tumors, surgery, or uveitis.

Congenital glaucoma: Includes juvenile or infantile glaucoma.

A. Assessment

Chronic simple glaucoma: Patient usually asymptomatic but may complain of tired eyes, progressive decreased peripheral acuity, colored halos around lights, and frequent changes in prescription eye glasses. There is increased intraocular pressure, and often a history of diabetes mellitus. There is no pain or headache associated with the decreased visual acuity.

Congestive glaucoma: Patient complains of seeing halos or rainbows, severe and spontaneous eye pain, cloudy or blurred vision, decreased vision with or without pain in darkened environments, headaches, nausea, vomiting, and poor night vision. There is increased intraocular pressure, bloodshot eyes, and midpositioned or dilated pupils. A history of diabetes is common.

Secondary glaucoma: Patient complains of progressive blurring of vision. Typically, there is history of eye trauma, tumors, surgery, uveitis, or use of corticosteroids. Intraocular pressure is increased.

Congenital glaucoma: Rapidly developing myopia, increased intraocular pressure, decreased visual acuity, and increased corneal diameter in infants. The infantile type is usually identified from birth to age 3, while the juvenile type can develop up to age 30.

B. Diagnostic Tests

1. <u>Darkened-room technique:</u> To differentiate between open-angle and narrow-angle glaucoma. It must be used cautiously as it can precipitate a narrow-angle attack from increased intraocular pressure and severe pain.

2. <u>Tonometry:</u> Use of a small instrument to measure intraocular pressure or tension in the eye.

3. <u>Tonography:</u> Uses electronic indentation tonometer and recording device to measure how well aqueous humor flows when a known amount of pressure is placed on the eye. A flat tracing indicates a decreased rate of outflow.

4. <u>Gonioscopy:</u> Uses a special lens light and microscope to view the trabecular structures and identify width of the drainage area, adhesions, undiagnosed trauma, and tumors. It is done prior to instillation of mydriatic or cycloplegic drug. This test differentiates open-angle from narrow-angle glaucoma.

5. <u>Fundoscopy:</u> Used if it is deemed safe after gonioscopy. The pupil is dilated to inspect the optic disk as well as the shape, color, and size of the fundus. This test can identify disk degeneration.

6. <u>Water-provocative test:</u> Performed after patient has been NPO from midnight the previous day. An initial tonometer reading is taken, and after patient has consumed approximately 1 L of fluid, the intraocular pressure is read q15min for 1 hour. This test identifies open-angle glaucoma.

7. <u>Ophthalmoscopic examination:</u> Identifies increased cupping of the disk.

8. <u>Visual field:</u> A map that is made of the total visual area the eye can see. It identifies blind spots and can be used as a baseline to identify subsequent degeneration.

C. Medical Management and Surgical Interventions

Medical management is the treatment of choice, and the regimen selected depends on disease etiology. Surgery is performed only when the disease progresses and medical management is ineffective.

1. **Open-angle glaucoma:** Usually treated with miotics and carbonic anhydrous inhibitors on a continuous cycle to decrease intraocular pressure. If pharmacotherapy is ineffective, surgery is usually indicated.

   □ *Trabeculectomy:* Building of a new channel for the aqueous humor.

   □ *Iridectomy:* Withdrawal of a portion of the iris via a small corneal incision (to improve aqueous drainage) or use of a laser, which bores a fine hole in the iris to provide an artificial channel for the aqueous humor.

   □ *Cyclocryosurgery:* Freezing of the ciliary body with a cryoprobe to reduce secretions.

   □ *Cyclodialysis:* Separation of the ciliary body from the sclera and its blood supply to decrease aqueous production.

2. **Congestive glaucoma:** Usually treated with miotic drugs such as pilocarpine to constrict the pupil, drawing the iris away from the cornea and facilitating flow of aqueous humor. Strong miotic drugs are not used, however, because they can increase eye congestion and narrow the angle.

The following surgeries may be performed:

□ *Iridectomy:* Procedure of choice (see preceding discussion, p. 474).

□ *Laser iridotomy:* Light energy from an argon laser allows the passage of aqueous fluid from the posterior chamber into the anterior chamber. This procedure can be performed on an outpatient basis.

3. **Congenital glaucoma:** Treated surgically, usually with a *trabeculectomy* (see preceding discussion, p. 474) because the response to pharmacotherapy is usually poor.

4. **Secondary glaucoma:** Causative factor is identified and eliminated. Either surgery or drug therapy is initiated, depending on the causative factor. Prognosis is often poor. Complications of surgery include retinal detachment, cataract development, hemolytic glaucoma, hemorrhage, decreased visual acuity, and light sensitivity. It must be emphasized to patients that surgery does not eliminate the need for eyedrops, and a lifetime pharmacologic regimen must be maintained.

D. Nursing Diagnoses and Interventions

Knowledge deficit: Diagnosis, surgery, and treatment plan

Desired outcome: Patient can verbalize (and demonstrate, as appropriate) understanding of the diagnosis, surgery, and treatment plan.

1. For primary interventions, see "Corneal Transplant," pp. 470–471.

2. Explain that patient will probably be able to ambulate within 24 hours after surgery as soon as the anesthetic has worn off. Ambulation will be increased gradually and slowly to prevent major and sudden eye movements.

Potential for noncompliance related to frustration secondary to extensiveness of pharmacologic regimen and lack of knowledge of its importance

Desired outcomes: Patient can verbalize understanding of the importance of frequent medication instillation and the consequence of noncompliance, and complies with the prescribed treatment plan. Patient and/or SOs can effectively return demonstration of medication administration technique.

1. Explain importance of timely administration of medications and the consequence of noncompliance: Blindness can occur if the condition is left untreated.

2. Assist patient and/or SOs with labeling each eyedrop bottle and writing out schedules for administration. This is especially important for patients with minimal visual acuity, to whom all bottles look alike. Color or texture-coding of the bottles may be effective for some patients.

3. Demonstrate technique for administration of eyedrops and/or ointment. Stress importance of asepsis. Have patient or SOs return the demonstration until their understanding is assured.

See "Cataract" for the following: **Sensory-Perceptual alterations**, p. 465, **Potential for infection**, p. 466, **Knowledge deficit:** Importance of avoiding increased intraocular pressure, p. 466, **Potential for injury** related to increased risk of bleeding, p. 467, and **Self-care deficit**, p. 467. See nursing diagnoses and interventions for the care of preoperative and postoperative patients, pp. 528–532 in "Appendix One."

E. Patient–Family Teaching and Discharge Planning

Provide patient and SOs with verbal and written information for the following:

1. Necessity of getting intraocular pressure checked frequently, at least four times a year.

2. Importance for family members over age 35 to get a complete eye exam every 2 years, including tonometry.

3. Necessity of providing extra lighting in darkened areas and need for extra caution when driving at night.

4. Importance of wearing a Medic-Alert bracelet identifying patient's glaucoma and eye medication used.

5. See teaching and discharge planning interventions in "Vitreous Disorders and Vitrectomy," p. 473, for other information

VII. Retinal Detachment

A detached retina is the partial or complete separation of the retina from the choroid. The retina is attached to the choroid in two places, at the optic nerve and at the ora serrata near the ciliary body. It is held in place by the gentle pressure of the vitreous body. Detachment is usually caused by a tear in the retina either from trauma or the aging process, but it also can be caused by a leak in the blood vessels as seen with choroidal tumors, malignant hypertension, central serous retinopathy, and some inflammatory conditions. A detachment is often spontaneous and usually occurs in persons over the age of 50. Myopic men and individuals with aphakia and eye trauma are especially susceptible to this disorder.

Approximately 80% of uncomplicated cases are cured with a surgical procedure. Ten percent require two or more operations, and 10% never achieve reattachment. One out of three patients with unilateral degenerative detachment eventually will have detachment in the second eye. Without treatment, a partial detachment becomes complete in 1–6 months, with eventual loss of vision.

A. Assessment

Signs and symptoms: Patient complains of flashing lights, floaters, blurred or "sooty" vision, unilateral loss of vision, and sensation of a veil over one eye. Usually, redness and pain are not present.

Physical exam: Ophthalmoscopic evaluation will reveal a retina that is hanging in a vitreous-like gray-white cloud. Crescent-shaped red-orange tear(s) will be present, and the retina may appear to be bulging. With a visual field and acuity examination, there will be decreased or limited central and peripheral vision, depending on location of the detachment.

B. Medical Management and Surgical Interventions

Surgery is the treatment of choice.

1. **Presurgical regimen:** Prior to surgery, patient will be on bed rest and may be placed in various positions to promote reattachment. Mydriatics and cycloplegics are often used to dilate the pupil and decrease movement of the intraocular structures.

2. **Surgery:** The procedure selected depends on the extent of detachment, MD preference, and patient's pre-existing medical condition. The goal of surgery is to induce inflammation, which will seal the retinal hole or tear. One of the following surgical procedures is used:

   ☐ *Cryotherapy:* A super-cooled metal probe is placed on the conjunctiva near the tear. Scleral inflammation occurs, leading to scar formation and reattachment in approximately 1 week.

   ☐ *Diathermy:* Uses heat rather than cold and is similar to cryotherapy but not as widely used.

   ☐ *Photocoagulation:* A xenon arc or argon laser emits a bright light onto the pigment epithelium, causing coagulation and attachment of the retina. Because it is not possible to reach all tears with this method, it is not frequently used.

   ☐ *Scleral buckling:* The sclera is shortened, creating a buckling of the choroid.

This brings the choroid and retina closer together and reattachment occurs. Many times, cryotherapy or photocoagulation is used in conjunction with this therapy to "weld" the retina to the choroid.

C. Nursing Diagnoses and Interventions

Knowledge deficit: Diagnosis, surgical procedure, and treatment plan

Desired outcomes: Patient can verbalize (and demonstrate, as appropriate) understanding of the diagnosis, surgical procedure, and treatment plan, and does not exhibit signs of harmful anxiety.

1. Assess patient's knowledge of the diagnosis and surgery. Clarify or provide explanation as appropriate. Allow time for patient to ask questions and express fears and anxiety.

2. Explain that both eyes may be patched for several days after surgery to rest the operative eye.

3. Explain that mydriatic and cycloplegic drops will be instilled to dilate the pupil, expose the retina, and decrease iris movement.

4. Explain that patient may be restricted to a specific position (sometimes prone) for several days after surgery.

5. To prevent increased intraocular pressure after surgery, explain that patient must not strain with bowel movements, cough or sneeze (unless done with the mouth and eyes open), or bend. Patient should notify staff of constipation, nausea, or need for assistance with putting on slippers, etc.

6. Explain that to minimize excessive movements of the eye muscles, shaving, face washing, and hair combing are contraindicated until approved by MD.

7. Demonstrate deep-breathing exercises to help prevent postsurgical pulmonary complications and passive ROM and limb movements, which are used after surgery to help promote venous return. Have patient return the appropriate demonstrations. Coughing exercises are contraindicated because they cause increased intraocular pressure.

Potential for injury related to increased risk of bleeding secondary to hypervascularity of ocular tissue

Desired outcomes: Patient does not exhibit signs of bleeding, or if it occurs, it is detected and reported promptly, resulting in immediate treatment and absence of injury to patient.

1. Inspect the outer dressing for the presence of bleeding. Notify MD of significant findings.

2. Once the initial dressing has been removed by MD, be alert to hyphema (bleeding in the anterior chamber of the eye), which can occur because of the high vascularity of the tissue. Teach patient to report to staff the presence of sudden severe pain, which can signal occurrence of hyphema.

3. If bleeding occurs, keep patient calm and in the prescribed position. Notify MD promptly.

Potential impairment of skin integrity related to vulnerability secondary to imposed immobility and positional restrictions

Desired outcome: Patient does not exhibit signs of skin irritation or breakdown.

Because it is essential that patient maintain prescribed position and avoid head (and eye) movements, logroll patient and provide skin care at frequent intervals to help prevent skin breakdown.

See "Cataract" for the following: **Sensory-Perceptual alterations**, p. 465, **Potential for infection**, p. 466, **Knowledge deficit:** Importance of avoiding increased intraocular pressure, p. 466, and **Self-care deficit**, p. 467. See nursing diagnoses and interventions for the care of preoperative and postoperative patients, pp. 528–532 in "Appendix One."

D. Patient–Family Teaching and Discharge Planning

Provide patient and SOs with verbal and written information for the following:

1. Medications, including drug name, purpose, dosage, schedule, precautions, and potential side effects. Stress the importance of keeping a spare bottle of eyedrops on hand.

2. Recognizing and reporting signs of infection to MD: purulent drainage, pain, persistent redness, and swelling.

3. Importance of avoiding the following: rubbing, touching, or bumping operative eye; contact sports for lifetime of patient (confirm with MD); sudden jarring and quick head movements; constipation and straining; heavy lifting (>5 lb) and strenous activity for 4–6 weeks, or as directed; and use of OTC ophthalmic drops and ointments unless approved by MD.

4. Importance of minimizing reading and TV viewing for several weeks after surgery to prevent eye fatigue.

5. Wearing dark glass to minimize photophobia when mydriatics are used.

6. Need for follow-up care; confirm date and time of next appointment if known.

7. Potential for detachment in opposite eye.

In addition,

8. Floaters, if present preoperatively, may also appear postoperatively and can disappear in weeks or last for years.

9. Continuing light flashes may indicate that complete vitreous traction was not relieved by surgery. Though this does not necessarily indicate unsuccessful surgery, it does necessitate careful follow-up.

VIII. Enucleation

Enucleation is the surgical removal of an eyeglobe without disturbance of orbital integrity. Because enucleation is a drastic measure that results in blindness in the affected eye, it is not considered until all other possible medical and surgical therapies have been utilized. Indications for enucleation include malignant tumor; a blind or disfiguring eye; absolute glaucoma; presence of a nonremovable, irritating foreign substance in the eye; severe infection; and as prophylaxis in sympathetic ophthalmia.

A. Medical Management and Surgical Interventions

1. **Medical treatment:** Removal of foreign body or treatment of tumor, infection, or pain is instituted initially. If treatment is ineffective or severe trauma or disfigurement exists, surgery is performed.

2. **Surgery:** Usually performed under general anesthesia. The goal of surgery is to maintain orbital integrity, and an attempt is made to preserve the muscles and tendons for later insertion of an ocular prosthesis. Once the globe is removed, an artificial globe made of gold, teflon, or plastic is usually inserted to improve cosmetic appearance.

3. **Fitting and insertion of an ocular prosthesis:** Often delayed until postoperative edema decreases, usually 4–6 weeks after surgery.

B. Nursing Diagnoses and Interventions

Knowledge deficit: Surgical procedure, postsurgical precautions, and function of the ocular prosthesis

Desired outcomes: Patient can verbalize knowledge of the surgical procedure, postsurgical precautions, and function of the ocular prosthesis, and does not exhibit signs of harmful anxiety.

1. Assess patient's knowledge of the diagnosis, surgery, and treatment plan; explain or clarify information as necessary.
2. Provide time for patient and SOs to express fears and anxieties and ask questions.
3. Inform patient that a pressure dressing will be applied for 4–5 days after surgery.
4. Caution patient that touching and rubbing the orbit or tightly squeezing the eyelid are contraindicated because these actions can cause injury and infection.
5. Explain that some discomfort after surgery is normal but a headache or sharp pain on operative side should be reported promptly (see #2, below).
6. Explain that to minimize intraorbital pressure, patient should not lie on the operative side, but rather maintain the prescribed position (usually supine to 30° elevation of the HOB), and that stooping, bending, lifting heavy objects, straining with bowel movements, and coughing or sneezing with a closed mouth are contraindicated.
7. Inform patient that there is usually no restriction of activities after the first postoperative day.
8. Teach patient the function of the ocular prosthesis and approximate schedule for insertion, if appropriate.

Alterations in comfort: Pain related to surgical procedure

Desired outcome: Patient relates a reduction in discomfort and does not exhibit signs of uncontrolled pain.

1. Explain to patient that discomfort after surgery is normal and that analgesia will be provided as needed.
2. Monitor for the presence of discomfort at frequent intervals, and ask patient to alert staff to severe pain or headache on enucleated side, which can signal complications such as hemorrhage, broken sutures, and/or infection.
3. Provide prescribed analgesia and other comfort measures such as backrubs. If patient desires, arrange for relaxing music or tapes if available.
4. There may be discomfort from the pressure dressing, which is used to minimize edema and ensure hemostasis. Provide rationale for this dressing to the patient, and explain that it is used for the first 4–5 postoperative days.
5. Use prescribed antibiotic ointment to decrease discomfort from drying of tissues, which can occur with excessive conjunctival edema.

See "Cataract" for the following: **Sensory-Perceptual alterations**, p. 465, and **Self-care deficit**, p. 467. See "Caring for Preoperative and Postoperative Patients," pp. 528–532, and "Caring for Patients with Cancer and Other Life-Disrupting Illnesses, pp. 544–551, in "Appendix One."

C. Patient–Family Teaching and Discharge Planning

Provide patient and SOs with verbal and written information for the following:

1. Medications, including drug name, purpose, dosage, schedule, precautions, and potential side effects.
2. Necessity of reporting signs of infection to MD: purulent drainage, swelling of orbit, pain, persistent orbital redness.
3. Importance of avoiding rubbing, touching, or bumping orbit or wearing eye makeup without MD approval.

4. Need for follow-up care; confirm date of next appointment if known.

5. Address and phone number of local agencies or programs that deal with visual deficits or blind individuals.

6. Referral to social worker or mental health nurse clinician as needed.

In addition, once ocular prosthesis is inserted:

7. Necessity of obtaining Medic-Alert bracelet and/or card that identifies patient as having ocular prosthesis.

IX. Otosclerosis (Otospongiosis)

Otosclerosis is a sclerotic disease of the bony labyrinth and stapes. With this disorder, normal bone tissue is absorbed and replaced by new, spongy bone that is highly vascular. Eventually, the footplate of the stapes becomes fixated, preventing the transmission of sound through the ossicles to the inner fluids of the ear. Although the etiology is unknown, 5–10% of the population is affected, and it is the most common cause of conductive hearing loss.

A. Assessment

Signs and symptoms: Tinnitus, slow and progressive loss of hearing.

Physical exam: Positive Schwartz's sign (pink blush in the inner ear caused by hypervascularity) and negative Rinne's test (bone conduction of sound waves greater than that of air conduction in the presence of conductive hearing loss). Weber's test will reveal lateralization of sound to the poorer ear.

Risk factor: Family history of the disease.

B. Medical Management and Surgical Interventions

1. **Hearing aid:** Medical treatment of choice.

2. **Stapedectomy:** Surgery of choice. It involves removal of all or part of the footplate and creation of a patent oval window using natural or synthetic materials. A stapedectomy is usually performed on the poorer ear first. If successful, the other ear can be treated after a year. The operation is not done when only one ear is affected, because the incidence of complications such as deafness or vertigo is high.

3. **Stapes mobilization:** Re-establishes normal pathway of sound to the cochlea by loosening the fixed stapes. Although hearing becomes greatly improved, there is a high risk that the stapes will refix.

4. **Fenestration:** Creation of a window in the labyrinth, allowing sound waves to reach the cochlea. It does not alter the disease process and it is rarely performed.

C. Nursing Diagnoses and Interventions

Knowledge deficit: Surgical procedure, postsurgical regimen, and expected outcomes

Desired outcomes: Patient can verbalize (and demonstrate, as appropriate) knowledge of the surgical procedure, postsurgical regimen, and expected outcomes, and does not exhibit signs of harmful anxiety.

1. Explain upcoming surgical procedure, postsurgical routine, and expected outcomes. Provide time for patient to ask questions and express fears and anxieties.

2. Stress that patient must maintain the position specified by MD both during and after surgery. After surgery the operative ear may be up—to maintain graft position and stability, or down—to facilitate drainage. Confirm with MD.

3. Explain that bed rest probably will be required for 24 hours and that it may be necessary to remain flat, even for meals, to prevent slipping of prosthesis.

4. Instruct patient to inform staff of headache, vertigo, or postoperative pain that increases or is sudden and severe. These can signal infection, hemorrhage, facial nerve encroachment, labyrinthitis, or irritation of the auditory nerve.

5. Explain that patient may have an earplug after surgery to absorb drainage in the operative ear. Caution patient not to remove this plug or get it wet.

6. Instruct patient not to blow nose because air forced into the eustachian tube can disturb the operative site. If blowing the nose is unavoidable, it should be done gently without restricting either nostril, and with the mouth and eyes open to minimize intracranial pressure.

7. Caution patient not to wash hair for 2 weeks after surgery or get water in the ear for 6 weeks, or as directed.

Potential for infection (and meningitis) related to increased susceptibility secondary to invasive procedure and proximity of surgical site to the brain

Desired outcome: Patient does not exhibit signs of infection.

1. After the earplug and bandage have been removed, monitor for drainage, redness and swelling in the canal, fever, and patient complaints of pain or headache, which can signal the presence of infection.

2. Assist patient with maintaining dry operative site, which will help prevent infection. Avoid hair washing and showers until approved by MD.

3. Be alert to the following indicators of meningitis, which is a rare but potential complication of this surgery: fever, chills, headache, nuchal rigidity, photophobia, nausea, and vomiting.

Potential for injury related to increased risk of falling secondary to vertigo

Desired outcome: Patient does not exhibit signs of injury caused by vertigo.

1. Monitor for the presence of vertigo or nausea. Advise patient to alert staff to the presence of nausea or vertigo so that appropriate medications can be administered.

2. To prevent falls, keep siderails up when patient is in bed.

3. Instruct patient to seek assistance with ambulation once it is allowed.

4. Instruct patient to maintain sitting position for a few moments before assuming a standing position. To minimize feelings of dizziness while ambulating, advise patient to look straight ahead rather than down.

Sensory-Perceptual alterations related to auditory deficit secondary to disease process, postoperative earplug, and/or tissue edema

Desired outcomes: Patient relates the ability to understand speaker and expresses satisfaction with sensory input.

1. Inform patient that hearing may be impaired for a few weeks after surgery because of tissue edema and ear packing.

2. Teach patient to maximize hearing by using lipreading, hearing aid in the nonoperative ear, or turning better ear toward the speaker.

3. Maintain quiet environment to minimize extraneous sounds during conversations.

4. Speak to patient slowly, in even tones; avoid turning away from patient or covering mouth while speaking.

5. Provide alternative sensory input such as books or puzzles.

See nursing diagnoses and interventions for the care of preoperative and postoperative patients, pp. 528–532 in "Appendix One."

D. Patient–Family Teaching and Discharge Planning

Provide patient and SOs with verbal and written information for the following:

1. Medications, including drug name, purpose, dosage, schedule, route, precautions, and potential side effects.

2. Need for medical follow-up; confirm date and time of next appointment if known. Usually, the inner earplug is removed 7 days after surgery.

3. Reporting the following indicators of ear infection to MD: persistent redness and swelling of canal, purulent drainage, vertigo, persistent pain, and fever.

4. Reporting to MD the sensation of fluid "sloshing" in ear, which is an indicator of serous fluid buildup.

5. Keeping ear covered with hat or cotton plug (depending on MD preference) for the first week while outdoors.

6. Avoiding blowing nose or sneezing. If unavoidable, explain that the mouth and eyes should be kept open in the process to minimize pressure buildup.

7. Avoiding changes in air pressure (air travel, diving, riding elevators) for at least 6 months after sugery.

8. Avoiding contact with individuals known to have URIs, which can lead to otitis media.

9. Keeping ear dry for at least 6 weeks.

10. Changing only the *outer* earplug as prescribed, using sterile technique.

11. Avoiding smoking, which is contraindicated because smoke may go up the eustachian tube and irritate the surgical site.

► Section Two   **Managing Wound Care**

A wound is a disruption of tissue integrity caused by trauma, surgery, or an underlying medical disorder. Wound management is directed at preventing infection and/or deterioration in wound status and promoting healing.

I. Wounds Closed by Primary Intention

Clean, surgical, or traumatic wounds whose edges are closed with sutures, clips, or sterile tape strips are referred to as wounds closed by primary intention. Impairment of healing most frequently manifests as dehiscence, evisceration, or infection. Individuals at high risk for disruption of wound healing include those who are obese, diabetic, elderly, malnourished, receiving steroids, or undergoing chemotherapy or radiation therapy.

A. Assessment

Optimal healing: Immediately after injury, the incision line is warm, reddened, indurated, and tender. After 1 or 2 days, wound fluid on the incision line dries, forming a scab that subsequently falls off and leaves a pink scar. After 5–9 days a healing ridge, a palpable accumulation of scar tissue, forms. In patients who undergo cosmetic surgery, scab formation and a healing ridge are purposely avoided to minimize scar formation.

Impaired healing: Lack of an adequate inflammatory response manifested by absence of initial redness, warmth, and/or induration; continued drainage from the incision line 2 days after injury (when no drain is present); absence of a healing ridge by the 9th day after injury; and/or presence of purulent exudate.

B. Diagnostic Tests

1. <u>WBC with differential:</u> To assess for infection.

2. <u>Gram stain of drainage:</u> If infection is suspected, to identify the offending organism and aid in the selection of preliminary antibiotics.

3. <u>Culture and sensitivity of drainage:</u> To determine optimal antibiotic. Infection is said to be present when there are 10^5 organisms per gram of tissue and/or fever and drainage.

C. Medical Management and Surgical Interventions

1. **Application of a sterile dressing in surgery:** To protect wound from external contamination, trauma, and/or provide pressure. Usually, surgeon changes the initial dressing.

2. **High-calorie/high-protein diet:** To promote positive nitrogen balance for optimal wound healing.

3. **Multivitamins, especially C:** To enhance tissue healing.

4. **Minerals,** especially zinc and iron: May be prescribed, depending on patient's serum levels.

5. **Supplemental oxygen:** Typically 2–4 L/min, in high-risk patients. After injury wound Pao_2 is low and administration of oxygen may enhance healing.

6. **Insulin:** As needed to control glucose levels in diabetics.

7. **Local and/or systemic antibiotics:** Given when infection is present and sometimes used prophylactically as well.

8. **Incision and drainage of the incision line:** When infection is present and localized. This allows healing by secondary intention. Often, the wound is irrigated with antiinfective agents such as dilute Dakin's solution or povidone-iodine.

D. Nursing Diagnoses and Interventions

Potential impairment of skin integrity: Wound site, related to risk of infection, metabolic alterations (eg, diabetes mellitus), impaired oxygen transport, altered tissue perfusion, dehydration, and nutritional alterations

Desired outcome: Patient exhibits signs of wound healing within an acceptable time frame.

1. Assess wound for indications of impaired healing, including absence of a healing ridge, presence of purulent exudate, and delayed inflammatory response. Monitor VS for signs of infection, including elevated temperature and pulse rate. Document findings.

2. Use aseptic technique when changing dressings. If a drain is present, keep it sterile, maintain patency, and handle it gently to prevent it from becoming dislodged. If wound care will be necessary after hospital discharge, teach the dressing change procedure to patient and SOs.

3. Maintain blood glucose within normal range for diabetics by performing serial monitoring of blood glucose and administering insulin on time, as indicated.

4. Explain to patient that deep breathing promotes oxygenation, which enhances wound healing. If indicated, provide incentive spirometry at least qid. Stress the importance of position changes and activity as tolerated to promote ventilation. Explain that if maximal inspiratory efforts are not sufficient to keep the lungs clear, coughing must be performed at frequent intervals to raise secretions.

5. Monitor perfusion status by checking BP, pulse, capillary refill time in the tissue adjacent to incision, moisture of mucous membranes, skin turgor, volume and specific gravity of urine, and I&O.

6. For nonrestricted patients, ensure a fluid intake of at least 2–3 L/day.

7. Encourage ambulation and/or ROM exercises as allowed to enhance peripheral circulation.

8. To promote positive nitrogen balance, which enhances wound healing, provide a diet high in protein and calories. Ensure sufficient dietary intake of vitamin C and encourage between-meal supplements that are high in protein. If patient complains of feeling full with three meals a day, give six small feedings instead.

9. Check protein status via serum protein and serum albumin levels. Optimal levels are 6–8 g/100 mL total protein and 3.5–5.5 g/100 mL serum albumin.

10. Obtain a dietary consult if intake is not adequate and/or will not be adequate during the first 7–10 days after the injury.

11. Provide prescribed vitamin supplements, as well as zinc and iron when indicated.

12. Weigh patient daily and evaluate trend of weight change.

13. Teach patient about nutrient needs for healing so that he or she can participate in the planning to meet requirements.

E. Patient–Family Teaching and Discharge Planning

Provide patient and SOs with verbal and written information for the following:

1. Local wound care, including type of equipment necessary, wound care procedure, and therapeutic and negative side effects of topical agents used. Have patient/SOs demonstrate dressing change procedure before hospital discharge.

2. Signs and symptoms that occur with improvement in wound status.

3. Signs and symptoms that signal deterioration in wound status, including those that necessitate notification of MD or clinic.

4. Diet that enhances wound healing.

5. Activities that maximize ventilatory status: a planned regimen for ambulatory patients and deep breathing and turning (at least q2h) for those on bed rest.

6. Importance of taking multivitamins, antibiotics, and supplements of iron and zinc as prescribed. For all medications to be taken at home, provide the following: name, purpose, dosage, schedule, precautions, and potential side effects.

7. Importance of follow-up care with MD; confirm time and date of next appointment if known.

In addition:

8. If needed, arrange for a visit by public health or visiting nurses before hospital discharge.

II. Surgical and/or Traumatic Wounds Healing by Secondary Intention

Wounds healing by secondary intention are those with tissue loss and/or heavy contamination that form granulation tissue and contract in order to heal. Most often, impairment of healing is caused by infection, which results in a delay in the healing process. Individuals at risk for impaired healing include those who are obese, diabetic, malnourished, elderly, taking steroids, or undergoing radiation or chemotherapy.

A. Assessment

Optimal healing: Initially, the wound edges are inflamed, indurated, and tender. At first, granulation tissue on the floor and walls is pink, progressing to a deeper pink and then to a beefy red; it should be moist. Epithelial cells from the tissue surrounding the wound gradually migrate across the granulation tissue. As healing occurs, the wound edges become pink, the angle between surrounding tissue and the wound becomes less acute, and wound contraction occurs. Occasionally a wound has a tract or sinus that gradually decreases in size as healing occurs.

Impaired healing: Exudate appears on the floor and walls of the wound and does not abate as healing progresses. It is important to note the distribution, color, odor, volume, and adherence of the exudate. The skin surrounding the wound should be assessed for signs of tissue damage, including disruption, discoloration, and increasing pain. When a drain is in place, the volume, color, and odor of the drainage should be evaluated. It is also important to note whether the drain is sutured in place.

B. Diagnostic Tests

1. <u>CBC with WBC differential:</u> To assess hematocrit level and for presence of infection. To maintain capillary osmotic pressure for optimal healing, the hematocrit should be >20%.

2. <u>Gram stain of drainage:</u> To determine the offending organism, if present, and aid in the selection of the preliminary antibiotic.

3. <u>Tissue biopsy or culture and sensitivity of drainage:</u> To determine presence of infection and the optimal antibiotic, if appropriate.

4. <u>Ultrasound, sonogram, or sinogram:</u> To determine wound size, especially when abscesses or tracts are suspected.

C. Medical Management and Surgical Interventions

1. **Debriding enzymes:** For example, fibrinolysin plus desoxyribonuclease (Elase), to soften and remove necrotic tissue.

2. **Dressings:** To provide mechanical debridement, keep healthy wound tissue moist, or provide antiseptic agent to decrease wound surface bacterial counts (see Tables 10-1 and 10-2).

3. **Hydrophylic agents:** For example, dextran beads or paste (Debrisan) or polymer flakes (Bard Absorption Dressing), to remove contaminants and excess moisture.

Table 10-1 Dressings Used for Debridement*

Dressing	Advantages	Limitations
Dry to Dry Insert dry and remove dry	Highly absorbant; good mechanical debridement	Excessively drying to tissue; disruption of new tissues; painful removal
Wet to Dry Insert wet and remove dry	Good absorption but not as absorptive as dry to dry. Good mechanical debridement	Drying of tissues but not as much as dry to dry; disruption of new tissue; painful removal
Wet to Damp (Moist to Moist) Insert and remove with moisture present	Provides topical anti-infective agent; no wound dessication; good debridement	Less effective removal of exudate. If excessively, wet can cause tissue maceration

*All dressings are sterile, coarse mesh gauze without cotton fiber fill and are covered with dry sterile outer layer to prevent ingress of organisms. When moisture is prescribed, it is provided with an anti-infective agent or physiologic solution.

Table 10-2 Examples of Dressings Used to Support Healthy New Tissue Growth

Dressing	Advantages	Limitations
Moist to Moist Coarse or fine mesh gauze	Keeps tissue hydrated; not painful; inexpensive	If it dries out, dressing must be moistened before removal
Xeroform Gauze	Provides topical antiseptic; keeps tissue hydrated; minimal pain with removal	Can cause tissue maceration if it is excessively moist
Porcine Skin Dressing	Can provide topical antibiotic; keeps tissue hydrated; not painful when removed; often used before closure of wound with tissue grafts	Expensive; usually stored in refrigerator until use
Transparent Dressing eg, Op-Site, Tegaderm, Bioocclusive	Prevents loss of wound fluid; protects wound from external contamination; minimal pain with removal	Must withdraw excessive drainage and reseal dressing. Appearance of drainage is unpleasant to some
Occlusive Opaque Dressing eg, Duoderm	Prevents loss of wound fluid while minimizing pooling; easy to apply; minimal pain with removal	Cannot directly assess wound without removing dressing; melts when used under radiant heat
Hydrophylic Gel eg, Vigilon	Nonadherent; absorbs exudate; compatible with topical medications; easy to apply; minimal pain with removal	Causes disruption when in direct contact with normal tissue; expensive; may require frequent changing

4. **Hydrotherapy:** To soften and remove debris mechanically.

5. **Wound irrigation with or without antiinfective agents:** To dislodge and remove bacteria and loosen necrotic tissue, foreign bodies, and exudate.

6. **IV fluids:** For patients unable to take adequate oral fluids.

7. **Topical or systemic vitamin A:** As needed to reverse adverse effects of steroids on healing.

8. **Drain(s):** To remove excess tissue fluid or purulent drainage.

9. **Surgical debridement:** To remove dead tissue and reduce debris and fibrotic tissue

10. **Skin graft:** To provide closure of wound if necessary.

11. **Tissue flaps:** To provide wound closure with its own blood supply.

12. **High-protein/high-calorie diet, supplemental oxygen, multivitamins and minerals, insulin, and incision and drainage:** See discussion in "Wounds Closed by Primary Intention," p. 483.

D. Nursing Diagnoses and Interventions

Impairment of skin integrity related to impaired wound healing

Desired outcomes: Patient's wound exhibits signs of healing within an acceptable time frame. Patient and/or SO can successfully demonstrate wound care procedure if appropriate.

1. Use dressings as prescribed. Insert dressing into all tracts to promote gradual closure of those areas. Use sterile technique for all dressing changes. Ensure good handwashing before and after dressing changes, and dispose of contaminated dressings appropriately.

2. When a drain is used, maintain its patency, prevent kinking of the tubing, and secure the tubing to prevent the drain from becoming dislodged. Always use aseptic technique when caring for drains.

3. To help prevent contamination, cleanse the skin surrounding the wound with a mild disinfectant, eg, soap and water. Friction with cleansing is essential in removing contaminants.

4. If irrigation is prescribed for reducing contaminants, use high-pressure irrigation with an ultrasonic water jet or a 35-mL syringe with an 18-gauge needle. If the tissue is friable or the wound is over a major organ or blood vessel, use extreme caution with the irrigation pressure. Both the patient and nurse should wear a surgical mask to prevent seeding of the nares with wound contaminants, thereby eliminating a potential reservoir for cross-contamination. To remove contaminants effectively, use a large volume of irrigant, for example, 100–150 mL.

5. Topically applied antiinfective agents such as neomycin and iodophors are absorbed by the wound and can produce systemic side effects. When these agents are used, be alert to side effects such as nephrotoxicity and acidosis.

6. When a hydrophilic agent such as Debrisan or Bard Absorption Dressing is prescribed, remove it with high-pressure irrigation. If the agent were to be removed with a 4×4 or surgical sponge, the friction would disrupt capillary budding and delay healing.

7. When topical enzymes are prescribed, use them on necrotic tissue only and follow package directions carefully. Do not use with topical agents, such as povidone-iodine, that interfere with the enzymatic activity. Protect surrounding undamaged skin with zinc oxide or aluminum hydroxide paste.

8. Teach patient and/or SOs the prescribed wound care procedure, if indicated.

Impairment of skin integrity: Wound, related to alterations in fluid volume and nutrition

Desired outcome: Patient exhibits signs of wound healing within an acceptable time frame.

1. Compare energy expenditure and nutrient intake with daily weights until stable, and then twice a week thereafter. If weight loss is progressive or intake insufficient to offset demands during the first 7–10 days after injury, discuss supplemental enteral or parenteral nutrition with MD and/or dietitian. For more information, see "Providing Nutritional Therapy," pp. 513–524, in Chapter 11, "Metabolic Disorders."

2. Be alert to fluid and electrolyte losses that can occur with draining wounds.

3. If patient exhibits signs of dehydration and/or is unable to consume adequate amounts of oral fluids, discuss with MD the possibility of IV fluids.

4. For other interventions, see **Potential impairment of skin integrity**, p. 483, in "Wounds Closed by Primary Intention."

E. Patient–Family Teaching and Discharge Planning

See teaching and discharge planning interventions in "Wounds Closed by Primary Intention," p. 484.

III. Pressure (Decubitus) Ulcers

Pressure ulcers result from a disruption in tissue integrity and are most often caused by excessive tissue pressure or shearing of blood vessels. High-risk patients include the elderly and those who have decreased mobility, decreased LOC, impaired sensation, debilitation, incontinence, sepsis/elevated temperature, and/or malnutrition.

A. Assessment

High-risk individuals should be identified upon admission assessment, with ongoing assessments during hospitalization. Assessment should include the patient's LOC, ability to perform ADLs, degree of sensation and mobility, status of nutrition and continence, body temperature, and age.

When pressure ulcers are present, their severity can be graded on a scale of I to IV.

Grade I: Irregular area of soft tissue swelling, pain, erythema, and heat. Erythema is not relieved by alleviation of pressure or stimulation of local circulation. In dark-skinned individuals, heat may be the only indication of a grade I pressure ulcer.

Grade II: Full-thickness skin damage with heat, erythema, pain, and induration. The skin may be attached to or removed from the ulcer.

Grade III: Involves subcutaneous tissue down to fat; often infected and/or necrotic; muscle under the fat frequently inflamed; and skin surrounding the ulcer often affected. Induration and pain are present.

Grade IV: Involves extensive soft tissue damage, extending to the bone; often associated with osteomyelitis, profuse drainage, tissue necrosis, and pain.

See "Surgical and/or Traumatic Wounds Healing by Secondary Intention," p. 485, for other assessment data.

B. Diagnostic Tests

See "Diagnostic Tests," p. 485, in "Surgical and/or Traumatic Wounds Healing by Secondary Intention."

C. Medical Management and Surgical Interventions

1. **Debriding enzymes:** To soften and remove necrotic tissue.
2. **Dressings:** To provide mechanical debridement, keep healthy tissue moist, or apply an antiinfective agent.
3. **Hydrophylic agents:** To remove contaminants and excess moisture.
4. **Wound irrigation with antiinfective agents:** To reduce contamination.
5. **Hydrotherapy:** To soften and remove debris mechanically.
6. **Diet:** Adequate protein and calories to promote positive nitrogen balance for rapid wound healing.
7. **Supplemental vitamins and minerals:** As needed.
8. **Supplemental oxygen:** Usually 2–4 L/min to promote wound healing for high-risk patients or those with delayed wound healing.
9. **Surgical debridement:** Removal of devitalized tissue with a scalpel to reduce the amount of debris and fibrotic tissue.
10. **Tissue flaps:** Provides closure of wound as well as its own blood supply.

D. Nursing Diagnoses and Interventions

Potential impairment of skin integrity related to excessive tissue pressure secondary to prolonged immobility (for patients without pressure ulcers who are at risk because of immobility)

Desired outcomes: Patient does not exhibit signs of impaired skin integrity. Patient participates in prevention measures and can verbalize knowledge of the rationale for these interventions.

1. Assist patient with position changes. There is an inverse relationship between pressure and time in ulcer formation; therefore, heavier patients need to change position more frequently. Position changes include turning the bed-bound patient q1–2h as well as having the wheelchair-bound patient perform pushups in the chair q20 min to ensure periodic relief from pressure on the buttocks. In addition, patients with history of previous tissue injury will require pressure relief measures more frequently. Use low Fowler's position and alternate supine position with side-lying and prone positions.

2. Establish and post a position-changing schedule.

3. Minimize friction on tissue during activity. Friction causes shearing of vessels, which leads to tissue disruption. Lift rather than drag patient during position changes and transferring; use a draw sheet to facilitate patient movement.

4. Use a mattress that minimizes tissue pressure, such as the Clinitron bed, water bed, or alternating pressure mattress.

5. When using egg-crate mattress, make sure patient's weight and sheets do not compress the mattress. When the mattress is compressed, it cannot effectively reduce tissue pressure.

6. With every position change, massage susceptible areas, especially bony prominences such as the sacrum and greater tuberosities. Be aware that massage of erythematous skin that does not blanch in response to digital pressure *may* exacerbate tissue damage. At this time, research does not indicate whether skin breakdown can be prevented with massage of blanchable erythematous skin or massage of skin surrounding the reddened areas.

7. To enhance circulation, encourage patient to perform ROM, ankle-circling, and isometric exercises unless contraindicated.

Impairment of skin integrity related to pressure ulcer (with increased risk of further breakdown)

Desired outcomes: Patient exhibits signs of healing within an acceptable time frame. Patient can verbalize causes and preventive measures for pressure ulcers and successfully participates in the plan of care to promote healing and prevent further breakdown.

1. Use barrier dressings such as Op-Site, Tegaderm, Duoderm, or Vigilon on grade I and grade II pressure ulcers. These dressings maintain a moist environment to promote epithelialization.

2. Be sure patient's skin is kept clean with regular bathing, and be especially conscientious about washing urine and feces from the skin. Soap should be used and then thoroughly rinsed from the skin.

3. If the patient has excessive perspiration, use sheepskin to absorb moisture.

4. To absorb moisture and prevent shearing when the patient is moved, apply heel and elbow covers as needed.

5. Use lambswool to keep the areas between the toes dry. Change it periodically, depending on the amount of moisture present.

6. Do not use a heat lamp, because it increases the metabolic rate of the tissues, resulting in increased demand for blood flow in an area with impaired perfusion. As a result, ulcer diameter and/or depth can be increased.

7. Teach patient and SOs the importance of and measures for preventing excess pressure as a means of preventing pressure ulcers.

See "Surgical and/or Traumatic Wounds Healing by Secondary Intention" for the following: **Impairment of skin integrity** related to impaired wound healing, p. 487, and **Impairment of skin integrity:** Wound, related to alterations in fluid volume and nutrition, p. 487.

▶ **Note:** Many products used on decubitus ulcers have not been scientifically evaluated. Before initiating therapy, understand the mechanism by which all drugs and treatments produce their effects. Follow directions for new products carefully and monitor healing progress.

E. Patient—Family Teaching and Discharge Planning

Provide patient and SOs with verbal and written information for the following:

1. Location of local medical supply stores that have pressure-reducing mattresses and wound care supplies.
2. Planning a schedule for changing patient positions.

For other teaching and discharge planning interventions, see "Wounds Closed by Primary Intention," p. 484.

▶ Section Three   Care of the Burn Patient

The functions of the skin include protection from infection, protection of the organs from external elements, regulation of temperature, secretion, excretion, maintenance of fluid balance, and production of vitamin D. After a burn injury any or all of these functions may be altered. Burns can be caused by chemicals, contact with hot surfaces, electricity, flames, flammable liquids, flashes from explosives, radioactive materials, hot liquids, and the sun. The American Burn Association categorizes burn injuries in the following way:

Major burn injury: Partial-thickness burns >25% total body surface area (TBSA) for adults and >20% for children; full-thickness burns 10% TBSA or greater; most deep-partial-thickness and full-thickness burns involving the hands, face, eyes, ears, feet, and perineum; most burns complicated by inhalation injury; most electrical and chemical burns; burns complicated by fractures or other major trauma; burns in poor-risk patients (extremes of age, intercurrent disease).

Moderate uncomplicated burn injury: Partial-thickness burns of 15–20% TBSA for adults and 10–20% for children; less than 10% full-thickness burns; burns not involving specific conditions identified above.

Minor burn injury: Partial-thickness burns of less than 15% TBSA for adults and less than 10% for children; burns less than 2% full thickness.

This classification is used to determine the appropriate medical facility for the burn injury victim. The American Burn Association advocates that major burns be treated in a specialized facility or hospital with special expertise in burn care. Moderate burns often require hospitalization, not necessarily in a burn center; minor burns are usually treated in an outpatient area.

A. Assessment

Severity of the burn is determined by the size and depth of the involved area, age of the patient, patient's medical history, and burn site. In addition, added complications such as infection and shock can cause tissue damage beyond that of the initial injury.

Size or extent of the burn area: May be measured according to the "rule of nines." Each area is assigned a percentage of body surface area to establish the percentage of involvement. The head and neck area is assigned 9%, each upper extremity 9%, anterior chest 18%, posterior chest 18%, each lower extremity18%, and the genitalia 1%.

Depth of the burn: Also significant (see Table 10-3). The depth is not always immediately evident, even to the experienced observer. Often it will take several days for the level of injury to become apparent.

Table 10-3 Classification of Burns

Classification	Skin Level	Indicators	Recovery
First Degree	Epidermis	Pain, erythema	Rapid, no sequelae
Second Degree	Epidermis, partial thickness of dermis	Blisters, erythema, moistness, pain	Scarring, depigmentation
Third Degree	Epidermis, dermis	Anesthesia; avascularity; skin white, black, or brown in color	Scarring, functional loss, requires skin grafting
Fourth Degree	Epidermis, dermis subcutaneous, muscle, bone	Charring, organ damage	Functional loss, skin grafting, amputation

The following body systems also should be evaluated for involvement:

Cardiovascular: With a burn injury involving >20% TBSA, there is a systemic response characterized by increased capillary permeability and shifting of plasma into the interstitial space. This can result in hypovolemia and edema formation. Assess for presence of disorientation, decreasing BP, tachycardia, and oliguria. Sealing of the capillary leak followed by cellular fluid mobilization back into vascular spaces with diuresis occurs 24–48 hours after the injury. Circumferential burns to the extremities combined with edema formation can compromise peripheral circulation. Close monitoring of peripheral pulses, skin temperature and color, and capillary refill is essential.

Respiratory: Carbon monoxide poisoning can result from inhalation of smoke. Laryngeal and/or oropharyngeal edema can be present; and any carbonaceous sputum, hoarseness, singed nasal hair, smoky breath, or stridor should be observed for and documented. Chemical pneumonitis and progressive adult respiratory distress syndrome (ARDS) can occur during the first 72 hours after inhalation of toxic particles and chemicals in smoke, and pneumonia can develop from prolonged bed rest and/or bacterial invasion of damaged lung tissue.

Neurologic: Alteration in status can signal presence of head trauma at the time of the accident, deficiency in circulating blood volume, hypoxia from inadequate ventilation, or impending sepsis. LOC, orientation, and pupillary reactions should be monitored routinely. Circumferential burns of the extremities and resulting edema may compromise peripheral neurologic status. Closely monitor peripheral sensorimotor function.

Gastrointestinal: Diversion of blood flow to vital organs can result in paralytic ileus during the first 24 hours after the injury. Sepsis and electrolyte (potassium) shifts also can cause ileus. Routine auscultation of the abdomen for bowel sounds is important.

Renal–Urinary: Urinary output should be maintained at a minimum 30–50 mL/h. Hydration status should be assessed routinely.

B. Diagnostic Tests

1. <u>CBC:</u> Will reveal elevated WBC in the presence of infection; hematocrit will reflect fluid volume status.

2. <u>Serum chemistry:</u> Will reflect the success of fluid management. Initially, slight elevation of potassium can occur with tissue destruction. Low serum albumin is sometimes seen with inadequate nutrition.

3. <u>Serial chest x-rays:</u> Performed for suspected inhalation injury. A true inhalation injury will present as progressive ARDS.

4. <u>ABG values:</u> Will help evaluate respiratory status.

5. <u>Carboxyhemoglobin (a measure of carbon monoxide in the blood):</u> Assessed on admission to determine severity of the smoke inhalation.

6. <u>Wound cultures:</u> Taken if the burn wound is believed to be infected.

C. Medical Management and Surgical Interventions

1. **IV therapy:** To restore circulating blood volume and maintain urine output at minimum of 30–50 mL/h. Typically, this is done for individuals with burns >20% TBSA. Use of IV dextrose solutions is contraindicated because osmotic diuresis can occur.

2. **Tetanus prophylaxis.**

3. **NG tube connected to suction:** In the presence of ileus.

4. **High-protein/high-calorie diet:** To promote positive nitrogen balance for optimal wound healing.

5. **Vitamin and mineral supplements:** Including vitamins C and A and zinc to promote wound healing.

6. **Systemic antibiotics:** If indicated to treat specific bacterial organisms.

7. **OT and PT consultation:** To provide exercise, splinting of affected joints and extremities, and fitting of pressure garments that will minimize scarring and prevent contractures.

8. **IV or oral medications during the edema phase:** When IM and SC routes are contraindicated.

9. **Wound care:** Involves cleansing, debridement, and topical antimicrobial therapy to control bacterial proliferation. Typically, silver sulfadiazine is applied twice daily. Use of biologic dressings (eg, porcine, amniotic membranes, and cadaver skin) may provide interim protection until grafting.

10. **Surgical debridement and/or tangential excision and split-thickness skin grafting:** To reduce debris and provide closure for full-thickness wounds. Fasciotomy or escharotomy may be required to relieve pressure from circumferential burns of the thorax or extremities.

11. **Oxygen therapy:** As determined by ABG values.

12. **Endotracheal intubation:** For patients with severe pharyngeal edema. Typically, these patients are in burn or critical care units.

D. Nursing Diagnoses and Interventions

▶ **Note:** Because patients with major burns are treated in special burn units, this section focuses on the care of patients with moderate, uncomplicated burn injuries.

Potential alteration in respiratory function related to distress secondary to smoke inhalation and inactivity secondary to prolonged bed rest

Desired outcome: Patient does not exhibit signs of respiratory dysfunction.

1. Assess VS and auscultate lung fields for the presence of adventitious breath sounds at least q shift; notify MD of significant findings, including crackles (rales) and rhonchi.
2. Monitor for evidence of inhalation injury: burns on the head and neck, soot in the oropharynx, singed nasal or facial hairs, carbonaceous sputum, hoarseness, and stridor.
3. Monitor ABG results, being alert to decreasing Pao_2 (<50), decreasing pH (acidosis), and increasing $Paco_2$ (>50), which can occur with smoke inhalation and developing pneumonia.
4. Instruct patient to cough and breathe deeply q2h; assist with turning after each coughing and deep-breathing exercise.
5. Encourage use of incentive spirometry q2h.
6. Perform tracheal suctioning as necessary.
7. Deliver oxygen as prescribed.

Alteration in tissue perfusion: Peripheral, related to edema secondary to burn injury or skin grafting

Desired outcome: Patient's physical findings are within acceptable limits.

1. Monitor peripheral pulses and capillary refill, color, and skin temperature of extremities; notify MD of significant changes.
2. Elevate burned extremities above the level of the heart.
3. Observe for increasing edema.
4. Before patient ambulates, use elastic bandages to double wrap lower extremities that have been burned, grafted, or used as donor sites.
5. Immobilize newly grafted areas for 3 days or as prescribed, to ensure optimum graft adherence.

Alteration in nutrition: Less than body requirements related to increased need secondary to hypermetabolic state associated with burn injury

Desired outcome: Patient does not exhibit signs of malnutrition or weight loss.

1. Monitor weight daily; report progressive loss.
2. Provide high-protein/high-calorie diet; record daily calorie count.
3. Encourage high-calorie nutritional supplements between meals.
4. Limit intake of water and foods low in calories, promoting high-calorie fluids and foods instead.
5. In the presence of progressive weight loss or slow wound healing, consult with MD and dietitian regarding need for enteral nutritional supplement via NG tube.

Potential for infection related to increased susceptibility secondary to loss of protective skin layer

Desired outcome: Patient does not exhibit signs of infection.

1. Monitor and record patient's temperature q4h.
2. If temperature is >102F, obtain prescription for culture of blood, sputum, urine, and/or wound drainage.

3. Be alert to early signs of wound infection, including change in wound color, increased pain, and redness at wound edges.

4. Monitor wound for evidence of cellulitis (tissue that is swollen, red, and warm to the touch), purulent drainage, and increasing wound depth. Document and report changes in appearance to MD.

5. Use strict aseptic technique for all wound care.

6. Apply prescribed topical antimicrobial agents to wound. If silver sulfadiazide is used, it is normal for the wound to have green-yellow drainage.

7. Shave hair from wounds and skin that is within 2 inches of wound margins.

8. Be alert to deterioration in mentation, an early indicator of sepsis.

9. Administer antibiotics as prescribed.

Potential impairment of physical mobility: Contractures and/or muscle atrophy related to inactivity secondary to discomfort and prolonged bedrest

Desired outcome: Patient does not exhibit signs of joint contractures or muscle atrophy.

1. Encourage self-care, to patient's tolerance.

2. To prevent joint contractures and promote maximum function, ensure that patient's joints are extended while on bed rest.

3. Apply splints as indicated by OT/PT.

4. Provide assistive devices such as a walker and modified eating utensils as necessary for performance of ADLs.

5. Encourage ambulation as prescribed by MD.

6. Provide for active, passive, resistive, and/or assisted ROM exercises as indicated.

7. Offer prescribed pain medications one-half hour before ambulation and planned exercise periods to enhance compliance.

Alteration in comfort: Pain related to burn injury

Desired outcome: Patient expresses relief of discomfort and does not exhibit signs of uncontrolled pain.

1. Assist patient with using nonpharmacologic methods of pain control such as relaxation breathing, guided imagery, and soothing music.

2. Provide prescribed pain medications throughout the day, as indicated, and one-half hour before procedures that may cause discomfort.

3. Recognize that anxiety can increase the perception of pain; relieve stress by providing supportive atmosphere, informing patient of procedures and progress made, and administering prescribed antianxiety medications as indicated.

See "Caring for Patients with Cancer and Other Life-Disrupting Illnesses," pp. 544–546, "Appendix One," as appropriate.

E. Patient–Family Teaching and Discharge Planning

▶ **Note:** Because every patient situation is unique, discharge plans must address problems specific to the individual. Begin discharge planning early in the hospital stay. Assessments of patient and family resources and the patient's ability to function independently are essential.

As appropriate, provide patient and SOs with verbal and written information for the following:

1. *Wound care:* Teach a simplified dressing procedure, or refer patient to an appropriate resource for outpatient care. Alert patient to the signs of infection, which necessitate prompt medical attention.

2. *Skin care:* Advise patient to expect itching and blistering of healed wounds. Instruct patient in the use of moisturizers and sunscreen lotions that are recommended by MD. Explain the scarring process.

3. *Medications:* Teach patient the drug name, purpose, dosage, schedule, route, precautions, and potential side effects.

4. *Use of pressure garments:* Explain application and laundering procedure and importance of monitoring skin under the garments.

5. *Exercise program:* Stress the importance of following program outlined by PT. Remind patient that pain medications should be taken a half-hour before exercise and wound care.

6. *Nutrition:* Explain dietary requirements to promote healing.

7. *Psychological adjustments after hospital discharge:* Advise patient there is a potential for boredom, being stared at by strangers, and difficulty with finding a role in the family again. Provide phone numbers of appropriate resource professionals.

8. *Phone number:* Of MD or nurse who can answer questions after patient is discharged from hospital.

9. *Long-term outcome and, if appropriate, future reconstructive surgery:* Ensure that patient discusses these topics with MD before discharge from hospital.

▶ Selected References

Boyd-Monk H: Screening for glaucoma. *Nursing 79* 1979; 9(8):42.

Brown M: Retinal vascular disorders: Nursing and medical implications. *Nurs Clin North Am* 1981; 16:415–432.

Carpenito LJ: *Nursing Diagnosis: Application to Clinical Practice.* Lippincott, 1983.

De Weese D, Saunders H: *Textbook of Otolaryngology,* 6th ed. Mosby, 1982.

Dineen P, Hildick-Smith G (editors): *The Surgical Wound.* Lea and Febiger, 1981.

Flaherty T et al: *Ophthalmology: A Nursing Perspective.* Stanford University Press, 1983.

Flint LM, Fry DE (editors): *Surgical Infections.* Medical Examination Publishing, 1982.

Goroll A et al: *Primary Care Medicine.* Lippincott, 1981.

Hayes P: Treatment and nursing care of corneal disease. *Nurs Clin North Am* 1981; 16:383–392.

Hummel R (editor): *Clinical Burn Therapy: A Management and Prevention Guide.* PSG/Wright Publishing, 1982.

Hunt TK, Dunphy JE (editors): *Fundamentals of Wound Management.* Appleton-Century-Crofts, 1979.

Kilroy J: Care and teaching of patients with glaucoma. *Nurs Clin North Am* 1981; 16:393–404.

Krupp M, Chatton M (editors): *Current Medical Diagnosis and Treatment*. Lange, 1984.

Lee K: *Essential Otolaryngology: Head and Neck Surgery*, 3rd ed. Medical Examination Publishing, 1983.

Mc Coy K: Cataracts and intraocular lenses: From cloudy to clear. *Nurs Clin North Am* 1981; 16:405–415.

Parish LC et al (editors): *The Decubitus Ulcer*. Masson Publishing USA, 1983.

Rooke F et al: *Ophthalmic Nursing—its Practice and Management*. Churchill Livingstone, 1980.

Rudolph R, Noe JM (editors): *Chronic Wound Problems*. Little, Brown, 1983.

Saxton D et al: *The Addison-Wesley Manual of Nursing Practice*. Addison-Wesley, 1983.

Stotts, NA: Impaired wound healing. In: *Pathophysiological Phenomena in Nursing: Clinical and Theoretical Perspectives*. Carrieri VL et al (editors). Saunders (in press).

Vaughn D, Asbury T: *General Ophthalmology*, 10th ed. Lange, 1983.

11

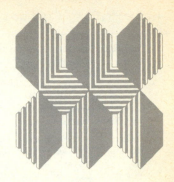

Metabolic Disorders

▶ Section One   **Fluid and Electrolyte Disturbances**

All bodily functions rely on the proper distribution of fluids and electrolytes between the intracellular and extracellular compartments. Fluid and electrolyte balance is maintained by the interaction of renal, hormonal, and metabolic mechanisms. Imbalances can occur secondary to other disorders or as complications of therapy. Major objectives of fluid and electrolyte therapy include maintenance of normal fluid and electrolyte distribution, replacement for prior deficits and continuing losses, and nutrition.

Fluids: Body fluids maintain blood volume, aid digestion, transport material to and from body cells, act as a medium for cellular metabolism and excretion of waste, and help regulate body temperature. Water is the largest single constituent of the human body. In the adult, 60% of body weight consists of water, of which 45% is intracellular fluid (ICF). The remaining 15% is distributed between the intravascular and interstitial compartments and is considered extracellular fluid (ECF). The concentration of particles in a fluid compartment is known as osmolality. Normal plasma osmolality is about 280–295 mOsm/L. Exogenously, water is obtained by drinking fluids, eating foods that contain water, and IV administration. Endogenously, food and body tissue are oxidized to produce carbon dioxide and water. Fluid balance can be assessed by determining volume of fluid intake versus volume of fluid output. Normal output ranges from 2–3 L/day. Losses occur via the urine, GI tract, skin, and lungs. Important homeostatic mechanisms include thirst and antidiuretic hormone (ADH). For example,

H_2O deficit → secretion of ADH → conservation of H_2O by kidney

H_2O deficit → thirst → ↑ H_2O ingestion

H_2O excess → ↓ ADH → ↑ H_2O loss in urine

H_2O excess → no thirst

Because acute changes in body weight are rarely caused by caloric excess or deficiency, daily weight measurement is the most reliable guide for assessing fluid balance. To ensure accuracy, the patient should wear the same amount of clothing and be weighed on a balance scale at the same time each day, preferably before breakfast.

Electrolytes: Electrolytes are chemicals that, when dissolved, dissociate into positively and negatively charged ions (cations and anions). Total cations always equals total anions. They are important constituents of intracellular and extracellular fluids, serving vital functions in maintaining fluid and acid–base balance, neuromuscular excitability, blood clotting, and protein and cellular metabolism. The composition and concentration of electrolytes in each fluid compartment vary. Measurement of electrolytes is usually expressed in milliequivalents per liter (mEq/L).

I. Fluid Disturbances

A. Hypervolemia

Hypervolemia is a condition in which the ECF compartment becomes expanded, and there is a surplus of circulating fluid with normal or near normal proportions of electrolytes.

  1. *Causes:*

  □ *Inability of the kidneys to excrete excess water and electrolytes:* Chronic renal disease, chronic liver disease with portal hypertension, congestive heart failure, or administration of oral or parenteral fluids at a rate beyond renal capacity for excretion.

  □ *Interstitial-to-plasma fluid shift:* Excessive administration of hypertonic solutions or large-molecular fluids, or the recovery phase of a plasma-to-interstitial fluid shift.

□ *Hormonal/metabolic disturbances:* Syndrome of inappropriate antidiuretic hormone (SIADH), hyperaldosteronism, or excessive glucocorticosteroid administration.

2. *Clinical indicators:*

□ Elevated BP, bounding pulse, distended neck veins, weight gain (1 L H_2O = 2.2 lb), dyspnea, crackles (rales), and pretibial and sacral edema. If overload becomes sufficiently severe to exceed the pumping capacity of the left ventricle, pulmonary edema will result.

□ *Laboratory findings* are variable. Serum osmolality usually remains unchanged, although hypo-osmolality can occur. Serum sodium values are not often affected, although they may be low. Hematocrit may be decreased, reflecting hemodilution; and urine sodium may be low because of sodium retention. Both serum osmolality and serum sodium will be decreased, and urine specific gravity will be elevated in SIADH.

3. *Medical management:* The goal is to obtain a definitive diagnosis of the underlying cause to determine appropriate treatment.

□ Restrict fluids and sodium.

□ Administer diuretics.

□ Replace potassium losses secondary to diuretic therapy.

□ Provide pulmonary hygiene.

□ Administer dialysis for patients with renal failure or life-threatening hypervolemia.

4. *Nursing diagnoses and interventions:*

Fluid volume excess: Edema related to surplus of circulating fluid

Desired outcome: Patient's VS, physical findings, and lab values are within acceptable limits.

□ Assess VS and monitor I&O; measure weight daily.

□ Observe for and report indicators of edema, which may not be clinically evident until 5–10 pounds of fluid have been retained. The elderly can develop dependent edema with relatively little fluid excess. Check sacral areas in patients on bed rest. Look for edema in the ankles and pretibial areas of ambulatory patients.

□ Maintain fluid and sodium restrictions (IV and PO) as prescribed.

□ Administer diuretics as prescribed.

□ Monitor lab values; be especially alert to decreased potassium in patients on diuretics.

□ Monitor for clinical indicators of potassium depletion during diuretic therapy: muscle weakness/cramping, nausea, anorexia, cardiac dysrhythmias. Alert MD to the development of an irregular pulse, which can be indicative of dangerous hypokalemia.

□ Replace potassium losses. Administer potassium supplements as prescribed, and teach patient about foods high in potassium, including oranges, tomatoes, and bananas. (For a list of these foods, see Table 3-2, p. 96.)

Impaired gas exchange related to tissue hypoxia secondary to pulmonary edema

Desired outcome: Patient does not exhibit signs of respiratory dysfunction.

□ Monitor character, rate, and depth of respirations; auscultate lung fields for adventitious breath sounds.

□ As necessary, place patient in semi-Fowler's position to facilitate respirations.

□ Teach patient deep-breathing exercises to enhance gas exchange.

See "Heart Failure" in Chapter 2, "Cardiovascular Disorders," for the following: **Fluid volume excess:** Edema related to retention secondary to decreased cardiac output, p. 49. See "Acute Renal Failure" in Chapter 3, "Renal–Urinary Disorders," for the following: **Fluid volume excess:** Edema related to fluid retention secondary to renal dysfunction: Oliguric phase, p. 108.

B. Hypovolemia

Hypovolemia is a condition in which depletion of ECF occurs as a result of water and sodium loss in varying proportions, depending on underlying pathology.

1. *Causes:*

   □ *GI losses:* Vomiting, diarrhea, fistulous drainage, ileostomy, gastric suction.

   □ *Urinary losses:* Diuretic administration, renal or adrenal disease, diabetes insipidus.

   □ *Sequestration of fluid (plasma-to-interstitial fluid shift):* Postoperative state, burns, peritonitis, ileus, ascites, acute pancreatitis.

   □ Profuse diaphoresis, hyperventilation, fever.

   □ Decreased intake of water and electrolytes.

2. *Clinical indicators:*

   □ Postural hypotension, weak pulse with tachycardia, flattened neck veins, increased respirations, poor skin turgor, longitudinal furrows in the tongue, absence of moisture in the groin and axillae, decreased tearing and salivation, anorexia, nausea, vomiting, weakness, apathy, weight loss, subnormal temperature, and decreased urine output. Shock and coma can ensue if volume depletion is severe.

   □ *Laboratory findings:* BUN elevated out of proportion to serum creatinine, and an elevated hematocrit and protein count, all reflective of hemoconcentration. Serum sodium may be high, normal, or low. Urinary sodium is decreased, and urine specific gravity is elevated.

3. *Medical management:* The goal is to restore ECF volume and correct the underlying pathology.

   □ Administer oral or IV fluids to replace prior and ongoing water and electrolyte losses while definitive diagnosis is being made.

4. *Nursing diagnosis and interventions:*

   Fluid volume deficit related to abnormal loss and/or decreased intake

   Desired outcome: Patient's VS, physical findings, and lab values are within acceptable limits.

   □ Monitor VS, lab values, and I&O for evidence of dehydration; measure weight daily. Check specific gravity of urine.

   □ As appropriate, encourage oral intake or administer prescribed replacement solutions. Observe for indications of fluid overload during rapid IV replacement. Provide oral hygiene at frequent intervals.

   □ Obtain accurate measurements of "third space" (interstitial) fluid accumulation areas such as the abdomen and limbs. Measure abdomen or limb(s) at the same place with each assessment. To ensure accuracy, mark the measurement site with indelible ink, and use the same tape measure for all assessments.

See "Acute Renal Failure" in Chapter 3, "Renal–Urinary Disorders," for the following: **Fluid volume deficit** related to abnormal loss secondary to excessive urinary output: Diuretic phase, p. 109.

II. Electrolyte Disturbances

Sodium: Sodium is the major cation of extracellular fluid and is primarily responsible for osmotic pressure in that compartment. Normal serum sodium concentration is approximately 137–147 mEq/L. Body water and electrolyte regulation by the kidneys is based in part on sodium concentration in the ECF. When ECF sodium concentration rises, the kidneys attempt to maintain normal sodium concentration by retaining water. When ECF water increases, sodium is retained. An elevated serum sodium level (hypernatremia) usually reflects a relative ECF water deficit rather than an increase in total body sodium. Hyponatremia exists when the serum sodium concentration in a given amount of plasma water falls below normal. Symptoms might not occur until the serum sodium level is <120–125 mEq/L. Sodium is also important in cellular functioning. It stimulates reactions in nerve and muscle tissues and is essential for maintaining normal acid–base balance. Aldosterone, which is secreted by the adrenal cortex, is essential in sodium regulation through its effect on renal tubular resorption of sodium.

A. Hypernatremia

1. *Causes:*

   □ *Decreased intake of water:* Inability to respond to thirst, such as in an unconscious state or infancy; less efficient functioning of the thirst center in the base of the brain, as is commonly seen with the elderly; hyperosmolar (eg, high protein) tube feedings with inadequate water supplements.

   □ *Increased output of water:* Severe hypotonic fluid losses through the GI and respiratory tracts, increased urinary water loss through osmotic diuresis, and diabetes insipidus.

   □ *Increased intake of sodium:* Excessive administration of concentrated electrolyte mixtures, salt-water drowning.

   □ *Primary hyperaldosteronism.*

2. *Clinical indicators:*

   □ Intense thirst; flushed skin; dry, sticky mucous menbranes; rough, reddened, dry tongue; firm, rubbery tissue turgor; elevated temperature if ambient temperature is >18C (65F); restlessness, excitement, mania, convulsions; decreased reflexes; oliguria or anuria. Symptomatic hypernatremia does not occur in the alert patient who has an intact thirst mechanism and access to water.

   □ *Laboratory findings:* Serum sodium >147 mEq/L, increased serum osmolality, urine specific gravity >1.030 (except in diabetes insipidus).

3. *Medical management:* The goal is to restore normal sodium concentration.

   □ Replace water: Plain water given by mouth may be sufficient in the early stages of sodium excess or if serum sodium is <160 mEq/L; IV infusion of hypotonic solution of water and electrolytes in advanced stages or if serum sodium is >160 mEq/L. **Note:** Rapid reduction of serum sodium (serum osmolality) may lead to cerebral edema, seizures, or death.

   □ Administer diuretics by mouth with plain water.

   □ Draw serum sodium levels q6h.

4. *Nursing diagnosis and interventions (one example):*

   Fluid volume deficit related to abnormal (hypotonic) loss or decreased intake

Desired outcome: Patient's VS, physical findings, and lab values are within acceptable limits.

☐ Monitor VS and I&O, and assess skin turgor and mucous membranes for evidence of dehydration. Check urine specific gravity and monitor serum sodium levels.

☐ As appropriate, encourage oral fluids or administer prescribed fluid replacement.

☐ Administer diuretics, if prescribed.

☐ Assess patient's sensorium; institute seizure precautions and notify MD if significant findings are noted.

See "Nursing Components" (for tube feedings) in "Providing Nutritional Therapy" for the following: **Potential fluid volume deficit or excess** related to abnormal loss or retention secondary to osmolality and substrate content of tube feeding solutions, p. 521.

B. Hyponatremia

1. *Causes:*

   ☐ *Loss of sodium-containing fluids:* Vomiting, diarrhea, profuse diaphoresis, salt-losing nephropathy, adrenal insufficiency, excessive diuretic use together with reduced sodium intake, and plasma-to-interstitial fluid shift in massive burns and trauma.

   ☐ *Impaired renal excretion of water:* Renal failure, nephrotic syndrome, CHF, and hepatic cirrhosis.

   ☐ *Increased intake of water, which dilutes serum sodium:* Excessive administration of electrolyte-free IV solutions, fresh-water drowning, or compulsive polydipsia.

   ☐ *Secretion of inappropriate antidiuretic hormone (SIADH).*

2. *Clinical indicators:*

   ☐ Variable: Can include anorexia, nausea, vomiting, cold and clammy skin, postural hypotension, apprehension, confusion, lethargy, coma, and seizures.

   ☐ *Laboratory findings:* Serum sodium below normal; urine specific gravity <1.010; urine sodium <20 mEq/L, except in salt-losing nephropathy, in which urinary sodium losses are very high. If SIADH is the cause, serum sodium will be <120 mEq/L, urine specific gravity >1.012, and urine osmolality will exceed serum osmolality.

3. *Medical management:* The goal is to restore normal serum sodium levels as quickly as possible without volume overload and to establish a definitive diagnosis to determine appropriate therapy.

   ☐ Replace salt and water orally in cases of mild deficit.

   ☐ Provide parenteral replacement with 3–5% sodium chloride in water if the deficit is severe.

   ☐ Restrict water if the hyponatremia is dilutional.

   ☐ In patients with SIADH, administer demeclocycline, 300–600 mg bid, which may eliminate the need for severe water restriction.

4. *Nursing diagnosis and interventions:*

   Fluid volume deficit or excess related to abnormal fluid loss, increased intake, or interstitial spacing of fluids

   Desired outcome: Patient's physical findings and lab values are within acceptable limits.

□ Monitor I&O and weigh patient daily.

□ Monitor serial sodium levels.

□ Maintain fluid restrictions, or administer oral or parenteral fluids as prescribed.

□ Provide safety measures as indicated for patients with altered LOC.

Potassium: Potassium is the major cation of intracellular fluid, and it plays a leading role in cellular metabolic activities. It is essential for neuromuscular function and is instrumental in maintaining normal cellular water content. Potassium is not stored in the body, nor is it conserved by the kidneys. Most of the daily potassium intake is excreted in the urine, with only small amounts lost through perspiration and feces. Potassium excess does not usually develop in the presence of normal renal function. Although only 2% of body potassium is extracellular, serum potassium concentration generally reflects total body potassium and is affected by the pH of ECF. In acidosis, extracellular hydrogen is exchanged for intracellular potassium. An opposite reaction occurs in alkalotic states. The body is intolerant of fluctuations from normal serum potassium concentration, which is 3.5–5.5 mEq/L; excess or deficit can cause a medical crisis.

A. Hyperkalemia

1. ***Causes:***

   □ *Decreased potassium excretion:* Renal failure; adrenal insufficiency (Addison's disease).

   □ *Increased potassium load:* Increased tissue breakdown, as in crush injuries, burns, major surgery, rhabdomyolysis, severe hemolysis, or GI bleeding; excessive administration of potassium-containing IV solutions or potassium supplements; potassium-sparing diuretics or high doses of penicillin in patients with renal failure; massive transfusions of stored blood.

   □ *Redistribution of intracellular potassium resulting from metabolic acidosis.*

2. ***Clinical indicators:***

   □ *Neuromuscular:* Irritability, weakness, paresthesia, areflexia, muscular or respiratory paralysis.

   □ *Gastrointestinal:* Nausea, diarrhea, cramping.

   □ *Cardiac:* Bradycardia, ventricular fibrillation, cardiac arrest (not usually seen with serum potassium concentrations below 6.5 mEq/L).

   □ *Laboratory findings:* Repeated serum potassium values >5.6 mEq/L; renal function tests usually show some degree of renal impairment.

   □ *EKG:* Tall, peaked T-waves progressing to disappearance of atrial activity; development of wide, bizarre QRS complexes culminating in ventricular fibrillation or asystole.

3. ***Medical management:*** The goal is the rapid restoration of normal serum potassium levels.

   □ Administer IV calcium gluconate or calcium chloride, 5–10 mL of a 10% solution, to quickly antagonize the toxic neuromuscular and cardiac effects of hyperkalemia, particularly if hypocalcemia is present. Serum potassium levels are not affected.

   □ Redistribute ECF potassium: IV injection of one ampule of sodium bicarbonate, which causes rapid movement of potassium into the cells; IV administration of hypertonic solutions of glucose and regular insulin, which causes intracellular potassium shift. These are temporary measures for the immediate reduction of serum potassium until potassium removal can be effected by other means.

   □ Administer cation-exchange resins (eg, Kayexalate) by mouth or rectum, which remove potassium ions from the body in exchange for sodium.

□ Perform dialysis to remove potassium from the blood.

□ Treat the underlying disease.

4. *Nursing diagnoses and interventions:*

Ineffective breathing patterns related to restricted chest movement secondary to impairment/paralysis of respiratory muscles

Desired outcome: Patient's respiratory rate and depth are within acceptable limits.

□ Monitor neuromuscular status; assess character, rate, and depth of respirations.

□ Reposition patient q2h to enhance aeration. Elevate HOB to facilitate respirations; ensure that patient deep breathes and coughs at frequent intervals.

□ Suction airway if patient is unable to expectorate secretions.

Potential alterations in cardiac output: Decreased: Risk of dysrhythmias and cardiac arrest secondary to hyperkalemia

Desired outcome: Patient's VS and lab and physical findings are within acceptable limits.

□ Monitor EKG, cardiac rate and rhythm, and serial serum potassium values. Notify MD if potassium levels exceed 6.0–6.6 mEq/L.

□ Administer IV calcium gluconate or calcium chloride as prescribed.

□ Administer prescribed IV or oral fluids and/or ion-exchange resins.

Knowledge deficit: Foods relatively high in potassium and diuretics that are potassium-sparing

Desired outcome: Patient can verbalize knowledge of foods that are relatively high in potassium and diuretics that are potassium-sparing.

□ Teach patient the importance of limiting dietary potassium intake. For a list of foods relatively high in potassium, see Table 3-2, p. 96.

□ As appropriate teach patient about diuretics that spare potassium. For information, see Table 3-1, p. 93.

B. Hypokalemia

1. *Causes:*

□ *GI losses:* Diarrhea, vomiting, NG suctioning, intestinal or biliary fistulas.

□ *Urinary losses:* Renal tubular disorders, osmotic diuresis, administration of potent diuretics, corticosteroid therapy, primary or secondary hyperaldosteronism, Cushing's syndrome.

□ *Inadequate intake:* Starvation, inadequate replacement during diuretic therapy, prolonged administration of potassium-free parenteral fluids.

□ *Redistribution of extracellular potassium* during correction of acidotic states or treatment for hyperkalemia. It also may occur during TPN because of hypersecretion of insulin.

2. *Clinical indicators:*

□ *Neuromuscular:* Fatigue, muscle weakness, hyporeflexia, paresthesias, flaccid paralysis, tetany (rare).

□ *GI:* Anorexia, nausea, vomiting, decreased bowel sounds, paralytic ileus.

□ *Cardiac:* Atrial and ventricular dysrhythmias, weak pulse, distant heart sounds, hypotension secondary to decreased stroke volume, enhanced response to digitalis.

□ *Laboratory findings:* Repeated serum potassium <3.5 mEq/L.

□ *EKG:* Prolonged P–R interval, flattened or inverted T wave, S–T segment depression, prominent U wave.

3. *Medical management:* The goal is to replenish potassium without inducing hyperkalemia.

□ Administer oral therapy: Dietary intake of potassium-rich foods; oral potassium supplements in liquid, tablet, or powder form.

□ Administer IV potassium chloride if hypokalemia is severe. Serum potassium levels should be determined after the first 50–100 mEq of potassium replacement and q6–12h thereafter until normal values are obtained. Evaluation of renal function should be made before beginning IV potassium replacement.

4. *Nursing diagnoses and interventions:*

Knowledge deficit: Foods high in potassium and diuretics that spare potassium

Desired outcome: Patient can verbalize knowledge of foods that are high in potassium and diuretics that spare potassium.

□ Teach patient the importance of eating foods high in potassium. For a list of foods relatively high in potassium, see Table 3-2, p. 96.

□ As appropriate teach patient about diuretics that spare potassium. For information, see Table 3-1, p. 93.

Potential alterations in cardiac output: Decreased: Risk of dysrhythmias secondary to hypokalemia

Desired outcome: Patient's VS and lab and physical findings are within acceptable limits.

□ Monitor VS. Assess cardiac rate and rhythm, noting character and intensity of pulse and heart tones.

□ Notify MD of EKG or pulse changes, which can signal dangerous dysrhythmias and/or complications. **Note:** Hypokalemia is especially likely to cause dysrhythmias in patients taking digitalis preparations.

□ Monitor serum potassium levels. Notify MD if K+ is below 3.5 mEq/L.

□ Administer oral potassium supplements with at least 4 ounces of water or fruit juice to minimize gastric irritation.

□ Administer prescribed parenteral potassium supplements; monitor flow rate precisely. **Note:** Rates >20 mEq/hr at concentrations >40 mEq/L require continuous cardiac monitoring.

□ Provide for undisturbed rest periods, especially after care activities.

Calcium: Calcium serum level is controlled by hormonal activity of the parathyroid glands and is inversely related to phosphate levels. Calcium is necessary for the formation of bones and teeth, blood clotting, maintenance of the normal transmission of nerve impulses, and muscle contraction. Sufficient vitamin D and protein are required for normal calcium utilization. Approximately half the circulating calcium is bound to albumin; the rest is ionized (free). Only the ionized calcium is physiologically active. Plasma determination of both calcium and albumin is necessary to interpret calcium values accurately. Serum pH also affects the percentage of calcium that is ionized. For example, as pH increases, protein binding increases. Excretion occurs via the feces (80%) and urine.

A. Hypercalcemia

1. *Causes:*

□ *Metabolic:* Hyperparathyroidism, parathyroid tumor, excessive administration of vitamin D.

□ *Release of calcium stores:* Prolonged immobility, multiple fractures, bone tumors, osteoporosis, osteomalacia.

□ *Ingestion of excessive amounts of dietary calcium* and/or calcium-containing antacids or prolonged use of thiazide diuretics.

2. *Clinical indicators:*

□ Anorexia, nausea, vomiting, constipation, pathologic fractures, deep bone pain, flank pain (related to kidney stone formation), polydipsia, polyuria, relaxed skeletal muscles, paranoia, personality changes, lethargy, stupor, coma.

□ *Laboratory findings:* Repeated serum calcium levels >5.8 mEq/L or 11 mg/dL; normal serum calcium values associated with marked decrease in serum albumin; elevated BUN caused by fluid volume deficit or renal damage. Sulkowitch's test of urine will reveal presence of precipitate.

□ *EKG:* Shortening of Q–T interval.

□ *Radiographic findings:* May demonstrate generalized osteoporosis, urinary calculi, bone cavitation.

3. *Medical management:* The goal is to restore normal serum calcium levels.

□ Promote renal calcium excretion: Rapidly infuse saline solution to induce calcium diuresis (sodium inhibits tubular reabsorption of calcium) and diuretics to prevent volume excess; replace urinary water, sodium, and potassium losses.

□ Restrict calcium intake.

□ Administer steroids to inhibit intestinal absorption of calcium and reduce inflammation and associated calcium-mobilizing stress response.

□ Administer oral or parenteral phosphates to alter the calcium–phosphorus equilibrium and IV mithramycin to inhibit bone resorption.

□ Administer calcitonin SC or IM to reduce serum calcium levels temporarily when hypercalcemia is caused by increased parathyroid hormone (PTH).

□ Monitor serial serum calcium values.

4. *Nursing diagnoses and interventions:*

Alteration in pattern of urinary elimination: Dysuria, urgency, or frequency related to presence of renal calculi

Desired outcome: Patient relates the return of a normal voiding pattern.

□ Encourage early mobility to prevent further mobilization of calcium from the bones. If patient is on bed rest, assist with ROM exercises, turn patient q2h, and encourage gastrocnemius, gluteal, and quadriceps muscle-setting exercises.

□ Administer prescribed fluids and medications, and encourage oral fluid intake to dilute urinary calcium, which can result in kidney stones.

□ Monitor I&O and serum calcium levels; strain all urine to check for renal stones.

□ Caution patient about intake of foods and medications high in calcium (eg, cheese, milk, spinach, eggs, peanuts, oysters, and calcium-containing antacids).

For related nursing diagnoses and interventions, see "Hyperparathyroidism," pp. 232–234, in Chapter 5, "Endocrine Disorders," and "Renal Calculi," pp. 101–102, in Chapter 3, "Renal–Urinary Disorders."

B. Hypocalcemia

1. *Causes:* Loss of calcium-rich secretions through diarrhea or wound exudate, vitamin D deficiency, hypoparathyroidism, hyperphosphatemia, hypomagne-

semia, mobilization and excretion of calcium during stress, massive subcutaneous infections and burns, diuretic and terminal phases of renal failure, and massive and rapid transfusions of citrated blood (rare cause). Hypocalcemia is also associated with alkalotic states.

2. *Clinical indicators:*

   □ *Neuromuscular:* Muscle cramps, hyperreflexia, circumoral paresthesia, numbness and tingling of the fingers, positive Trousseau's and Chvostek's signs, laryngeal stridor, tetany, convulsions.

   □ *Cardiovascular:* Hypotension, bleeding if hypocalcemia is severe.

   □ *Laboratory findings:* Repeated serum calcium values <4.5 mEq/L or 8.5 mg/dL (provided that albumin level is within normal range).

   □ *EKG:* Prolonged Q–T interval.

3. *Medical management:* The goal is to restore serum calcium level to normal with minimal hypercalciuria.

   □ Administer IV calcium: 100–200 mg calcium (10–20 mL 10% calcium gluconate) over 10–15 minutes in acute symptomatic hypocalcemia, followed by IV administration of 600–800 mg calcium gluconate in 1000 mL D_5W (5% dextrose in water), which is titrated until the need can be met orally.

   □ Administer oral calcium supplements in less acute conditions.

   □ Administer vitamin D to enhance calcium absorption from the GI tract.

   □ Administer oral or parenteral magnesium if calcium deficit is caused by magnesium depletion.

   □ Monitor serial serum calcium.

4. *Nursing diagnoses and interventions:*

   Potential for injury related to increased risk of seizure activity secondary to hypocalcemia

   Desired outcome: Patient's physical findings are within acceptable limits, or if positive findings of tetany are noted, they are detected and reported immediately, resulting in immediate treatment and absence of injury to patient.

   □ Administer prescribed calcium, vitamin D, and magnesium supplements. Teach patient about foods containing calcium (see "Hypercalcemia," **Alteration of pattern of urinary elimination**, p. 506). Caution patient about use of laxative preparations that contain phosphate and alter metabolism of calcium.

   □ Monitor patient for numbness and tingling around the mouth, an early indicator of hypocalcemia, and be alert to signs and symptoms of tetany: muscle twitching, facial spasms, and painful tonic muscle spasms.

   □ Monitor serum calcium values.

   □ Assess for Trousseau's sign: carpopedal spasm when blood supply to hand is decreased.

   □ Assess for Chvostek's sign: spasm of lip and cheek when the facial nerve is tapped.

   □ If significant findings are noted, minimize environmental stimuli, notify MD, and initiate seizure precautions.

   For related nursing diagnoses and interventions, see "Hypoparathyroidism," pp. 235–236, in Chapter 5, "Endocrine Disorders;" "Acute Renal Failure," pp. 108–110, in Chapter 3, "Renal–Urinary Disorders;" and "Osteoporosis," p. 400, in Chapter 8, "Musculoskeletal Disorders."

► Section Two **Acid–Base Imbalance**

The human body maintains a relatively constant internal environment, of which the balance between acids and bases is one vital aspect. Optimally, cellular processes occur within a narrow range of pH values (concentration of free hydrogen ions). When an imbalance occurs, compensatory mechanisms engage to bring the pH into normal range. Arterial blood gas (ABG) analysis is a clinical tool that can reveal a variety of acid–base disturbances. A sample of arterial blood is taken from the radial or femoral artery and immediately placed on ice to slow the blood's metabolism of oxygen. To ensure accurate results, data regarding the amount of oxygen delivered at the time of the blood draw and patient's temperature must accompany the sample. Oxygen, carbon dioxide, bicarbonate, and pH levels are determined.

I. Acids and Bases

A. Acids

There are two categories of acids found in the body: nonfixed (volatile) and fixed (nonvolatile).

1. *Nonfixed acids:* Those that can change easily between a liquid and gas state. Carbonic acid (carbon dioxide dissolved in water) is the most prevalent nonfixed acid and is primarily controlled and excreted by the respiratory system.

2. *Fixed acids:* Produced by metabolic processes within the body and buffered and excreted by the kidneys. The three predominant categories include the following:

   □ Sulfuric, phosphoric, and other acids that are produced from dietary intake.

   □ Lactic acid, produced by RBCs, WBCs, skeletal muscles, and the brain, and during periods of anaerobic metabolism (eg, vigorous exercise, cardiac/respiratory arrest).

   □ Ketoacids, produced as byproducts of fatty acid oxidation. Fatty acids are an alternate energy source for cell metabolism in glucose-deficient states such as starvation and insulin-deficient states such as diabetes mellitus.

B. Bases

These are substances that are capable of accepting free hydrogen ions. Bicarbonate is the body's predominate base.

II. Maintenance of Acid–Base Balance

There are three ways the body maintains acid–base balance: the buffer system response, respiratory response, and renal response.

Buffer system response: The most immediate. A buffer is a combination of two or more compounds that can combine either with acids or bases to maintain pH. One common combination is carbonic acid and sodium bicarbonate. Others are the plasma proteins, hemoglobin, phosphate, and ammonium complexes.

Respiratory system response: The change in rate and depth of ventilation. Increased respirations will cause CO_2 levels to decrease, and decreased respirations will increase CO_2 levels.

Renal response: Occurs over a 2–3 day period and is the slowest of the three responses. When sustained imbalances tax the abilities of the above two systems, the kidneys begin either eliminating or conserving bicarbonate or hydrogen ions.

III. Components of Arterial Blood Gases

A. Normal Values for Arterial Blood Gases

pH—7.40	range 7.38–7.42
$Paco_2$—40 mm Hg	range 36–44
HCO_3—24 mEq/L	range 22–26
Pao_2—90 mm Hg	range 80–100 (room air)

▶ **Note:** For the elderly, the minimum Pao_2 can be calculated by subtracting 1 mm Hg from 80 mm Hg for every year over 60. This does not apply to the patient over 90 (Shapiro et al, 1977, p.130).

1. ***pH:*** The concentration of hydrogen and hydroxyl ions in equivalents per liter, or in the commonly known scale of pH. An increase in hydrogen ions will cause a more acidic environment, and a decrease will cause a more alkaline environment. pH is inversely proportional to the number of hydrogen ions. As they increase in number, the pH decreases (acidosis occurs); as they decrease in number, pH increases (alkalosis occurs).

2. ***$Paco_2$:*** The partial pressure of dissolved CO_2 in arterial blood. Along with water, CO_2 is an end-product of cell metabolism; therefore, $Paco_2$ can be considered an index of the effectiveness of ventilation in relation to the metabolic rate. Carbon dioxide is highly soluble and can rapidly diffuse into plasma to form carbonic acid, which breaks down to form hydrogen and bicarbonate ions. Most CO_2 is transported via the RBCs, where it combines with water to form carbonic acid, which again breaks down to form hydrogen and bicarbonate ions. The formation of hydrogen and bicarbonate ions plays an important role in diffusing O_2 and CO_2 in the lungs and in maintaining electrical neutrality within the RBCs.

3. ***HCO_3:*** The measurement of bicarbonate ion concentration in the blood. The bicarbonate system is the major and most immediate buffer response. Bicarbonate is a base, and is capable of accepting hydrogen ions. Increased amounts of bicarbonate or other bases can cause an alkaline environment. The kidneys regulate bicarbonate excretion and reabsorption.

4. ***Pao_2:*** The partial pressure of dissolved oxygen in arterial blood. Oxygen is dissolved and carried in the plasma and combined with hemoglobin in the RBCs. Hemoglobin plays a key role in the transport of CO_2 and O_2 from the lungs and tissue. Generally, hemoglobin has a strong affinity for oxygen, but this affinity can be altered by hydrogen ion concentration, CO_2 concentration, and body temperature.

IV. System for Reading ABG Results

A. Step 1

Look at the pH, and determine whether acidosis or alkalosis is present.

$$acidosis \longleftarrow 7.38-7.42 \longrightarrow alkalosis$$
$$\text{low} \qquad \text{normal} \qquad \text{high}$$

B. Step 2

Look at the $Paco_2$. An abnormal value represents a respiratory cause if the HCO_3 is within normal range. A normal $Paco_2$ value in the presence of other abnormal ABG results is indicative of a metabolic cause.

$$alkalosis \longleftarrow 36-44 \longrightarrow acidosis$$
$$\text{low} \qquad \text{normal} \qquad \text{high}$$

C. Step 3

Look at the HCO_3. If the $Paco_2$ is normal, an abnormal HCO_3 value is indicative of a metabolic cause.

$$\text{acidosis} \longleftarrow \underset{\text{low} \quad\quad \text{normal} \quad\quad \text{high}}{22-26} \longrightarrow \text{alkalosis}$$

D. Step 4

Look at the Pao_2. Normally, it is 80–100 mm Hg at room air. Changes in this range can occur with disease as well as with increasing age and high altitude. An individual with a Pao_2 below 80 mm Hg is considered to be hypoxemic and requires supplemental oxygen therapy.

V. Acid–Base Imbalance

There are two categories of acid–base imbalance. A *simple imbalance* is characterized by a change in pH as well as one abnormal value of either $Paco_2$ or HCO_3. *Compensated imbalances* are characterized by a near-normal pH and abnormal values of both $Paco_2$ and HCO_3. In compensated imbalances, the first-line buffer responses cannot rectify the imbalance. The long-term buffer responses come into play and attempt to add the needed substance, either acid or base, to bring the pH to normal range. Because the underlying problem is not corrected, the values of $Paco_2$ and HCO_3 remain abnormal. The pH rarely becomes overcompensated; a compensated pH will be on the side of the initial imbalance state.

A. Respiratory Acidosis

1. *Sample values:*

Simple		Compensated
7.26	pH	7.37
56	$Paco_2$	56
26	HCO_3	40

2. *Causes:* Reduced ventilation states found with respiratory arrest, head/brain trauma, pneumonia, hypoventilation caused by sedation or anesthesia, atelectasis, Guillain-Barré syndrome, chronic obstructive pulmonary disease (COPD).

3. *Signs and symptoms:* Early signs include weakness, headache, SOB, fatigue, anxiety, and tremors. Progressive signs include dehydration and confusion, leading ultimately to coma if untreated.

4. *Medical management:*

   ☐ Find the cause to determine appropriate treatment.

   ☐ Administer bicarbonate.

   ☐ Provide pulmonary hygiene measures.

   ☐ Initiate intubation and mechanical ventilation for patients exhibiting signs of respiratory failure.

   ☐ Begin antibiotic therapy for patients with pneumonia.

   ☐ Administer naloxone hydrochloride for patients who are oversedated.

   ☐ Replace potassium chloride (because acidosis causes potassium ions to leave and hydrogen ions to enter the cells).

   ☐ No measures are taken if the patient is asymptomatic and the underlying cause cannot be treated.

4. *Nursing diagnoses and interventions:*

See "Atelectasis" in Chapter 1, "Respiratory Disorders," for the following:
Potential alteration in respiratory function related to prolonged inactivity

and/or omission of deep breathing, p. 12. See "Caring for Preoperative and Postoperative Patients" in "Appendix One" for the following: **Ineffective Breathing Pattern** related to decreased respiratory depth secondary to anesthesia, immobility, and guarding with painful surgical incision, p. 530. (These are only a few examples of related nursing diagnoses in this manual.)

B. Metabolic Acidosis

1. *Sample values:*

Simple		Compensated
7.24	pH	7.37
38	$Paco_2$	18
12	HCO_3	10

2. *Causes:* Build up of fixed acids, as in cardiac arrest, renal failure, ketoacidosis, or ingestion of acidic substances; loss of base, as in diarrhea.

3. *Signs and symptoms:* Kussmaul's respirations, dehydration, lethargy, malaise, fatigue, nausea/vomiting, headache, SOB, vasodilation, tremors, coma.

4. *Medical management:*

☐ Find the cause to determine appropriate treatment.

☐ If ketoacidosis is the cause, administer glucose, insulin, or IV potassium chloride.

☐ Replace fluid losses.

☐ Administer bicarbonate.

☐ If renal failure is the cause, prescribe diet low in protein and high in carbohydrates.

☐ Replace phosphates.

5. *Nursing diagnoses and interventions:*

Fluid volume deficit related to abnormal losses

Desired outcome: Patient's VS, physical findings, and lab values are within acceptable limits.

☐ Monitor I&O, LOC, and VS; evaluate laboratory results for abnormal values of glucose and potassium; monitor EKG for evidence of cardiac dysrhythmias.

☐ Assess for signs of dehydration and decreased sensorium.

☐ Test urine pH and specific gravity.

☐ Encourage intake of fluids and/or administer fluids such as IV lactate and $NaHCO_3$ as prescribed.

☐ Institute seizure precautions if patient exhibits signs of decreased sensorium.

As appropriate, see related nursing diagnoses and interventions in "Acute Renal Failure," pp. 108–110, in Chapter 3, "Renal–Urinary Disorders."

C. Respiratory Alkalosis

1. *Sample values:*

Simple		Compensated
7.52	pH	7.46
24	$Paco_2$	28
24	HCO_3	12

2. *Causes:* Hyperventilation states, as in mechanical overventilation, pain, anxiety, brain injury, fever, pulmonary edema, acute asthma.

3. *Signs and symptoms:* Restlessness, dizziness, tingling, spasms, tetany, anxiety.

4. *Medical management:*

   □ Find the cause to determine appropriate treatment.

   □ Decrease ventilations, for example, with sedation or rebreathing apparatus.

   □ Replace sodium and/or chloride.

   □ Replace potassium chloride.

5. *Nursing diagnoses and interventions:*

   Ineffective breathing patterns related to hyperventilation

   Desired outcome: Patient's respiratory rate and depth are within acceptable limits.

   □ Monitor VS and LOC.

   □ Place patient in semi-Fowler's position to enhance ventilation.

   □ Provide paper bag in which patient can rebreathe exhaled CO_2.

   □ Allay patient's anxieties.

   □ Sedate patient as prescribed.

As appropriate, see related nursing diagnoses and interventions in "Asthma," p. 19, in Chapter 1, "Respiratory Disorders," and "Pulmonary Edema," p. 69, in Chapter 2, "Cardiovascular Disorders."

D. Metabolic Alkalosis

1. *Sample values:*

Simple		*Compensated*
7.54	pH	7.48
44	$Paco_2$	66
36	HCO_3	34

2. *Causes:* Buildup of bicarbonate or base by ingestion of bicarbonate in the form of antacids; loss of chloride or hydrogen ions as with long-term NG suctioning, diuretic therapy, and/or vomiting; and corticosteroid treatment.

3. *Signs and symptoms:* Dizziness, lethargy, weakness, dysrhythmias, tetany, hypoventilation, convulsions, irritability, disorientation.

4. *Medical management:*

   □ Find the cause to determine appropriate treatment.

   □ Replace fluids; administer acidifying IV fluids.

   □ Replace potassium, sodium, and/or chloride, if needed.

   □ Administer acetazolamide to increase excretion of HCO_3.

5. *Nursing diagnosis and interventions:*

   Fluid volume deficit related to abnormal losses

   Desired outcome: Patient's VS, physical findings, and lab values are within acceptable limits.

   □ Monitor I&O; monitor for indicators of hypokalemia, such as dysrhythmias and tetany.

   □ Ensure minimal bicarbonate administration or ingestion.

- □ Administer potassium chloride, sodium chloride, and fluids as prescribed.
- □ Use saline rather than water to irrigate NG tube.
- □ Institute seizure precautions if indicated.

▶ Section Three **Providing Nutritional Therapy**

Malnutrition is a functional disease that is found in 25% of all hospitalized patients. Approximately half of medical-surgical admissions have some evidence of protein-calorie malnutrition, while 10% have advanced forms. Malnourished patients have longer hospital stays, higher morbidity and mortality rates, poorer wound healing, and increased susceptibility to infection.

High-risk patients: Those who are grossly underweight (below 80% of ideal body weight); grossly overweight (120% or more above ideal body weight); alcoholics; elderly; pregnant adolescents; persons experiencing excessive nutrient losses (as with malabsorption, short bowel syndrome/fistulas, and dialysis); patients receiving steroids, immunosuppressants, antineoplastic drugs, or radiation therapy; patients with chronic diseases such as arthritis or COPD; patients with disorders that increase metabolic needs, such as sepsis, burns, trauma, or fever; and those who have recently lost 10% or more of their usual body weight.

I. Basic Components

A. Protein-Calorie Malnutrition (PCM)

Three major types of malnutrition are classicially recognized.

1. *Marasmus:* Seen in individuals with prolonged starvation. Total dietary intake is inadequate but contains both protein and calories. The individual has experienced weight loss and fat and muscle wasting. Laboratory values measuring visceral protein status, eg, albumin or transferrin, may appear normal. However, depressed cellular immunity (measured by skin test antigens) and decreased anthropometric measurements (triceps skinfold, midarm circumference, arm muscle area) can support the diagnosis. Clinical conditions that can lead to marasmus include anorexia, partial small bowel obstruction, chronic illness, and old age.

2. *Kwashiorkor-like:* Seen in individuals with adequate calorie intake but little or no protein intake. The individual may appear obese while visceral protein status and cellular immunity are significantly depressed. Predisposing conditions include fad diets, nutritionally incomplete liquid diets, and IV glucose administration without protein supplementation.

3. *Kwashiorkor-marasmus mix:* Occurs when both major types of malnutrition exist concurrently.

▶ **Note:** Because pure marasmus or kwashiorkor is rarely seen in clinical practice, the term *protein-calorie malnutrition* (PCM) has been adopted to describe the type of malnutrition seen in the majority of hospitalized patients.

B. Basal Energy Expenditure (BEE)

BEE is the energy expended by a fasting, unstressed person lying quietly in bed. The Harris-Benedict equation is a method used to determine the BEE in calories per day for a healthy individual. The equations are as follows:

$$\text{Female} = 655 + (9.6 \times W) + (1.7 \times H) - (4.7 \times A)$$

$$\text{Male} = 66 + (13.7 \times W) + (5 \times H) - (6.8 \times A)$$

W = weight in kg; H = height in cm; A = age in years. Determining the BEE is the initial step in estimating a patient's calorie requirements. Accurate documentation of the patient's age, weight, and height is essential. An individual's BEE in kilocalories per day can be quickly and roughly estimated by multiplying 20–25 kcal by the individual's weight in kilograms (20–25 kcal × kg). This method may not be as accurate as the Harris-Benedict formula or other methods of calculating a BEE. Some hospitals use sophisticated equipment to determine accurate resting energy expenditure via indirect calorimetry. This method measures heat production based on oxygen consumption and carbon dioxide production.

C. Estimating Calorie and Protein Needs

Energy needs include the following:

BEE + metabolic stress + activity + weight gain (if desirable)

Metabolic stress: Fever, infection, long-bone fractures, major surgery, and burns, any of which increases energy needs by varying degrees. In general, the needs of the hypermetabolic, hypercatabolic patient do not exceed 100% over the calculated BEE. *Activity:* Paralyzed, weak, or critically ill patients expend little or no energy on movement, while patients on bed rest and those ambulating may use 10–20% over their BEE. *Weight gain:* 500 kcal/day above energy needs will provide for a gain of approximately 1 pound per week. Severely stressed and injured patients should be nutritionally maintained during the stressful period to prevent further weight loss. Attempts to replace lean body mass and achieve weight gain in such patients are usually futile and can be dangerous. In general, protein needs are estimated separately from caloric needs. Hospitalized patients can require 1–4 g/kg/day of protein to meet needs for stress and repletion. Evaluation of protein tolerance versus needs must be considered in patients with impaired renal or hepatic function. In general, the goal of estimating calorie and protein needs is to provide a therapy that will maintain positive nitrogen balance. (See p. 518 for a discussion of nitrogen balance studies.)

D. Substrates and Essential Nutrients

Substrates are the fuel for metabolic pathways and result in the production of energy.

1. *Protein:* Constitutes 15% of the typical American diet. US recommended daily allowance (RDA) is 0.8 g/kg/day. Of 22 amino acids, 8 are essential for endogenous protein synthesis. Insufficient caloric intake results in diversion of amino acids for energy rather than for maintenance of lean body mass and circulating proteins.

2. *Carbohydrates:* Constitute 50% of the typical American diet. The brain, renal medulla, and RBCs have an obligatory need for approximately 500 kcal/day.

3. *Fat:* Constitutes 35% of the typical American diet and enhances fat-soluble vitamin absorption. Two fatty acids, linoleic and arachidonic, are essential. Linoleic acid must be supplied exogenously, while arachidonic acid can be synthesized from linoleic acid. Currently, linolenic acid is being studied to determine whether or not it is essential. Essential fatty acids should comprise approximately 4% of daily caloric intake.

4. *Vitamins:* US RDA of fat- and water-soluble vitamins is necessary for regulation of metabolic processes in healthy individuals and is based on dietary intake. Parenteral requirements are less well defined.

5. *Trace elements:* Adequate amounts are provided in ordinary diet. Parenteral requirements are less certain, and special consideration is needed for patients receiving long-term IV nutritional support. Essential trace elements include zinc, copper, chromium, manganese, selenium, iodine, and iron. Undiagnosed/untreated deficiencies impair bodily functions. For example, patients

with ileostomies or other small bowel fluid losses can lose up to 17 mg/L of zinc. If not replaced, deficiency can result, leading to poor wound healing and impaired ability to taste. Replenishing deficiencies prevents and/or cures clinical symptoms.

E. Metabolic Adaptation

Metabolic adaptation occurs with early and prolonged starvation, in response to stress associated with various catabolic states, and during recovery/repletion. When starvation occurs, carbohydrate reserves are limited to approximately a 24-hour supply.

1. *Early starvation:* Because of limited carbohydrate reserves and the obligatory need of certain tissues for glucose, skeletal muscle protein becomes the fuel for gluconeogenesis. Protein breakdown results in the loss of about 0.5 lb/day of lean body mass. The exogenous provision of 100 g/day of carbohydrate (approximately 400 kcal) aids in decreasing the rate of muscle protein breakdown.

2. *Prolonged starvation:* After several days, the brain converts to the utilization of ketone bodies (oxidized free fatty acids) as an alternative fuel. This decreased requirement for glucose results in decreased rate of muscle protein breakdown. Additionally, there is an increased efficiency of amino acid utilization for protein synthesis.

3. *Catabolic states:* Stress increases the body's demand for energy and protein. Increased levels of corticosteroids and catecholamines result in catabolism of protein, which provides amino acids for gluconeogenesis and tissue repair. Catabolic states, including major burns, sepsis, fever, bone fractures, major surgery, and multiple trauma, are often characterized by hyperglycemia and insulin resistance.

4. *Refeeding syndrome:* Extremely malnourished patients are at increased risk of cardiovascular collapse during the initial 3–5 days of therapy. Fluid overload, intracellular shifts of potassium and phosphorus (hypokalemia, hypophosphatemia), and the effects of increased cardiac output and metabolic rate on a decreased left ventricular mass can be life-threatening. Careful assessment and identification of these patients (eg, for loss of >30% of normal body mass), slow refeeding (providing less than the calculated basal requirements for several days with a slow advance to goals over a few weeks), and intensive metabolic monitoring with fluid and electrolyte adjustments are essential for successful refeeding.

5. *Recovery/repletion:* Metabolic and endocrine changes associated with acute stress or trauma usually begin to subside within approximately a week. With aggressive nutritional support after this period, patients usually can be converted to an anabolic state. Anabolism can be more difficult to achieve when acute stress or trauma is superimposed on malnutrition. Protein and caloric requirements are increased during this period and body fat supplies are repleted only after nitrogen losses have been restored.

F. Fluid and Electrolytes

For general discussion, refer to "Fluid and Electrolyte Disturbances," pp. 498–507.

1. *Sodium:* The exact daily requirement is unknown. Dietary intake is usually obtained in the form of sodium chloride and varies greatly with the individual.

2. *Potassium:* Average daily requirement is 40–100 mEq/day, and it increases as the patient becomes anabolic. See Table 3-2, p. 96.

3. *Calcium:* The daily requirement varies widely. It is found in milk, milk products, vegetables, sesame seeds, edible bones (salmon, sardines), and meats.

4. *Magnesium:* The daily requirement is about 25 mEq/day, and normal plasma

Table 11-1 Composition of Gastrointestinal Secretions

Type of Secretion	Na (mEq/L)	K (mEq/L)	Cl (mEq/L)	HCO₃ (mEq/L)
salivary	10	26	10	30
gastric	60	10	130	—
duodenal	140	5	80	—
ileal	140	5	104	30
colonic	60	30	40	—
pancreatic	140	5	75	115
biliary	145	5	100	35

concentration is about 2 mEq/L. It is an important coenzyme in carbohydrate and protein metabolism, and is involved in neuromuscular irritability. Approximately 35% of plasma magnesium is bound to protein. Its regulation depends on renal function and plasma concentration of calcium and phosphorus, and it is found in virtually all foods. Excretion occurs primarily via the kidneys.

5. *Phosphorus:* Daily requirements vary, but increase as anabolism occurs. It is a major intracellular anion, required for tissue synthesis, and is present in virtually all foods. Metabolism resembles that of calcium. Normal plasma concentration is about 2 mEq/L. Resorption occurs in the renal tubules, and urinary excretion is affected by dietary intake, acid–base status, and the secretion of parathyroid hormone.

6. *Chloride:* Daily requirements vary, and increase as anabolism occurs. Primarily, it is found in interstitial and lymph fluid compartments. It aids in the preservation of osmotic pressure and water balance and buffers the exchange of carbon dioxide and oxygen in RBCs. Concentration changes affect acid–base status. Normal plasma concentration is about 103 mEq/L. Deficiency leads to potassium deficiency. Losses follow those of sodium and can be compensated for by bicarbonate. Excretion occurs via output of urine and other body fluids.

7. *Bicarbonate:* A byproduct of carbon dioxide production and always present in the body. Concentration depends on kidney function. Its presence or absence determines metabolic acidosis or alkalosis. Normal plasma concentration is about 24 mEq/L.

G. Assessment

Evaluation of nutritional status is a fundamental part of patient assessment. It should include dietary, medical, and social history; physical examination; anthropometric measurements; and laboratory test results. Extremely valuable clues of subclinical malnutrition may be obtained and further evaluated during dietary history and a thorough physical exam.

1. *Dietary history:* May identify the patient at high risk for having or developing a nutritional problem. Nutritional problems can arise from nutrient excess or deficiency. Suspect possible malnutrition and evaluate further if the patient responds positively to any of the following:

☐ History of recent weight gain or loss (eg, >5 kg over several weeks).

☐ Recurrence of nausea, vomiting, diarrhea.

☐ Presence of chronic illness such as cancer; diabetes mellitus; hyperlipidemia; ulcers; hypertension; or liver, heart, or kidney failure.

☐ Presence of digestive disorders such as pancreatic disease, inflammatory bowel disease, intolerance to milk, intestinal bypass or resection, fistulas, strictures.

☐ Alcohol or drug addiction.

☐ Living alone, elderly, impoverishment.

☐ Presence of abnormal dietary habits such as fad diet, loss of taste or smell, allergies to food, recent change in diet, ill-fitting dentures.

☐ Consumption of drugs that alter dietary intake or utilization of drugs such as analgesics, antacids, antibiotics, anticonvulsants, diuretics, antineoplastic agents, oral contraceptives, or laxatives.

2. *Physical assessment:* May reveal findings suggestive of protein, calorie, vitamin, or mineral deficiencies. Assessment should include the following components:

☐ *General appearance:* eg, thinness, obesity.

☐ *Head:* eg, bossing, deformities, temporal wasting.

☐ *Hair:* eg, easy pluckability, sparseness, lackluster appearance, depigmentation, dryness.

☐ *Eyes:* eg, night blindness, pale conjunctiva, xerosis (congenital or corneal), retinal hemorrhage, Bitot's spots, cataracts.

☐ *Nose:* eg, anosmia, dysosmia, nasolabial seborrhea.

☐ *Mouth:* eg, angular stomatitis, cheilosis, glossitis, gingivitis, caries/periodontal disease, ageusia, dysgeusia.

☐ *Neck:* eg, goiter, enlarged parotid gland.

☐ *Skin:* eg, pallor, abnormal pigmentation, flaky-paint dermatitis, follicular hyperkeratosis, perifollicular petechiae, bruises, edema, fistula, open wounds, decubiti.

☐ *Nails:* eg, friability, presence of bands and lines, concavity.

☐ *Cardiovascular system:* eg, cardiomegaly, resting tachycardia. With prolonged starvation, bradycardia, hypotension, and hypothermia can occur.

☐ *Respiratory system:* eg, SOB, use of accessory muscles.

☐ *Gastrointestinal system:* eg, hepatomegaly, ascites, distention, masses, scaphoid abdomen.

☐ *Genitourinary system:* eg, delayed onset of puberty, secondary sexual characteristics, hypogonadism.

☐ *Musculoskeletal system:* eg, osteoporosis, bowed limbs, atrophy, pain, weakness.

☐ *Nervous system:* eg, listlessness, mental confusion, confabulation, hyperreflexia, hyporeflexia, irritability, improper position and vibratory sense.

3. *Anthropometric measurements*

☐ Obtain weight and height on admission, and compare them to ideal weight (see Table 11-2, p. 518) and patient's usual weight. Body weight is one of the most convenient and useful indicators of nutritional status.

☐ Measure triceps skinfold thickness, which is a good indicator of body fat or calorie stores. Measurements can be compared to HANES (Health and Nutrition Examination Survey) reference values for the patient's sex and age range. Average triceps skinfold measurements are 12.5 mm (male) and 16.5 mm (female).

☐ Measure midarm circumference as an indicator of skeletal muscle mass. Measurements can be compared to HANES reference values for patient's sex and age range. Average midarm circumference measurements are 25.5 cm (male) and 16.5 cm (female).

Table 11-2 Ideal Weights*

Height	Men			Women		
	Small Frame	Medium Frame	Large Frame	Small Frame	Medium Frame	Large Frame
4 ft 10 in	—	—	—	102–111	109–121	118–131
4 ft 11 in	—	—	—	103–113	111–123	120–134
5 ft	—	—	—	104–115	113–126	122–137
5 ft 1 in	—	—	—	106–118	115–129	125–140
5 ft 2 in	128–134	131–141	138–150	108–121	118–132	128–143
5 ft 3 in	130–136	133–143	140–153	111–124	121–135	131–147
5 ft 4 in	132–138	135–145	142–156	114–127	124–138	134–151
5 ft 5 in	134–140	137–148	144–160	117–130	127–141	137–155
5 ft 6 in	136–142	139–151	146–164	120–133	130–144	140–159
5 ft 7 in	138–146	142–154	148–168	123–136	133–147	143–163
5 ft 8 in	140–148	145–157	152–172	126–139	136–150	146–167
5 ft 9 in	142–151	148–160	156–176	129–142	139–153	149–170
5 ft 10 in	144–154	151–163	158–180	132–145	142–156	152–173
5 ft 11 in	146–157	154–166	161–184	135–148	145–159	155–176
6 ft	149–160	157–170	164–188	138–151	148–162	158–179
6 ft 1 in	152–164	160–174	168–192	—	—	—
6 ft 2 in	155–168	164–178	172–197	—	—	—
6 ft 3 in	158–172	167–182	176–202	—	—	—
6 ft 4 in	162–176	171–187	181–207	—	—	—

*Ages 25 through 59, for 5 lb of indoor clothing for men and 3 lb of indoor clothing for women, and 1-inch heels for both. Data for 1983. Courtesy of the Metropolitan Life Insurance Company.

4. **Laboratory test results:** Can provide accurate information about patient's nutritional status. Decreased serum levels of albumin, transferrin, and total lymphocytes can indicate decreased visceral protein. Cellular immunity is determined by the patient's ability to respond to skin tests such as PPD, mumps, and *Candida*. A 24-hour urine collection for urine urea nitrogen (UUN) excretion is one method used to calculate nitrogen balance. Nitrogen balance calculations provide an assessment of adequate protein intake:

$$\text{Nitrogen (N) balance} = \text{N in} - \text{N out}$$

$$\text{N in} = \frac{\text{grams protein}}{6.25}$$

$$\text{N out} = \text{grams excreted in 24-hour collection UUN} + 20\% \text{ UUN} + 2$$

Healthy individuals are usually in neutral or slightly positive nitrogen balance. The goal of nutrition therapy in hospitalized patients is to provide adequate nitrogen to prevent a negative nitrogen state. When nitrogen balance studies are in progress, critical nursing goals include accurate collection, measurement, and recording of I&O for the designated period. Laboratory values must be used in conjunction with nutritional history, physical findings, and anthropometrics to provide a complete and accurate nutritional assessment.

H. Nutritional therapy

Nutritional therapy should entail the delivery of utilizable nutrients into the body via the route that is most natural, safe, efficient, and cost-effective. The primary goals of specialized nutritional support include prevention of further depletion of body protein stores, maintenance of nitrogen balance, promotion of protein synthesis for tissue repair and wound healing, and promotion of synthesis of hormones and enzymes that are necessary for regulation of metabolic processes. Treatment modalities include the following:

1. *Oral diet:* A wide variety of standard and specialized hospital diets are available and appropriate for many patients with poor dentition; fluid, electrolyte, and substrate restrictions; or chronic disease such as diabetes mellitus, renal/ cardiac/liver failure, short bowel syndrome, and cystic fibrosis.

2. *Supplements and liquid diets:* A variety of liquid diets are available commercially; most are lactose-free. Special care should be given in the selection of such products because they are marketed to supply extra calores, fat, and protein while not necessarily being nutritionally complete (eg, lacking in vitamins, trace minerals, and electrolytes).

3. *Modular components:* Individual carbohydrate, fat, and protein modules are available commercially in liquid and powder forms. Generally, they are used to fortify other solutions, but can be mixed together to provide highly individualized feeding regimens.

4. *Tube feedings:* Liquid diets are administered through a variety of feeding tubes. Feeding tubes can be placed temporarily (eg, oro/nasogastric, nasoduodenal/jejunal) or on a long-term basis (eg, in pharyngostomy, gastrostomy, cervical esophagostomy, jejunostomy). Methods of administration include continuous, intermittent, and bolus. Feedings are delivered by syringe, gravity drip, or infusion management device. Regardless of the method of administration or delivery, progression to protein and energy needs should be governed by patient tolerance. In general, isotonic solutions (approximately 300 mOsm/L) are started at full strength (undiluted) and delivered initially at low rates of administration. Hypertonic solutions (>600 mOsm/L) are diluted with tap water to half strength and delivered at low rates of administration (25 mL/h). Advance either the rate or concentration independently, not simultaneously. For example, advance half strength at 25 mL/h to full strength at 25 mL/h or to half strength at 50 mL/h. However, do *not* directly advance half strength at 25 mL/h to full strength at 50 mL/h.

5. *Intravenous nutrition:* Few patients can meet their total caloric and protein needs with peripheral parenteral nutrition because of the large volume of fluid required to supply nutrients. In general, peripheral vein therapy requires good venous access and low metabolic needs; and it should be for short-term (7–10 day) therapy only. Central vein therapy should be restricted to those patients with high nutritional requirements needing therapy longer than 7–10 days and to those with exhausted peripheral access. Fat emulsions are isotonic solutions administered with parenteral nutrition to prevent or correct essential fatty acid deficiency and/or provide an additional, concentrated source of calories.

II. Nursing Components

A. General Nursing Interventions

For all nutritional treatment modalities:

1. Explain purpose and plans for feedings to patient; provide time for questions and answers.

2. Encourage participation of patient and SOs in patient care.

3. Encourage and provide means for exercise, recreation, personal hygiene, and other activities as indicated and tolerated. These measures provide distractions and enhance a personal sense of well-being while maintaining lean body mass.

4. Document types of nutritional support, route and frequency of administration, IV catheter or feeding tube care, patient's weight, I&O, VS, patient tolerance to the diet, and patient teaching.

B. Specific Nursing Diagnoses and Interventions

For oral diet:

Alteration in nutrition: Less than body requirements related to increased need or decreased intake

Desired outcome: Patient does not exhibit signs of malnutrition or weight loss.

1. Maximize patient's oral dietary intake potential by assisting with positioning the bed or chair and setting up food tray and utensils for patients who are incapable of doing so on their own.
2. When appropriate, encourage SOs to assist with feedings.
3. Allow favorite foods that comply with the prescribed diet to be brought in from outside the patient care setting.
4. Respond to and honor patient's food preferences when feasible.
5. Create an attractive environment to enhance oral intake.
6. Offer smaller, more frequent meals.

For oral supplements:

Alteration in nutrition: Less than body requirements related to increased need or decreased intake

Desired outcome: Patient does not exhibit signs of malnutrition or weight loss.

1. When appropriate, refrigerate solutions or pour over ice before serving, to enhance the flavor.
2. Pour solutions into an attractive container to enhance patient's appetite.
3. When appropriate, offer small amounts of the solution between meals.
4. Solicit and honor patient's preferences, and provide a variety of solutions when feasible.
5. Encourage patient's efforts with normal dietary intake.

For tube feedings:

Potential impairment of skin integrity related to mucosal and skin surface irritation secondary to presence of the feeding tube

Desired outcome: Patient's skin does not exhibit signs of irritation or breakdown.

1. Minimize patient discomfort and help prevent skin breakdown by providing, at frequent intervals, oral and nasal hygiene or skin care around ostomies.
2. Secure tubes to patient to help prevent irritation to the skin and mucous membranes. As an alternative to adhesive tape and to minimize body image disturbances, use semipermeable transparent dressing materials.
3. When irrigating the tube, use a 50-mL bulb syringe, which creates less pressure during irrigation than a piston syringe, and hence, minimizes the risk of tissue and mucosal trauma.
4. When tube-feeding therapy has been discontinued, remove the tube slowly, using gentle tension to prevent trauma to tissues and mucosa.

Potential alterations in bowel elimination: Diarrhea or constipation related to contamination and/or side effects of the feeding solution

Desired outcome: Patient does not experience diarrhea or constipation.

1. Assess patient for intolerance to the feeding solution as evidenced by distention, cramping, nausea, flatulence, and/or diarrhea. Report significant findings to MD.
2. Whenever possible, hang a 24-hour supply of feeding solution unless manufacturer's recommendations differ. Risk of contamination is decreased by

using clean technique and ensuring that the solution enters the administration system in the least amount of time possible. Check institutional procedures for specific policies.

3. Attach a three-way stopcock with an injection port between the administration tubing and feeding tube to minimize the risk of contamination during irrigation or administration of medications.

4. Improve patient tolerance to the feeding solution and minimize metabolic and mechanical complications by utilizing infusion management devices whenever possible. Carefully monitor gravity-drip administration rates.

5. Administer additional prescribed electrolytes and trace minerals (eg, potassium, phosphorus, magnesium) slowly and diluted in at least 1 hour's feeding to minimize the risk of diarrhea from bolus administration of these hyperosmolar solutions.

6. Because most enteral solutions are low in residue, assess patient for constipation. If indicated, consult with MD regarding patient's need for laxative assistance.

Potential alteration in respiratory function related to increased risk of aspiration secondary to tube-feeding therapy

Desired outcome: Patient does not exhibit signs of respiratory dysfunction.

1. Prevent instillation of feeding solution into the airway by testing for correct position of tube in the stomach before administering *any* solution into the tube as well as at 4–6 hour intervals for continuous feedings. For intermittent tube feedings, proper tube position can be determined when aspirating and measuring stomach contents to evaluate absorption of previous feeding.

▶ **Note:** Check the hospital's aspiration precaution policy to determine whether or not to withhold feeding because of a high residual. Reinstill residual stomach contents into the tube to minimize disturbance of fluid and electrolyte status.

---

2. Elevate HOB at least 30° to minimize the risk of aspiration. For patients receiving intermittent feedings, maintain this position for 45–60 minutes after each feeding. A slightly elevated right-side-lying position can be used for patients intolerant of higher positions.

3. Monitor for indicators of aspiration, including SOB, discolored tracheal aspirate, and fever. If found, stop the feeding and report findings to MD.

4. Before removal of orogastric or NG tube, irrigate the tube and then clamp or pinch the tube back on itself to minimize the risk of aspiration as the tube is being pulled out.

Potential fluid volume deficit or excess related to abnormal loss or retention secondary to osmolality and substrate content of tube-feeding solutions

Desired outcome: Patient does not exhibit signs of dehydration or overhydration.

1. Osmolality and substrate content of solutions can contribute to the development of fluid and electrolyte disturbances. Be alert to the following indicators of dehydration: thirst, poor skin turgor, dryness of mucous membranes, tachycardia, hypotension, and I&O imbalance. Overhydration can be detected by SOB, digital/sacral/pretibial edema and, in extreme cases, by anasarca. Serum sodium values may coincide with the above physical assessments.

2. If patient appears dehydrated, instill water into NG tube. Unless contraindicated, instill a minimum of 1 L over a 24-hour period for optimal hydration and to ensure tube patency. For continuous feedings, irrigate tube with 30–50 mL water q4–6h, or irrigate after each intermittent feeding and/or as often as indicated.

3. The carbohydrate composition of some feeding solutions may result in glycosuria. Perform urine glucose tests q6–8h to test patient's tolerance to the feeding.

For intravenous nutrition:

Potential for infection related to increased susceptibility secondary to invasive procedure and parenteral delivery of nutrients

Desired outcome: Patient does not exhibit signs of infection.

1. Ensure that the peripheral needle or cannula is inserted by a trained staff member.

2. Precede all entries into the IV system by thorough handwashing and preparation of the site with povidone-iodine. Allow the solution to dry completely before inserting needle or cannula.

3. If a needle or cannula is already present, initiate nutritional therapy through the existing device. If the previous solution is incompatible, irrigate the device with 10 mL normal saline and hang a new administration system and tubing.

4. Change, label, and date tubing and administration system q24–48h, according to institutional policy.

5. Be alert to glycosuria and indicators of infection, such as fever and warmth, redness, swelling, pain, and purulent drainage at the insertion site. Glucose intolerance can occur secondary to increasing glucose load or infectious process.

Potential for injury related to risk of metabolic abnormalities secondary to peripheral-vein nutritional therapy

Desired outcome: Patient does not exhibit signs of metabolic abnormalities; or, if they occur, they are detected and reported promptly, resulting in immediate treatment and absence of injury to the patient.

1. Be alert to metabolic abnormalities, which can occur within 24–72 hours after administering IV nutritional therapy. These include hyperglycemia (eg, polyuria, headache, fatigue), hypokalemia (eg, weakness, anorexia, dysrhythmias), hypophosphatemia (eg, parathesias, respiratory distress), and hyponatremia (eg, headache, anxiety, abdominal cramps). Review routine serum laboratory test results (including sodium, potassium, chloride, bicarbonate, BUN, creatinine, glucose, calcium, phosphorus, magnesium, liver enzymes, CBC, and prothrombin time).

2. Maintain I&O records for all fluids; measure VS q4h; and weigh patient daily until stable and then twice a week thereafter. Monitor for *dehydration:* thirst, poor skin turgor, dry mucous membranes, tachycardia, hypotension; and for *overhydration:* SOB, digital/sacral/pretibial edema.

3. Ensure that final amino acid concentrations do not exceed 5%. In some institutions, 10% dextrose is allowed if fat emulsions are infusing continuously.

4. Deliver prescribed volume, provided it is within patient's tolerance. Stop the therapy as prescribed; it is not necessary to taper the delivery.

Potential for injury related to risk of metabolic abnormalities secondary to central-vein nutritional therapy

Desired outcome: Patient does not exhibit signs of metabolic abnormalities; or, if they occur, they are detected and reported promptly, resulting in immediate treatment and absence of injury to the patient.

1. Initiate nutritional therapy slowly, and increase it gradually to meet the prescribed goals for the patient. Hyperosmolar solutions are diluted by rapid blood flow in the central veins.

2. Advance the rate of glucose adminstration only when patient is stable on the current regimen.

3. Perform urine/serum testing for glucose at least q6h.

4. Do not stop the delivery abruptly unless 5% dextrose solution has been infusing via another route. Solutions can be tapered over approximately 6 hours by decreasing the rate of administration to one-half of the current administration rate. Solutions, when cycled, are oftentimes stopped after a 1-hour taper (in stable patients) without encountering rebound hypoglycemia.

5. For additional information, see interventions 1 and 2 with the preceding nursing diagnosis.

Potential alteration in tissue perfusion: Cardiopulmonary, related to impaired circulation secondary to complications of central-vein nutritional therapy

Desired outcome: Patient demonstrates circulatory status and physical findings within acceptable limits.

1. Be aware of the following potential complications of central-vein therapy: perforation of vascular structures; pneumothorax; inappropriate position of the catheter tip (into the internal jugular vein, pleural space, mediastinum, pulmonary or carotid artery, hepatic vein); thrombosis of the great veins; or air embolus.

2. Deliver isotonic solutions at a "keep open" rate until chest x-ray confirms correct catheter placement.

3. Minimize the risk of air embolus, clotting, and loss of IV access by using Luer-Lok and/or securely taping all tubing connections.

4. When changing central venous access tubing, instruct patient to perform the Valsalva maneuver to prevent air embolus.

5. If patient exhibits evidence of air embolus (eg, severe chest pain and/or coughing), turn patient into a left-side-lying position. This displaces the air into the apex of the heart, which helps prevent its movement into the pulmonary artery. Remove the pillow, and lower the HOB into Trendelenburg's position, which increases intrathoracic pressure. Administer oxygen if it is at the bedside. Notify MD immediately.

Potential for infection related to increased susceptibility secondary to invasive procedure and delivery of nutrients into central vein

Desired outcome: Patient does not exhibit signs of infection.

1. Using aseptic technique, provide central access site care and dressing changes qod, or according to institution policy. Change the administration system and tubing q24–48 hours, according to institution policy.

2. Be alert to glycosuria and indicators of infection, such as fever and warmth, redness, swelling, pain, and purulent drainage at the insertion site. Glucose intolerance can occur secondary to increasing glucose load or infectious process.

3. Common organisms that invade access sites include *Staphyloccoccus* species (eg, *S aureus*) and fungi (eg, *Candida*). Refer to institution policy for specific criteria and methods of culturing IV catheters and insertion sites.

Potential for injury related to risk of complications secondary to fat-emulsion therapy

Desired outcomes: Patient does not demonstrate evidence of fat-emulsion therapy complications, or if they occur, they are detected and reported promptly, resulting in immediate treatment and absence of injury to patient.

1. Use the special administration set that is provided with the fat-emulsion container. When gravity infusion is used, hang fat-emulsion (low-density solution) container higher than amino acid/dextrose (high-density solution) container.

2. Initiate the delivery slowly (1 mL/min for 15 min) or as prescribed by MD. Assess patient for adverse reactions (eg, fever, chills, sensation of warmth, shivering, vomiting, diaphoresis, and drowsiness). If any occur, stop the infusion and notify MD.

3. Follow these general guidelines for infusion:
   - □ Infuse 500 mL of a 10% emulsion over 4 hours or more.
   - □ Infuse 500 mL of a 20% emulsion over 8 hours or more.

4. Minimize the risk of bacterial growth by discarding solution that has not infused within 12 hours of hanging.

5. Do not add anything to a fat-emulsion container, and avoid blood drawing and CVP readings from the access site and the administration of medications, blood products, and maintenance fluids into the access site.

6. In general, incompatibility must be assumed unless scientific documentation proves otherwise. Physical and chemical incompatibilities result in loss of IV access and waste of nutritional fluids. The following are *compatible:* insulin, heparin, and albumin. The following are *incompatible:* sodium bicarbonate, diazepam, phenytoin, and amphotericin.

7. Assess laboratory values for results of serum triglycerides and liver function tests. Abnormalities can reflect patient's inability to metabolize the lipids.

C. Patient–Family Teaching and Discharge Planning

Specific instructions related to specialized home nutritional therapy should begin as early as possible in the patient's hospital stay. Discussion of dietary modifications and printed instructions for home use will suffice for many patients. Patients dependent on tube feeding or IV support will require more sophisticated and involved training before they can function safely and independently at home. Multidisciplinary coordination (nurse, dietitian, social worker, pharmacist, MD) is essential for providing comprehensive home care planning. Easy transition from hospital to home and arrangements for follow-up care should be primary goals of discharge planning. Arrangements and adequate time for teaching may require 3–4 days for patients on home tube feedings and 10–14 days for those on home IV therapy. Optimally, the following should be accomplished before discharge:

1. Determination of the suitability of the patient and patient's home for the specific treatment modality.

2. Documentation of the failure or futility of alternative means of support, such as supplements and tube feedings.

3. Teaching patient and SOs all skills required to deliver safe home therapy.

4. Documentation of caregiver's abilities, understanding, level of proficiency, and competence to deliver safe home therapy.

5. Review of the indicators of potential complications, such as infection (redness, swelling, pain, fever, malaise, purulent discharge) and air embolus (SOB, chest pain, confusion).

6. Arrangement for the patient to receive all the supplies necessary for care. These may be provided by the following: hospitals, local pharmacies, durable medical equipment suppliers, and home health care agencies. Supplies should include infusion management devices, dressings and site care products, and enteral or parenteral nutrition solutions

► Selected References

Brunner LS, Suddarth DS: *Textbook of Medical-Surgical Nursing*, 5th ed. Lippincott, 1984.

Burton GG, Hodgkin JE: *Respiratory Care: A Guide to Clinical Practice*, 2nd ed. Lippincott, 1984.

Campbell JW, Frisse M (editors): *Manual of Medical Therapeutics*, 24th ed. Little, Brown, 1983.

Carpenito LJ: *Nursing Diagnosis: Application to Clinical Practice*. Lippincott, 1983.

Ellerbe SE (editor): *Fluid and Blood Component Therapy in the Critically Ill and Injured*. Churchill-Livingstone, 1981.

Elwyn D: Nutritional requirements of the adult surgical patient. *Critical Care Medicine* 1980; 8:15.

Emanuelsen KL, Densmore MJ: *Acute Respiratory Care*. Fleschner, 1981.

Flomenbaum N: Acid-base disturbance. *Emergency Medicine* 1984; 16(3):59–61, 65–66, 71–72.

Frisancho AR: New norms of upper limb fat and muscle areas for assessment of nutritional status. *Am J Clin Nutr* 1981; 34:2540–2545.

Grant JP, Custer PB, Thurlow J: Current techniques of nutritional assessment. *Surg Clin North Am* 1981; 61:437–463.

Guyton AC: *Textbook of Medical Physiology*, 6th ed. Saunders, 1981.

Halpern SL: *Quick Reference to Clinical Nutrition*. Lippincott, 1979.

Harper RE: *A Guide to Respiratory Care: Physiology and Clinical Applications*. Lippincott, 1981.

Hincker EA, Malasanos L: *The Little, Brown Manual of Medical-Surgical Nursing*. Little, Brown, 1983.

Holloway NM: *Nursing the Critically Ill Adult*, 2nd ed. Addison-Wesley, 1984.

Hudak CM, Lohr T, Gallo BM: *Critical Care Nursing*, 3rd ed. Lippincott, 1982.

Lewis SM, Collier IC: *Medical-Surgical Nursing: Assessment and Management of Clinical Problems*. McGraw-Hill, 1983.

Metheny NM, Snively WD Jr: *Nurses' Handbook of Fluid Balance*, 4th ed. Lippincott, 1983.

Miller WE: The ABC's of blood gases. *Emergency Medicine* 1984; 16(3):37–38, 43–45, 48.

Nursing '83 Books: *Monitoring Fluid and Electrolytes Precisely*. Springhouse, 1983.

Ravel R: *Clinical Laboratory Medicine*, 4th ed. Yearbook, 1984.

Saxton DF, et al: *The Addison-Wesley Manual of Nursing Practice*. Addison-Wesley, 1983.

Shapiro BA, Harrison RA, Walton JR: *Clinical Application of Blood Gases*, 2nd ed. Yearbook, 1977.

Spence AP, Mason EB: *Human Anatomy and Physiology*, 2nd ed. Benjamin/Cummings, 1983.

Stedman LW: Nursing Aspects of the Tube-Fed Patient. *Nutr Supp Serv* 1984; 4:36–39.

Stroot VR, Lee CA, Schaper CA: *Fluids and Electrolytes: A Practical Approach*, 3rd ed. F A Davis, 1984.

Swearingen PL: *The Addison-Wesley Photo-Atlas of Nursing Procedures*. Addison-Wesley, 1984.

Tilkian SM, Conover MB, Tilkian AG: *Clinical Implications of Laboratory Tests*, 3rd ed. Mosby, 1983.

Vander AJ: *Renal Physiology*, 2nd ed. McGraw-Hill, 1980.

Wade JF: *Respiratory Nursing Care*, 3rd ed. Mosby, 1982.

Weinsier RL, Butterworth CE: *Handbook of Clinical Nutrition*. Mosby, 1981.

Weisberg HF (editor): *The Fundamentals of Body Water and Electrolytes*. Travenol Laboratories, 1967.

Appendixes

Appendix One   **Patient Care**

► Section One   **Caring for Preoperative and Postoperative Patients**

Knowledge deficit: Surgical procedure, preoperative routine, and postoperative care

Desired outcome: Patient can verbalize knowledge of the surgical procedure, including preoperative and postoperative care, and does not exhibit signs of harmful anxiety.

1. Assess patient's understanding of the diagnosis and surgical procedure; clarify or explain as appropriate.

2. Explain both the preoperative routine and expected postoperative regimen, discussing the following, as appropriate: preoperative preparation and medications; application of antiembolic hose; placement of indwelling catheters, drains, and tubes; and the potential for postoperative discomfort and availability of analgesia. Provide preoperative instructions for deep-breathing exercises. Also teach the technique for effective coughing, if appropriate. **Caution:** Patients for whom increased intracranial or intra-abdominal pressure is contraindicated (eg, those undergoing eye and ear surgery, spinal fusion, transphenoidal hypophysectomy, and many cranial operations) should not cough. In addition, if coughing is allowed after a herniorrhaphy, it should be done in a controlled manner, with the incision carefully supported to protect the repair.

3. Teach patient calf-pumping and ankle-circling exercises to enhance postoperative circulation in the lower extremities.

4. Provide patient with a written handout that reviews the main components of the postoperative routine.

5. Provide time for patient to ask questions and express feelings of anxiety; be reassuring and supportive.

Alteration in comfort: Pain and nausea related to surgical procedure

Desired outcome: Patient relates a reduction in discomfort and does not exhibit signs of uncontrolled pain or nausea.

1. Monitor patient for the presence of pain and nausea.

2. Administer prescribed analgesics and antiemetics before pain and discomfort become severe. Discuss effectiveness of the medications with patient; document effective pain-relief measures in the nursing care plan.

3. Encourage relaxation with slow, deep breaths to minimize pain and nausea.

4. Use other nonpharmacologic methods of relieving discomfort, such as repositioning, backrubs and massage, distraction, guided imagery, relaxation tapes, and transcutaneous electrical nerve stimulation (TENS) device. Keep patient's environment quiet to promote rest.

5. To help minimize or prevent nausea and distention once oral fluids are allowed, provide small quantities at frequent intervals (30 mL q30 min) for the specified total.

Potential alteration in tissue perfusion: Gastrointestinal, related to altered peristalsis secondary to general anesthesia and surgical procedure

Desired outcome: Patient's physical findings and GI function are within acceptable limits.

1. Assess for abdominal findings that can occur with ileus, including distention, tenderness, and absence of bowel sounds.

2. Monitor for and document the elimination of flatus or stool, which indicates returning intestinal motility. Bowel sounds and bowel function normally return within 48–72 hours following surgery.

3. To stimulate peristalsis, encourage in-bed position changes, exercises, and ambulation to patient's tolerance unless contraindicated.

4. If NG tube is in place, perform the following:

   □ Measure and record the quantity and quality of output. Typically, the color will be green. For patients who have undergone gastric surgery it may be brownish initially, due to small amounts of bloody drainage, but should change to green after about 12 hours. Guaiac-test reddish or brown output for the presence of blood, which can signal the development of a stress ulcer or indicate that a tube opening is compressed against the stomach lining. Reposition tube as necessary.

   □ Maintain patency of NG tube with gentle instillation of normal saline as prescribed. **Caution:** For patient with a gastroplasty or gastrectomy, irrigation can perforate the incision line and should be avoided except by explicit request of the surgeon.

   □ When the NG tube is removed, monitor patient for the presence of nausea or vomiting.

5. Monitor and document patient's reponse to diet advancement from clear liquids to a regular unrestricted, low-residue, or other prescribed diet.

6. Document and report significant findings to MD.

Potential fluid volume deficit related to abnormal loss secondary to vomiting or gastric decompression; and/or decreased intake secondary to nausea and/or NPO status

Desired outcome: Patient does not exhibit signs of dehydration.

1. Assess for the presence of nausea. If present, determine whether it occurs after the administration of narcotics. As appropriate, consult with MD regarding the potential need for a change in patient's analgesia.

2. If needed, medicate patient with prescribed antiemetic. Document patient's response to the medication.

3. Evaluate and document patient's hydration status by assessing for excessive thirst and the presence of parched lips and tongue. Assess skin turgor by lifting a section of skin along either the forearm, abdomen, or calf. Release the skin and watch its return to the original position. With good hydration, it will return quickly; with dehydration, the skin will remain in the lifted position (tenting) or return slowly. **Note:** This test may be less reliable in the elderly due to loss of skin elasticity and subcutaneous fat.

4. Monitor patient's VS and be alert to hypotension and tachycardia, which can signal dehydration. Notify MD if BP is significantly below patient's baseline.

5. Ensure patency of the NG tube, and record quality and quantity of the output.

6. Monitor patient's weight on a daily basis, which can be used as an indicator of hydration and nutrition. Always weigh the patient at the same time every day, using the same scale and same type and amount of bed clothing.

7. Measure and record urinary output, and report any changes from the normal (usually 60 mL/h or 1400–1500 mL/day) output. In addition, note and record output from drains and ostomies, if present.

8. Measure, describe, and document any emesis; be alert to and document excessive perspiration. Both should be included with documentation of urinary, fecal, and NG output for a total picture of the patient's hydration status.

9. Monitor serum electrolytes. Be alert to low potassium levels and the following signs and symptoms of hypokalemia: lethargy, irritability, anorexia, vomiting, muscle weakness and cramping, paresthesia, weak and irregular pulse, and respiratory dysfunction. Also assess for low calcium levels and the following signs and symptoms of hypocalcemia: Trousseau's sign, Chvostek's sign, tetany, muscle cramps, fatigue, irritability, and personality changes.

10. Administer and regulate IV fluids and electrolytes as prescribed until patient is able to resume oral intake. When IV fluids are discontinued, encourage intake of oral fluids, at least 2–3 L/day in the nonrestricted patient.

Potential alterations in fluid volume: *Deficit* related to risk of third (interstitial) spacing of fluids after anesthesia and surgery (particularly abdominal); *excess* related to retention secondary to compensatory mechanisms following surgery

Desired outcome: Patient does not exhibit signs of dehydration or overhydration.

1. Maintain records of 8-hour and 24-hour I&O. Report deficits or excess.

2. Assess for and report any indicators of fluid overload, such as dyspnea, tachycardia, crackles (rales), and edema (pretibial, sacral).

3. Assess for indicators of decreasing vascular volume, including decreasing urinary output, postural hypotension, decreasing BP, or increased heart rate.

4. As prescribed, administer plasma expanders to increase intravascular volume and albumin to increase colloid osmotic pressure.

5. Anticipate postoperative diuresis at approximately 48–72 hours after surgery due to the mobilization of third-space (interstitial) fluid.

6. Administer diuretics (usually 20–40 mg furosemide) if prescribed, to mobilize interstitial fluid.

7. Monitor VS for significant indicators of hypovolemic shock.

Potential fluid volume deficit related to abnormal loss secondary to postsurgical bleeding

Desired outcome: Patient does not exhibit signs of excessive bleeding or hypovolemia.

1. Monitor VS at frequent intervals during the first 24 hours of the postoperative period. Be alert to indicators of internal hemorrhage and impending shock, including decreasing BP, increased pulse and respiratory rates, pallor, increasing agitation, and diaphoresis.

2. Inspect the dressing for evidence of frank bleeding, eg, saturation of the dressing with bright red blood. Record the number of saturated dressings.

3. If a gastric tube is being used for decompression, note the amount and character of the drainage at least q shift. If it appears to contain blood (eg, bright red, burgundy, coffee ground appearance), perform a guaiac test to confirm its presence. After gastric surgery, the patient will have small amounts of bloody red drainage that should change to greenish yellow after the first 12 hours. Be alert to large amounts of bloody drainage.

4. Review CBC values for evidence of bleeding: decreases in hemoglobin and hematocrit.

5. Notify MD of significant findings.

Ineffective breathing pattern related to decreased respiratory depth secondary to immobility, anesthesia, and guarding from painful surgical incision

Desired outcome: Patient exhibits respiratory rate and depth within acceptable limits.

1. Assess patient preoperatively for history of pulmonary disease, smoking habits, and current drug and/or respiratory therapies.

2. Perform a baseline assessment of patient's respiratory system preoperatively, noting rate, rhythm, degree of chest expansion, quality of breath sounds, and cough and sputum production.

3. If appropriate, encourage patient to refrain from smoking for at least 1 week after surgery. Explain the effects of smoking on the body.

4. Perform respiratory system assessments at least q4h after surgery, comparing the postoperative assessment to the baseline. Be alert to indicators of pulmonary dysfunction, including dyspnea, tachypnea, pallor, adventitious breath sounds, and restlessness. Often, a low-grade fever (100F or less) is a signal of the need for pulmonary exercises and mobilization. Notify MD of significant findings.

5. Assist patient with turning and deep-breathing exercises q2h for the first 72 hours postoperatively to promote lung aeration. In the presence of crackles (rales), and if not contraindicated, have patient cough to expectorate secretions. Facilitate deep breathing and coughing by demonstrating how to splint the incision with the hands or a pillow. If indicated, medicate patient a half-hour before deep breathing, coughing, or ambulation to enhance compliance. Be aware that narcotic use depresses the respiratory system.

6. If patient has an incentive spirometer, provide instructions and encourage its use q2h.

7. Unless contraindicated, assist patient with ambulation by the second postoperative day to enhance ventilation.

8. Ensure adequate hydration (at least 2–3 L/day) in nonrestricted patients. Explain that secretions will be thinner and easier to expectorate if patient is well hydrated.

9. For other interventions, see **Potential alteration in respiratory function** related to prolonged inactivity and/or omission of deep breathing (for all patients on bed rest and/or at risk for atelectasis), p. 12 in "Atelectasis," Chapter 1, "Respiratory Disorders."

Potential alteration in respiratory function related to aspiration or airway obstruction secondary to the presence of an NG tube

Desired outcome: Patient does not exhibit signs of respiratory dysfunction.

1. Check placement of the tube after insertion, before *any* instillation, and q4h. Either insert air into the proximal end of the tube to elicit a "whoosh" sound, which can be heard while auscultating over the epigastric area, or aspirate gastric contents. If the tube is in the trachea, the patient will exhibit signs of respiratory distress.

2. Prevent migration of the tube by keeping it securely taped to the patient's nose and reinforcing placement by attaching the tube to the patient's gown with a safety pin or tape.

Potential impairment of skin integrity related to continuous mucosal and skin surface irritation secondary to the presence of NG tube

Desired outcome: Patient's skin and mucosa do not exhibit signs of irritation or breakdown.

1. Ensure that the suction apparatus is decompressing at the prescribed pressure (usually low, intermittent). High-vacuum pressure can result in damage to the mucosal lining.

2. Provide oral care and nasal hygiene q4h and prn. Arrange for patient to gargle, brush the teeth, and cleanse the mouth with swabs as necessary to prevent excoriation and excessive dryness. A cotton-tipped applicator can be used to lubricate the nares and remove encrustations. Lubricate the lips and nares with a water-soluble lubricant. If patient's throat is irritated from the tube, obtain a prescription for a lidocaine gargling solution.

Potential for infection related to vulnerability secondary to the presence of an indwelling urethral catheter

Desired outcome: Patient does not exhibit signs of UTI.

1. Prevent reflux of urine into the bladder by keeping drainage collection container below the level of patient's bladder.

2. Do not open closed urinary drainage system unless absolutely necessary; irrigate catheter only with MD prescription and when obstruction is the known cause.

3. Never open the drainage system to obtain urine specimen for analysis. Either use the sampling port, which is at the proximal end of the drainage tube, or in its absence, aspirate from the catheter just distal to the bifurcation. Cleanse either area with an antimicrobial wipe, and use a sterile syringe with a 25-gauge needle to aspirate the urine.

4. Wash your hands before and after handling the patient's urinary drainage system; use aseptic technique for all procedures that require manipulation of the catheter or opening of the closed drainage system.

5. Assess for indicators of UTI, including chills, high-grade fever (>100F), flank or labial pain, and cloudy or foul-smelling urine.

6. Help prevent urinary stasis by avoiding kinks or obstructions in the drainage tubing.

7. Encourage intake of 2–3 L/day in nonrestricted patients to minimize the potential for UTI by diluting the urine and maximizing urinary flow.

8. Minimize the potential for infection by providing juices (eg, cranberry, plum, or prune) that leave an acid ash in the urine to lower the urinary pH. **Note:** This intervention is contraindicated for patients known to develop calculi in the presence of acidic urine.

9. Ensure that the patient's perineum and meatus are cleansed during the daily bath and that the perianal area is cleansed after bowel movements. Do not hesitate to remind patient of these hygiene measures. Be alert to indicators of meatal infection, including swelling, purulent drainage, and persistent meatal redness. Intervene for the patient if he or she is unable to perform self-care.

10. Change the catheter according to established protocol, or sooner if sandy particles can be felt in the distal end of the catheter and/or patient develops a UTI. Change the drainage collection container according to established protocol, or sooner, if it becomes foul-smelling or leaks.

Potential impairment of skin integrity related to irritation of skin around percutaneous drains and tubes

Desired outcome: Patient does not exhibit signs of skin irritation or breakdown.

1. Change dressings as soon as they become wet. (MD may prefer to perform the first dressing change.)

2. Keep the area around drain and/or T-tube as clean as possible. The presence of bile, for example, can quickly lead to skin excoriation.

3. If drainage is a problem, position a pectin-wafer skin barrier around the drain or tube. Ointments such as zinc oxide, petrolatum, and aluminum paste also may be used.

For the care of patients with surgical incisions, see "Wounds Closed by Primary Intention," p. 483, and "Surgical and/or Traumatic Wounds Healing by Secondary Intention," p. 486, in "Managing Wound Care," in Chapter 10, "Sensory Disorders."

▶ Section Two   **Caring for Patients on Prolonged Bed Rest**

Potential alteration in tissue perfusion: Peripheral, related to compromised circulation secondary to prolonged immobility

Desired outcome: Patient's physical findings are within acceptable limits.

1. Teach patient that pain, swelling, warmth in the involved area, coolness distal to the involved area, superficial venous dilation, and persistent redness are all indicators of deep-vein thrombosis (DVT) and should be reported to staff promptly if they occur.

2. Monitor for the same indicators listed in preceding paragraph, along with routine VS checks. If patient is *a*symptomatic of DVT, assess for a positive Homan's sign: Flex the knee 30° and dorsiflex the foot. Pain elicited with the dorsiflexion may be a sign of DVT, and patient should be referred to MD for further evaluation.

3. Teach patient calf-pumping (ankle dorsiflexion-plantarflexion) and ankle-circling exercises. Instruct patient to repeat each movement 10 times, performing each exercise hourly during extended periods of immobility, provided that patient is *a*symptomatic of DVT. Help promote circulation by performing passive ROM or encouraging active ROM exercises.

4. Encourage deep breathing, which increases negative pressure in the lungs and thorax to promote emptying of large veins.

5. When not contraindicated by peripheral vascular disease, ensure that patient wears antiembolic hose. Remove them for 10–20 minutes q8h and inspect underlying skin for evidence of irritation or breakdown. Reapply hose after elevating patient's legs 10–15° for 10 minutes.

6. Instruct patient not to cross the feet at the ankles or knees while in bed because doing so may cause venous stasis. If patient is at risk for DVT, elevate the foot of the bed 10° to increase venous return.

7. In nonrestricted patient, increase fluid intake to at least 2–3L/day to reduce hemoconcentration, which can contribute to the development of DVT. Educate patient about the need to drink large amounts of fluid.

8. Patients at risk for DVT, including those with chronic infection and a history of peripheral vascular disease, as well as the aged, obese, and anemic, may require pharmacologic interventions such as aspirin, sodium warfarin, or heparin. Administer medication as prescribed and monitor appropriate lab values (eg, PT, PTT).

Diversional activity deficit related to monotony of confinement secondary to prolonged bed rest

Desired outcome: Patient engages in diversional activities and relates the absence of boredom.

1. Be alert to patient indicators of boredom, including wishing for something to read or do, daytime napping, and expressed inability to perform usual hobbies because of hospitalization.

2. Collect a data base by assessing patient's normal support systems and relationship patterns with SOs. Question patient about his or her interests, and explore diversional activities that may be suitable for the hospital setting.

3. Obtain appropriate diversional activities such as puzzles, model kits, and handicrafts; encourage patient to use them.

4. Encourage SOs to visit within limits of patient's endurance and to involve patient in activities that are of interest to him or her, such as playing cards or backgammon. Encourage SOs to stagger their visits throughout the day.

5. Spend extra time with patient.

6. Suggest that SOs bring in a radio, or, if appropriate, rent a TV or radio from the hospital if not part of the standard room charge.

7. If appropriate for patient, arrange for hospital volunteers to visit, play cards, read books, and/or play board games.

8. As appropriate for patient who desires social interaction, consider relocation to a room in an area of high traffic.

9. Request consultation from social services, occupational therapy, pastoral services, and/or psychiatric nurse for interventions as appropriate.

10. Increase patient's involvement in self-care to provide a sense of purpose and accomplishment. Performing in-bed exercises (eg, deep breathing, ankle circling, calf pumping), keeping track of I&O, and similar activities, can and should be accomplished routinely by these patients.

Ineffective individual coping related to depression secondary to prolonged confinement

Desired outcome: Patient is able to identify and verbalize his or her feelings and does not demonstrate ineffective coping mechanisms.

1. Assess patient's coping mechanisms, and determine those that have been effective for patient in the past. Interview SOs, discuss patient's situation with other nurses or counselors, and solicit suggestions for assisting patient with developing effective coping mechanisms.

2. Evaluate with patient the effectiveness of coping mechanisms that he or she is using. Provide reinforcement for those that are positive. Assist patient with changing those that are ineffective or inappropriate.

3. Encourage patient to verbalize anxieties about the current problem; provide an accepting atmosphere for patient's verbalization, which might promote a catharsis for the anxiety.

4. Clearly define or isolate patient's current problems. For example, is the patient just acting out, or is the negative behavior caused by pain?

5. Develop a collaborative approach with patient, assuring him or her that together you can solve the problem

6. Explore available support systems with patient and develop new support systems when needed, such as chaplain, friends, family, counselors, or health care staff.

Sexual dysfunction related to actual or perceived physiologic limitations on sexual performance secondary to disease, therapy, or prolonged hospitalization

Desired outcome: Patient relates satisfaction with sexual activity.

1. Assess patient's normal sexual function, including the importance placed on sex in the relationship, frequency of interaction, normal positions used, and the couple's ability to adapt or change to meet requirements of patient's limitations.

2. Identify patient's problem diplomatically, and clarify it with patient. Indicators of sexual dysfunction can include regression, acting-out with inappropriate behavior such as grabbing or pinching, sexual overtures toward the hospital staff, self-enforced isolation, and other similar behaviors.

3. Encourage patient and SO to verbalize their feelings and anxieties about sexual abstinence, having sexual relations in the hospital, hurting the patient, or having to use new or alternative methods for sexual gratification. Develop strategies collaboratively among the patient, SO, and yourself.

4. Inform patient and SO that it is possible to have time alone together for intimacy. Provide that time accordingly by putting a "Do Not Disturb" sign on

the door, enforcing privacy by restricting staff and visitors from the room, and/or arranging for temporary private quarters.

5. Encourage patient and SO to seek alternate methods of sexual expression when necessary. This may include mutual masturbation, altered positions, vibrators, and identification of other erotic areas for the partner.

6. Refer patient and SO to professional sexual counselling as necessary.

Potential impairment of physical mobility related to inactivity secondary to prolonged bed rest

Desired outcome: Patient does not exhibit signs of joint contractures or muscle atrophy.

1. Be alert to the following areas that are especially prone to joint contracture: *shoulder*, which can become "frozen," limiting abduction and extension; *wrist*, which can "drop," prohibiting extension; *fingers*, which can develop flexion contractures that limit extension; *hips*, which can develop flexion contractures that affect the gait by shortening the limb; *knees*, in which flexion contractures can develop that limit extension and alter the gait; and *feet*, which can "drop" as a result of plantarflexion, limiting dorsiflexion and altering the gait.

2. Ensure frequent position changes. If not contraindicated, assist patient into prone position periodically to help prevent hip contractures. Keep the body in proper alignment.

3. To maintain the joints in neutral position, use the following as indicated: pillows, rolled towels, blankets, sandbags, antirotation boots, splints, and orthotics. When using adjunctive devices, monitor the involved skin at frequent intervals for alterations in integrity, and implement measures to prevent skin breakdown.

4. Teach patient the rationale and procedure for ROM exercises, and have patient return the demonstrations. Provide passive exercises for patients unable to perform active or active-assistive exercises. Ensure that joints especially prone to contracture are exercised more stringently. Provide patient with a handout that reviews the exercises and lists the repetitions for each.

5. Perform and document limb girth measurements, dynamography, and exercise baseline limits to assess patient's existing muscle mass and strength.

6. Explain to patient that muscle atrophy occurs because of disuse or failure to use the joint, often due to immediate or anticipated pain. Eventually, this may result in a decrease in muscle mass and blood supply, which in turn can lead to increased muscle fatigue with use.

7. Emphasize the importance of maintaining or increasing muscle strength through exercise. If unsure about patient's complicating pathology, consult with MD about the appropriate form of exercise for patient.

8. Explain the necessity of participating maximally in self-care to help maintain muscle strength and enhance a sense of participation and control.

9. For patients needing greater help with muscle strength, assist with resistive exercises, eg, moderate weight lifting to increase the size, endurance, and strength of the muscles. For patients in beds with Balkan frames, provide the means for resistive exercise by implementing a system of weights and pulleys. First, determine patient's baseline level of performance on a given set of exercises, and then set realistic goals with the patient for repetitions. For example, if the patient can do 5 repetitions of lifting a 5-pound weight with the biceps muscle, the goal may be to increase the repetitions to 10 within a week, to an ultimate goal of 20 within 3 weeks, and then advance to 7.5-pound weights.

10. If the joints require rest or need to avoid fatigue, isometric exercises can be used. With these exercises, teach the patient to contract a muscle group and

hold the contraction for a count of five or ten. The sequence is repeated for increasing numbers of repetitions until an adequate level of endurance has been achieved. Thereafter, maintenance levels are performed.

11. Provide a chart to show patient's progress, and combine this with large amounts of positive reinforcement.

12. As appropriate, teach transfer and/or crutchwalking techniques and/or use of a walker, wheelchair, or cane so that patient can maintain the highest level of mobility possible. Include SOs in the demonstrations, and stress the importance of good body mechanics.

13. Seek a referral to a physical or occupational therapist as appropriate

Potential alteration in tissue perfusion: Cerebral, related to orthostatic hypotension secondary to prolonged bed rest

Desired outcomes: Patient's VS and physical findings are within acceptable limits and patient relates the absence of symptoms of orthostatic (postural) hypotension.

1. Explain the cause of orthostatic hypotension and measures for preventing it.

2. Application of antiembolic hose, which are used to prevent deep-vein thrombosis, may be useful in preventing orthostatic hypotension once the patient is mobilized. For patients who continue to have difficulty with orthostatic hypotension, it may be necessary to supplement these hose with elastic wraps during the period of time the patient is out of bed. Ensure that these wraps encompass the entire surface of the legs.

3. When patient is in bed, provide instructions for leg exercises, including ankle circling, calf pumping, and isometrics of the gastrocnemius, gluteal, and quadriceps muscles. In addition to helping prevent orthostatic hypotension, these exercises will maintain muscular and vascular tone and decrease pooling of blood.

4. Prepare patient for getting out of bed by encouraging position changes within necessary confines. It is sometimes possible and advisable to use a tilt table to reacclimate patient to upright positions.

5. Follow these guidelines for mobilization:

   □ Begin by having patient dangle legs at the bedside. Be alert to indicators of orthostatic hypotension, including diaphoresis, pallor, tachycardia, hypotension, and syncope. Question patient about the presence of lightheadedness or dizziness.

   □ If indicators of orthostatic hypotension do occur, check the VS. Low BP and increased pulse rate, combined with symptoms of vertigo and impending syncope, signal the need for return to a supine position.

   □ If leg dangling is tolerated, have patient stand at the bedside with two staff members in attendance. If no adverse signs or symptoms occur, have patient progress to ambulation as tolerated.

Alteration in bowel elimination: Constipation related to immobility, changes in normal bowel habits during hospitalization, alteration in the diet, and use of narcotic analgesics

Desired outcomes: Patient can verbalize knowledge of measures that promote bowel elimination. Patient relates the return of his or her normal pattern of bowel elimination.

1. Assess patient's bowel history to determine normal bowel habits and interventions that are used successfully at home.

2. Monitor and document patient's bowel movements, diet, and I&O. Be alert to the following indications of constipation: fewer than usual number of bowel movements, abdominal discomfort and/or distention, straining at stool, and patient complaints of rectal pressure or fullness.

3. Teach patient the importance of a high-roughage diet and a fluid intake of at least 2–3 L/day (unless this is contraindicated by a renal or cardiac disorder). High-roughage foods include bran, whole grains, nuts, raw and coarse vegetables, and fruits with skins.

4. Maintain patient's normal bowel habits whenever possible by offering the bedpan; ensuring privacy; providing warm oral fluids; and timing medications, enemas, or suppositories so that they take effect at the time of day patient normally has a bowel movement.

5. Maximize patient's activity level within the limitations of therapy and pain.

6. Request pharmacologic interventions from MD when necessary. To help prevent rebound constipation, prioritize pharmacologic interventions to ensure minimal disruption of patient's normal bowel habits. A suggested hierarchy of interventions is the following:

   □ Bulk-building additives (psyllium), bran.

   □ Mild laxatives (apple or prune juice, milk of magnesia).

   □ Stool softeners (docusate sodium).

   □ Potent laxatives and cathartics (bisacodyl, cascara sagrada).

   □ Medicated suppositories.

   □ Enemas.

Ineffective individual coping related to depression secondary to perceived role change: Dependence versus independence

Desired outcome: Patient collaborates with caregivers in planning goals for independence and does not demonstrate ineffective coping mechanisms.

1. Encourage patient to be as independent as possible within limitations of the therapy and pain.

2. Ensure that all health care providers are consistent in conveying their expectations of independence.

3. Alert patient to areas of overdependence, and involve him or her in collaborative goal-setting to achieve independence.

4. If indicated, provide self-help devices to increase patient's independence with self-care.

5. Provide positive reinforcement when patient meets or advances toward goals.

See "Atelectasis" in Chapter 1, "Respiratory Disorders," for the following: **Potential alteration in respiratory function** related to prolonged inactivity and/or omission of deep breathing (for all patients on bed rest and/or at risk for atelectasis), p. 12. See "Pressure (Decubitus) Ulcers" in Chapter 10, "Sensory Disorders," for the following: **Potential impairment of skin integrity** related to excessive tissue pressure secondary to prolonged immobility (for patients without pressure ulcers who are at risk because of immobility), p. 488.

▶ Section Three   **Caring for Patients with Neurologic Problems**

Potential for injury related to unsteady gait secondary to motor deficit

Desired outcomes: Patient does not exhibit signs of injury due to gait unsteadiness. Patient can demonstrate proficiency with assistive devices, if appropriate.

1. Evaluate patient's gait, and assess for motor deficit such as weakness or paralysis. Document baseline neurologic and physical assessments so that changes in status can be detected promptly.

2. To minimize the risk of injury, assist patient as needed when unsteady gait, weakness, and/or paralysis are noted.

3. Orient patient to new surroundings. Keep necessary items (including water, telephone, and call light) within easy reach of patient. Assess patient's ability to use these items. The patient who is very weak or partially paralyzed may require a tap bell instead of a call light.

4. Maintain an uncluttered environment to minimize the risk of tripping. Ensure adequate lighting at night (eg, a night light) to help prevent falls in the dark. In addition, keep siderails up and the bed in its lowest position.

5. For unsteady, weak, or partially paralyzed patient, encourage use of low-heel, non-skid shoes for walking. Teach the use of a wide-based gait to provide a broader base of support. Teach, reinforce, and encourage use of canes, walkers, and crutches to provide patient with added stability. Teach exercises that strengthen arm and shoulder muscles for using walkers and crutches. Teach patients in wheelchairs how and when to lock and unlock the wheels.

6. Seek a referral to a physical therapist as appropriate.

Potential for injury related to impaired pain, touch, and temperature sensations secondary to sensory deficit and/or decreased LOC

Desired outcome: Patient does not exhibit signs of injury due to sensory impairment.

1. Assess patient for indicators of sensory deficits, such as decreased or absent vision and impaired temperature and pain sensation. Document baseline neurologic and physical assessments so that changes in status can be detected promptly.

2. Protect patient from exposure to hot food or equipment that can burn the skin. Avoid use of heating pads.

3. Always check the temperature of heating devices and bath water before patient is exposed to them. Teach patient and SOs about these precautions.

4. Inspect patient's skin daily for evidence of irritation. Teach coherent patient to perform self-inspection daily, and provide a mirror for inspecting posterior aspects of the body.

Potential for injury related to risk of corneal irritation/abrasion secondary to diminished blink reflex and/or inability to close the eyes

Desired outcome: Patient does not exhibit signs of corneal injury.

1. Normally, blinking occurs every 5–6 seconds. If patient has a diminished blink reflex and/or is stuporous or comatose, assess the eyes for irritation or the presence of foreign objects. Instill prescribed eye drops to prevent corneal irritation. Instruct coherent patients to make a conscious effort to blink the eyes several times an hour to help prevent corneal irritation.

2. For patient who is unable to close the eyes completely, apply an eyeshield or tape the eyes shut.

Alteration in nutrition: Less than body requirements related to decreased intake secondary to chewing and swallowing deficits, fatigue, weakness, paresis, paralysis, visual neglect, and/or decreased LOC

Desired outcomes: Patient does not exhibit signs of malnutrition or weight loss. Patient can demonstrate measures that enhance chewing and swallowing.

1. For patient with chewing or swallowing difficulties, assess alertness, ability to cough, and swallow and gag reflexes before all meals. Keep suction equipment at the bedside if indicated. If patient cannot chew or swallow effectively

or safely, enteral or parenteral nutrition may be necessary. Alert MD to your findings.

2. For patient with some chewing or swallowing ability, request soft, semi-solid, or chopped foods. Although a pureed diet may be needed eventually, this type of food can be unappealing to many people and may have a negative impact on patient's self-concept.

3. To help patient focus on swallowing, reduce other stimuli in the room (eg, turn off the TV or radio).

4. Teach patient to break down the act of swallowing, which will help prevent choking and/or the fear of choking: Place food on the tongue, use tongue to transfer food so it is directly under the teeth on the unaffected side of the mouth, chew the food thoroughly, hold the breath, and then swallow.

5. Evaluate patient's food preferences and offer small, frequent servings. Plan mealtimes for periods during which the patient is rested; use a warming tray or microwave oven to keep the food warm and appetizing until the patient is able to eat.

6. Cut up foods, unwrap silverware, and otherwise "set up" the food tray so that patients with a weak or paralyzed arm can manage the tray one-handed.

7. For patient with "visual neglect," place food within patient's unaffected visual field and return during the meal to make sure she or he has eaten from both sides of the plate. Turn the plate around so that any remaining food is in patient's visual field.

8. Feed or assist very weak or paralyzed patients. If not contraindicated, position patient in a chair or elevate HOB. Ensure that patient's head is flexed slightly forward to close the airway. Begin with small amounts of food. Do not hurry patient. Be sure that each bite is completely swallowed before giving another.

9. If appropriate, provide assistive devices such as built-up utensil handles, broad-handled spoons, spill-proof cups, sectionalized plates, and other devices that promote self-feeding and independence.

10. Provide materials for oral hygiene after meals to minimize risk of aspiration of food particles. Good oral hygiene will also help maintain integrity of the mucous membranes to minimize risk of stomatitis, which may prevent adequate oral intake.

11. Weigh patient regularly (at least weekly) to assess for loss/gain. If indicated, notify MD of the potential need for high-protein/high-calorie supplements.

12. For the weak, debilitated, or partially paralyzed patient, assess support systems such as family or friends who can assist patient with meals. Consider referral to an organization that will deliver a daily meal to patient's home.

13. If appropriate for patient's diagnosis (eg, multiple sclerosis), consider referral to a speech pathologist for exercises that enhance the ability to swallow.

Potential fluid volume deficit related to decreased intake secondary to dysphagia, weakness, paresis, paralysis, or decreased LOC

Desired outcomes: Patient does not exhibit signs of dehydration. Patient can verbalize knowledge of the signs of dehydration and the importance of a fluid intake of at least 2–3 L/day. Patient can demonstrate measures that enhance intake and minimize the potential for choking.

1. Monitor I&O to assess for fluid volume imbalance; ensure that weight is measured daily if patient is at risk for sudden fluid shifts or imbalances. Patients with neurologic deficits may have great difficulty attaining adequate intake of fluids. Alert MD to a significant I&O imbalance, which may signal the need for enteral or IV therapy to prevent dehydration.

2. Assess for and teach patient the indicators of dehydration, including thirst,

poor skin turgor, decreased BP, increased pulse rate, dry skin and mucous membranes, increased body temperature, and decreased urinary output.

3. Evaluate patient's fluid preferences and offer fluids q1–2h. For nonrestricted patients, encourage a fluid intake of at least 2–3 L/day.

4. If not contraindicated, assist patient into high Fowler's position to facilitate oral fluid intake. Instruct patient to flex the head slightly forward, which closes the airway and helps prevent aspiration. Teach patient with hemiparalysis or paresis to tilt the head toward the unaffected side to facilitate intake.

5. If patient has difficulty swallowing, provide nectars and other thick fluids, which are better tolerated than thin fluids. Instruct patient to sip rather than gulp fluids.

6. For patients at risk of increased ICP, maintain fluid restrictions.

Ineffective airway clearance related to coughing and swallowing deficits secondary to facial and throat muscle weakness and/or decreasing LOC

Desired outcome: Patient does not exhibit signs of aspiration or URI. Alert patients demonstrate effective coughing.

1. Monitor patient for the presence of dyspnea, pallor, restlessness, diaphoresis, and a change in the rate or depth of respirations. Auscultate lung fields for breath sounds. Note the presence of crackles (rales), rhonchi, or wheezes, and diminished or adventitious breath sounds. Assess effectiveness of patient's cough and the quality, amount, and color of the sputum. Measure body temperature q4h. Often, a low-grade fever (100F or less) is indicative of the need for aggressive pulmonary hygiene.

2. Teach patient to deep breathe and cough, and assist with repositioning at least q2h. **Caution:** Instruct patients at risk of increased ICP not to cough, as it increases intra-abdominal and intrathoracic pressures, which in turn increase ICP. Explain that if sneezing is unavoidable, it should be done with an open mouth to minimize the increase in ICP.

3. Assess swallow and gag reflexes. If poor or absent, withhold oral fluids and foods, and inform MD of the possible need for IV therapy and/or enteral or parenteral nutrition.

4. Keep HOB elevated after meals or assist patient into a right-side-lying position to minimize the potential for regurgitation and aspiration. Provide oral hygiene after meals to prevent aspiration of food particles.

5. Assist with prescribed postural drainage (for patients *not* at risk of increased ICP), chest physiotherapy, and IPPB. Provide incentive spirometry as indicated.

6. Keep oxygen and/or suction apparatus available as indicated.

Self-care deficit: Inability to perform ADLs related to spasticity, tremors, weakness, paresis, paralysis, or decreasing LOC secondary to sensorimotor deficits

Desired outcomes: Patient can perform care activities independently and demonstrates the ability to use adaptive devices for successful completion of ADL. Totally dependent patients express satisfaction with activities that are completed for them.

1. Assess patient's ability to perform ADLs.

2. As appropriate, demonstrate use of adaptive devices such as long-, and/or broad-handled combs, brushes, and eating utensils; nonspill cups; and/or stabilized plates, all of which may assist the patient with maintaining independence of care. For self-care interventions for oral hygiene, see the same nursing diagnosis in "Stomatitis," p. 273, in Chapter 6, "Gastrointestinal Disorders."

3. To facilitate dressing and undressing, encourage patient and/or SOs to buy

shoes without laces and loose-fitting clothing or clothing with snaps or Velcro closures.

4. Place a stool in the shower if sitting down will enhance self-care with bathing. Provide a commode chair or elevated toilet seat if it will facilitate self-care with elimination. Teach self-transfer techniques that will enable patient to get to the commode or toilet.

5. Some individuals may have difficulty with perineal care after elimination. For many patients with limited hand or arm mobility, a long-handled reacher that can hold tissues or wash cloth may help patient maintain independence with perineal care.

6. For patient with hemiparesis or hemiparalysis, teach use of the stronger or unaffected hand and arm for dressing, eating, bathing, and grooming.

7. Obtain a referral to an OT if indicated.

8. Provide care to the totally dependent patient and assist those who are not totally dependent. Do not hurry patient. Involve SOs with care activities if they are comfortable doing so.

9. If indicated, teach patient self-catheterization, or teach the technique to the caregiver. Provide instructions for catheter care if patient is to be discharged with an indwelling catheter.

Impaired verbal communication related to dysarthria secondary to facial/throat muscle weakness, intubation, or tracheostomy

Desired outcome: Patient communicates effectively, either verbally or nonverbally.

1. If appropriate, obtain referral to a speech therapist/pathologist to assist patient with strengthening muscles used in speech.

2. Provide a supportive and relaxed environment for those patients who are unable to form words or sentences or who are unable to speak clearly or appropriately. Acknowledge patient's frustration over the inability to communicate. Maintain a calm, positive attitude. Ask patient to repeat unclear words. Observe for nonverbal cues. Anticipate needs, and phrase questions to allow simple answers such as yes or no.

3. Provide alternative methods of communication if patient is unable to speak, for example, a language board, flash cards, or a system that uses eyeblinks, bell signal taps, or gestures such as hand signals and head nods. Document method of communication used.

4. If patient's voice is very weak and difficult to hear, reduce environmental noise to enhance listener's ability to hear words. Suggest that patient take a deep breath before speaking; provide a voice amplifier if appropriate for patient.

5. If patient has swallowing difficulties that result in the accumulation of saliva, suction the mouth to promote clearer speech.

6. If patient has a tracheostomy, ensure that a tap bell is within reach. It may be necessary to place the bell on the pillow near the patient's head so that patient can activate the device with head movement. Reassure tracheostomy patient that the inability to speak is only temporary.

Alteration in bowel elimination: Constipation related to inability to chew and swallow a high-roughage diet, side effects of medications, and immobility

Desired outcome: Patient complies with the anticonstipation regimen and relates the return of normal pattern of bowel elimination.

1. Although a high-roughage diet is ideal for the patient who is immobilized or on prolonged bed rest, the individual with chewing and swallowing difficulties may be unable to consume such a diet. For these patients, encourage use of natural fiber laxatives such as psyllium (eg, Metamucil).

2. A bowel-elimination program may include the following elements: setting a regular time of day for attempting a bowel movement, preferably 30 minutes after eating a meal; using a medicated suppository 15–30 minutes before a scheduled attempt; bearing down by contracting the abdominal muscles or applying manual pressure to the abdomen to help increase intra-abdominal pressure; and drinking 4 oz of prune juice nightly. **Caution:** Spinal-cord injury (SCI) patients with involvement at T-6 and above should employ *extreme* caution if use of an enema or suppository is unavoidable, because either can precipitate life-threatening autonomic dysreflexia. Liberal application of anesthetic jelly into the rectum should precede their use. In addition, instruct patient at risk of increased ICP not to bear down with bowel movements because this action can cause increased intra-abdominal pressure, which in turn increases ICP.

3. If indicated by patient's diagnosis (eg, multiple sclerosis), provide instructions for digital stimulation of the anus to promote reflex bowel evacuation. **Caution:** This intervention is contraindicated for SCI patients with involvement at T-6 or above because it can precipitate life-threatening autonomic dysreflexia.

4. For other interventions, see **Alteration in bowel elimination:** Constipation, in "Caring for Patients on Prolonged Bed Rest," p. 536.

Potential for injury related to risk of increased ICP secondary to positional factors, increased intrathoracic or intra-abdominal pressure, fluid volume excess, hyperthermia, and/or discomfort

Desired outcomes: Patient does not exhibit signs of increased ICP. However, if they appear, they are detected and reported promptly, resulting in immediate treatment and absence of injury to patient.

1. Monitor for and report any of the following indicators of increased ICP: sudden onset of or worsening of headache, renewed or worsening nuchal rigidity/stiffness, renewed or persistent nausea and vomiting, increasing BP, widening pulse pressure, decreased pulse rate (may initially increase), transient loss of vision, seizures, alteration in LOC ranging from irritability and restlessness to confusion to coma, and onset of or increase in sensorimotor changes or deficits.

2. Monitor for and report any of the following indicators of brain stem herniation, which can signal that brain tissue has shifted because of the increased pressure: alteration in LOC (see preceding paragraph); Cheyne-Stokes respirations; hemiparesis; and pupillary changes such as inequality, inability to react to light, or dilation and fixation (as ICP increases further).

3. If changes occur, prepare to transfer patient to ICU. Insertion of ICP sensors for continuous monitoring, barbiturate therapy, and/or ventricular drainage may be necessary.

4. For patients at risk for increased ICP, prevention of hypoxia and CO_2 retention is essential for preventing vasodilation of cerebral arteries. Preventive measures include ensuring a patent airway, delivering oxygen as prescribed, hyperventilating ("sighing") patient before suctioning, and limiting suction to 10–15 seconds. Reduce $Paco_2$ by instructing conscious patients to take deep breaths on their own or by providing manual ventilation when patient is intubated or has a tracheostomy.

5. Promote venous blood return to the heart to reduce cerebral congestion by keeping HOB elevated at 15–30° (unless otherwise directed); maintaining head-and-neck alignment to avoid hyperextension, flexion, or turning; ensuring that tracheostomy and endotracheostomy ties do not compress the jugular vein; and avoiding Trendelenburg position for any reason.

6. Take precautions against increased intra-abdominal and intrathoracic pressures in the following ways: Teach patient to exhale when turning; provide passive ROM exercises rather than allow active or assistive exercises; admin-

ister prescribed stool softeners or laxatives to prevent straining; avoid enemas and suppositories because they can cause straining; instruct patient not to push against the bed with hands or feet when changing positions; assist patient with sitting up; instruct patient to avoid coughing and sneezing, or if unavoidable, to do so with an open mouth; instruct patient to avoid hip flexion (increases intra-abdominal pressure); and avoid using restraints (straining against them increases ICP). In addition, rather than have patient perform the Valsalva maneuver to prevent an air embolism during insertion of central venous catheter, MD should use a syringe to aspirate air from the catheter lumen.

7. Help reduce cerebral congestion by enforcing fluid limitations as prescribed, typically to <1500 mL/day. Keep accurate I&O records. When administering additional IV fluids, for example with IV drugs, avoid using D_5W because its hypotonicity can increase cerebral edema.

8. Because fever increases metabolic requirements and aggravates hypoxia, help maintain patient's body temperature within normal limits by giving prescribed antipyretics, keeping patient's trunk warm to prevent shivering, and administering tepid sponge baths or hypothermia blanket to reduce fever.

9. Administer prescribed osmotic diuretics to reduce cerebral edema and produce a state of dehydration, and glucocorticoids to reduce edema and inflammation. Because pain can increase BP and consequently increase ICP, administer prescribed analgesics promptly and as necessary. Barbiturates and narcotics are usually contraindicated because of the potential for masking the signs of increased ICP and causing respiratory depression.

10. Because multiple procedures and nursing care activities can increase ICP by increasing discomfort and anxiety, individualize care to ensure optimal spacing of activities.

Potential for injury related to visual disturbance secondary to diplopia

Desired outcome: Patient does not exhibit signs of injury due to the presence of double vision.

1. Assess patient for the presence of diplopia.

2. If patient has diplopia, provide an eye patch or eyeglasses with frosted lenses. Alternate the eye patch q4h.

Alteration in comfort: Pain, spasms, headache, and photophobia related to neurologic dysfunction

Desired outcomes: Patient relates a reduction in discomfort and does not exhibit signs of uncontrolled pain. Patient and SOs can verbalize knowledge of preventive measures and demonstrate methods for controlling pain and spasms.

1. Assess duration and intensity of patient's pain and/or spasms. Administer analgesics and antispasmodics as prescribed; document effectiveness of the medication. Teach patient and SOs the importance of timing the pain medication so that it is taken before the pain becomes too severe and prior to major moves.

2. Instruct patient and SOs in the use of nonpharmacologic pain management techniques such as repositioning; backrubs, massage, and tactile distraction; auditory distraction such as soothing music; guided imagery; relaxation tapes and techniques; biofeedback; and a transcutaneous electrical nerve stimulation (TENS) device, as appropriate.

3. Teach patient about the relationship between anxiety and pain as well as other factors that enhance pain and spasms, eg, staying in one position for too long, fatigue, and chilling.

4. If patient has photophobia, provide a quiet and dark environment. Close the door and curtains; avoid artificial lights whenever possible.

▶ Section Four **Caring for Patients with Cancer and Other Life-Disrupting Illnesses**

Fear related to threat to biologic integrity secondary to grave diagnosis

Desired outcomes: Patient does not demonstrate ineffective coping mechanisms. Patient discusses feelings and relates the presence of psychologic comfort.

1. Encourage patient and SOs to verbalize feelings regarding the diagnosis of cancer and/or grave prognosis. Provide a nonthreatening, unhurried atmosphere; use communication techniques such as open-ended statements and reflective questions.

2. Besides verbal communications of feelings of fear, be alert to somatic complaints such as frequent urination; abdominal discomfort; and behaviors such as repetitive questioning, irritability, inability to concentrate, appetite changes, and/or sleeplessness.

3. Provide calm, realistic assurance to patient.

4. Assess patient's and SOs' normal pattern of coping to determine sources of strength that may be utilized. Encourage and support patient's positive and effective coping mechanisms.

5. Assess patient's knowledge of the disorder, and answer questions regarding the disease, its diagnosis, and treatment. Refer patient and SOs to MD for clarification as necessary, and provide educational pamphlets such as those distributed by American Cancer Society or National Cancer Institute.

6. Because fear tends to inhibit learning, provide recurring instruction and obtain validation of learning to ensure that appropriate information has been retained.

7. Keep patient and SOs well informed of activities, therapy, or procedures patient will participate in.

8. Provide continuity of care by assigning a regular staff member.

9. Assist patient with assessing availability of, and using, a support system. Supportive individuals may include friends, relatives, clergy.

10. Recognize that anger, withdrawal, demanding behavior, or inappropriate affect may be adaptive responses to fear. Be supportive to SOs who may misinterpret patient's coping mechanisms.

11. A sense of safety may be enhanced when patient can identify with another individual who has survived with a similar diagnosis. Consult MD regarding feasibility of such a visitor.

12. Assess your own feelings about cancer (or other grave prognosis). If you feel that the diagnosis is a death sentence, your attitude may be reflected to the patient. Recognize that your own positive attitude can be very therapeutic.

Disturbance in self-concept related to alteration in body image secondary to loss of body part or body function

Desired outcome: Patient does not verbalize or demonstrate negative self-attitudes.

1. Encourage patient to ask questions about the disease, treatment, and prognosis. Answer questions and clarify misconceptions.

2. Provide time for patient to verbalize feelings regarding actual or perceived changes in body function as well as perceived changes in lifestyle, fear of rejection from others, and feelings of helplessness, hopelessness, guilt, and shame. Encourage patient to share these feelings with SOs.

3. Allow patient to grieve.

4. Emphasize patient's remaining strengths, abilities, or functions, and assist him or her with exploring realistic future goals.

5. Give patient the opportunity to accomplish activities at which he or she can succeed. Have patient participate in as much self-care as possible to enhance a feeling of control. Acknowledge and reinforce patient's grooming efforts, which may be a first step in patient's attainment of a positive body image.

6. Recognize that patient will attempt to view wounds or altered body part when he or she is psychologically prepared. Offer support and reassurance as appropriate

7. If appropriate for patient, consult with MD regarding visitation by an individual who has successfully undergone a similar surgery (eg, amputation, mastectomy, ileostomy).

Grieving related to loss of body part or change in body function

Desired outcome: Patient verbalizes feelings of grief and shares feelings with SOs.

1. Because of the loss of body part (and/or function) and perceived mutilation of the body, expect and accept patient's behavioral reponses. Reassure patient that these responses are normal and similar to those experienced upon facing death.

2. Expect initial shock and disbelief upon patient's first awareness and view of the wound (eg, stoma, amputation). Few patients are fully prepared for the reality of changes that occur with a surgical procedure such as an amputation or fecal or urinary diversion, regardless of the amount of preoperative information given. Assist patient with assuming self-care and decision making. Provide a calm and accepting environment.

3. Expect sad and angry feelings and statements expressing resistance and dislike. Anger or rejection may be expressed by crying. Permit patient's expressions of sadness and anger; provide an open, nonjudgmental environment.

4. Expect patient to begin to participate in self-care upon resolution of the loss. Anticipate that patient will continue to experience feelings of sadness and anger, which are normal.

Ineffective individual coping related to depression secondary to severity of the diagnosis

Desired outcome: Patient verbalizes feelings and exhibits effective coping mechanisms within an acceptable time frame.

1. Encourage patient to express feelings, fears, and anxieties and to verbalize and discuss these feelings with SOs.

2. Assess patient's normal pattern of coping; encourage and support coping mechanisms that are positive and effective for the patient.

3. Seek referrals to social services, chaplains, and psychiatric nurses as appropriate.

4. Another patient with the same disease who has successfully adapted may be a useful role model in some instances. Consult with MD regarding the advisability of such a visitor.

5. Inform patient and SOs that emotions and alterations in behavior such as increased dependency, mood swings, depression, denial, grief, and anger are normal following a grave diagnosis; encourage patient to express feelings openly.

6. Give patient as much control over his or her environment as possible; encourage self-care as appropriate.

7. Provide a referral to hospice or similar organization, if appropriate.

8. When necessary, ensure that the patient is assisted with bringing closure to

his or her affairs and relationships. For example, provide privacy for SOs, call patient's attorney if needed, and request that patient's chaplain visit.

Alteration in family processes related to grave illness and/or impending death of a family member

Desired outcomes: SOs participate in patient's care, if appropriate, and are assisted with seeking appropriate outside support systems.

1. Encourage patient and SOs to verbalize fears and concerns regarding patient's illness, impaired level of functioning, and/or impending death. Assist patient with recognizing and understanding patient's behavior as it relates to the disease process and/or disability.

2. Provide accurate information when it is requested, and/or encourage patient and SOs to speak openly with MD.

3. Assess SOs for ineffective coping mechanisms, such as denial of patient's diagnosis or its severity, intolerance, rejection, feelings of abandonment, and hostility.

4. Provide an atmosphere of trust and concern. Explore with SOs the need to restructure short-term and long-term goals and plans.

5. Provide opportunities for patient and SOs to spend time alone. Allow SOs to administer care to the patient if they choose.

6. Encourage patient and SOs to continue making patient-care decisions, which will help combat feelings of powerlessness.

7. Support and acknowledge SOs' contributions to patient's care.

8. When indicated, initiate outside support systems, eg, clergy, hospice, psychiatric healthworker, or structured support groups composed of individuals confronted with the same problem.

9. Monitor SOs for exhaustion of supportive capacity. Encourage rest and scheduled respites from the care of the patient.

Grieving: Individual/family related to anticipated or actual loss secondary to terminal illness

Desired outcome: Patient and SOs verbalize feelings and share grief with one another.

1. Assess patient and SOs for the stage of the grieving process currently being experienced.

2. Give patient and SOs the opportunity to explore and communicate feelings regarding anticipated or actual loss of significant relationships.

3. Provide an open and supportive environment; be as comfortable as possible with crying, anger, and regressive behavior. Advise SOs that patient's behavior is not directed at them personally.

4. For some individuals, attaining an intellectual grasp of the grieving process may provide a means for understanding their feelings. Provide these individuals with a cursory explanation of the grieving process.

5. When appropriate, assist patient and SOs through the grieving process by providing a referral to a therapist trained in this process, eg, a psychologist or psychiatric nurse.

6. As appropriate, arrange for a visit by patient's clergy.

Social isolation related to imposed restrictions secondary to presence of radioactive implants

Desired outcomes: Patient can verbalize knowledge of the rationale for the isolation. Patient relates the absence of boredom.

1. Explain the rationale for the private room and isolation and the need for

limiting staff and family visits. Reassure patient that the isolation is only temporary.

2. Encourage diversional activities such as reading books, watching television, listening to the radio, writing letters, knitting, and working crossword puzzles.

3. To minimize feelings of isolation, encourage patient to use the intercom system or telephone for contacting staff and SOs.

4. Maximize the quality of the time spent in patient's room. Work quickly but do not ignore patient's need for socialization.

5. Evaluate patient's emotional status with each visit. Be alert to indicators of withdrawal and negative comments about self.

Potential for injury to patient, staff, and visitors related to risk of exposure to radiation secondary to proximity of the radiation implant

Desired outcome: Patient, staff, and visitors can verbalize knowledge about the potential dangers of radiation therapy and the measures that must be taken to ensure safety.

1. Place a warning sign on patient's door, notifying staff and visitors that radiation therapy is in process.

2. Follow radiologist or agency protocol for restricting or limiting visitors and staff from patient's room. Usually, only the spouse or SO is allowed to visit for limited periods of time.

3. Ensure that pregnant women do not enter the room.

4. Attach a radiation badge (dosimeter) to your clothing before entering the room to monitor the amount of radiation exposure. According to federal regulations, radiation exposure should not exceed 400 mrem/mo. Nurses who care for patients with radiation implants rarely receive this much exposure.

5. Perform care activities at the side of the bed opposite patient's implant to minimize the amount of exposure. For example, if the implant is in the pelvic region, perform care activities from the head of the bed as much as possible.

6. Be aware that the patient' secretions and excretions are *not* radioactive.

7. Check position of the implant at least q shift. If it has migrated or is lying in the bed, *do not* touch it. Notify radiation department for replacement. MD or radiation therapist will use long-handled forceps to replace it.

8. Monitor patient for and report signs of radiation cystitis, including severe urgency, burning on urination, and frequency. Medicate with prescribed antispasmodics and analgesics and encourage a fluid intake of at least 2–3 L/day.

Impairment of physical mobility related to imposed activity and positional limitations/restrictions secondary to the presence of a radium implant

Desired outcomes: Patient can verbalize knowledge of the imposed activity and positional limitations and/or restrictions. Patient does not exhibit signs of skin impairment or other problems of immobility.

1. Explain the rationale and importance of inactivity during the period of time the implant will be indwelling.

2. As indicated, instruct patient to remain flat and limit movements to prevent dislodging the implant.

3. Because patient movement is limited, keep frequently used items within easy reach.

4. Position patient on sheepskin or pressure-relief mattress to help prevent skin impairment, especially areas most prone to breakdown, eg, scapulae, sacrum, and iliac crests.

5. For patient with a radium implant in the pelvis, encourage active ROM of shoulders, elbows, and wrists. If the implant is in the upper part of the body, encourage active ROM of the lower extremities.

6. Do not turn patient from side to side unless it is approved by MD. For patient with a pelvic implant, use pillows to prop the shoulders, and change position of the pillows q2h. Massage the upper back and shoulders, but do not turn patient for a full back rub if the supine position has been prescribed to prevent dislodging of the implant. Logroll patient if turning from side to side is allowed.

Potential alterations in bowel elimination: *Constipation* related to low-residue diet and immobility; and *diarrhea* related to presence of radium implant

Desired outcome: Patient does not experience bowel elimination while the radium implant is indwelling.

▶ **Note:** Patients with radium implants will have had cleansing enemas prior to implant insertion; low-residue diets and an antidiarrheal are given while the implant is in place to prevent diarrhea, which is a common occurrence with a radium implant. The medical goal is to minimize bowel stimulation to prevent disruption of the implant.

---

1. Auscultate the abdomen for frequent bowel sounds, and question patient about the urge to defecate. Notify MD accordingly.

2. For interventions for constipation after the implant has been removed, see **Alteration in bowel elimination:** Constipation, in "Caring for Patients on Prolonged Bed Rest," p. 536.

Knowledge deficit: Potential for severe side effects from radiation and chemotherapy

Desired outcome: Patient can verbalize knowledge of the potential side effects from radiation and/or chemotherapy and measures that can be taken to prevent injury.

1. Teach patient the signs of infection (eg, fever, cough, sore throat, burning with urination), which can occur as a consequence of bone marrow depression and subsequent leukopenia. Explain the importance of undergoing scheduled laboratory work-ups to assess for bone marrow depression. Caution patient to avoid exposure to individuals known to have infections.

2. Teach patient signs and symptoms of an increased bleeding tendency (eg, ecchymosis, petechiae, bleeding gums, hematuria, blood in the stool) that can occur secondary to a depressed platelet count associated with bone marrow depression. Advise patient to avoid situations that can cause physical trauma and to use a soft-bristled toothbrush and an electric razor.

3. Explain that GI side effects (eg, diarrhea, nausea, vomiting) and subsequent dehydration can accompany treatment. Advise the intake of small, frequent meals. Explain that carbonated beverages, gelatins, and Popsicles are especially well tolerated. Reassure patient that antiemetics are helpful for reducing nausea.

4. With cellular destruction, which occurs with radiation and chemotherapy, purines are released, and they in turn become uric acid. Uric acid may precipitate as crystals in the kidney, causing renal failure. Explain the importance of laboratory follow-up assessment for hyperuricemia and altered kidney function (as evidenced by elevated serum uric acid, BUN, and creatinine). Remind patient of the importance of maintaining fluid intake of at least 2–3 L/ day to flush the renal–urinary system.

5. For other interventions, see Table A-1, "Potential Side Effects of Common Cancer Chemotherapeutic Agents," p. 549; **Knowledge deficit:** Potential for

Table A-1 Potential Side Effects of Common Cancer Chemotherapeutic Agents

Generic Name	Acute Toxicity	Delayed Toxicity	Special Precautions
doxorubicin	Nausea, red urine	Bone marrow depression; stomatitis, alopecia, development of secondary cancers	
carmustine	Nausea, vomiting (onset within 2–4 h, and can last several days)	Hepatic, renal toxicity; granulocyte and platelet suppression, development of secondary cancers	
cyclo-phosphamide	Nausea, vomiting	Bone marrow depression, alopecia, stomatitis, hemorrhagic cystitis, amenorrhea, development of secondary cancers	Drink at least 2–3 L/day of fluids after treatment and void frequently to prevent bladder irritation
fluorouracil	Nausea	Stomatitis, GI ulceration, diarrhea, development of secondary cancers	
lomustine	Severe nausea and vomiting, anorexia	Alopecia, confusion, ataxia, lethargy, thrombocytopenia, development of secondary cancers	
mechlor-ethamine	Severe nausea and vomiting (rapid onset of 1–2 h; can last several days)	Skin rash, alopecia, amenorrhea, bone marrow depression, secondary cancers	
methotrexate	Diarrhea, nausea, and vomiting	Stomatitis; mucositis of the esophagus, GI tract, vagina; hyper-pigmentation; alopecia; renal failure; bone marrow depression; development of secondary cancers	Perform oral hygiene at frequent intervals; keep urine alkaline to prevent renal damage from precipitation of the drug in the kidney. Avoid the following drugs, which potentiate side effects: salicylates, phenytoin, tetracycline, sulfonamides, and penicillins
procarbazine hydrochloride	Nausea, vomiting, anorexia	Bone marrow depression, leukopenia, alopecia, CNS depression, secondary cancers	Avoid alcoholic beverages while taking this medication
vincristine sulfate		Numbness, tingling of extremities, muscle weakness, loss of deep tendon reflexes, paralytic ileus, constipation, jaw pain, decrease in sperm count, plantar-flexion, development of secondary cancers	

alopecia due to chemotherapy, p. 550; and nursing diagnoses in "Stomatitis," pp. 273–274 in Chapter 6, "Gastrointestinal Disorders."

Knowledge deficit: Potential for alopecia due to chemotherapy

Desired outcomes: Patient can verbalize knowledge of the potential for alopecia as well as measures that can be taken to disguise the problem.

1. Advise patient in advance that alopecia can occur secondary to treatment with certain chemotherapeutic agents (see Table A-1, p. 549), but that after therapy the condition reverses itself.

2. Explain that hair loss can begin within a few days or weeks of treatment and result in partial or complete baldness within a short period of time.

3. Encourage use of wigs, hairpieces, and/or hats. Advise women that scarves also can help disguise this problem.

4. If prescribed, explain that scalp tourniquets or ice packs may be used to limit alopecia.

5. Refer patient to the American Cancer Society for assistance with wig purchase, if appropriate.

Alteration in nutrition: Less than body requirements related to decreased intake secondary to anorexia, nausea, and stomatitis (side effects of chemo/radiation therapy)

Desired outcomes: Patient does not exhibit signs of malnutrition or weight loss. Patient can verbalize knowledge of the type of diet necessary for tissue healing.

1. Encourage a diet high in protein and calories. Emphasize the importance of a balanced diet and good eating habits for optimal tissue repair. For some patients, tube feeding and total parenteral nutrition may be necessary to ensure a high calorie count.

2. If possible, schedule chemotherapy treatments so that episodes of nausea do not occur during mealtimes.

3. For many patients with stomatitis, foods and liquids are better tolerated if they are served at room temperature. Instruct patient accordingly.

4. If indicated, obtain a prescription for a bland diet for patients with stomatitis.

5. For further information, see nursing diagnoses and interventions in "Stomatitis," pp. 273–274 in Chapter 6, "Gastrointestinal Disorders."

Knowledge deficit: Effects of radiation and/or chemotherapy on skin integrity

Desired outcomes: Patient can verbalize knowledge of the effects of radiation and chemotherapy on skin integrity and measures that improve the condition of the skin and prevent further breakdown.

▶ **Note:** Radiation therapy disrupts cellular DNA in the process of cell division. Cancer cells divide faster than normal cells, and they are more susceptible to radiation. Normal cells also recover more quickly than cancer cells. However, normal cells are affected by radiation to some degree.

---

1. Explain to patient that to prevent friction or trauma, the skin should be patted rather than rubbed dry. Massage and scratching should be avoided.

2. Advise patient to avoid all skin ointments, creams, and powders unless MD approves them. The following are often prescribed: ointment containing vitamins A and D for dryness/itching, hydrocortisone cream for reducing inflammation, and cornstarch for absorbing moisture. All prescribed creams should be applied *gently*.

3. Caution patient to avoid the following: irritating shampoos, hair dyes, or permanents; applying adhesive tapes or dressings to the skin; and exposing skin

to direct sunlight, strong winds, extreme heat or cold (including heating or cooling devices), salt water, and chlorinated water.

4. Caution patient to avoid shaving with a razor; however, MD may approve use of an electric shaver.
5. Purple marks are used to identify area of irradiation. Instruct patient not to remove these marks or use soap directly on the outlined areas.
6. Suggest use of lukewarm water and a mild soap for washing the skin.
7. Explain the need for a well-balanced diet to ensure optimal tissue healing.
8. Instruct patient to assess skin for breakdown and delayed wound healing, and stress the importance of reporting any open areas or scabs to MD.

Appendix Two   **Nursing Diagnoses Used in this Manual**

Activity Intolerance related to fatigue secondary to inflammatory process, *"Pneumonia," p. 6;* related to fatigue secondary to infectious process, *"Tuberculosis," p. 28;* related to fatigue and weakness secondary to right and left ventricular failure, *"Pulmonary Hypertension," p. 37;* related to weakness and fatigue secondary to decrease in cardiac muscle contractility, *"Cardiomyopathy," p. 39;* related to weakness and fatigue secondary to tissue ischemia (myocardial infarction), *"Coronary Artery Disease," p. 42;* related to fatigue and weakness secondary to decreased strength of cardiac contraction, *"Myocardial Infarction," p. 46;* related to weakness and fatigue secondary to decreased strength of cardiac contraction, *"Heart Failure," p. 48;* related to weakness and dyspnea secondary to inflammation of the cardiac muscle and restriction of contraction, *"Pericarditis," p. 52;* related to weakness and fatigue secondary to dysfunction of myocardial muscle, *"Myocarditis," p. 54;* related to fatigue and weakness secondary to decreased left ventricular filling, *Mitral Stenosis," p. 58;* related to fatigue and weakness secondary to decreased cardiac output with valvular regurgitation, *"Mitral Regurgitation and Mitral Valve Prolapse," p. 61;* related to weakness secondary to cardiac surgery, *"Cardiac Surgery," p. 75;* related to lost endurance secondary to prolonged bed rest and weakness secondary to renal dysfunction, *"Glomerulonephritis," p. 93;* related to fatigue and weakness secondary to uremia and anemia, *"Acute Renal Failure," p. 109;* related to fatigue and weakness secondary to anemia and uremia, *"Chronic Renal Failure," p. 113;* related to weakness and fatigue secondary to slowed metabolism and decreased cardiac output associated with pericardial effusions, atherosclerosis, and decreased adrenergic stimulation, *"Hypothyroidism," p. 227;* related to neuromuscular weakness and joint pain secondary to increased serum calcium and altered phosphate levels, *"Hyperparathyroidism," p. 232;* related to weakness and fatigue secondary to decreased cardiac contractility, *"Hypoparathyroidism," p. 235;* related to fatigue and weakness secondary to decreased cardiac output, *"Addison's Disease," p. 238;* related to weakness and fatigue secondary to intestinal inflammatory process, *"Crohn's Disease," p. 312;* related to fatigue secondary to decreased oxygen-carrying capacity of the blood, *"Pernicious Anemia," p. 341;* related to fatigue and weakness secondary to decreased oxygen-carrying capacity of the blood, *"Hypoplastic Anemia," p. 349;* related to fatigue and weakness secondary to decreased oxygen-carrying capacity of the blood, *"Acute Leukemia," p. 361.*

Anxiety related to perceived threat to biologic integrity secondary to sensation of suffocation, *"Asthma," p. 19;* related to actual or perceived threats or changes secondary to degeneration of intellectual functioning, *"Alzheimer's Disease," p. 163;* related to untoward response secondary to sympathetic nervous system stimulation, *"Hyperthyroidism," p. 222.*

Bowel Elimination, Alterations in: Constipation related to negative side effects of drugs, restriction of fresh fruit and fluids, and prolonged bed rest, *"Acute Renal Fail-*

ure," p. 110; related to immobility and decreased peristalsis, atonic bowel, and loss of voluntary function secondary to sensorimotor deficit, *"Spinal Cord Injury," p. 174;* related to decreased peristalsis secondary to slowed metabolism, *"Hypothyroidism," p. 226;* related to decreased peristalsis secondary to increased serum calcium level, *"Hyperparathyroidism," p. 233;* related to fear of pain with postoperative defecation, *"Hemorrhoids," p. 299;* related to gastrointestinal mucosal atrophy secondary to reduced hematocrit, *"Pernicious Anemia," p. 341;* related to restriction against straining, low-residue diet, and/or pain with defecation secondary to surgical procedure, *"Rectocele," p. 440;* related to contamination and/or side effects of tube-feeding solution, *"Providing Nutritional Therapy," p. 520;* related to immobility, changes in normal bowel habits during hospitalization, alteration in diet, and use of narcotic analgesics, *"Caring for Patients on Prolonged Bed Rest," p. 536;* related to inability to chew and swallow a high-roughage diet, side effects of medications, and immobility, *"Caring for Patients with Neurologic Problems," p. 541;* related to low-residue diet and immobility, *"Caring for Patients with Cancer and other Life-Disrupting Illnesses," p. 548.*

Bowel Elimination, Alterations in: Diarrhea, bloating, excessive flatus, and abdominal cramping related to specific malabsorption disorder, *"Malabsorption/Maldigestion," p. 287;* related to intestinal inflammatory process, *"Ulcerative Colitis," p. 308;* related to intestinal inflammatory process and/or malabsorption, *"Crohn's Disease," p. 312;* related to gastrointestinal mucosal atrophy secondary to reduced hematocrit, *"Pernicious Anemia," p. 341;* related to contamination and/or side effects of tube-feeding solution, *"Providing Nutritional Therapy," p. 520;* related to presence of radiation implant, *"Caring for Patients with Cancer and other Life-Disrupting Illnesses," p. 548.*

Bowel Elimination, Alterations in related to disruption of normal function secondary to ureterosigmoidostomy, *"Urinary Diversions," p. 131;* related to disruption of normal function secondary to fecal diversion, *"Fecal Diversions," p. 316.*

Cardiac Output, Alterations in: Decreased: Impaired oxygen transport secondary to cardiac arrest, *"Cardiac Arrest," p. 67;* Fluid loss and serum electrolyte imbalance secondary to osmotic diuresis associated with hyperglycemia, *"Diabetic Ketoacidosis," p. 264;* Fluid loss and serum electrolyte imbalance secondary to osmotic diuresis associated with hyperglycemia, *"Hyperosmolar Hyperglycemic Nonketotic Coma," p. 265;* Risk of cardiac arrest secondary to hyperkalemia, *"Electrolyte Disturbances," p. 504;* Risk of dysrhythmias secondary to hypokalemia, *"Electrolyte Disturbances," p. 505.*

Comfort, Alteration in : Pain related to pneumothorax and/or chest tube insertion, *"Pneumothorax," p. 4;* Pain related to surgical incision or disease process, *"Atelectasis," p. 13;* Angina related to decreased oxygen supply to the myocardium, *"Coronary Artery Disease," p. 42;* Pain related to ischemia and infarction of myocardial tissue, *"Myocardial Infarction," p. 45;* Chest (pericardial) pain related to friction rub, *"Pericarditis," p. 53;* Pain related to pacemaker insertion, *"Pacemakers," p. 72;* Chronic pain related to ischemia secondary to atherosclerotic obstructions, *"Atherosclerotic Arterial Occlusive Disease," p. 79;* Pain related to inflammatory process secondary to thrombus formation, *"Venous Thrombosis/Thrombophlebitis," p. 85;* Pain related to preoperative venous engorgement and/or surgical procedure, *"Vericose Veins," p. 88;* Dysuria related to infection, *"Acute Pyelonephritis," p. 99;* Acute pain related to calculus or surgical procedure to remove it, *"Ureteral Calculi," p. 123;* Pain related to bladder spasms, *"Urinary Tract Obstruction," p. 127;* Pain and spasms related to motor nerve tract damage, *"Multiple Sclerosis," p. 148;* Headache related to head injury, *"Head Injury," p. 180;* Pain related to tumor growth, *"Spinal Cord Tumors," p. 187;* Malaise and nausea related to sedative-hypnotic withdrawal, *"Sedative-Hypnotic Abuse," p. 212;* Malaise and other physiologic symptoms related to withdrawal from opioid substance, *"Opioid Abuse," p. 215;* Pain related to surgical procedure, *"Hyperthyroidism," p. 224;* Pain/arthralgia related to bone demineralization and/or surgery, *"Hyperparathyroidism," p. 233;* Pain related to inflammatory process of the pancreas, *"Pancreatitis," p. 250;* Pain related to major abdominal surgery, *"Pancreatic Tumors,"* *p. 254;* Pain, nausea, and feeling of fullness related to gastrointestinal reflux and increase in intra-abdominal pressure, *"Hiatal Hernia and Reflux Esophagitis," p. 276;* Acute epigastric pain related to ulcerations, *"Peptic Ulcers," p. 282;* Abdominal fullness, weakness, and diaphoresis related to postgastrectomy dumping syndrome, *"Peptic Ulcers," p. 283;* Nausea, distention, and pain related to abdominal visceral disorder and gastrointestinal obstructive process, *"Obstructive Processes," p. 289;* Pain related to hernia condition and/or surgical intervention, *"Hernia," p. 291;* Pain, abdominal distention, and nausea related to inflammatory process, *"Peritonitis," p. 293;* Acute pain and nausea related to inflammatory process, *"Appendicitis," p. 297;* Postoperative pain and itching, *"Hemorrhoids," p. 298;* Pain, abdominal cramping, and nausea related to intestinal inflammatory process, *"Ulcerative Colitis," p. 307;* Pain, abdominal cramping, and nausea related to intestinal inflammatory process, *"Crohn's Disease," p. 311;* Pain and nausea related to surgical procedure, *"Obesity," p. 323;* Pain, spasms, nausea, and itching related to obstructive and/or inflammatory process, *"Cholelithiasis and Cholecystitis," p. 335;* Pain related to hemolysis in joints, *"Hemolytic Anemia," p. 344;* Headache, angina, and abdominal and joint pain related to decreased circulation secondary to hyperviscosity of the blood, *"Polycythemia," p. 351;* Malaise and joint pain related to hemorrhagic episodes and/or blood extravasation into the tissues, *"Thrombocytopenia," p. 353;* Pain related to swollen joints, *"Hemophilia," p. 355;* Pain related to inflammatory process or corrective therapy, *"Osteoarthritis," p. 367;* Pain related to phantom limb sensations, *"Amputation," p. 407;* Pain related to surgical procedure, *"Breast Augmentation," p. 420;* Pain related to biopsy, *"Benign Breast Disease," p. 425;* Pain related to surgical procedure, *"Malignant Disorders of the Breast," p. 429;* Pain related to surgery or radiation implant, *"Cancer of the Cervix," p. 432;* Acute pain related to uterine contractions, *"Spontaneous Abortion," p. 444;* Pain related to bladder spasms, *"Benign Prostatic Hypertrophy," p. 450;* Pain related to infectious process, *"Prostatitis," p. 452;* Pain related to scrotal swelling secondary to orchiectomy and/or lymphadenectomy, *"Testicular Neoplasm," p. 458;* Pain related to surgical procedure, *"Penile Implants," p. 460;* Pain related to corneal ulceration/surgical procedure, *"Corneal Ulceration," p. 469;* Pain related to surgical procedure, *"Corneal Transplant," p. 471;* Pain related to surgical procedure, *"Enucleation," p. 479;* Pain related to burn injury, *"Care of the Burn Patient," p. 494;* Pain and nausea related to surgical procedure, *"Caring for Preoperative and Postoperative Patients," p. 528;* Pain, spasms, headache, and photophobia related to neurologic dysfunction, *"Caring for Patients with Neurologic Problems," p. 543.*

Communication, Impaired Verbal related to aphasia and/or dysarthria secondary to cerebrovascular insult, *"Cerebrovascular Accident," p. 195;* related to dysarthria secondary to facial/throat muscle weakness, intubation, or tracheostomy, *"Caring for Patients with Neurologic Problems," p. 541.*

Coping, Ineffective Individual related to anger, denial, and poor self-esteem secondary to inability to manage stressors without alcohol, *"Alcohol Abuse," p. 209;* related to dysphoria, poor self-esteem, and denial secondary to inability to manage stressors without cocaine, *"Cocaine Abuse," p. 214;* related to denial, poor self-esteem, and depression secondary to inability to manage stressors without opioids, *"Opioid Abuse," p. 216;* related to depression secondary to diagnosis of breast cancer, *"Malignant Disorders of the Breast," p. 428;* related to depression secondary to prolonged confinement, *"Caring for Patients on Prolonged Bed Rest," p. 534;* related to depression secondary to perceived role change: Dependence versus independence, *"Caring for Patients on Prolonged Bed Rest," p. 537;* related to depression secondary to severity of the diagnosis, *"Caring for Patients with Cancer and other Life-Disrupting Illnesses," p. 545.*

*Coping, Ineffective Family

Diversional Activity Deficit related to monotony of confinement secondary to prolonged bed rest, *"Caring for Patients on Prolonged Bed Rest," p. 533.*

Family Processes, Alterations in related to illness of family member, *"Alzheimer's Disease," p. 164;* related to grave illness and/or impending death of a family member, *"Caring for Patients with Cancer and other Life-Disrupting Illnesses," p. 546.*

Fear related to life-threatening situation, *"Pulmonary Edema," p. 69;* related to threat to biologic integrity, *"Guillain-Barré Syndrome," p. 151;* related to the possibility of cancer, change in body image, surgical or diagnostic procedure, and pain, *"Benign Breast Disease," p. 425;* related to the possibility of cancer and its treatment, *"Malignant Disorders of the Breast," p. 428;* related to threat to biologic integrity secondary to grave diagnosis, *"Caring for Patients with Cancer and other Life-Disrupting Illnesses," p. 544.*

Fluid Volume Deficit related to increased need secondary to infection and/or loss secondary to diaphoresis, *"Pneumonia," p. 6;* related to decreased intake secondary to fatigue and/or prescribed limitations, *"Acute Respiratory Failure," p. 17;* related to decreased intake and/or fluid restriction, *"Chronic Bronchitis," p. 22;* related to loss secondary to hemorrhage/hematoma formation after arterial puncture, *"Cardiac Catheterization," p. 73;* related to loss secondary to postsurgical bleeding/hemorrhage, *"Aneurysms," p. 82;* related to vascular dehydration secondary to pharmacotherapy, *"Nephrotic Syndrome," p. 96;* related to decreased intake secondary to anorexia and abnormal loss secondary to vomiting and diaphoresis, *"Acute Pyelonephritis," p. 100;* related to abnormal loss secondary to postoperative bleeding, *"Renal Calculi," p. 101;* related to abnormal loss secondary to postobstructive diuresis, *"Hydronephrosis," p. 104;* related to abnormal loss secondary to excessive urinary output: Diuretic phase, *"Acute Renal Failure," p. 109;* related to abnormal loss secondary to hypertonicity of the dialysate, *"Care of the Peritoneal Dialysis Patient," p. 118;* related to excessive fluid removal secondary to dialysis, *"Care of the Hemodialysis Patient," p. 120;* related to excessive urinary loss and/or hemorrhage secondary to rapid bladder decompression during catheterization procedure, *"Urinary Tract Obstruction," p. 127;* related to loss secondary to postsurgical hemorrhage (after TUR or segmental resection), *"Cancer of the Bladder," p. 129;* related to abnormal blood loss secondary to surgical procedure, *"Urinary Diversions," p. 133;* related to abnormal loss secondary to osmotic diuresis, vomiting, or diarrhea caused by oral phosphate supplements, *"Hyperparathyroidism," p. 232;* related to abnormal loss secondary to diuresis, *"Addison's Disease," p. 238;* related to abnormal loss secondary to polyuria, *"Diabetes Insipidus," p. 244;* related to abnormal loss secondary to NG suctioning, vomiting, diaphoresis, or pooling of fluids in the abdomen and retroperitoneum, *"Pancreatitis," p. 250;* related to loss secondary to postsurgical hemorrhage (due to high vascularity of surgical site or multiple anastomosis sites) and/or risk of fluid shift to third-space (interstitial) compartments, *"Pancreatic Tumors," p. 253;* related to abnormal loss secondary to osmotic diuresis, *"Diabetic Ketoacidosis," p. 263;* related to increased need secondary to impaired absorption and/or abnormal loss secondary to diarrhea, *"Malabsorption/Maldigestion," p. 288;* related to abnormal losses secondary to vomiting and/or gastric decompression of large volumes of GI fluids and decreased intake secondary to fluid restrictions, *"Obstructive Processes," p. 289;* related to abnormal blood loss secondary to slipped ligatures, *"Hemorrhoids," p. 299;* related to abnormal loss secondary to diarrhea, *"Ulcerative Colitis," p. 308;* related to abnormal loss secondary to diarrhea and/or GI fistula, *"Crohn's Disease," p. 312;* related to decreased intake secondary to dietary restrictions and/or postsurgical regimen, *"Obesity," p. 322;* related to loss secondary to postsplenectomy bleeding/hemorrhage, *"Thrombocytopenia," p. 354;* related to abnormal loss secondary to postsurgical hemorrhage or hematoma formation, *"Torn Anterior Cruciate Ligament," p. 383;* related to abnormal loss secondary to postsurgical hemorrhage, *"Amputation," p. 407;* related to abnormal loss secondary to postsurgical hemorrhage or hematoma formation, *"Breast Reconstruction," p. 422;* related to abnormal loss secondary to postoperative or post-implant bleeding, *"Cancer of the Cervix," p. 433;* related to abnormal loss secondary to postsurgical or post-abortion bleeding, *"Spontaneous Abortion," p. 444;* related to abnormal loss secondary to bleeding/hemorrhage with ectopic rupture, *"Tubal Preg-*

nancy," *p. 446;* related to abnormal loss secondary to bleeding/hemorrhage due to surgical procedure and/or pressure on the prostatic capsule, *"Benign Prostatic Hypertrophy," p. 449;* related to abnormal loss secondary to postsurgical bleeding, *"Testicular Neoplasm," p. 458;* related to abnormal loss and/or decreased intake, *"Fluid Disturbances," p. 500;* related to abnormal (hypotonic) loss or decreased intake, *"Electrolyte Disturbances," p. 501;* related to abnormal fluid loss or interstitial spacing of fluids, *"Electrolyte Disturbances," p. 502;* related to abnormal losses, *"Acid–Base Imbalances," p. 511* and *512;* related to abnormal loss secondary to osmolality and substrate content of tube feeding solutions, *"Providing Nutritional Therapy," p. 521;* related to abnormal loss secondary to vomiting or gastric decompression and/or decreased intake secondary to nausea and/or NPO status, *"Caring for Preoperative and Postoperative Patients," p. 529;* related to risk of fluid shift to third space (interstitial) compartments after major (particularly abdominal) surgery, *"Caring for Preoperative and Postoperative Patients," p. 530;* related to abnormal loss secondary to postsurgical bleeding, *"Caring for Preoperative and Postoperative Patients," p. 530;* related to decreased intake secondary to dysphagia, weakness, paresis, paralysis, or decreased LOC, *"Caring for Patients with Neurologic Problems," p. 539.*

Fluid Volume Excess: Edema related to retention secondary to decreased cardiac output, *"Chronic Bronchitis,"* p. 22; related to retention secondary to decreased cardiac output, *"Myocardial Infarction," p. 45;* related to retention secondary to decreased cardiac output, *"Heart Failure," p. 49;* related to retention secondary to right-sided heart failure, *"Mitral Stenosis," p. 59;* related to retention secondary to decreased cardiac output, *"Pulmonary Edema," p. 70;* related to retention secondary to decreased renal function, *"Glomerulonephritis," p. 93;* related to retention secondary to decreased serum albumin or renal retention of sodium and water, *"Nephrotic Syndrome," p. 96;* related to fluid retention secondary to renal dysfunction: Oliguric phase, *"Acute Renal Failure," p. 108;* related to retention or inadequate exchange secondary to catheter problems and/or peritonitis, *"Care of the Peritoneal Dialysis Patient," p. 118;* related to retention secondary to renal failure, *"Care of the Hemodialysis Patient," p. 120;* related to retention secondary to irrigation, *"Cancer of the Bladder," p. 129;* related to retention secondary to decreased metabolic rate and adrenal insufficiency, *"Hypothyroidism," p. 228;* and ascites related to retention secondary to portal hypertension and hepatocellular failure, *"Cirrhosis," p. 332;* related to retention secondary to administration of high volumes of irrigating fluid, *"Benign Prostatic Hypertrophy," p. 450;* related to surplus of circulating fluid, *"Fluid Disturbances," p. 499;* related to increased intake, *"Electrolyte Disturbances," p. 502;* related to retention secondary to osmolality and substrate content of tube feeding solutions, *"Providing Nutritional Therapy," p. 521.*

Grieving related to anticipated or actual fetal loss, *"Spontaneous Abortion," p. 445;* related to sexual dysfunction secondary to radical prostatectomy, *"Prostatic Neoplasm," p. 456;* related to loss of body part or change in body function, *"Caring for Patients with Cancer and other Life-Disrupting Illnesses," p. 545;* Individual/family related to anticipated or actual loss secondary to terminal illness, *"Caring for Patients with Cancer and other Life-Disrupting Illnesses," p. 546.*

*Health Maintenance, Alterations in

*Home Maintenance Management, Impaired

Infection, Potential for (recurring URIs) related to vulnerability secondary to ongoing lung tissue inflammation and destruction, *"Pneumoconioses," p. 26;* (for other patients and staff members) related to susceptibility secondary to communicable nature of the disease, *"Tuberculosis," p. 28;* (with concomitant endocarditis) related to increased susceptibility secondary to valvular disorder, *"Mitral Stenosis," p. 59;* related to increased susceptibility secondary to corticosteroid therapy, immobility, invasive procedures, and impaired skin integrity, *"Glomerulonephritis," p. 94;*

related to vulnerability secondary to treatment with immunosuppressive agents, prolonged immobility, invasive procedures, and disease process, *"Nephrotic Syndrome," p. 97;* related to increased susceptibility secondary to disease process, *"Acute Pyelonephritis," p. 99;* related to increased susceptibility secondary to uremia, *"Acute Renal Failure," p. 110;* related to increased susceptibility secondary to invasive procedures, risk of exposure to infected individuals, and immunosuppression, *"Care of the Renal Transplant Patient," p. 116;* related to increased vulnerability secondary to direct access of the catheter to the peritoneum, *"Care of the Peritoneal Dialysis Patient," p. 118;* related to vulnerability secondary to presence of suprapubic catheter and opening of a closed drainage system, *"Cancer of the Bladder," p. 129;* related to vulnerability secondary to invasive procedures, reflux of feces into the urinary tract, and contact of pouch with the suture line, *"Urinary Diversions," p. 132;* related to increased susceptibility secondary to penetrating or open head injuries and/or surgical wounds, *"Head Injury," p. 180;* related to increased susceptibility secondary to repeated IV drug injections and/or antitussive effects of opioids, *"Opioid Abuse," p. 216;* related to increased susceptibility secondary to alterations in adrenal function, *"Hypothyroidism," p. 227;* related to lowered resistance secondary to decreased adrenal function, *"Addison's Disease," p. 237;* related to increased susceptibility secondary to disease process, *"Diabetes Mellitus—General Discussion," p. 259;* related to risk of rupture, peritonitis, and abscess formation secondary to inflammatory process, *"Appendicitis," p. 296;* related to increased susceptibility secondary to decreased leukocyte production, *"Pernicious Anemia," p. 341;* related to increased susceptibility scondary to decreased leukocytes, *"Hypoplastic Anemia," p. 348;* related to increased susceptibility secondary to myelosuppression from disease process or therapy, *"Acute Leukemia," p. 360;* (for others) related to risk of cross-contamination; (for patient) related to susceptibility secondary to disease chronicity, *"Osteomyelitis," p. 387;* related to increased susceptibility secondary to retention of some or all of the products of conception, *"Spontaneous Abortion," p. 444;* related to increased susceptibility secondary to ectopic rupture, *"Tubal Pregnancy," p. 447;* related to increased susceptibility secondary to invasive and therapeutic procedures, *"Cataract," p. 466;* related to increased susceptibility secondary to invasive procedure and proximity of surgical site to the brain, *"Otosclerosis," p. 481;* related to increased susceptibility secondary to loss of protective skin layer, *"Care of the Burn Patient," p. 493;* related to increased susceptibility secondary to invasive procedure and parenteral delivery of nutrients, *"Providing Nutritional Therapy," p. 522;* related to increased susceptibility secondary to invasive procedure and delivery of nutrients into central vein, *"Providing Nutritional Therapy," p. 523;* related to vulnerability secondary to presence of an indwelling urethral catheter, *"Caring for Preoperative and Postoperative Patients," p. 532*

Injury, Potential for related to increased risk of bleeding secondary to anticoagulant therapy, *"Pulmonary Embolism," p. 9;* related to risk of complications secondary to insertion/presence of nephrostomy tube, *"Hydronephrosis," p. 103;* related to sensorimotor and mentation alterations secondary to uremia, electrolyte imbalance, and metabolic acidosis, *"Acute Renal Failure," p. 109;* related to sensorimotor and mentation alterations secondary to electrolyte and acid-base imbalances, *"Chronic Renal Failure," p. 114;* related to sensorimotor and mentation alterations secondary to uremia and serum electrolyte imbalance, *"Care of the Peritoneal Dialysis Patient," p. 119;* related to increased risk of bleeding secondary to heparinization with dialysis, *"Care of the Hemodialysis Patient," p. 120;* related to risk of complications secondary to creation of the vascular access, *"Care of the Hemodialysis Patient," p. 120;* related to alterations in mentation and/or motor function secondary to reabsorption of electrolytes through the urinary diversion (ureterosigmoidostomy) or loss of sodium and potassium (ileal conduit), *"Urinary Diversions," p. 132;* related to unsteady gait secondary to bradykinesis, tremors, and rigidity, *"Parkinsonism," p. 159;* related to lack of awareness of environmental hazards secondary to cognitive deficit, *"Alzheimer's Disease," p. 161;* related to risk of autonomic dysreflexia secondary to noxious stimulus, *"Spinal Cord Injury," p. 173;* related to lack of access for external cardiac compression, incorrect neck position, irritation of cranial nerves, and impaired lateral vision secondary to use of halo vest traction, *"Spinal Cord Injury," p. 175;* related to oral, musculoskeletal, and airway vulnerability secondary to seizure activity, *"Seizure Disorders," p. 203;* related to tremors, disorientation, and hallucinations secondary to withdrawal from alcohol, *"Alcohol Abuse," p. 208;* related to tremors, disorientation, and hallucinations secondary to withdrawal from CNS depressant, *"Sedative-Hypnotic Abuse," p. 212;* related to risk of corneal damage secondary to exophthalmos, *"Hyperthyroidism," p. 222;* related to risk of thyrotoxic crisis secondary to emotional stress, trauma, infection, or surgical manipulation of the gland, *"Hyperthyroidism," p. 223;* related to risk of myxedema coma secondary to inadequate response to treatment of hypothyroidism or stressors such as infection, *"Hypothyroidism," p. 228;* related to risk of tetany, thyroid storm, and hypercalcemia secondary to surgical procedure and/or manipulation of the gland, *"Hyperparathyroidism," p. 232;* related to risk of pathologic fractures secondary to bone demineralization, *"Hyperparathyrodism," p. 232;* related to risk of seizures, tetany, and respiratory distress secondary to hypocalcemia, *"Hypoparathyroidism," p. 235;* related to risk of Addisonian crisis or negative side effects from the drug therapy used to treat it, *"Addison's Disease," p. 238;* related to negative side effects of vasopressin, *"Diabetes Insipidus," p. 244;* related to risk of increased intracranial pressure, cerebrospinal leak, hemorrhage, infection, and/or diabetes insipidus secondary to transphenoidal hypophysectomy, *"Pituitary Tumors," p. 246;* related to risk of complications secondary to hyperglycemia and acid–base imbalance, *"Diabetic Ketoacidosis," p. 264;* related to risk of complications secondary to hypoglycemia, *"Hypoglycemia," p. 267;* related to alteration in LOC and risk of seizures secondary to hypoglycemia, *"Hypoglycemia," p. 266;* related to risk of gastrointestinal complications (obstruction, recurring reflux, esophageal tear, or perforation) secondary to surgery, *"Hiatal Hernia and Reflux Esophagitis," p. 277;* related to risk of gastrointestinal complications (bleeding, obstruction, and perforation) secondary to ulcerative process, *"Peptic Ulcers," p. 282;* related to risk of GI complications secondary to inflammatory process, *"Peritonitis," p. 294;* related to risk of septic shock secondary to infectious process, *"Peritonitis," p. 294;* related to risk of complications secondary to intestinal inflammatory disorder, *"Ulcerative Colitis," p. 307;* related to negative side effects of pharmacotherapy, *"Crohn's Disease," p. 312;* related to risk of gastrointestinal complications secondary to bariatric surgery, *"Obesity," p. 322;* related to increased risk of bleeding secondary to decreased vitamin-K absorption, *"Hepatitis," p. 328;* related to increased risk of bleeding secondary to altered clotting factors and portal hypertension, *"Cirrhosis," p. 332;* related to risk of hepatic coma secondary to cerebral accumulation of ammonia and/or GI bleeding, *"Cirrhosis," p. 332;* related to risk of complications secondary to surgical procedure, use of T-tube, and/or recurrence of biliary obstruction, *"Cholelithiasis and Cholecystitis," p. 335;* related to risk of sensorimotor deficit secondary to inability to absorb and utilize vitamin B_{12}, *"Pernicious Anemia," p. 342;* related to risk of sensorimotor deficit secondary to peripheral nerve hypoxia, *"Hemolytic Anemia," p. 344;* related to increased risk of bleeding secondary to decreased platelet count, *"Thrombocytopenia," p. 353;* related to increased risk of bleeding secondary to clotting factor deficiency, *"Hemophilia," p. 355;* related to increased risk of bleeding secondary to decreased platelet count, *"Acute Leukemia," p. 360;* related to increased risk of bleeding secondary to high vascularity of the ocular tissue, *"Cataract," p. 467;* related to increased risk of bleeding secondary to hypervascularity of the ocular tissue, *"Retinal Detachment," p. 477;* related to increased risk of falling secondary to vertigo, *"Otosclerosis," p. 481;* related to increased risk of seizure activity secondary to hypocalcemia, *"Electrolyte Disturbances," p. 507;* related to risk of metabolic alterations secondary to peripheral vein nutritional therapy, *"Providing Nutritional Therapy," p. 522;* related to risk of metabolic alterations secondary to central vein nutritional therapy, *"Providing Nutritional Therapy," p. 522;* related to risk of complications secondary to fat emulsion therapy, *"Providing Nutritional Therapy," p. 523;* related to unsteady gait secondary to motor deficit, *"Caring for Patients with Neurologic Problems," p. 537;* related to impaired pain, touch, and temperature sensations secondary to sensory deficit and/or decreased LOC, *"Caring for Patients with Neurologic Problems," p. 538;* related to risk of corneal irritation/abrasion secondary to diminished blink reflex and/or inability to close the eyes, *"Caring for Patients with Neurologic Problems," p. 538;* related to risk of increased ICP secondary to positional factors, increased intrathoracic or intra-abdominal pressure, fluid volume excess, hyperthermia, and/or discomfort, *"Caring for Patients with Neurologic Problems," p. 542;* related to visual disturbance secondary to diplopia, *"Caring for Patients with Neurologic Problems," p. 543;* to patient, staff, and visitors related to risk of exposure to radiation secondary to proximity of the radiation implant, *"Caring for Patients with Cancer and other Life-Disrupting Illnesses, p. 547.*

Knowledge Deficit: Disease process and treatment, *"Pulmonary Hypertension," p. 37;* Precautions and negative side effects of nitrates, *"Coronary Artery Disease," p. 43;* Precautions and negative side effects of beta blockers, *"Coronary Artery Disease," p. 43;* Precautions and negative side effects of diuretic therapy, *"Heart Failure," p. 49;* Precautions and negative side effects of digitalis therapy, *"Heart Failure," p. 49;* Precautions and negative side effects of vasodilators, *"Heart Failure," p. 50;* Disease process and therapeutic regimen, *"Infective Endocarditis," p. 56;* Potential for development of endocarditis, *"Mitral Stenosis," p. 59;* Pacemaker insertion procedure and pacemaker function, *"Pacemakers," p. 71;* Catheterization procedure and postcatheterization regimen, *"Cardiac Catheterization," p. 73;* Diagnosis, surgical procedure, preoperative routine, and postoperative course, *"Cardiac Surgery," p. 75;* Interventions that increase peripheral circulation, *"Atherosclerotic Arterial Occlusive Disease," p. 78;* Potential for infection and impaired skin integrity due to decreased arterial circulation, *"Atherosclerotic Arterial Occlusive Disease," p. 79;* Potential for aneurysmal rupture, *"Aneurysms," p. 81;* Surgical procedure and postoperative regimen, *"Aneurysms," p. 82;* Signs and symptoms of fluid and electrolyte imbalance, *"Glomerulonephritis," p. 94;* Negative side effects of corticosteroids and cytotoxic agents, *"Glomerulonephritis," p. 94;* Technique for measuring BP and the rationale for frequent assessments after angioplasty, *"Renal Artery Stenosis," p. 105;* Need for frequent BP checks and compliance with antihypertensive therapy and the potential for change in insulin requirements for diabetics, *"Chronic Renal Failure," p. 114;* Signs and symptoms of rejection, negative side effects of immunosuppressive agents, and importance of protecting the fistula, *"Care of the Renal Transplant Patient," p. 116;* Diet and its relationship to stone formation, *"Ureteral Calculi," p. 125;* Procedure for bladder training and/or Kegel exercise program, *"Urinary Incontinence," p. 137;* Use of external (condom) catheter, *"Urinary Incontinence," p. 137;* Care of long-term indwelling catheters after continent vesicostomy, *"Neurogenic Bladder," p. 142;* Factors that aggravate and/or exacerbate MS symptoms, *"Multiple Sclerosis," p. 147;* Precautions and potential side effects of prescribed medications, *"Multiple Sclerosis," p. 148;* Side effects and precautions for the prescribed antibiotics, *"Bacterial Meningitis," p. 154;* Rationale and procedure for respiratory isolation and/or secretion precautions, *"Bacterial Meningitis," p. 154;* Precautions for taking levodopa, *"Parkinsonism," p. 159;* Facial and tongue exercises that enhance verbal communication and help prevent choking, *"Parkinsonism," p. 159;* Proper body mechanics and other measures that prevent back injury, *"Herniated Nucleus Pulposus," p. 167;* Pain control measures, *"Herniated Nucleus Pulposus," p. 168;* Surgical procedure, preoperative routine, and postoperative regimen, *"Herniated Nucleus Pulposus," p. 169;* Caretaker's responsibilities for observing the patient who is sent home with a concussion, *"Head Injury," p. 179;* Potential for rebleeding, rupture, vasospasm, and negative side effects of drug therapy (aminocaproic acid), *"Cerebral Aneurysm," p. 190;* Life-threatening environmental factors and preventive measures for seizures, *"Seizure Disorders," p. 203;* Purpose, precautions, and side effects of anticonvulsant medications, *"Seizure Disorders," p. 204;* Potential for side effects from iodides or taking or abruptly stopping thioamides, *"Hyperthyroidism," p. 223;* Potential for negative side effects from steroids, phosphate supplements, and mithramycin, *"Hyperparathyroidism," p. 233;* Procedure for insulin administration, *"Diabetes Mellitus—General Discussion," p. 260;* Disease process, diagnostic testing, indicators of hypoglycemia, and therapeutic regimen, *"Hypoglycemia," p. 267;* Disease process, treatment, and factors that potentiate bleeding, *"Stomatitis," p. 273;* Disease process and treatment for hiatal hernia and reflux esophagitis, *"Hiatal Hernia and Reflux Esophagitis," p. 276;* Disease process and therapeutic regimen for achalasia, *"Achalasia," p. 279;* Potential for GI complications and measures that can prevent their occurrence, *"Hernia," p. 291;* Potential for recurrence of hemorrhoids and measures that can help prevent it, *"Hemorrhoids," p. 300;* Colostomy irritation procedure, *"Fecal Diversions," p. 318;* Healthy dietary behaviors and patterns, *"Obesity," p. 321;* Dietary regimen after bariatric surgery, *"Obesity," p. 323;* Causes of hepatitis and modes of transmission, *"Hepatitis," p. 327;* Factors that precipitate or aggravate cirrhosis, *"Cirrhosis," p. 333;* Factors that can precipitate hemolytic crisis and measures that can help prevent it, *"Hemolytic Anemia," p. 345;* Potential for bleeding and measures that can help prevent it, *"Hypoplastic Anemia," p. 349;* Proper use of a heating device, *"Osteoarthritis," p. 368;* Disease process, medication regimen, and potential drug side effects, *"Gouty Arthritis," p. 370;* Proper care of inflamed joints, *"Gouty Arthritis," p. 371;* Signs and symptoms and preventive measures for uric acid renal calculi, *"Gouty Arthritis," p. 371;* Need for elevation of the involved extremity, use of thermotherapy, and exercise regimen, *"Ligamentous Injuries," p. 376;* Care and assessment of the casted extremity, *"Ligamentous Injuries," p. 377;* Potential for joint weakness and the techniques for applying elastic wraps and assessing neurovascular status, *"Ligamentous Injuries," p. 378;* Adverse side effects from prolonged use of potent antibiotics, *"Osteomyelitis," p. 387;* Potential for infection and air embolus related to use of Hickman catheter or similar device for long-term intermittent antibiotic therapy, *"Osteomyelitis," p. 389;* Potential for disuse osteoporosis, *"Fractures," p. 394;* Potential for infection related to orthopedic procedure and/or presence of internal or external device, *"Fractures," p. 395;* Potential for refracture due to vulnerability from presence of internal fixator, *"Fractures," p. 395;* Function of external fixator, pin care, and signs and symptoms of pin site infection, *"Fractures," p. 395;* Disease process and potential for recurrence, *"Benign Neoplasms," p. 397;* Disease process and importance of compliance with the prescribed therapy, *"Malignant Neoplasms," p. 400;* Potential complications of Paget's disease, *"Paget's Disease," p. 402;* Disease process and therapeutic regimen, *"Bunionectomy," p. 403;* Postsurgical exercise regimen, *"Amputation," p. 406;* Care of the stump and prosthesis; signs and symptoms of skin irritation or pressure necrosis, *"Amputation," p. 406;* Potential for and mechanism of THA dislocation, preventive measures, positional restrictions, prescribed ambulation regimen, and use of assistive devices, *"Total Hip Arthroplasty," p. 413;* Potential for infection caused by foreign body reaction to endoprosthesis, *"Total Hip Arthroplasty," p. 413;* Incisional site care and the potential for postoperative capsular contracture, *"Breast Augmentation," p. 421;* Surgical procedure, preoperative care, and postoperative regimen, *"Breast Reconstruction," p. 422;* Potential for postoperative fibrotic capsular contracture and the technique for breast massage, *"Breast Reconstruction," p. 422;* Potential for infection/shock after cystoscopy or TURP, *"Benign Prostatic Hypertrophy," p. 449;* Side effects of estrogen therapy and/or bilateral orchiectomy, *"Prostatic Neoplasm," p. 455;* Diagnosis, treatment plan, and surgical procedure, *"Cataract," p. 465;* Importance of avoiding increased intraocular pressure and activities that can cause it, *"Cataract," p. 466;* Diagnosis and treatment plan, *"Corneal Ulceration," p. 469;* Diagnosis, surgery, precautionery measures, and treatment plan, *"Corneal Transplant," p. 470;* Diagnosis, surgery, and treatment plan, *"Vitreous Disorders and Vitrectomy," p. 472;* Diagnosis, surgery, and treatment plan, *"Glaucoma," p. 475;* Diagnosis, surgical procedure, and treatment plan, *"Retinal Detachment," p. 477;* Surgical procedure, postsurgical precautions, and function of the ocular prosthesis, *"Enucleation," p. 479;* Surgical procedure, postsurgical regimen, and expected outcomes, *"Otosclerosis," p. 480;* Foods relatively high in potassium and diuretics that are potassium-sparing, *"Electrolyte Disturbances," p. 504* and *505;* Surgical procedure, preoperative routine, and postoperative care, *Caring for Preoperative and Postoperative Patients," p. 528;* Potential for severe side effects from radiation and chemotherapy, *"Caring for Patients with Cancer and other Life-Disrupting Ilnesses," p. 548;* Potential for alopecia due to chemotherapy, *"Caring for Patients with Cancer and other Life-Disrupting Illnesses," p. 550;* Effects of radiation and/or chemotherapy on skin integrity, *"Caring for Patients with Cancer and other Life-Disrupting Illnesses," p. 550.*

Mobility, Impaired Physical related to inactivity and/or spasticity secondary to sensorimotor deficits, *"Spinal Cord Injuries," p. 175;* related to prolonged inactivity secondary to sensorimotor deficits and decreased LOC, *"Head Injury," p. 180;* related to imposed activity restrictions secondary to risk of aneurysm or rebleeding, *"Cerebral Aneurysm," p. 191;* related to alterations in the upper and lower limbs secondary to hemiparesis or hemiplegia, *"Cerebrovascular Accident," p. 195;* related to adjustment to a new walking gait with an assistive device, *"Osteoarthritis," p. 368;* related to immobilization device and/or nonweightbearing secondary to bunionectomy, *"Bunionectomy," p. 403;* related to contracture secondary to disuse of the extremity, *"Amputation," p. 405;* related to altered stance secondary to amputation of the lower limb, *"Amputation," p. 405;* related to risk of alterations in the upper extremity secondary to postmastectomy complications, *"Malignant Disorders of the Breast," p. 428;* Contractures and/or muscle atrophy related to inactivity secondary to discomfort and prolonged bed rest, *"Care of the Burn Patient," p. 494;* related to inactivity secondary to prolonged bed rest, *"Caring for Patients on Prolonged Bed Rest," p. 535;* related to imposed activity and positional limitations/restrictions secondary to the presence of a radium implant, *"Caring for Patients with Cancer and other Life-Disrupting Illnesses," p. 547.*

Noncompliance with the therapy related to frustration secondary to negative side effects of anticonvulsant medications and difficulty with making necessary lifestyle changes and/or denial of the illness, *"Seizure Disorders," p. 204;* related to reluctance secondary to need for major lifestyle change and disappointment secondary to slow weight loss, *"Obesity," p. 321;* related to frustration secondary to frequency of antibiotic administration and lack of knowledge of its importance, *"Corneal Ulceration," p. 469;* related to frustration secondary to extensiveness of pharmacologic regimen and lack of knowledge of its importance, *"Glaucoma," p. 475.*

Nutrition, Alterations in: Less Than Body Requirements related to decreased intake secondary to anorexia, *"Pneumonia," p. 6;* related to decreased intake secondary to fatigue and anorexia, *"Asthma," p. 19;* related to decreased intake secondary to fatigue and anorexia, *"Tuberculosis," p. 28;* related to decreased intake secondary to fatigue and anorexia, *"Pulmonary Fibrosis," p. 30;* related to decreased intake secondary to anorexia and increased need secondary to urinary losses of protein, *"Nephrotic Syndrome," p. 97;* related to decreased intake secondary to nausea and/or anorexia, *"Acute Pyelonephritis," p. 100;* related to increased need secondary to protein loss in the dialysate, *"Care of the Peritoneal Dialysis Patient," p. 119;* related to decreased intake secondary to NPO status with adynamic ileus, *"Guillain-Barre Syndrome," p. 151;* related to decreased intake secondary to cognitive and motor deficit; and increased nutritional need secondary to constant pacing and restlessness, *"Alzheimer's Disease," p. 162;* related to history of poor intake and malabsorption secondary to alcoholism, *"Alcohol Abuse," p. 209;* related to increased need secondary to hypermetabolic state, *"Hyperthyroidism," p. 222;* related to decreased intake secondary to anorexia and dietary restrictions and increased need secondary to digestive dysfunction, *"Pancreatitis," p. 250;* related to decreased intake secondary to discomfort with chewing and swallowing, *"Stomatitis," p. 274;* related to decreased intake secondary to dysphagia and/or surgery, *"Achalasia," p. 279;* related to decreased intake secondary to nausea, vomiting, bloating, and anorexia, *"Gastric Neoplasm," p. 284;* related to losses secondary to vomiting and intestinal suctioning and increased need secondary to GI dysfunction, *"Peritonitis," p. 294;* related to decreased intake secondary to dietary restriction and/or postsurgical regimen, *"Obesity," p. 322;* related to decreased intake secondary to anorexia, nausea, and gastric distress, *"Hepatitis," p. 327;* related to decreased intake secondary to anorexia and nausea, *"Cirrhosis," p. 331;* related to decreased intake secondary to fatigue, impairment of oral mucosa, and/or anorexia, *"Pernicious Anemia," p. 342;* related to decreased intake secondary to feelings of fullness (associated with congestion of organ systems), *"Polycythemia," p. 351;* related to increased need for calcium and vitamin D, *"Osteoporosis," p. 400;* related to increased need secondary to hypermetabolic state associated with burn injury, *"Care of the Burn Patient," p. 493;* related to increased need or decreased intake, *"Providing Nutritional Therapy," p. 520;* related to decreased intake secondary to chewing and swallowing deficits, fatigue, weakness, paresis, paralysis, visual neglect, and/or decreased LOC, *"Caring for Patients with Neurologic Problems," p. 538;* related to decreased intake secondary to anorexia, nausea, and stomatitis (side effects of chemo/radiation therapy), *"Caring for Patients with Cancer and other Life-Disrupting Illnesses," p. 550.*

Nutrition, Alterations in: More Than Body Requirements related to excessive intake of calories, sodium, and /or fats, *"Coronary Artery Disease," p. 42;* related to hyperphagia secondary to cocaine withdrawal, *"Cocaine Abuse," p. 214;* related to decreased need secondary to slowed metabolism, *"Hypothyroidism," p. 227;* related to excessive intake of purines and/or alcohol, *"Gouty Arthritis," p. 371.*

Oral Mucous Membrane, Alterations in related to stomatitis, *"Stomatitis," p. 273.*

**Respiratory Function, Alterations in related to blockage, air leak, or dislodging of chest tube, *"Pneumothorax," p. 3;* related to blockage or dislodging of chest tube, *"Hemothorax," p. 11;* related to prolonged inactivity and/or omission of deep breathing, *"Atelectasis," p. 12;* related to decreased lung expansion secondary to fluid accumulation in the pleural space, *"Pleural Effusion," p. 14;* related to decreased lung capacity secondary to thoracotomy, *"Bronchogenic Carcinoma," p. 32;* related to immobility, embolus, and/or increased secretions secondary to paresis or plegia of the respiratory muscles, and/or restriction of chest expansion secondary to halo vest traction, *"Spinal Cord Injuries," p. 175;* related to imposed inactivity secondary to the risk of aneurysm rupture or rebleeding, *"Cerebral Aneurysm," p. 190;* related to edema and/or laryngeal nerve damage secondary to surgical procedure, *"Hyperthyroidism," p. 224;* related to decreased ventilatory drive or upper airway obstruction secondary to myxedematous infiltration, *"Hypothyroidism," p. 227;* related to diminished oxygen transport secondary to loss of circulating volume, and/or guarding secondary to severe abdominal pain, *"Peritonitis," p. 293;* related to distress secondary to smoke inhalation and inactivity secondary to prolonged bed rest, *"Care of the Burn Patient," p. 492;* related to increased risk of aspiration secondary to tube-feeding therapy, *"Providing Nutritional Therapy," p. 521;* related to aspiration or airway obstruction secondary to presence of an NG tube, *"Caring for Preoperative and Postoperative Patients," p. 531.*

Ineffective Airway Clearance related to pain and fatigue secondary to lung consolidation, *"Pneumonia," p. 5;* related to ineffective coughing, *"Acute Respiratory Failure," p. 17;* related to excessive mucus production and ineffective coughing, *"Asthma," p. 19;* related to coughing and swallowing deficits secondary to weakness or paralysis of the facial, throat, and respiratory muscles, *"Guillain-Barré Syndrome," p. 151;* related to coughing and swallowing deficits secondary to facial and throat muscle weakness and/or decreasing LOC, *"Caring for Patients with Neurologic Problems," p. 540.*

Ineffective Breathing Patterns related to guarding secondary to pain at the affected lung site, *"Pleurisy," p. 7;* related to hyperpnea secondary to infectious process, *"Tuberculosis," p. 28;* related to hyperpnea secondary to decreased lung compliance, *"Pulmonary Fibrosis," p. 30;* related to guarding secondary to pericardial pain, *"Pericarditis," p. 53;* related to hypoventilation secondary to respiratory depression with use of narcotics, and/or guarding secondary to painful abdominal incision, *"Pancreatic Tumors," p. 254;* related to guarding secondary to pain of thoracic incision and/or chest tube insertion, *"Hiatal Hernia and Reflux Esophagitis," p. 276;* related to decreased inspiratory depth secondary to anesthesia and/or guarding from painful abdominal incision, *"Obesity," p. 323;* related to restricted chest movement secondary to impairment/paralysis of respiratory muscles, *"Electrolyte Disturbances," p. 504;* related to hyperventilation, *"Acid–Base Imbalances," p. 512;* related to decreased respiratory depth secondary to anesthesia, immobility, or guarding with painful surgical incision, *"Caring for Preoperative and Postoperative Patients," p. 530.*

Impaired Gas Exchange related to tissue hypoxia secondary to decreased lung capacity, *"Pneumothorax," p. 3;* related to tissue hypoxia secondary to inflammatory process, *"Pneumonia," p. 6;* related to chronic tissue hypoxia secondary to disease process, *"Acute Respiratory Failure," p. 16;* related to chronic tissue hypoxia secondary to obstructive process in the bronchioles and bronchi, *"Asthma," p. 19;* related to chronic tissue hypoxia secondary to bronchiole obstruction, *"Chronic Bronchitis," p. 21;* related to decreased lung capacity and trapping of CO_2 secondary to pulmonary tissue destruction and/or cystic tissue formation, *"Emphysema," p. 24;* related to decreased lung capacity secondary to ongoing lung tissue destruction, *"Pneumoconioses," p. 26;* related to altered oxygen transport secondary to pulmonary capillary constriction and restricted blood flow, *"Pulmonary Hypertension," p. 37;* related to tissue hypoxia secondary to fluid accumulation in the lungs, *"Myocardial Infarction," p. 46;* related to tissue hypoxia secondary to decreased circulating blood volume, *"Cardiac and Noncardiac Shock," p. 66;* related to tissue hypoxia secondary to fluid accumulation in the alveoli, *"Pulmonary Edema," p. 69;* related to decreased lung expansion secondary to pressure on the diaphragm caused by ascites, *"Cirrhosis," p. 331;* related to tissue hypoxia secondary to pulmonary edema, *"Fluid Disturbances," p. 499.*

Self-Care Deficit: Inability to perform ADLs related to memory loss and coordination problems secondary to cognitive and motor deficits, *"Alzheimer's Disease," p. 163;* Inability to perform ADLs related to imposed activity restrictions secondary to risk of aneurysm rupture or rebleeding, *"Cerebral Aneurysm," p. 191;* Inability to perform oral hygiene related to sensorimotor deficit or decreased LOC, *"Stomatitis," p. 273;* Inability to perform ADLs related to physical limitations secondary to cast and/or surgical procedure, *"Fractures," p. 393;* Inability to perform ADLs related to imposed activity restrictions and visual deficit, *"Cataract," p. 467;* Inability to perform ADLs related to spasticity, tremors, weakness, paresis, paralysis, or decreasing LOC secondary to sensorimotor deficits, *"Caring for Patients with Neurologic Problems," p. 540.*

Self-Concept, Disturbance in related to odor and discomfort secondary to incontinence, *"Urinary Incontinence," p. 136;* related to altered body image secondary to exophthalmos and/or surgical scar, *"Hyperthyroidism," p. 222;* related to altered body image secondary to physical changes associated with increased ACTH production, *"Cushing's Disease," p. 241;* related to alteration in body image secondary to fecal diversion, *"Fecal Diversions," p. 317;* related to alteration in body image secondary to jaundice, *"Hepatitis," p. 328;* related to alteration in body image and role performance secondary to amputation, *"Amputation," p. 407;* related to body image secondary to small breast size, *"Breast Augmentation," p. 420;* related to altered body image secondary to breast reconstruction surgery, *"Breast Reconstruction," p. 423;* related to altered body image secondary to loss of a breast, *"Malignant Disorders of the Breast," p. 429;* related to altered body image and role performance expectations secondary to diagnosis of cancer, *"Cancer of the Cervix," p. 433;* related to changes in body image and role performance expectations secondary to hysterectomy, *"Uterine Prolapse," p. 442;* related to altered expectations for role performance secondary to loss of fetus, *"Spontaneous Abortion," p. 445;* related to actual and perceived changes in sexual function secondary to impending orchiectomy, *"Testicular Neoplasm," p. 458;* related to altered body image secondary to the presence of a penile implant, *"Penile Implants," p. 460;* related to alteration in body image secondary to loss of body part or body function, *"Caring for Patients with Cancer and other Life-Disrupting Illnesses," p. 544.*

Sensory-Perceptual Alterations related to inability to evaluate reality secondary to degeneration of intellectual functioning, *"Alzheimer's Disease," p. 163;* related to sensory overload secondary to degeneration of intellectual functioning, *"Alzheimer's Disease," p. 163;* related to neglect of the affected side secondary to neurologic deficit, *"Cerebrovascular Accident," p. 194;* related to confusion secondary to cerebral retention of water, *"Hypothyroidism," p. 228;* related to confusion secondary to infectious process, *"Prostatitis," p. 453;* related to visual deficit secondary to disease process and/or presence of cataract glasses, eye shield, eye patch, or other measure that distorts or diminishes vision, *"Cataract," p. 465;* related to auditory deficit secondary to disease process, postoperative earplug, and/or tissue edema, *"Otosclerosis," p. 481.*

Sexual Dysfunction related to physiologic limitations secondary to abnormal hormone levels, *"Pituitary Tumors," p. 246;* related to fear of impotence secondary to lack of knowledge of postsurgical sexual function, *"Benign Prostatic Hypertrophy," p. 450;* related to actual or perceived physiologic limitations on sexual performance secondary to disease, therapy, or prolonged hospitalization, *"Caring for Patients on Prolonged Bed Rest," p. 534.*

Skin Integrity, Impairment of related to vulnerability secondary to venous stasis and rupture of small veins, *"Venous Thrombosis/Thrombophlebitis," p. 86;* related to irritation secondary to wound drainage (pyelolithotomy), *"Renal Calculi," p. 101;* related to pruritus secondary to uremia, *"Chronic Renal Failure," p. 113;* related to irritation secondary to postoperative wound drainage, *"Ureteral Calculi," p. 125;* Stoma and peristomal area related to erythema, improper appliance, or sensitivity to appliance material, *"Urinary Diversions," p. 133;* related to irritation of perineum secondary to incontinence of urine, *"Urinary Incontinence," p. 136;* related to irritation or pressure secondary to cervical or pelvic traction, *"Herniated Nucleus Pulposus," p. 170;* related to irritation and pressure secondary to presence of halo vest traction, *"Spinal Cord Injuries," p. 176;* related to vulnerability secondary to thinning of skin and fragility of capillaries, *"Cushing's Disease," p. 241;* related to irritation secondary to wound drainage and/or pressure on the incision, *"Pancreatic Tumors," p. 254;* related to increased susceptibility secondary to peripheral neuropathy and vascular pathology, *"Diabetes Mellitus—General Discussion," p. 259;* Perineal/perianal area related to irritation secondary to persistent diarrhea, *"Ulcerative Colitis," p. 308;* Stoma and peristomal area related to erythema, improper appliance, or sensitivity to appliance material, *"Fecal Diversions," p. 315;* (with concomitant risk of poor wound healing) related to vulnerability secondary to sedentary lifestyle, *"Obesity," p. 323;* related to pruritus secondary to hepatic dysfunction, *"Hepatitis," p. 328;* related to vulnerability secondary to occlusion of the vessels and impaired oxygen transport to the tissues and skin, *"Hemolytic Anemia," p. 343;* related to irritation secondary to presence of a cast, *"Fractures," p. 393;* related to maceration of the axillary skin secondary to shoulder immobilization, *"Repair of Recurrent Shoulder Dislocation," p. 411;* related to irritation secondary to wound drainage, *"Benign Prostatic Hypertrophy," p. 450;* related to vulnerability secondary to imposed immobility and positional restrictions, *"Retinal Detachment," p. 477;* Wound site, related to risk of infection, metabolic alterations, impaired oxygen transport, altered tissue perfusion, and nutritional alterations, *"Wounds Closed by Primary Intention," p. 483;* related to impaired wound healing, *"Surgical and/or Traumatic Wounds Healing by Secondary Intention," p. 486;* Wound, related to alterations in fluid volume and nutrition, *"Surgical and/or Traumatic Wounds Healing by Secondary Intention," p. 487;* related to excessive tissue pressure secondary to prolonged immobility, *"Pressure Ulcers," p. 488;* related to pressure ulcer, *"Pressure Ulcers," p. 489;* related to mucosal and skin surface irritation secondary to presence of feeding tube, *"Providing Nutritional Therapy," p. 520;* related to continous mucosal and skin surface irritation secondary to presence of NG tube, *"Caring for Preoperative and Postoperative Patients," p. 531;* related to irritation of skin around percutaneous drains and tubes, *"Caring for Preoperative and Postoperative Patients," p. 532.*

Sleep Pattern Disturbance related to awakening secondary to pain and dyspnea, *"Pleurisy," p. 8;* related to awakening secondary to dyspnea and treatment schedule, *"Acute Respiratory Failure," p. 16;* related to awakening for VS assessment or medication administration, *"Myocardial Infarction," p. 46;* related to agitation secondary to withdrawal from short-acting CNS depressant, *"Alcohol Abuse," p. 209;* related to agitation secondary to accelerated metabolism, *"Hyperthroidism," p. 221;* related to agitation secondary to hepatic dysfunction, *"Hepatitis," p. 327.*

Social Isolation related to imposed restrictions secondary to presence of radioactive implants, *"Caring for Patients with Cancer and Other Life-Disrupting Illnesses," p. 546.*

Tissue Perfusion, Alteration in: Cardiopulmonary and peripheral related to impaired circulation secondary to embolus formation, *"Cardiomyopathy," p. 40;* Peripheral, cardiopulmonary, and cerebral related to impaired circulation secondary to dysfunctional cardiac muscle, *"Pericarditis," p. 52;* Peripheral, cardiopulmonary, cerebral, and renal related to impaired circulation secondary to decreased circulating blood volume, *"Cardiac and Noncardiac Shock," p. 65;* Cardiopulmonary, peripheral, and cerebral related to impaired circulation secondary to decreased cardiac output, *"Pulmonary Edema," p. 69;* Peripheral and cardiopulmonary related to impaired circulation secondary to pacemaker malfunction, *"Pacemakers," p. 71;* Peripheral, cardiopulmonary, and cerebral related to impaired circulation secondary to the catheterization procedure, *"Cardiac Catheterization," p. 73;* Peripheral related to impaired circulation secondary to embolization, *"Cardiac Catheterization," p. 74;* Renal related to impaired circulation secondary to decreased cardiac output or reaction to contrast dye, *"Cardiac Catheterization," p. 74;* Peripheral related to impaired circulation secondary to graft occlusion, *"Atherosclerotic Arterial Occlusive Disease,". p. 79;* Renal related to impaired circulation secondary to decreased blood supply during surgery, *"Atherosclerotic Arterial Occlusive Disease," p. 80;* Peripheral related to impaired circulation secondary to postoperative embolization, *"Aneurysms," p. 82;* Peripheral related to impaired circulation secondary to embolization (preoperative period), *"Arterial Embolism," p. 83;* Peripheral related to impaired circulation secondary to embolization, *"Venous Thrombosis/Thrombophlebitis," p. 85;* Peripheral related to impaired circulation secondary to venous engorgement, *"Venous Thrombosis/Thrombophlebitis," p. 86;* Peripheral, cardiopulmonary, renal, cerebral, and gastrointestinal related to impaired circulation and sensation secondary to development and progression of macroangiopathy and microangiopathy, *"Diabetes Mellitus—General Discussion," p. 258;* Renal related to impaired circulation secondary to hemolytic obstruction, *"Hemolytic Anemia," p. 344;* Peripheral and cardiopulmonary related to decreased circulation secondary to inflammatory process and occlusion of blood vessels with RBCs, *"Hemolytic Anemia," p. 344;* Peripheral and cerebral related to tissue hypoxia secondary to decreased production of erythrocytes, *"Hypoplastic Anemia," p. 349;* Peripheral and cerebral related to decreased circulation secondary to phlebotomy, *"Polycythemia," p. 351;* Peripheral and renal related to decreased circulation secondary to hyperviscosity of the blood, *"Polycythemia," p. 351;* Peripheral, cerebral, and renal related to altered circulation secondary to coagulation/fibrinolysis processes, *"Disseminated Intravascular Coagulation," p. 357;* Renal related to decreased circulation secondary to destruction of RBCs and their precipitation in kidney tubules, *"Acute Leukemia," p. 361;* Peripheral, cerebral, or cardiopulmonary related to impaired circulation secondary to fat embolization, *"Fractures," p. 394;* Peripheral related to impaired circulation secondary to compression from circumferential cast or dressing, *"Bunionectomy," p. 404;* Peripheral, related to impaired circulation and compression of the musculocutaneous nerve secondary to pressure from the immobilization device, *"Repair of Recurrent Shoulder Dislocation," p. 411;* Peripheral, related to impaired circulation secondary to compression from traction or abduction device, *"Total Hip Arthroplasty," p. 414;* Peripheral related to edema secondary to burn injury or skin grafting, *"Care of the Burn Patient," p. 493;* Cardiopulmonary, related to impaired circulation secondary to complications of central vein nutritional therapy, *"Providing Nutritional Therapy," p. 523;* Gastrointestinal, related to altered peristalsis secondary to general anesthesia and surgical procedure, *"Caring for Preoperative and Postoperative Patients," p. 528;* Peripheral, related to compromised circulation secondary to prolonged immobility, *"Caring for Patients on Prolonged Bed Rest," p. 533;* Cerebral, related to orthostatic hypotension secondary to prolonged bed rest, *"Caring for Patients on Prolonged Bed Rest," p. 536.*

Urinary Elimination, Alteration in Patterns of: Dysuria, urgency, or frequency related to the presence of a ureteral calculus, *"Ureteral Calculus," p. 124;* related to obstruction or positional problems of the ureteral catheter, *"Ureteral Calculus," p. 124;* related to obstruction of suprapubic catheter or anuria/dysuria secondary to removal of the catheter, *"Cancer of the Bladder," p. 130;* related to postoperative use of catheters, stents, and/or rectal tube, *"Urinary Diversions," p. 134;* related to acute retention, *"Urinary Retention," p. 139;* related to retention secondary to bladder dysfunction, *"Neurogenic Bladder," p. 140;* related to incontinence or retention secondary to cognitive deficit, *"Alzheimer's Disease," p. 162;* Anuria or dysuria related to local swelling and/or presence of rectal packing secondary to hemorrhoidectomy, *"Hemor-rhoids," p. 299;* related to inadequate intake or obstruction of indwelling catheter, *"Cancer of the Cervix," p. 433;* related to dysuria or anuria secondary to obstructive process associated with prostatitis, *"Prostatitis," p. 453;* Dysuria, urgency, or fre-quency related to presence of renal calculi, *"Electrolyte Disturbances," p. 506.*

Violence, Potential for related to irritability, frustration, and disorientation second-ary to degeneration of cognitive thinking, *"Alzheimer's Disease," p. 164;* related to hal-lucinations/paranoia secondary to cocaine use/withdrawal, *"Cocaine Abuse," p. 213.*

*NANDA-approved nursing diagnoses that are not discussed in this manual.

**Nursing diagnosis not approved by NANDA.

Appendix Three Abbreviations Used in this Manual

AA: Alcoholics Anonymous
ABG: arterial blood gas
AC: before meals
ACL: anterior cruciate ligament
ACTH: adrenocorticotropic hormone
ADH: antidiuretic hormone
ADL: activity of daily living
ALL: acute lymphoblastic leukemia
A P: anterior posterior
ARF: acute respiratory failure
ASA: acetylsalicylic acid
ATN: acute tubular necrosis
A-V: atrioventricular

BEE: basal energy expenditure
BP: blood pressure
BSE: breast self-examination
BUN: blood urea nitrogen
bid: twice a day

C: cervical
CABG: coronary artery bypass grafting
CAD: coronary artery disease
CBC: complete blood count
CBI: continuous bladder irrigation
CCU: coronary care unit
CHF: congestive heart failure
CNS: central nervous system
CO₂: carbon dioxide
COPD: chronic obstructive pulmonary disease
CPK: creatinine phosphokinase
CPM: continuous passive movement
CRF: chronic renal failure
CSF: cerebrospinal fluid
CT: computerized axial tomography
CVA: cerebrovascular accident
CVP: central venous pressure

Cl: chloride
cm: centimeter

DJD: degenerative joint disease
DKA: diabetes ketoacidosis
D₅W: 5% dextrose in water
DTs: delirium tremens
DTR: deep tendon reflex
dL: deciliter

ECF: extracellular fluid
EEG: electroencephalogram
EKG: electrocardiogram
EMG: electromyography
ESR: erythrocyte sedimentation rate
ESRD: end-stage renal disease
ET: enterostomal therapy
eg: for example

FSH: follicle-stimulating hormone

GH: growth hormone
GI: gastrointestinal
GN: glomerulonephritis
g: gram

HCG: human chorionic gonadotropin
HCO₃: bicarbonate
HHNC: hyperosmolar hyperglycemic non-ketotic coma
HOB: head of bed
h: hour
hct: hematocrit
hgb: hemoglobin
hs: hour of sleep

I&O: intake and output
ICF: intracellular fluid

ICP: intracranial pressure
ICU: intensive care unit
IDDM: insulin-dependent diabetes mellitus
IM: intramuscular
IPPD: intermittent positive pressure breathing
IUD: intrauterine device
IV: intravenous
IVP: intravenous pyelogram

K: potassium
KUB: kidney, ureter, bladder
kg: kilogram

L: liter; lumbar
LDH: lactate dehydrogenase
LES: lower esophageal sphincter
LH: luteinizing hormone
LLQ: left lower quadrant
LOC: level of consciousness
lb: pound

MI: myocardial infarction
MR: magnetic resonance
MS: multiple sclerosis
MSG: monosodium glutamate
mEq: milliequivalent
mg: milligram
min: minute
mL: milliliter
mm Hg: millimeters of mercury
mOsm: milliosmol
μg: microgram

N: nitrogen
NG: nasogastric
NIDDM: non-insulin-dependent diabetes mellitus
NPO: nothing by mouth
Na: sodium
ng: nanogram

O$_2$: oxygen
ORIF: open reduction with internal fixation
OT: occupational therapist
OTC: over-the-counter

PCM: protein-calorie malnutrition
PIP: proximal interphalangeal
PMI: point of maximal impulse
PT: physical therapist; prothrombin time
PTH: parathyroid hormone
PTT: partial thromboplastin time

Paco$_2$: partial pressure of dissolved carbon dioxide in arterial blood
Pao$_2$: partial pressure of dissolved oxygen in arterial blood
pc: after meals
pg: picogram
po: by mouth
prn: as needed

q: every

RA: rheumatoid arthritis
RBC: red blood cell
RDA: recommended daily allowance
RLQ: right lower quadrant
RUQ: right upper quadrant
ROM: range of motion

SC: subcutaneous
SGOT: serum glutamic oxaloacetic-acid-transaminase
SGPT: serum glutamic pyruvic transaminase
SIADH: secretion of inappropriate anti-diuretic hormone
SO: significant other
SOB: shortness of breath
stat: immediately

T: thoracic
TB: tuberculosis
TBSA: total body surface area
THA: total hip arthroplasty
TIA: transient ischemic attack
TKA: total knee arthroplasty
TKO: to keep open
TOPS: Take Off Pounds Sensibly
TPN: total parenteral nutrition
TPR: temperature, pulse, respirations
TRH: thyrotropin-releasing hormone
TSH: thyroid-stimulating hormone
TUR: transurethral resection

U: unit
UA: urinalysis
URI: upper respiratory infection
UTI: urinary tract infection
UUN: urine urea nitrogen

VMA: vanillamandelic acid
VS: vital signs

WBC: white blood cell

Appendix Four **Normal Values for Laboratory Tests Discussed in This Manual**

Whole Blood, Serum, and Plasma (Chemistry)

Test	Specimen	Normal Values*
ACTH	Plasma	8 AM–10 AM: <80 pg/mL
Albumin	Serum	3.5–5.5 g/dL
Aldosterone	Serum	Female: 4–31 ng/dL
		Male: 6–22 ng/dL
α_1-Antitrypsin	Serum	210–500 mg/mL
α_1-Fetoprotein (AFP)	Serum	Males and nonpregnant females: <25 ng/mL
Ammonia	Whole blood	70–200 μg/dL*
	Plasma	56–150 μg/dL
Amylase	Serum	60–180 Somogyi units/dL
Antidiuretic hormone (ADH)	Plasma	0–2 pg/mL: serum osmolality <285 mOsm/kg
		2–12 pg/mL: serum osmolality >290 mOsm/kg
Base, total	Serum	145–160 mEq/L
Bicarbonate	Plasma	22–26 mEq/L
Bilirubin	Serum	Direct: 0.1–0.4 mg/dL
		Indirect: 0.2–1.0 mg/dL
		Total: 0.3–1.4 mg/dL
Blood gases, arterial	Whole blood	
pH		7.38–7.42
$Paco_2$		36–44 mm Hg
Pao_2		80–100 mm Hg
Bromsulphthalein (BSP) 5 mg/kg	Serum	<0.4 mg/dL or 5% retention after 45 minutes
Calcitonin	Serum or plasma	<425 pg/mL
Calcium	Serum	Adults:
		8.5–10.5 mg/dL
		4.3–5.3 mEq/L
Carcinoembryonic antigen (CEA)	Plasma	0–2.5 ng/mL
Carotene	Serum	50–300 μg/dL (varies with diet)
Chloride	Serum	95–108 mEq/L
Cholesterol, fractionated	Plasma	
HDL cholesterol		29–77 mg/dL
LDL cholesterol		62–185 mg/dL
VLDL cholesterol		0–40 mg/dL
Cortisol	Plasma	8 AM–10 AM: 5–25 μg/dL
		4 PM–midnight: 2–18 μg/dL
Creatine phosphokinase (CPK)	Serum	Male:
		55–170 U/L*
		5–35 U/mL
		Female:
		30–135 U/L*
		5–25 U/mL

*Normal values may vary significantly with different laboratory methods.

Adapted from Byrne, C. J. et al. 1986. *Laboratory Tests: Implications for Nursing Care*, 2nd ed. Menlo Park, Calif.: Addison-Wesley Publishing Co.

Whole Blood, Serum, and Plasma (Chemistry) *continued*

Test	Specimen	Normal Values*
Creatinine	Serum	0.6–1.5 mg/dL
Creatinine clearance	Serum or plasma and urine	Male: 107–141 mL/min Female: 87–132 mL/min
Estradiol	Serum or plasma	Male: 8–50 pg/mL Female: (menstrual cycle) 1–10 days: 20–170 pg/mL 11–20 days: 70–500 pg/mL 21–30 days: 45–340 pg/mL
Estrogens, total	Serum or plasma	Male: 35–130 pg/mL Female: (menstrual cycle) Follicular: 60–250 pg/mL Midcycle: 120–570 pg/mL Luteal: 75–450 pg/mL
Fats, neutral	Serum or plasma	0–200 mg/dL
Fatty acids, free	Serum	<25 mg/dL; 0.3–1.0 mEq/L
Fibrinogen	Plasma	200–400 mg/dL
Follicle-stimulating hormone (FSH)	Seru	Male: 4–25 mIU/mL Female: Premenopausal: 4–30 mIU/mL Midcycle peak: 2 × baseline Postmenopausal: 40–250 mIU/mL
Globulins, total	Serum	1.5–3.5 g/dL
Glucose, fasting	Serum	"True glucose": 65–110 mg/dL All sugars: 80–120 mg/dL
Glucose, 2-hour postprandial	Serum	<145 mg/dL
Glucose tolerance, intravenous	Serum or plasma	Fasting: 65–110 mg/dL 5 minutes: maximum of 250 mg/dL 60 minutes: significant decrease 120 minutes: below 120 mg/d' 180 minutes: fasting level
Glucose tolerance, oral	Serum or plasma	Fasting: 65–110 mg/dL 30 minutes: <155 mg/dL 60 minutes: <165 mg/dL 120 minutes: <120 mg/dL 180 minutes: fasting level or less
Growth hormone (GH)	Serum	Male: <10 ng/mL Female: <15 ng/mL
Human chorionic gonadotropin (HCG)	Serum	<3 mIU/mL Pregnancy: >10mIU/L by 10 days after implantation
17-Hydroxycortico-steroids (17-OCHS)	Plasma	Male: 7–19 µg/dL Female: 9–21 µg/dL After administration of 25 units of ACTH intramuscularly: 35–55 µg/dL
Immunoglobulins IgG IgA IgM	Serum	 Adults: 80%; 800–1600 mg/dL Adults: 15%; 50–250 mg/dL Adults: 0.5%; 40–120 mg/dL
Insulin	Plasma	11–240 µIU/mL* 4–24 µU/mL
Iron, total	Serum	60–200 µg/dL Male average: 125 µg/dL Female average: 100 µg/dL Elderly: 60–80 µg/dL

Whole Blood, Serum, and Plasma (Chemistry) *continued*

Test	Specimen	Normal Values*
Iron-binding capacity	Serum	Adult: 250−420 μg/dL
Iron saturation	Serum	Male: 35%−40% Female: 30%−35%
Ketone bodies	Serum	2−4 μg/dL
Lactate dehydro- genase (LDH)	Serum	80−120 Wacker units* 150−450 Wroblewski units 71−207 IU/L
Lipase	Serum	Less than 1.5 U/mL* 14−280 mIU/mL
Lipids Total Cholesterol Triglycerides Phospholipids Phospholipid phosphorus Fatty acids, free Neutral fat	Serum	 400−800 mg/dL 120−260 mg/dL (varies with age) 0−190 mg/dL 150−380 mg/dL 8−11 mg/dL Less than 25 mg/dL 0−200 mg/dL
Luteinizing hormone (LH)	Plasma	Male: <11 mIU/mL Female: Midcycle peak <3 × baseline value Premenopausal: <25 mIU/mL Postmenopausal: >25 mIU/mL
Magnesium	Serum	1.8−3.0 mg/dL 1.5−2.5 mEq/L
Methotrexate	Serum or plasma	Toxic level: >41 μg/dL
Nitrogen (NPN)	Whole blood	25−40 mg/dL
Osmolality	Serum	275−300 mOsm/kg
Parathyroid hormone	Serum	<2000 pg/mL
Phosphatase, acid	Serum	0−1.1 U/mL (Bodansky)* 1−4 U/mL (King-Armstrong) 0.13−0.63 U/mL (Bessey-Lowery)
Phosphatase, alkaline	Serum	Adults: 1.5−4.5 U/dL (Bodansky)* 4−13 U/dL (King-Armstrong) 0.8−2.3 U/mL (Bessey-Lowery)
Phosphorus	Serum	Adults: 3.0−4.5 mg/dL 1.8−2.6 mEq/L
Potassium	Serum	3.6−5.0 mEq/L
Progesterone	Serum or plasma	Male: <100 ng/mL Female: Follicular phase: 0.3−0.8 ng/mL Luteal phase: 1.2−25.8 ng/mL Normal pregnancy >28 weeks: 45−286 ng/mL Hypertensive pregnancy: 22−210 ng/mL
Prolactin	Serum	Male: 0−28 ng/mL Female: Follicular phase: 4−28 ng/dL Luteal phase: 5−40 ng/dL

*Normal values may vary significantly with different laboratory methods.

Whole Blood, Serum, and Plasma (Chemistry) *continued*

Test	Specimen	Normal Values
Renin	Plasma	Normal salt intake (100–180 mEq of sodium): Supine (4–6 hours): 0.5–1.6 ng/mL/hr Upright (4 hours): 1.8–3.6 ng/mL/hr Low salt intake (10 mEq of sodium for 4 days): Supine (4–6 hours): 2.2–4.4 ng/mL/hr Upright (4 hours): 4.0–8.1 ng/mL/hr With diuretic: 6.8–15.1 ng/mL/hr
Testosterone	Serum or plasma	Male: 400–1200 ng/dL Female: 30–120 ng/dL
Thyroid-stimulating hormone (TSH)	Serum	Adult: <4.6 μU/mL
Thyroid tests Protein-bound iodine	Serum	4.0–8.0 μg/dL
T_4 (radio-immunoassay)		Adult: 4.5–12.0 μg/dL
T_4 free	Serum	0.9–2.3 ng/dL
T_4 (by column)		4.5–11.0 μg/dL of thyroxine 3.2–7.2 μg/dL of thyroxine iodine
T_4 (Murphy-Pattee)		6.0–11.8 μg/dL of thyroxine 3.9–7.7 μg/dL of thyroxine iodine
T_3 (radio-immunoassay)		1.10–2.30 ng/dL
T_3 uptake		25%–35%
T_3 free		250–390 pg/dL
T_7 (free thyroxine index)		1.3–4.4
Thyroid-binding globulin (TBG)		10–26 μg/dL
Transferrin	Serum	200–400 mg/dL
Triglycerides	Serum	0–29 years: 10–140 mg/dL 30–39 years: 10–150 mg/dL 40–49 years: 10–160 mg/dL 50–59 years: 10–190 mg/dL
Urea clearance	Serum and 24-hour urine	64–99 mL/min (maximum clearance) 41–65 mL/min (standard clearance) or more than 75% of normal clearance
Urea nitrogen (BUN)	Serum	6–20 mg/dL
Uric acid	Serum	Male: 2.1–7.5 mg/dL Female: 2.0–6.6 mg/dL
Vitamin A	Serum	15–60 μg/dL
Vitamin B_{12}	Serum	Male: 200–800 pg/mL Female: 100–650 pg/mL
Vitamin C (ascorbic acid)	Whole blood Plasma	0.7–2.0 mg/dL 0.6–1.6 mg/dL
Vitamin D 25 hydroxy-cholecalciferol	Serum	10–60 ng/mL (lack of exposure to sunlight may reduce range)
Vitamin E	Serum	5–20 μg/mL
Zinc	Serum	50–150 μg/dL

Urine

Test	Specimen	Normal Values
Albumin	Random	Negative
	24-hour	10–100 mg/24 hr
Amylase	2-hour	35–260 Somogyi units/hr
	24-hour	80–5000 U/24 hr
Bence-Jones protein	Random	Negative
Bilirubin	Random	Negative: 0.02 mg/dL
Calcium	Random	1+ turbidity
		10 mg/dL
	24-hour	50–300 mg/24 hr (depends on diet)
		25–200 mEq/24 hr
Catecholamines	Random	0–18 μg/dL
	24-hour	Less than 100 μg/24 hr (varies with activity)
Concentration test	Random, after fluid restriction	1.025–1.035
Cortisol, free	24-hour	Men: 20–69 μg/24 hr
		Women: 8–63 μg/24 hr
Creatinine	24-hour	Male:
		20–26 mg/kg/24 hr
		1.0–2.0 g/24 hr
		Female:
		14–22 mg/kg/24 hr
		0.6–1.8 g/24 hr
Creatinine clearance	Serum or plasma and urine	Male: 107–141 mL/min
		Female: 87–132 mL/min
Glucose	Random	Negative: 15 mg/dL
	24-hour	130 mg/24 hr
Ketone	Random	Negative: 0.3–2.0 mg/dL
17-Ketosteroids (17-KS)	24-hour	Male: 8–25 mg/24 hr
		Female: 5–15 mg/24 hr
		Over 65: 4–8 mg/24 hr
		After 25 units of ACTH IM: 50%–100% increase
Microscopic examination	Random	RBC: 2–3/high-power field
		WBC: 4–5/high-power field
		Hyaline casts: occasional
		Bacteria: fewer than 1000/mL
Osmolality	Random	Male: 390–1090 mOsm/kg
		Female: 300–1090 mOsm/kg
	24-hour	Male: 770–1630 mOsm/24 hr
		Female: 430–1150 mOsm/24 hr
pH	Random	4.6–8.0
Phenolsulfon-phthalein (PSP)	Timed collection after 6 mg of PSP dye IV	15 minutes: 25%–35% of dye excreted
		30 minutes: 15%–25% of dye excreted
		60 minutes: 10%–15% of dye excreted
		120 minutes: 3%–10% of dye excreted
Phosphorus	24-hour	0.9–1.3 g/24 hr
		0.2–0.6 mEq/24 hr
Protein	Random	Negative: 2–8 mg/dL
	24-hour	40–150 mg/24 hr
Specific gravity	Random	1.016–1.022 (normal fluid intake)
		1.001–1.040 (range)
Sugar	Random	Negative

Urine *continued*

Test	Specimen	Normal Values
Urea clearance	Serum and 24-hour urine	64–99 mL/min (maximum clearance) 41–65 mL/min (standard clearance) or more than 75% of normal clearance
Urea nitrogen	24-hour	6–17 g/24 hr
Urobilinogen	2-hour	0.3–1.0 Ehrlich units
	24-hour	0.5–4.0 Ehrlich units/24 hr 0.05–2.5 mg/24 hr
Vanillylmandelic acid (VMA)	24-hour	0.5–14 mg/24 hr

Hematology

Complete Blood Count (CBC)	Normal Values, Adults
Hemoglobin	Male: 14–18 g/dL Female: 12–16 g/dL
Hematocrit	Male: 40%–54% Female: 37%–47%
Red blood cell count	Male: 4.5–6.0 million/μL Female: 4.0–5.5 million/μL
White blood cell count	4500–11,000/μL
Neutrophils	54%–75% (3000–7500/μL)
Band neutrophils	3%–8% (150–700/μL)
Lymphocytes	25%–40% (1500–4500/μL)
Monocytes	2%–8% (100–500/μL)
Eosinophils	1%–4% (50–400/μL)
Basophils	0%–1% (25–100/μL)
Erythrocyte indices	
Mean corpuscular volume (MCV)	76–100 fL
Mean corpuscular hemoglobin (MCH)	25–35 pg
Mean corpuscular hemoglobin concentration (MCHC)	30%–38%
Platelet count	150,000–400,000/μL

Hematology *continued*

Other Hematologic Studies	Specimen	Normal Values
Coagulation studies		
Bleeding time	Capillary blood	Duke method: 1–3 minutes
		Ivy method: 1–7 minutes
Fibrinogen assay	Plasma	200–400 mg/dL
Partial thromboplastin time (PTT)	Plasma	Activated: 30–40 seconds
		Nonactivated: 40–100 seconds
Platelet count	Whole blood	150,000–400,000/μL
Prothrombin time	Plasma	11–15 seconds
Whole blood clotting time	Whole blood	Siliconized tubes: 24–45 minutes
		Plain tubes: 5–15 minutes
Eosinophil count	Whole blood	50–400/μL
Erythrocyte sedimentation rate (ESR)	Whole blood	
Wintrobe method		Male: 0–9 mm/hr
		Female: 0–20 mm/hr
Westergren method		Male:
		Under 50 years, 0–15 mm/hr
		Over 50 years, 0–20 mm/hr
		Female:
		Under 50 years, 0–20 mm/hr
		Over 50 years, 0–30 mm/hr
Volume, blood	Whole blood	Male: 69 mL/kg
		Female: 65 mL/kg
Volume, plasma	Whole blood	Male: 39 mL/kg
		Female: 40 mL/kg

Cerebrospinal Fluid

Test	Normal Values
Appearance	Clear and colorless
Cell count	0–10 WBC/μL (60%–100% lymphocytes)
Glucose	Adults:
	40–80 mg/dL
	50%–80% of blood glucose
Immunoglobulin	
IgA	0–0.6 mg/dL
IgG	0–5.5 mg/dL
IgM	0–1.3 mg/dL
Protein	Adult: 15–50 mg/dL
Protein electrophoresis	Prealbumin: 3%–6%
	Albumin: 45%–68%
	α_1-globulin: 3%–9%
	α_2-globulin: 4%–10%
	β-globulin: 10%–18%
	γ-globulin: 3%–11%

Index

ddison-Wesley Health Sciences books are available at fine health sciences
ookstores everywhere, but you may also order direct from us.

ease send _____ copies of THE MANUAL OF NURSING
                    THERAPEUTICS #12940

          _____ copies x $19.95 = (TOTAL AMOUNT) _____

◻ my check is enclosed

◻ bill my MasterCard   # _____ expiration date _____

◻ bill my Visa   # _____ expiration date _____

 your check accompanies your order, Addison-Wesley will ship your book/s
ee.

illing address: _____
                   name

         ·   _____
                   address

                   _____
                   city/state/zip

hipping address: _____
f different)   name

                   _____
                   address

                   _____
                   city/state/zip

_____
thorized charge card signature

✳ ✳ ✳ ✳ ✳ ✳ ✳ ✳ ✳ ✳ ✳ ✳ ✳ ✳ ✳ ✳ ✳ ✳ ✳ ✳

Iave you seen the CARE PLANNING POCKET GUIDE? This convenient
eference will save you hours of planning time. It's the first book to offer both
omplete care plans for nursing diagnostic categories and groupings of possible
ursing diagnoses under common medical and surgical disorders. Now you can
uickly identify diagnoses for a particular patient, and then look up a complete
lan of care for each diagnosis in the same book! Developed by a team of
rofessional nurses from El Camino Hospital, Mountain View, CA, this handy
piral book is both comprehensive and easy to individualize. 160 pp., 1986

lease send me _____ copies of the CARE PLANNING POCKET GUIDE
#16305 at $9.95 and I'll pay as indicated above.

Return this form to: Order Department, Addison-Wesley Publishing Com-
any, One Jacob Way, Reading, MA 01867.

'rices indicated will be honored through June 1, 1987.